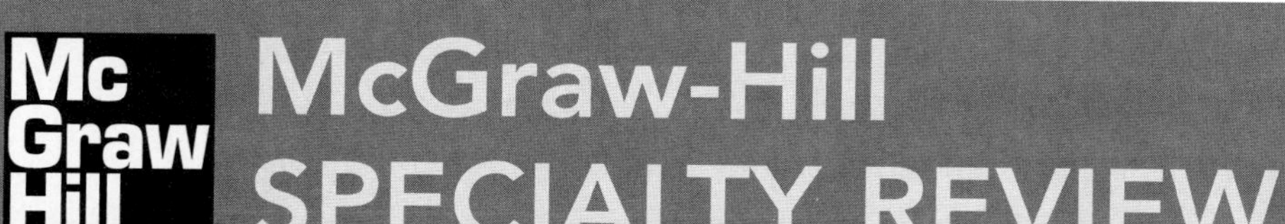

# Obstetrics and Gynecology

## Cases, Questions, and Answers



**Ricardo Azziz, MD, MPH, MBA**
Chair
Department of Obstetrics & Gynecology
Cedars-Sinai Medical Center
Los Angeles, California
Professor and Vice Chair
Department of Obstetrics & Gynecology
The David Geffen School of Medicine
University of California, Los Angeles

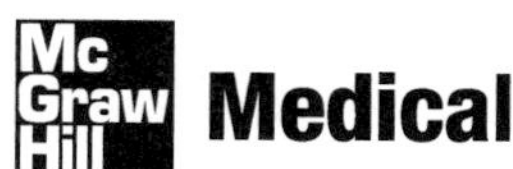

New York Chicago San Francisco Lisbon London Madrid Mexico City Milan
New Delhi San Juan Seoul Singapore Sydney Toronto

The **McGraw·Hill** Companies

**McGraw-Hill Specialty Review:**
**Obstetrics and Gynecology: Cases, Questions, and Answers**



1 2 3 4 5 6 7 8 9 0 QPD/QPD 0 9 8 7 6

ISBN-13: 978-0-07-145820-7
ISBN-10: 0-07-145820-4

**Notice**

Medicine is an ever-changing science. As new research and clinical experience broaden our knowledge, changes in treatment and drug therapy are required. The authors and the publisher of this work have checked with sources believed to be reliable in their efforts to provide information that is complete and generally in accord with the standards accepted at the time of publication. However, in view of the possibility of human error or changes in medical sciences, neither the authors nor the publisher nor any other party who has been involved in the preparation or publication of this work warrants that the information contained herein is in every respect accurate or complete, and they disclaim all responsibility for any errors or omissions or for the results obtained from use of the information contained in this work. Readers are encouraged to confirm the information contained herein with other sources. For example and in particular, readers are advised to check the product information sheet included in the package of each drug they plan to administer to be certain that the information contained in this work is accurate and that changes have not been made in the recommended dose or in the contraindications for administration. This recommendation is of particular importance in connection with new or infrequently used drugs.

This book was set in Times by International Typesetting and Composition.
The editors were Anne M. Sydor and Karen Edmonson.
The production supervisor was John Williams.
Project management was provided by International Typesetting and Composition.
Quebecor World was printer and binder.

This book is printed on acid-free paper.

**Cataloging-in-Publication Data for this title is on file with the Library of Congress.**

International Edition ISBN-13: 978-0-07-110005-2; ISBN-10: 0-07-110005-9

*To my patients, who have taught me so much and for whose trust I am eternally grateful.*

Ricardo Azziz

# CONTENTS

*Contributors* x
*Preface* xiii
*Acknowledgments* xiv

***Section 1***
OFFICE MANAGEMENT: PRIMARY CARE

**1** Management of a Breast Mass *Alison Axtell* 1
**2** Domestic Violence *John Williams III* 2
**3** General Medical Screening *Christine Walsh* 3
**4** Medical Ethics *Alison C. Madden* 5
**5** Obesity *Alison C. Madden* 7
**6** Smoking Cessation *Alison C. Madden* 8
**7** Hypothyroidism *John Kuo* 10

***Section 2***
OFFICE MANAGEMENT: GYNECOLOGY

**8** Abnormal Pap Smear *Alison Axtell* 15
**9** Abnormal Uterine Bleeding *Ashim Kumar* 16
**10** Contraception: Intrauterine Device *Jane L. Davis* 18
**11** Contraception: Tubal Sterilization *Jane L. Davis* 20
**12** Contraception: Depo-Provera *John Kuo* 21
**13** Emergency Contraception *Susan Sarajari* 24
**14** Oral Contraception *Susan Sarajari* 26
**15** Hidradenitis Suppurativa *Jane L. Davis* 29
**16** Menopause: Osteoporosis Prevention and Treatment *John Kuo* 31
**17** Menopause: Perimenopause *Margareta D. Pisarska* 33
**18** Menopause: Hormone Therapy Counseling *Margareta D. Pisarska* 35

**19** Chronic Pelvic Pain Causes *Ricardo Azziz* 37
**20** Interstitial Cystitis *Cynthia D. Hall* 40
**21** Chronic Pelvic Pain Treatments *Lee Kao* 42
**22** Sexual Assault *Alison C. Madden* 44
**23** Syphilis *Alison C. Madden* 45
**24** Salpingitis *Neil S. Silverman* 48
**25** Nonsurgical Management of Pelvic Organ Prolapse *Cynthia D. Hall* 49
**26** Diagnosis, Differential, and Treatment of Anal Incontinence *Cynthia D. Hall* 52
**27** Vaginitis: Recurrent Candida *Alison C. Madden* 54
**28** Vaginitis: Bacterial Vaginosis and Trichomonas *Alison C. Madden* 56
**29** Vulvar Disease: Lichen Sclerosus *Andrew John Li* 59

***Section 3***
OFFICE MANAGEMENT: OBSTETRICS

**30** Breast Feeding and Mastitis *Jane L. Davis* 61
**31** Hyperemesis Gravidarum *John Williams III* 63
**32** Syphilis *Marguerite Lisa Bartholomew* 66
**33** Herpes Simplex Virus *Marguerite Lisa Bartholomew* 69
**34** Hepatitis C *Neil S. Silverman* 71
**35** Human Immunodeficiency Virus *Neil S. Silverman* 73
**36** Parvovirus *Neil S. Silverman* 76
**37** Purified Protein Derivative Testing in Pregnancy *Neil S. Silverman* 78
**38** Varicella *Neil S. Silverman* 80
**39** Hepatitis B *Neil S. Silverman* 82
**40** Chronic Hypertension *Jasvant Adusumalli* 85
**41** Thyroid Disease in Pregnancy: Hyperthyroidism *Marguerite Lisa Bartholomew* 87
**42** Ovarian Masses in Pregnancy *Marguerite Lisa Bartholomew* 90
**43** Cholestasis of Pregnancy *Marguerite Lisa Bartholomew* 92
**44** Adnexal Masses During Pregnancy *Ilana Cass* 95
**45** Pregnancy After Breast Cancer *Ilana Cass* 96
**46** Asthma *Jane L. Davis* 97
**47** Depression and Postpartum Psychological Reactions *Jane L. Davis* 99
**48** Seizure Disorders *Jane L. Davis* 102
**49** Appendicitis *Kimberly D. Gregory* 104
**50** Cardiac Disease in Pregnancy *John Williams III* 105

## *Section 4*
## OBSTETRICS

**51** Abnormal Labor *Calvin J. Hobel* 109
**52** Abruption *Kimberly D. Gregory* 111
**53** Anesthesia Complications *Marguerite Lisa Bartholomew* 112
**54** Chorioamnionitis *Kevin R. Justus* 116
**55** Diabetic Ketoacidosis in Pregnancy *Marguerite Lisa Bartholomew* 118
**56** Acute Fatty Liver of Pregnancy *Jasvant Adusumalli* 120
**57** Fetal Heart Rate Patterns *Kimberly D. Gregory* 122
**58** HELLP Syndrome *Kimberly D. Gregory* 124
**59** Postpartum Hemorrhage *John Williams III* 126
**60** Nonimmune Hydrops *Kimberly D. Gregory* 128
**61** Incompetent Cervix/Cerclage *Calvin J. Hobel* 129
**62** Induction of Labor and Cervical Ripening *Jane L. Davis* 132
**63** Intrauterine Growth Restriction *Jane L. Davis* 133
**64** Meconium *Kimberly D. Gregory* 135
**65** Operative Vaginal Delivery *Kevin R. Justus* 136
**66** Placenta Accreta *Ilana Cass* 138
**67** Placenta Previa *Kimberly D. Gregory* 140
**68** Preeclampsia, Eclampsia, and HELLP Syndrome *Marguerite Lisa Bartholomew* 142
**69** Obesity and Bariatric Surgery *Kimberly D. Gregory* 144
**70** Shoulder Dystocia *Kimberly D. Gregory* 146
**71** Trauma During Pregnancy *Marguerite Lisa Bartholomew* 148
**72** Uterine Inversion *Calvin J. Hobel* 151
**73** Vaginal Birth After Cesarean and Uterine Rupture *Kevin R. Justus* 153
**74** Midtrimester Abortion *Jane L. Davis* 155

## *Section 5*
## GYNECOLOGY/UROGYNECOLOGY

**75** Adenomyosis *Ricardo Azziz* 159
**76** Bartholin's Gland Mass *Ilana Cass* 162
**77** DES Exposure *Lee Kao* 164
**78** Ectopic Pregnancy: Methotrexate versus Surgery *Margareta D. Pisarka* 166
**79** Endometrial Ablation *Lee Kao* 169
**80** Fibroids: Cause of Recurrent Abortion *Shahin Ghadir* 170
**81** Fibroids: Hysteroscopic Treatment *Amer K. Karam* 171

**82** Fibroids: Myomectomy versus Uterine Artery Embolization and Cryomyolysis *Susan Sarajari* 173
**83** Supracervical Hysterectomy *Ilana Cass* 175
**84** Complications of Hysteroscopy *Lee Kao* 177
**85** Laparoscopic Complications: Prediction and Avoidance *Ricardo Azziz* 180
**86** Adnexal Torsion *Shahin Ghadir* 182
**87** Urethral Diverticulum *Cynthia D. Hall* 183
**88** Stress Urinary Incontinence *Cynthia D. Hall* 186
**89** Urge and Overflow Urinal Incontinence *Cynthia D. Hall* 188
**90** Urinary Tract Infections *Cynthia D. Hall* 191
**91** Urodynamic Studies *Cynthia D. Hall* 194
**92** Uterine Prolapse *Alison C. Madden* 196
**93** Vaginal Vault Prolapse *Cynthia D. Hall* 199
**94** Vulvar Laceration in Pediatric Patients *Alison C. Madden* 201

***Section 6***
REPRODUCTIVE DISORDERS

**95** Recurrent Abortion *Margareta D. Pisarska* 205
**96** Amenorrhea Evaluation *Margareta D. Pisarska* 207
**97** Hypothalamic Amenorrhea *Margareta D. Pisarska* 209
**98** Hirsutism *Ricardo Azziz* 210
**99** 21-Hydroxylase Deficient Nonclassic Adrenal Hyperplasia *Ricardo Azziz* 214
**100** Polycystic Ovary Syndrome: Insulin Resistance and Use of Insulin Sensitizers *Ricardo Azziz* 217
**101** Polycystic Ovary Syndrome: Ovulation Induction *Ashim Kumar* 220
**102** Asherman's Syndrome *Ashim Kumar* 222
**103** Cushing's Syndrome *Ricardo Azziz* 223
**104** Galactorrhea *Shahin Ghadir* 226
**105** Gonadal Dysgenesis: Turner's Syndrome *Ricardo Azziz* 227
**106** Hyperprolactinemia *Lee Kao* 230
**107** In Vitro Fertilization *Margareta D. Pisarska* 232
**108** Endometriosis and Infertility *Lee Kao* 235
**109** Basic Evaluation for Female Infertility *Lee Kao* 237
**110** Lifestyle Implications (Smoking) for Infertility *Lee Kao* 239
**111** Hydrosalpinx/Tubal Damage *Ashim Kumar* 240
**112** Fibroids *Catherine M. DeUgarte* 242
**113** Advanced Reproductive Age *Margareta D. Pisarska* 243
**114** Male Infertility *Catherine M. DeUgarte* 246

**115** Menopause: Sexuality and Androgen Deficiency *Catherine M. DeUgarte* 247
**116** Clomiphene and Ovulation Induction *Lee Kao* 249
**117** Premature Ovarian Failure *Margareta D. Pisarska* 250
**118** Uterine Anomaly *Ricardo Azziz* 253

***Section 7***
GYNECOLOGIC ONCOLOGY

**119** Atypical Glandular Cells of Uncertain Significance *Alison Axtell* 257
**120** Adnexal Masses in Young Women *Ilana Cass* 258
**121** Borderline Ovarian Tumor *Andrew John Li* 259
**122** Squamous Cell Carcinoma of the Cervix *Andrew John Li* 261
**123** Neoadjuvant Chemotherapy *Christine Walsh* 262
**124** Endometrial Cancer *Andrew John Li* 264
**125** Gestational Trophoblastic Disease *Andrew John Li* 265
**126** Ovarian Teratomas *Ilana Cass* 267
**127** Hereditary Ovarian Cancer Syndrome *Andrew John Li* 268
**128** Granulosa Cell Tumor *Andrew John Li* 270
**129** Pelvic Exenteration *Ilana Cass* 272
**130** Primary Peritoneal Cancer *Amer K. Karam* 274
**131** Uterine Sarcoma *Amer K. Karam* 275
**132** Vulvar Carcinoma *Andrew John Li* 276
**133** Vulvar Intraepithelial Neoplasia *Christine Walsh* 278

*List of Abbreviations* 281
*Index* 283

# CONTRIBUTORS

**Ricardo Azziz, MD, MPH, MBA**
Chair, Department of Obstetrics & Gynecology
Cedars-Sinai Medical Center
Professor and Vice Chair
Department of Obstetrics & Gynecology
The David Geffen School of Medicine
University of California, Los Angeles
Los Angeles, California

**Jasvant Adusumalli, MD**
Clinical Fellow
Division of Maternal-Fetal Medicine
Department of Obstetrics & Gynecology
Cedars-Sinai Medical Center
Los Angeles, California

**Alison Axtell, MD**
Fellow, Gynecologic Oncology
Department of Obstetrics & Gynecology
The David Geffen School of Medicine
University of California, Los Angeles
Department of Obstetrics & Gynecology
Cedars-Sinai Medical Center
Los Angeles, California

**Marguerite Lisa Bartholomew, MD**
Assistant Professor
Department of Obstetrics & Gynecology
The David Geffen School of Medicine
University of California, Los Angeles
Department of Obstetrics & Gynecology
Cedars-Sinai Medical Center
Los Angeles, California

**Ilana Cass, MD**
Assistant Clinical Professor
Department of Obstetrics & Gynecology
The David Geffen School of Medicine
University of California, Los Angeles
Division of Gynecologic Oncology
Department of Obstetrics & Gynecology
Cedars-Sinai Medical Center
Los Angeles, California

**Jane L. Davis, MD**
Professor, Department of Obstetrics
& Gynecology
The David Geffen School of Medicine
University of California, Los Angeles
Associate Director, Residency Training
Department of Obstetrics & Gynecology
Cedars-Sinai Medical Center
Los Angeles, California

**Catherine M. DeUgarte, MD**
Reproductive Endocrinology and Infertility
Department of Obstetrics & Gynecology
The David Geffen School of Medicine
University of California, Los Angeles
Department of Obstetrics & Gynecology
Cedars-Sinai Medical Center
Los Angeles, California

**Shahin Ghadir, MD**
Fellow
Reproductive Endocrinology
Department of Obstetrics & Gynecology
The David Geffen School of Medicine
University of California, Los Angeles
Department of Obstetrics & Gynecology
Cedars-Sinai Medical Center
Los Angeles, California

**Kimberly D. Gregory, MD**
Associate Professor
Departments of Obstetrics & Gynecology, and
School of Public Health
Department of Heath Sciences
The David Geffen School of Medicine
University of California, Los Angeles
Vice Chair
Women's Healthcare Quality and
Performance Improvement
Department of Obstetrics & Gynecology
Cedars-Sinai Medical Center
Los Angeles, California

**Cynthia D. Hall, MD**
Assistant Professor
Department of Obstetrics & Gynecology
The David Geffen School of Medicine
University of California, Los Angeles
Director
Urogynecology and Pelvic Reconstruction
Surgery
Department of Obstetrics & Gynecology
Cedars-Sinai Medical Center
Los Angeles, California

**Calvin J. Hobel, MD**
Professor
Departments of Obstetrics & Gynecology, and
Pediatrics
The David Geffen School of Medicine
University of California, Los Angeles
Vice Chairman
Department of Obstetrics & Gynecology
Cedars-Sinai Medical Center
Los Angeles, California

**Kevin R. Justus, MD**
Fellow
Division of Maternal-Fetal Medicine
Department of Obstetrics & Gynecology
Cedars-Sinai Medical Center
Los Angeles, California

**Lee Kao, MD, PhD**
Assistant Professor
Department of Obstetrics & Gynecology
The David Geffen School of Medicine
University of California, Los Angeles
Co-Director
Center for Fertility and Reproductive Medicine
Department of Obstetrics & Gynecology
Cedars-Sinai Medical Center
Los Angeles, California

**Amer K. Karam, MD**
Fellow
Gynecologic Oncology
Department of Obstetrics & Gynecology
The David Geffen School of Medicine
University of California, Los Angeles
Department of Obstetrics & Gynecology
Cedars-Sinai Medical Center
Los Angeles, California

**Ashim Kumar, MD**
Fellow
Reproductive Endocrinology and Infertility
Department of Obstetrics & Gynecology
The David Geffen School of Medicine
University of California, Los Angeles
Department of Obstetrics & Gynecology
Cedars-Sinai Medical Center
Los Angeles, California

**John Kuo, MD**
Fellow
Reproductive Endocrinology and Infertility
Department of Obstetrics & Gynecology
The David Geffen School of Medicine
University of California, Los Angeles
Department of Obstetrics & Gynecology
Cedars-Sinai Medical Center
Los Angeles, California

**Andrew John Li, MD**
Assistant Professor
Department of Obstetrics & Gynecology
The David Geffen School of Medicine
University of California, Los Angeles
Department of Obstetrics & Gynecology
Cedars-Sinai Medical Center
Los Angeles, California

**Alison C. Madden, MD**
Assistant Clinical Professor
Department of Obstetrics & Gynecology
The David Geffen School of Medicine
University of California, Los Angeles
Associate Director, Residency Training
Department of Obstetrics & Gynecology
Cedars-Sinai Medical Center
Los Angeles, California

**Margareta D. Pisarska, MD**
Assistant Professor
Department of Obstetrics & Gynecology
The David Geffen School of Medicine
University of California, Los Angeles
Co-Director
Center for Fertility and Reproductive Medicine
Department of Obstetrics & Gynecology
Cedars-Sinai Medical Center
Los Angeles, California

**Susan Sarajari, MD, PhD**
Fellow
Reproductive Endocrinology and Infertility
Department of Obstetrics & Gynecology
The David Geffen School of Medicine
University of California, Los Angeles
Department of Obstetrics & Gynecology
Cedars-Sinai Medical Center
Los Angeles, California

**Neil S. Silverman, MD**
Clinical Professor
Department of Obstetrics & Gynecology
The David Geffen School of Medicine
University of California, Los Angeles
Medical Director
Inpatient Obstetric Services
Division of Maternal-Fetal Medicine
Department of Obstetrics & Gynecology
Cedars-Sinai Medical Center
Los Angeles, California

**Christine Walsh, MD**
Fellow
Gynecologic Oncology
Department of Obstetrics & Gynecology
The David Geffen School of Medicine
University of California, Los Angeles
Department of Obstetrics & Gynecology
Cedars-Sinai Medical Center
Los Angeles, California

**John Williams III, MD**
Clinical Professor
Department of Obstetrics & Gynecology
The David Geffen School of Medicine
University of California, Los Angeles
Director Reproductive Genetics
Maternal-Fetal Medicine
Department of Obstetrics & Gynecology
Cedars-Sinai Medical Center
Los Angeles, California

# PREFACE

The past decade has seen a number of changes in residency training, including limited work hours, changing demographics of the residents, the onslaught of the electronic and internet ages, and a growing recognition that most physicians today aim to achieve the elusive balance between professional and personal life. This transformation in the academic landscape requires both teachers and trainees to reassess how we learn. Among the many innovations possible (e.g., internet-based learning, personal digital assistant-based references, virtual patients), a relatively cost-effective technique for both self learning and teaching is the use of short, vignette-driven case reviews, as used in present text.

For over a decade, the faculty of the Department of Obstetrics & Gynecology at Cedars-Sinai Medical Center has conducted a weekly Morbidity and Mortality Conference for the residents in Obstetrics and Gynecology. The faculty prepares detailed questions to two cases, selected from the weekly case list for all services. These are cases that serve as the basis for *Obstetrics and Gynecology: Cases, Questions, and Answers*.

This text will provide brief, referenced reviews of many of the critical topics encountered in the field of Obstetrics and Gynecology, formatted as clinical vignettes with questions and referenced answers directed towards the vignette. This book was designed to serve as a practical reference and review summary for residents, medical students, practicing physicians, nurse practitioners, and a number of allied health professionals, such as physicians' assistants. It is our hope that the reader will find these vignettes educational and enlightening, in an easy to read format.

Ricardo Azziz, MD, MPH, MBA

# ACKNOWLEDGMENTS

First, I would like to thank the past and present faculty of the Department of Obstetrics & Gynecology at Cedars-Sinai Medical Center without whose persistent dedication to the teaching of residents and medical students the Morbidity and Mortality conferences on which this text is based would have never existed. I am also indebted to many of these same faculty members who gave freely their time and effort to write these chapters, and who endured my frequent requests for revisions under a tight and unforgiving timeline. Special thanks go to Drs. Alison C. Madden and Jane L. Davis for their inexhaustible effort to assist in the writing and editing of this text. I would like to thank our staff who helped in the preparation and formatting of the many drafts involved, particularly acknowledging the expert assistance of Lois Dollar, April Moore, James Morrow, and Fay Shapiro. Also greatly appreciated is the support, patience, and guidance offered to us by the editorial staff at McGraw-Hill, notably Anne M. Sydor and Karen Edmonson. Finally, I am grateful to the many medical students and residents who have afforded me the privilege of training and mentoring them into what I know are and will be quality and caring physicians.

Ricardo Azziz, MD, MPH, MBA

# Section 1

# OFFICE MANAGEMENT: PRIMARY CARE

## 1 MANAGEMENT OF A BREAST MASS

*Alison Axtell*

### LEARNING POINT

Appropriate triage of women who present with complaints of a breast mass.

## VIGNETTE

A 42-year-old, G3 P2012, presents to the office complaining of a new right breast mass. She noticed it on self-breast examination approximately 2 weeks ago. She denies pain or abnormal nipple discharge and has not palpated any axillary masses. The patient has no significant past medical or surgical history, exercises regularly, and does not smoke or drink. Her mother died of ovarian cancer at age 65, and she has a maternal aunt who was diagnosed with breast cancer at age 48. On examination, a 1.5 cm irregular lesion is appreciated in the upper outer quadrant of her right breast. There is no nipple discharge and no axillary adenopathy. The left breast is palpably normal as is the rest of her physical examination.

### QUESTION 1

*What risk factors for breast cancer do you look for when obtaining the history of a patient presenting with a new breast mass?*

### ANSWER 1

Factors which place patients at an increased risk for breast cancer include age, family history, use of hormone replacement therapy or questionably oral contraceptives, age at menopause/first birth/menarche, history of a breast biopsy, and known early on set breast cancer (BRCA) gene mutations. Protective factors include parity, breast-feeding, exercise, reduced body mass index (BMI), and oophorectomy before age 35.

### QUESTION 2

*What specific findings on physical examination are concerning for breast cancer?*

### ANSWER 2

Malignant breast lesions are often characterized as being firm, fixed, isolated, and irregular. However, 90% of benign lesions are also isolated, and 60% of malignant lesions are mobile, while 40% are regular. In addition, symptoms, such as pain and nipple discharge, which are more often associated with benign lesions, occur in about 15% of patients with breast cancer. Larger malignant lesions are often associated with overlying skin changes, such as dimpling.

### QUESTION 3

*How do you initiate evaluation of a patient with a palpable breast mass?*

### ANSWER 3

The answer to this question depends on the patient's age. In women over 35 years, a diagnostic mammogram should be the first step in evaluating a palpable mass, while a breast ultrasound would be recommended in women under the age of 35. Since breast tissue in young women is often too dense to evaluate by mammography. In women with a palpable breast lump, the sensitivity of diagnostic mammography is 87.3%, while the specificity is 84.5%. The negative predictive value of a normal mammogram and ultrasound in this setting is 97%. Some experts recommend that all women with a palpable mass should be referred directly for a fine needle aspiration (FNA). If an FNA is performed in the office, clear fluid does not need to be sent for cytology. However, bloody fluid and tissue from solid lesions need to be evaluated for malignancy. Most importantly, all palpable breast lesions should be followed to resolution.

## BIBLIOGRAPHY

Barlow WE, et al. Performance of diagnostic mammography for women with signs or symptoms of breast cancer. *J Natl Cancer Inst.* 2002;94:1151.

Barton MB, et al. Breast symptoms among women enrolled in a health maintenance organization: frequency, evaluation, and outcome. *Ann Intern Med.* 1999;130:651.

Ciatto S, et al. The value of routine cytologic examination of breast cyst fluids. *Acta Cytol.* 1987;31:301.

Clemons M, et al. Estrogen and the risk of breast cancer. *N Engl J Med.* 2001;344:276.

Donegan WL. Evaluation of a palpable breast mass. *N Engl J Med.* 1992;327:937.

Moy L, et al. Specificity of mammography and US in the evaluation of a palpable abnormality: retrospective review. *Radiology.* 2002;225:176.

Venet L, et al. Adequacies and inadequacies of breast examinations by physicians in mass screening. *Cancer.* 1971;28:1546.

# 2 DOMESTIC VIOLENCE

*John Williams III*

## LEARNING POINT

To understand the definition and prevalence of domestic violence, as well as the screening tools available to detect domestic violence.

## VIGNETTE

A 24-year-old, G3P1011, woman at 23-2/7 weeks' gestational age presents to her obstetrician's office for a follow-up prenatal visit. She is accompanied by her mother-in-law. The patient has visible left periorbital bruising and contusions over her left zygomatic arch and on both forearms. On questioning, she states that she tripped and fell against the kitchen counter. Her obstetrician perceives that she is not being truthful and suspects that she is being abused by her husband. The obstetrician informs the patient and her mother-in-law that she plans to perform a vaginal examination and asks the mother-in-law to leave the examination room for a moment. In privacy and upon further questioning, the patient confides to her obstetrician that her injuries were inflicted by her husband during an argument and that he has physically and verbally abused her on several occasions during their 3-year relationship.

## QUESTION 1

*How is domestic violence defined? What is the prevalence of domestic violence in the general population? What is the short-term and long-term impact of domestic violence?*

## ANSWER 1

Domestic violence is a pattern of assaultive and coercive behaviors, including physical, sexual, and psychological attacks, and economic coercion that adults or adolescents use against their intimate partners. Victims of domestic violence can include men and same-sex partners. However, domestic violence most frequently involves males abusing their female partners. Domestic violence is statistically the most common crime against women. Nearly 25% of women report that they have been raped and/or physically assaulted by a current partner or former spouse, cohabiting partner, or date at some time in their life. Each year, 8–12% of women in an ongoing relationship experience at least one episode of violence. Domestic violence accounts for ~21% of all violent crime against women. Among female murder victims, ~30% are killed by an intimate partner. Domestic violence is a major cause of physical injuries among females. Injuries are often severe, repetitive, and most commonly involve the head, face, breasts, or abdomen. Most victims will not report abuse to health-care workers or to law enforcement personnel. Instead they may offer vague somatic complaints. Often explanations are inconsistent with the nature of the injury. In addition to short- and long-term physical consequences, there are long-term psychological consequences due to the stress of living in an ongoing abusive relationship (i.e., chronic headache, chronic pelvic pain, sleep and appetite disorders, sexual dysfunction, and the like). Domestic violence not only affects families but also

**TABLE 2-1. Simple Behaviorally Specific Questions regarding Domestic Violence**

- Has anyone close to you ever threatened to hurt you?
- Has anyone ever hit, kicked, choked, or hurt you physically?
- Has anyone, including your partner, ever forced you to have sex?
- Are you ever afraid of your partner?

social services, legal and educational systems, workplace, and society at large.

## QUESTION 2

*What is the prevalence of domestic violence in pregnancy? Who is most likely to be the perpetrator? What are the risks of domestic violence in pregnancy? Is there an increased risk for abuse in the postpartum period?*

## ANSWER 2

The prevalence of domestic violence in pregnancy ranges from 1% to 20% with most studies reporting a rate of 3–9%. The perpetrator is usually a current or former intimate partner. Among younger women, it may be a parent or other family member. Domestic violence is associated with an increased risk for spontaneous abortion, preterm labor, poor maternal weight gain, low birth weight, and fetal death. The postpartum period is a very stressful time for any family coping with the demands of a newborn. The first 6 weeks postdelivery is when a couple's coping skills are stretched to the limit, which can lead to increased risk of domestic abuse.

## QUESTION 3

What are the potential barriers to detection of domestic violence? Who should be screened? What is the obstetrician-gynecologist's responsibility in screening for and intervention in domestic violence?

## ANSWER 3

In spite of increasing recognition of the problem of violence against women, there are still many barriers to screening. Lack of recognition of the widespread prevalence of domestic violence is one of the main obstacles to screening. All patients should be screened for domestic violence (universal screening). Asking each patient directly about prior or ongoing abuse increases the likelihood of disclosure. Simple behaviorally specific questions should be asked in private (specifically not in the presence of the partner or family). Examples are shown in Table 2-1. Screening should occur at the first prenatal visit, at least once per trimester and at the postpartum follow-up visit. The physician's responsibility in addressing domestic violence is listed in Table 2-2.

**TABLE 2-2. The Physician's Responsibility in Addressing Domestic Violence**

- Implement universal screening
- Acknowledge the trauma
- Assess immediate safety
- Help establish a safety plan
- Review options
- Offer educational materials
- Offer a list of community and local resources
- Provide referrals
- Document interactions
- Provide ongoing support at subsequent visits

## BIBLIOGRAPHY

ACOG Educational Bulletin No. 257. Domestic Violence. December 1999.

Gazmararian J, et al. Prevalence of violence against pregnant women. A review of the literature. *JAMA*. 1996;275:1915–1920.

Hedin LW. Physical and sexual abuse against women and children. *Curr Opin Obstet Gynecol*. 2000;12:349–355.

Mezey G, Bacchus L, Bewley S, White S. Domestic violence, lifetime trauma and psychological health of childbearing women. *BJOG*. 2005;112:197–204.

# 3 GENERAL MEDICAL SCREENING

*Christine Walsh*

## LEARNING POINT

Characteristics of effective screening tests and recommendations for screening in women.

## VIGNETTE

A 58-year-old postmenopausal woman comes into your office for an annual physical examination. She asks for the appropriate screening tests for her age group.

## QUESTION 1

*What is the purpose of a screening test and when are they appropriately used?*

## ANSWER 1

To be effective, a screening test should reduce morbidity and mortality from a particular disease, in a defined population, at a reasonable cost. These tests are appropriately used only when effective strategies exist for earlier intervention that are of greater benefit than the interventions at a later stage of the disease process. The disease that the screening test is trying to detect should have sufficient burden in terms of morbidity and mortality, and should have an available treatment that does more good than harm. An ideal screening test is sensitive, specific, has a high positive predictive value, and is safe, affordable, and reasonable to the patient. The Preventive Services Task Force has analyzed the effectiveness of various screening tests based on the quality of evidence available. Based on these recommendations, a number of groups have made recommendations for the use of particular screening tests in particular populations.

## QUESTION 2

*What are the opportunities for an obstetrician/gynecologist to provide preventive health care to women?*

## ANSWER 2

Preventive health care is oriented toward health maintenance, prevention, early detection of disease, availability of services, and continuity of care. For women in different stages of their reproductive lives, this encompasses screening, identification of risk factors, and counseling regarding a number of health behaviors including family planning, sexual practices, sexually transmitted diseases, and habits such as smoking, alcohol, drug use, exercise, and diet. Components of the periodic visit should include history, physical examination, laboratory evaluations, and counseling regarding issues of sexuality, fitness and nutrition, interpersonal relationships, and modification of cardiovascular and high-risk health behaviors. The goal of these efforts is the prevention or early detection of causes of morbidity and mortality in women.

## QUESTION 3

*What are the top three major causes of mortality that affect women in different age groups?*

## ANSWER 3

Ages 13–18

1. Motor vehicle accidents
2. Homicide
3. Suicide

Ages 19–39

1. Accidents and adverse effects
2. Cancer
3. Human immunodeficiency virus infection

Ages 40–64

1. Cancer
2. Cardiovascular disease
3. Cerebrovascular disease

Ages 65 and older

1. Cardiovascular disease
2. Cancer
3. Cerebrovascular disease

**TABLE 3-1. American College of Obstetricians and Gynecologists Recommendations for Periodic Evaluation and Screening**

| | |
|---|---|
| Cervical cancer screening | Pap smear when sexually active or beginning at age 18, yearly or at patient/physician discretion after three consecutive normal tests if low risk |
| Breast cancer screening | Mammogram every 1–2 years from ages 40 to 50, then every year beginning at age 50 |
| Colon cancer screening | Beginning at age 50, yearly fecal occult blood test plus one of the following:<br>• Flexible sigmoidoscopy every 5 years<br>• Colonoscopy every 10 years<br>• Double contrast barium enema every 5–10 years |
| Cholesterol screening | Beginning at age 45, cholesterol level every 5 years |
| Diabetes screening | Beginning after age 45, fasting glucose testing every 3 years |

QUESTION 4

*When should screening for cervical cancer, breast cancer, colon cancer, cholesterol, and diabetes begin and how often should the screening occur?*

ANSWER 4

The current recommendations of the American College of Obstetricians and Gynecologists are summarized in the following Table 3-1.

## BIBLIOGRAPHY

American College of Obstetricians and Gynecologists. *The Obstetrician-Gynecologist and Primary-Preventive Health Care.* Washington, DC: ACOG; 1993.

American College of Obstetricians and Gynecologists Committee on Gynecologic Practice. Committee Opinion No. 246. *Primary and Preventive Care: Periodic Assessments.* Washington, DC: ACOG; 2000.

Hillard PJA. Preventive health care and screening. In: Berek JS (ed.). *Novak's Gynecology.* 13th ed. Philadelphia, PA: Lippincott Williams & Wilkins; 2002:175–198.

Holzman GB (ed.). Precis: an update in obstetrics and gynecology. In: *Primary and Preventive Care.* 2nd ed. Danvers, MA: ACOG; 1999:15–22.

Woo BJ. Screening and immunization guidelines. In: Carlson KJ, Eisenstat SA (eds.). *Primary Care of Women.* St. Louis, MO: Mosby; 1995:514.

# 4 MEDICAL ETHICS

*Alison C. Madden*

## LEARNING POINT

Patient care is inextricably intertwined with concepts of medical ethics.

## VIGNETTE

A 56-year–old, G4P4, woman with Stage 3B cervical cancer is brought to the emergency department (ED) by her family for mental status changes. The patient was seen by the gyn oncology clinic 6 months ago and diagnosed with Stage 3B cervical cancer. She failed to follow-up or respond to any attempts to reach her. On initial visit, a thorough discussion of risks/benefits/alternatives for treatment of her cancer occurred. The patient declined all interventions, saying she would go home and pray with her family. Now, in the ED, she is not oriented, and the question of mental competency arises. Evaluation by the emergency room physician shows evidence of urosepsis. The family demands that her ureters be stinted and that radiation therapy begin at once. She is admitted to the intensive care unit (ICU) by gyn oncology, and discussion of plan of care and prognosis is begun with the family.

QUESTION 1

*What is autonomy, and how does it relate to informed consent?*

ANSWER 1

Pellegrino, defines an autonomous person as "one who, in his thoughts, work, and actions, is able to follow those norms he chooses as his own without external constraints or coercion by others." Autonomy is a person's right to self-rule, and to choose a course of action based on that person's own sense of values and principles.

Informed consent is based on the concept of autonomy. Informed consent is a process, not a document. A patient gives informed consent by accepting an intervention after full disclosure of the nature of the intervention, and an adequate discussion of the risks, benefits, and alternatives to the intervention. This discussion should take into account the patient's level of "health literacy;" for example, a discussion of collagen synthesis to explain risk of cervical stenosis after cervical biopsy would be inappropriate for most patient's level of understanding. The discussion of informed consent should be conducted in the patient's native language, if possible, or with an appropriate translator.

QUESTION 2

*What is informed refusal?*

ANSWER 2

In obtaining informed consent, a physician must discuss with the patient the risks, benefits, and alternatives that a reasonable person in the patient's position would want to know to make an informed decision. In this discussion, the patient's autonomy, level of health literacy, and cultural

**TABLE 4-1. Health Care Proxy, Living Will, and DNR Advance Directives in the State of New York**

| TYPE OF ADVANCE DIRECTIVE | HEALTH CARE PROXY | LIVING WILL | DO NOT RESUSCITATE (DNR) |
|---|---|---|---|
| Established under New York Law | Yes | No, but accepted as evidence of health care wishes by New York courts | Yes |
| Allows written statement about desired medical treatment decisions in advance | Yes | Yes | No, only cardio pulmonary resuscitation (CPR) decisions |
| Allows appointment of health care agent | Yes | No | No |

SOURCE: Planning Your Health Care in Advance; How to Make Your End-of-Life Wishes Known and Honored. State of New York, Office of the Attorney General. http://www.oag.state.ny.us/health/EOLGUIDE012605.pdf.

background should be taken into account. Informed refusal occurs when the patient then elects to decline or refuse the intervention the physician is recommending. Documentation of the informed refusal process is essential. The physician should document that the need for the intervention as well as risks, benefits, and alternatives to the intervention were discussed and the patient expressed understanding. Discussion of the possible consequences of refusal should also be documented. The patient's reason for refusal should be documented.

## QUESTION 3

*What are beneficence and nonmaleficence?*

## ANSWER 3

Beneficence is the obligation to promote the well-being of others. Nonmaleficence is the obligation to avoid doing harm (Hippocrates' classic "first do no harm" comes from this concept). Although these concepts are on first read quite straightforward, these issues are often intertwined and decisions may become quite complex. For example, an intervention might prolong a patient's life, but in the context of a terminal illness, perhaps the patient would exercise autonomy and argue that quality of life is more important than quantity of time alive. In this case, does one promote well-being by prolonging life, or by making the life that is left pain-free? In this case, does one do more harm by intervening or not intervening?

## QUESTION 4

*What is a surrogate decision maker? What is a living will?*

## ANSWER 4

Both are considered *advanced directives*, but there are important differences between a living will and a surrogate decision maker:

- A *living will* is documentation of an individual's wishes concerning future care in the event she becomes incompetent. The wishes of the patient are expressed by giving very specific instructions to the health care provider in specific circumstances.
- A *health care proxy* appoints an agent (surrogate decision maker) to act on the patient's behalf should she become incompetent. This agent knows the principal's wishes and desires.

The surrogate decision maker must make every attempt to make decisions as the patient would have wanted (see Table 4-1).

For children, parents are the surrogate decision makers, except in circumstances where the decision is life-threatening and might not reflect the decision the child would make for themselves later as an adult. The classic example of this special circumstance is a parent who is a Jehovah's Witness refusing blood transfusion for the child.

The legal age at which an adolescent child may legally make their own decisions varies from state to state.

## BIBLIOGRAPHY

ACOG Committee Opinion, No. 306, December 2004.

*Ethics in Obstetrics and Gynecology*, 2nd ed. Part II End of Life Decision Making. *Novack's Gynecology*, 13th edition Chapter 2.

Pellegrino ED. Patient and physician autonomy: conflicting rights and obligations in the physician-patient relationship. *J Contemp Health Law Pol.* 1994;10:47–68.

Dash & Mailleux. UpToDate. Ethical issues in the care of the patient with end-stage renal disease. In: Rose BD (ed.). *UpToDate.* Waltham, MA: UpToDate;2006. www.Uptodate.com

# 5 OBESITY

*Alison C. Madden*

## LEARNING POINT

To define obesity and learn the health risks and options for treatment.

## VIGNETTE

A 35-year-old, G4P4, obese Caucasian female presents to her primary care physician's office for her a physical examination for the new job she is starting the following week. Her only complaints are increasing shortness of breath when she walks upstairs and feeling sleepy during the day despite adequate hours of sleep. She rarely has seen a physician except during her previous pregnancies. Her previous visit was over 3 years ago when she had her last child. She has not had any medical problems except for gestational hypertension and gestational diabetes. All of her children were born vaginally without complications. She has had regular menses every month since menarche. She has never had any surgeries and she is not currently on any medications. Family history is significant for diabetes, hypertension, and colon cancer in her maternal grandfather. On examination, this is an obese White female in no acute distress. Weight is 235 lb and height is 5 ft/3 in. Her vitals are stable and the rest of the examination is unremarkable.

## QUESTION 1

*What is the definition of obesity and how is it measured?*

## ANSWER 1

Overweight refers to an excess of body weight while obesity refers to an excess of fat. The body mass index (BMI) is used by the National Heart, Lung, and Blood Institute (NHLBI) and the World Health Organization (WHO) to evaluate the degree of obesity. BMI is defined as body weight in kilograms divided by height in meters squared. WHO and the National Center for Health Statistics define overweight as a BMI between >25 and ≤29.9. Obesity is defined as a BMI >30 kg/m$^2$. Severe or morbid obesity is defined as a BMI >40 kg/m$^2$ (or ≥35 kg/m$^2$ in the presence of comorbidities).

## QUESTION 2

*What is the prevalence and mortality associated with obesity?*

## ANSWER 2

The prevalence of obesity is increasing in United States and worldwide. United States has one of the highest national levels of obesity in the world; the prevalence of obesity in adults between 1999 and 2000 was 30.5%. Mortality depends on the degree of obesity. One study estimated that between 280,000 and 325,000 deaths in United States annually could be attributed to obesity. Most of these deaths occur in adults with a BMI >30 kg/m$^2$. The risk of death is greater in smokers, Whites compared to Blacks, and those with other diseases.

## QUESTION 3

*What are the health risks associated with obesity?*

## ANSWER 3

Increased fat is associated with an increased risk of diabetes, hypertension, hypercholesterolemia, cardiovascular disease, gallbladder disease, some cancers, and osteoarthritis as well as other diseases. The risk for hypertension, hypercholesterolemia, and diabetes is greater in overweight adults aged 20–44 than in overweight adults aged 45–74 (see Table 5-1). This risk increases with increasing BMI. Obesity is also a major risk factor for the development of sleep apnea.

**TABLE 5-1. Relative Risk of Hypertension, Diabetes, and Hypercholesterolemia in Overweight Patients**

| | RELATIVE RISK | |
|---|---|---|
| | AGE 20–24, YEARS | AGE 45–74, YEARS |
| Hypertension | 5.6 | 1.9 |
| Hypercholesterolemia | 2.1 | 1.1 |
| Diabetes mellitus | 3.8 | 2.1 |

Overweight was defined as a BMI ≥27.8 kg/m$^2$ for men and ≥27.3 kg/m$^2$ for women.

SOURCE: Adapted from Van Itallie TB. Health implications of overweight and obesity in the United States. *Ann Int Med* 1985;103:983–988.

The health risk is increased with increasing abdominal fat (an increased waist-to-hip ratio) and the presence of comorbid conditions at any given level of BMI.

## QUESTION 4

*What are the therapeutic options for obesity?*

## ANSWER 4

Treatments for obesity depend upon either increasing energy expenditure, decreasing caloric intake, or both. The goal of therapy is to prevent the complications associated with obesity. Treatments include diet, exercise, medications, behavior modifications, surgery, or a combination of the above. The choice of therapy depends on the degree of obesity and patient preference. The most effective interventions combine nutrition, education, and diet—exercise counseling with behavioral strategies to help patients acquire the skills and supports needed to change eating patterns and become physically active. More aggressive therapy, including pharmacological, may be indicated for moderate to high-risk categories. Patients with severe obesity and who have failed previous nonsurgical techniques may be candidates for bariatric surgery.

## QUESTION 5

*What are the current screening recommendations?*

## ANSWER 5

The US Preventive Services Task Force (USPSTF) released recommendations in December 2003 regarding screening for obesity, as well as a review of the evidence for screening. USPSTF recommends that "clinicians screen all adult patients for obesity and offer intensive counseling and behavioral interventions to promote sustained weight loss for obese adults."

## BIBLIOGRAPHY

Allison DB, et al. Annual deaths attributable to obesity in the United States. *JAMA.* 1999;282:1530.

Calle EE, et al. Body mass index and mortality in a prospective cohort of U.S. adults. *N Eng J Med.* 1999;341:1097.

Flegal KM, et al. Prevalence and trends in obesity among US adults, 1999–2000. *JAMA.* 2003;289:76.

Must A, et al. The disease burden associated with overweight and obesity. *JAMA.* 1999;282:1523.

National Heart, Lung, and Blood Institute. Clinical guidelines on the identification, evaluation, and treatment of overweight and obesity in adults: the evidence report. *Obes. Res.* 1998; 6(suppl. 2):515.

National Heart, Lung, Blood Institute and the North American Association for the Study of Obesity. *Practical Guide Identification, Evaluation and Treatment of Overweight and Obesity in Adults.* Publication No. 00-4084. National Institutes of Health, Washington, DC; 2000.

Stevens J, et al. The effect of age on the association between body-mass index and mortality. *N Eng J Med.* 1998;338:1.

US Preventive Services Task Force. *Screening for Obesity in Adults.* December 2003. Available at: http://www.ahrq.gov/clinic/uspstf/uspsobes.htm.

WHO Consultation on Obesity. *Obesity: Preventing and Managing the Global Epidemic.* Geneva June 3–5, 1997. World Health Organization, Geneva, 1998.

Yanovski SZ, Yanovski JA. Obesity. *N Eng J Med.* 2002;346:591.

# 6 SMOKING CESSATION

*Alison C. Madden*

## LEARNING POINT

To describe the various strategies to help patients quit smoking.

## VIGNETTE

A 50-year-old Caucasian female, G0, with a history of type 2 diabetes and hypertension presents for her annual physical examination. She currently complains of a chronic nonproductive cough and shortness of breath when walking upstairs. Her diabetes has been well controlled with glyburide. Her blood pressure, however, continues to be a problem despite being on an ACE-inhibitor and a beta-blocker. She has never had any surgery. Her family history is significant for diabetes, hypertension, and colon cancer. She is married and works cleaning houses. She has smoked 1–2 packs/d for the last 32 years and has tried to quit "cold turkey" twice. She does not perform any exercise except for what is required at work. She is scheduled for colonoscopy in 2 months and her cholesterol is slightly elevated at 215. Physical examination reveals a moderately heavy white female in no acute distress. Her vitals are currently stable. Weight is 200 lb and height 5 ft/5 in. Her examination is remarkable only for decreased air movement in bilateral lung fields with rare diffuse crackles.

## QUESTION 1

*What is the prevalence of smoking and smoking related-deaths?*

## ANSWER 1

Smoking prevalence has steadily decreased from 42% of adults in the 1960s to 22% of adults in 2003. Earlier in the 1930–1950s, men predominately smoked, with steadily decreasing rates. However, women experienced a slight increase in the prevelance of smoking during the same period, which declined during the 1980s. Smoking results in approximately 400,000 deaths annually in United States and nearly 5 million worldwide.

## QUESTION 2

*What are the benefits of cessation?*

## ANSWER 2

For both genders of all ages with and without a prior history of cardiovascular disease, smoking cessation is associated with a rapid decrease in the risk of new myocardial events. Patients with chronic obstructive pulmonary disease (COPD) can expect an improvement in cough and sputum production and decreases the rate of decline of forced expiratory volume in one second ($FEV_1$). Smoking cessation has been associated with remission of pulmonary Langerhans cell histiocytosis and improvement of respiratory bronchiolitis. Smoking cessation can decrease the risk of a second smoking-related malignancy in individuals who already have one smoking-related malignancy. Smoking cessation decreases the risk of developing peptic ulcer disease and accelerates healing. Smoking increases the risk of several types of lung infections and is a major risk factor for many types of cancer. Smoking is associated with infertility, spontaneous abortion, ectopic pregnancy, and premature menopause. Smoking also accelerates bone loss and is a risk factor for hip fracture in women.

## QUESTION 3

*Which social attitudes and policies toward smoking have had a major impact on smoking cessation and smoking initiation?*

## ANSWER 3

Smoking behavior is strongly influenced by restriction of minor's access to tobacco products, restriction of smoking in public areas, restriction of advertisements promoting smoking behavior, and decreasing access by increasing pricing through taxation.

## QUESTION 4

*What are the major behavioral and pharmacological methods of cessation?*

## ANSWER 4

Behavioral approaches including physician and group counseling have shown to be of benefit. Abrupt cessation (selecting a *quit day*) is the preferred strategy. Simple physician advice, especially combined with a personalized health message can increase the rate of quitting. The National Cancer Institute has developed the five 'A's for the physicians which encourages physicians to: Ask patients about their smoking status, Assess their readiness to quit and their personal health-related risks, Advise smokers to quit, Assist them in their efforts, and Arrange follow-up visits.

Nicotine replacement therapy is designed to ameliorate the symptoms of nicotine withdrawal while allowing the patient to deal with the behavioral aspects of smoking cessation. The only other effective drug that is not nicotine replacement is buproprion, which is marketed as an antidepressant. See Table 6-1 for current pharmacological therapies. No nicotine replacement therapy is superior to the other and all are similarly effective.

## QUESTION 5

*What are the symptoms and signs of smoking withdrawal?*

## ANSWER 5

The symptoms related to nicotine withdrawal include depressed mood, insomnia, irritability, anxiety, difficulty concentrating, agitation, decreased heart rate, and increased appetite or weight gain.

**TABLE 6-1. Current Pharmacological Therapies**

| DRUG | DOSE | DURATION |
|---|---|---|
| Buproprion HCl | 150 mg PO bid starting 2 days prior to quit date | 7–12 weeks (optimal duration not defined) |
| Nicotine polacrilex (gum or lozenge) | 1–2 tabs/hour<br>Start on quit date<br><25 cig/day: 2 mg tabs<br>≥25 cig/day: 4 mg tabs | 6 weeks; taper over 6 weeks |
| Nicotine patch | Nicoderm CQ:<br>21 mg/day for 6 weeks, 14 mg/day for 2 weeks, 7 mg/day for 2 weeks<br>Nicotrol:<br>Single dose patch for 16 hours/day for 6 weeks | See dose; precaution in pregnant women (Category D), recent myocardial infarctions (within 4 weeks), or serious arrhythmia |
| Nicotine nasal spray | 1 to 2 doses/hour (most require 7–40 sprays over 24 hours | 3 months |
| Nicotine inhaler | 10 mg cartridges used over 20 minutes (6–16 cartridges per day) | Optimal not defined |

## BIBLIOGRAPHY


Behavioral Risk Factor Surveillance System. Survey data, 2000. Centers for Disease Control and Prevention. Available at: http://apps.nccd.cdc.gov/brfss/.

Cigarette smoking among adults—United States, 2001. *Morb Mortal Wkly Rep.* 2003;52:953.

Coleman T. ABC of smoking cessation. Use of simple advice and behavioural support. *Br Med J.* 2004;328:397.

Department of Health and Human Services. *Health Benefits of Smoking Cessation.* A report of the Surgeon General. Washington, DC: DHHS Publication No. (CDC) 90-8416, 1990.

Hughes JR, et al. Recent advances in the pharmacotherapy of smoking. *JAMA.* 1999;281:72.

Jamrozik K. Population strategies to prevent smoking. *Br Med J.* 2004;328:397.

Molyneux A. Nicotine replacement therapy. *Br Med J.* 2004;328:454.

Stillman FA, et al. Evaluation of the American stop smoking intervention study (ASSIST): a report of outcomes. *J Natl Cancer Inst.* 2003;95:1681.

U.S. Department of Health and Human Services. *Smoking Cessation: Information for Specialists.* Rockville, MD: Agency for Health Care Policy and Research. Publication No. 96-0694, 1996.

U.S. Department of Health and Human Services (USDHHS). *The Health Consequences of Smoking.* A report of the Surgeon General. Washington, DC: U.S. Department of Health and Human Services, Public Health Service, CDC; 2004. CDC Publication No. 7829. Available online at: http://www.cdc.gov/tobacco/sgr/sgr_2004/index.htm.

Vineis P, et al. Tobacco and cancer: recent epidemiological evidence. *J Natl Cancer Inst.* 2004;96:99.


# 7 HYPOTHYROIDISM

*John Kuo*

## LEARNING POINT

Understanding how to diagnose and treat hypothyroidism.

## VIGNETTE

A 55-year-old, G3P3003, Asian female presents for a routine annual examination. She has been postmenopausal for 6 years and has never been on hormone replacement therapy. Her past medical history is significant for insulin-dependent diabetes mellitus with good control. She denies any hot flashes, abnormal vaginal bleeding, or urinary incontinence. However, she does complaint of increasing fatigue, muscle cramping, hair loss, and forgetfulness over the last 1 year.

Physical examination reveals a slightly obese Asian woman. Her vital signs are blood pressure 110/70, pulse 64/min, and respiratory rate 12/min, and temperature 98.4°F. Examination reveals: Skin—dry and coarse, Scalp—diffuse alopecia, Thyroid—mild diffuse goiter, Lungs—clear, Heart—regular rate and rhythm, Back—nontender, Abdomen—soft, nontender, nondistended, Pelvic—normal vagina, cervix, uterus, and adnexa, Extremities—cool, mild edema, decreased deep tendon reflexes, decreased sensation to light touch on feet.

## QUESTION 1

What are the causes of hypothyroidism?

## ANSWER 1

Iodine deficiency remains the most common cause of hypothyroidism worldwide. In areas of iodine sufficiency, autoimmune (Hashimoto's) thyroiditis and iatrogenic causes are the most common. The cause of hypothyroidism should be identified since it may be transient and require no or only short-term therapy, may be caused by a drug that disappears upon discontinuation, or may be the first or only manifestation of hypothalamic or pituitary disease. See Table 7-1 for principal causes of hypothyroidism.

**TABLE 7-1. Principal Causes of Hypothyroidism**

**Causes of Primary Hypothyroidism**

- Autoimmune hypothyroidism: Hashimoto's thyroiditis, atrophic thyroiditis
- Iatrogenic: $^{131}$I treatment, subtotal or total thyroidectomy, external irradiation of neck for lymphoma or cancer
- Drugs: iodine excess (including iodine-containing contrast media and amiodarone), lithium, antithyroid drugs, p-aminosalicyclic acid, interferon-a and other cytokines, aminoglutethimide
- Congenital hypothyroidism: absent or ectopic thyroid gland, dyshormonogenesis, thyroid-stimulating hormone (TSH)-receptor mutation
- Iodine deficiency
- Infiltrative disorders: amyloidosis, sarcoidosis, hemo-chromatosis, scleroderma, cystinosis, Riedel's thyroiditis
- Overexpression of Type 3 deiodinase in infantile hemangioma

**Causes of Transient Hypothyroidism**

- Silent thyroiditis, including postpartum thyroiditis
- Subacute thyroiditis
- Withdrawal of thyroxine treatment in individuals with an intact thyroid
- Following $^{131}$I treatment or subtotal thyroidectomy for Graves' disease

**Causes of Secondary Hypothyroidism**

- Hypopituitarism: tumors, pituitary surgery or irradiation, infiltrative disorders, Sheehan's syndrome, trauma, genetic forms of combined pituitary hormone deficiencies
- Isolated TSH deficiency or inactivity
- Bexarotene treatment
- Hypothalamic disease: tumors, trauma, infiltrative disorders, idiopathic

## QUESTION 2

*What are the major signs and symptoms of hypothyroidism?*

## ANSWER 2

Symptoms include:

- Fatigue, lethargy, weakness
- Dry skin
- Cold intolerance
- Hair loss
- Difficulty concentrating and poor memory
- Constipation
- Muscle cramps
- Weight gain with poor appetite
- Dyspnea on exertion
- Hoarse voice
- Menorrhagia (later oligomenorrhea or amenorrhea)
- Myalgia, arthralgia, and paresthesia
- Impaired hearing
- Depression

Signs include:

- Dry coarse skin; cool peripheral extremities
- Puffy face, hands, and feet (myxedema)
- Diffuse alopecia
- Thin, brittle nails
- Slowed movement and speech
- Bradycardia
- Peripheral edema
- Delayed tendon reflex relaxation
- Goiter
- Carpal tunnel syndrome
- Serous cavity effusions
- Galactorrhea

## QUESTION 3

*How is hypothyroidism diagnosed?*

## ANSWER 3

Evaluation of a patient with suspected hypothyroidism should start with a detailed history and physical examination directed toward confirming the presence and identifying the cause of the hormone deficiency. Laboratory confirmation consists of measuring serum TSH and free thyroxine ($T_4$). Primary hypothyroidism is characterized by a high TSH and low free $T_4$. Secondary

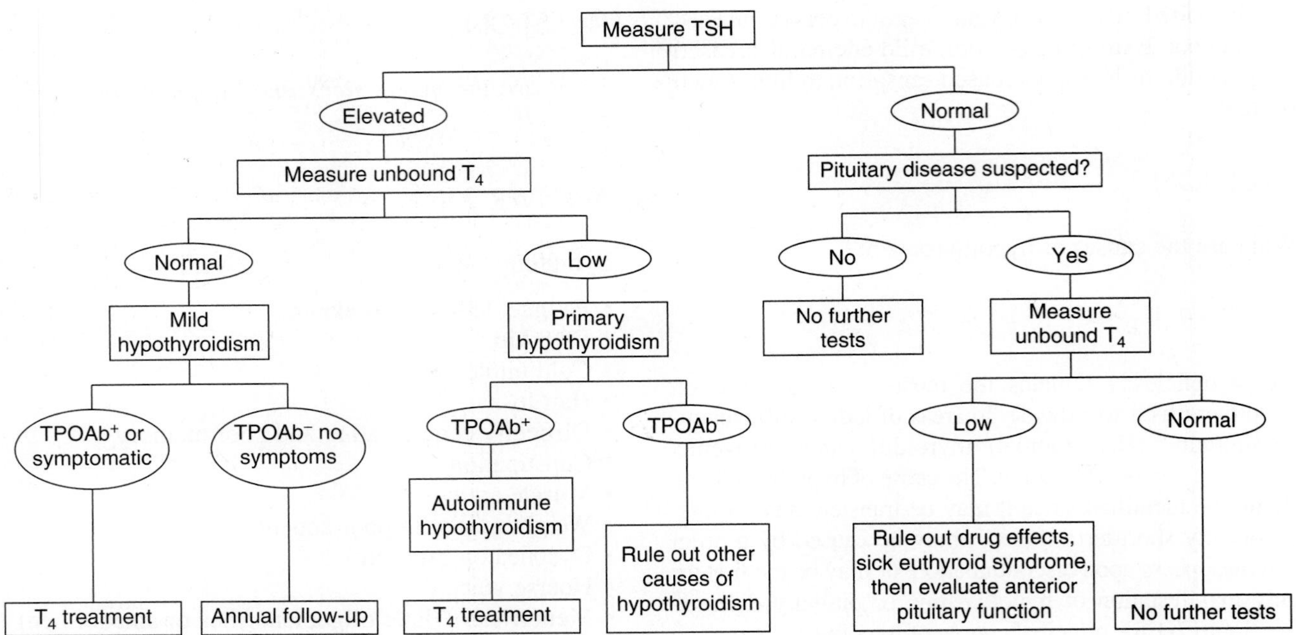


TPOAb$^+$, thyroid peroxidase antibodies present; TPOAb$^-$, thyroid peroxidase antibodies not present.

**FIG. 7-1** Evaluation of hypothyroidism.
SOURCE: From Jameson JL, Weetman AP. Disorders of the thyroid gland. In: Kasper DL, Braunwald E, Fauci AS, et al. (eds.). *Harrison's Principles of Internal Medicine.* 16th ed. New York: McGraw-Hill; 2005.

hypothyroidism is characterized by a low $T_4$ and a TSH level that is not appropriately elevated. Subclinical hypothyroidism is characterized by a high TSH but normal free $T_4$.

Once clinical or subclinical hypothyroidism is confirmed, the etiology is usually established by demonstrating the presence of thyroid peroxidase antibodies, which are present in 90–95% of patients with autoimmune hypothyroidism. If there is any doubt about the cause of a goiter associated with hypothyroidism, ultrasound and/or fine needle aspiration (FNA) biopsy can be used to confirm the etiology. A summary of the investigations used to determine the existence and cause of hypothyroidism is shown in Fig. 7-1. Free $T_3$ measurements are normal in about 25% of patients with hypothyroidism and therefore not usually indicated.

## QUESTION 4

*What is the treatment for hypothyroidism?*

## ANSWER 4

The treatment of choice for hypothyroidism is synthetic $T_4$ (levothyroxine) replacement. Approximately 80% of a dose of levothyroxine is absorbed when taken on an empty stomach with a plasma half-life of 7 days. The average adult replacement dose is about 1.6 μg/kg/d (range 50–200 μg/d). Older patients should be started on a lower dose. After initiating or changing levothyroxine therapy, serum $T_4$ and TSH levels should be measured in 3–8 weeks (depending upon the symptoms), and the dosage adjusted in 12.5–25 μg/d increments to achieve a normal TSH, ideally in the lower half of the reference range. However, it takes about 6 weeks to reach a steady state after therapy is initiated or changed. Patients may not experience full relief from symptoms until 3–6 months after normal TSH levels are restored. Once TSH levels are stable, TSH measurement is recommended at annual intervals and may be extended to every 2–3 years if a normal TSH is maintained over several years.

Levothyroxine requirements typically decrease in elderly patients and dosages should be monitored and adjusted accordingly. In pregnancy, about 50% of women required a 25–100% increase in levothyroxine dosage. Consequently, TSH levels should be measured every 4 weeks until stable, followed by TSH monitoring every trimester.

There are no universally accepted guidelines for the treatment of subclinical hypothyroidism. As long as excessive treatment is avoided, there is little risk in correcting a slightly increased TSH. Treatment is administered by starting with a low dose of levothyroxine (25–50 μg/d) to normalize TSH levels. If not treated, thyroid function should be evaluated annually.

## BIBLIOGRAPHY

ACOG Practice Bulletin No. 37. Thyroid Disease in Pregnancy, August 2002.

Jameson JL, Weetman AP. Disorders of the thyroid gland. In: Kasper DL, Braunwald E, Fauci AS, et al. (eds.). *Harrison's Principles of Internal Medicine*. 16th ed. New York, McGraw-Hill; 2005.

Mandel SJ, Larsen PR, Seely EW, et al. Increased need for thyroxine during pregnancy in women with primary hypothyroidism. *N Engl J Med.* 1990;323;91.

Ross DS. Diagnosis of and Screening for Hypothyroidism. In: Rose BD (ed.). *UpToDate*. Waltham, MA: UpToDate;2006. www.Uptodate.com

Ross DS. Disorders that cause hypothyroidism. In: Rose BD (ed.). *UpToDate*. Waltham, MA: UpToDate;2006. www.Uptodate.com

Ross DS. Treatment of Hypothyroidism. In: Rose BD (ed.). *UpToDate*. Waltham, MA: UpToDate;2006. www.Uptodate.com

Surks MI: Clinical manifestations of hypothyroidism. In: Rose BD (ed.). *UpToDate*. Waltham, MA: UpToDate;2006. www.Uptodate.com

# Section 2

# OFFICE MANAGEMENT: GYNECOLOGY

## 8 ABNORMAL PAP SMEAR

*Alison Axtell*

### LEARNING POINT

Appropriate triage and management of abnormal Pap smears.

### VIGNETTE

A 24-year-old, G0, presents for an annual exam and contraceptive counseling. This is her first gynecologic exam. She has no complaints at this time. She denies vaginal discharge, odor, abnormal vaginal bleeding, or abdominal pain. Currently, she is sexually active with one partner for the last 3 months and describes five lifetime partners. She denies a history of STDs, although she admits she has never been tested. Her menstrual cycles are regular every 28–30 days and last for approximately 4–5 days. The patient states that she smokes cigarettes and drinks alcohol in social situations, but she does not use drugs. She has no significant medical or surgical history. On physical exam, she has a nulliparous cervix that is slightly friable when the Pap smear is performed. One week later, the results of her Pap smear return as atypical squamous cells of undetermined significance (ASC-US).

### QUESTION 1

***Describe the Bethesda Classification of Cervical Cytology.***

### ANSWER 1

The Pap smear was introduced in 1941 as a screening test for cervical cancer and, in 1988, the Bethesda System was developed to standardize reporting of Pap smear results. This system was recently updated in 2001 and includes the following in result reports:

1. Specimen type: conventional smear versus liquid-based prep
2. Specimen adequacy: satisfactory or unsatisfactory (based on the number of squamous cells, endocervical cells, and presence of blood and/or inflammation)
3. General categorization: Negative, epithelial cell abnormality, or other
4. Interpretation/result: negative for intraepithelial lesion or malignancy, epithelial cell abnormality (see next), infection, atrophy, or inflammation.
5. Epithelial cell abnormalities: ASC-US cannot exclude high grade (ASC-H), low grade squamous intraepithelial lesion (LGSIL), high grade squamous intraepithelial lesion (HSIL), squamous cell carcinoma, atypical glandular cells of undetermined significance (AGC-US) or of endometrial/endocervical origin, endocervical adenocarcinoma in situ, and adenocarcinoma.
6. Educational notes and suggestions by the pathologist.

### QUESTION 2

*What are the relative frequencies of Pap smear cytologic abnormalities? What is the chance of having cervical intraepithelial neoplasia (CIN) II–III of invasive cancer on colposcopic biopsy based on Pap smear cytology?*

**TABLE 8-1. Prevalances of Cytologic Abnormalities on Papsmear and Correlation with Colposcopic Findings**

| CYTOLOGY | FREQUENCY | CIN II–III | CA |
|---|---|---|---|
| ASC-US | 3–5% | 5–179% | 0.1–0.29% |
| ASC-H | N/A | 24–949% | 0.1–0.29% |
| LSIL | 1.5–3.9% | 15–309% | <19% |
| HSIL | 0.3–0.69% | 70–759% | 1–29% |
| AGC | 0.4–0.79% | 9–549%* | 1–99%* |
| SCCA | 0.1–0.29% | – | – |
| Adeno CA | 0.29% | – | – |

*Higher if referred to as AGC—"favor neoplasia."

## ANSWER 2

ASC-US and LGSIL are the most common diagnoses found on cytology. Pap smear cytology does not always correlate with colposcopic findings (Table 8-1).

## QUESTION 3

*Describe the evaluation of ASC-US and AGC Pap smears.*

## ANSWER 3

ASC-US

1. Human papillomavirus (HPV) testing: refer to colposcopy if positive for high risk types, if negative, repeat Pap in 1 year. All smears with ASC-US cytology should be screened routinely for HPV.
2. Repeat cytology in 4–6 months until two consecutive normal results if HPV testing is not available.
3. Postmenopausal women with atrophy can be treated with topical estrogen followed by repeat testing after treatment.
4. Immunosuppression and ASC-H should be immediate referrals to colposcopy.

AGC-US

1. Immediate referral to colposcopy with biopsies and endocervical curettage (ECC).
2. Women over 35 and those with abnormal bleeding should also have an endometrial biopsy.

## QUESTION 4

*What is current role of HPV testing?*

## ANSWER 4

The ALTS trial was designed to evaluate the management of ASC-US Pap smears by randomizing 3488 women to follow up with immediate colposcopy, colposcopy only if positive for high risk HPV, or conservative management with colposcopy referral for HSIL only. All patients received liquid-based cytology smears every 6 months for 24 months. HPV testing was 96% sensitive for detecting CIN III and HPV testing confirms absence of disease with a negative predictive value of 99%.

## BIBLIOGRAPHY

Goodman A, Holschneider C. Management of the abnormal papanicolaou smear. *Up to Date*, 2004.

Adapted from 2001 Bethesda System, NIH consensus development conference statement, 2001.

Diaz-Rosario LA, et al. Performance of a fluid-based, thin-layer Papanicolaou smear method in the clinical setting of an independent laboratory and an outpatient screening population in New England. *Arch Pathol Lab Med*. 1999;123:817–821.

Results of a randomized trial on the management of cytology interpretations of atypical squamous cells of undetermined significance. *Am J Obstet Gynecol*. 2003 188(6):1383–1392.

Wright TC, Cox TC, Stewart-Massad I, et al. 2001:consensus guidelines for the management of women with cervical cytological abnormalities. *JAMA*. 2002;287:2120–2129.

# 9 ABNORMAL UTERINE BLEEDING

*Ashim Kumar*

## LEARNING POINT

To understand the definition and treatment of dysfunctional uterine bleeding (DUB).

## VIGNETTE

A 15-year-old female, body mass index of 25, P0, presents with complaints of a 14-month history of irregular and heavy menses every 2–3 months. Patient states that she is virginal and denies dysmenorrhea. Menarche was at 14 years of age. Patient does not have any medical problems. She underwent knee surgery 2 months ago due to a motor vehicle accident. The surgery was not complicated by excessive bleeding. She denies drug allergies and is not currently using any medications. She exercises for 45 minutes three times a week. She denies excessive emotional stress. She is in the 9th grade and obtains above average grades. Family history is noncontributory. Physical exam reveals a well-developed, well-nourished female with blood pressure of 110/70 mm Hg and pulse of 105 beats/min. Conjunctiva are pale. Pelvic exam reveals normal external genitalia, vaginal mucosa, and cervix without evidence of lesions except for moderate bleeding from the cervical os. Bimanual exam reveals a nulliparous-size, regularly-shaped uterus and normal adnexa.

## QUESTION 1

*What is the definition of abnormal uterine bleeding and DUB? How often is abnormal endometrial histology found in the setting of DUB?*

## ANSWER 1

Abnormal uterine bleeding encompasses all diagnoses that would lead to excessive or irregular bleeding including tumors (benign and malignant), infection, drugs, systemic disease, inherited disorders, and the like. DUB infers anovulatory cycles as the etiology and is a diagnosis made after excluding all other probable causes of abnormal bleeding. The differential diagnoses for abnormal uterine bleeding is dependent on the age of the patient. Anovulatory cycles are most frequently encountered at the extremes of reproductive age, perimenarche and perimenopause. In the older population, endometrial pathology is often associated with anovulatory cycles; the lack of progestin facilitates the trophic effects of estrogen on the endometrium. Fourteen to twenty-four percent of women with DUB will exhibit histological abnormalities.

## QUESTION 2

*What is the differential diagnosis of an adolescent with DUB? What is the incidence of anovulatory cycles in the first several years after menarche?*

## ANSWER 2

Although this patient's surgical history would be evidence against blood dyscrasias, they must be included in the differential diagnosis as they account for almost 20% of adolescents requiring acute medical care due to menorrhagia. However, the majority of DUB in the adolescent is due to anovulatory cycles. Approximately 50% of adolescent females will have anovulatory cycles in the first 2 years following menarche. This most likely occurs due to immaturity of the hypothalamic-pituitary-ovarian axis with inadequate regulation of gonadotropin secretion. The majority of these teenagers will progress to regular ovulatory cycles. Polycystic ovary syndrome (PCOS) should be considered as its onset is with menarche and the patient may benefit from additional evaluation aimed at the assement and treatment of metabolic parameters and hirsutism.

## QUESTION 3

*What are the acute and chronic treatment options for DUB in an adolescent? What are the differences for perimenopausal women?*

## ANSWER 3

In an urgent or emergent situation, estradiol is the quickest path to stabilization of the endometrium and therefore to cessation of bleeding. Estradiol can be administered intravenously, if the patient is hemodynamically stable oral administration can be used. After the acute bleeding has resolved, a progestin must be added to synchronize and add structural support to the endometrium. Iron and folic acid supplementation will help to restore the blood count.

The chronic treatment of anovulatory cycles in the adolescent is oral contraceptive pills (OCPs). Serial estrogen and progestin should be similar in efficacy. If PCOS is confirmed, additional pharmacological options should be discussed with the patient. Viable choices for use in teenagers include insulin sensitizers (e.g., metformin) for insulin resistance and antiandrogens (e.g., spironolactone) for hirsutism. OCPs may be discontinued empirically after 1–2 years to determine if patient is eumenorrheic/ normoulatory or they may be continued for other indications/benefits, such as the need for contraception.

Other options to consider in mature women include cyclic progestin, gonadotropin-releasing hormone agonists with add-back therapy, nonsteroidal anti-inflammatory agents, and antifibrinolytics (e.g., tranexamic acid). In patients who have completed childbearing, surgical options may also be considered. Endometrial ablation is a minimally invasive option that may be accomplished with a resectoscope, balloon thermal ablation, laser, cryoablation, and the like with similar overall efficacy. The definitive, but more invasive option is hysterectomy (total or supracervical).

## BIBLIOGRAPHY

Ash SJ, Farrell SA, Flowerdew G. Endometrial biopsy in DUB. *J Reprod Med.* 1996;41:892–896.

Bongers MY, Mol BW, Brolmann HA. Current treatment of dysfunctional uterine bleeding. *Maturitas.* 2004;47:159–174.

Claessens EA, Cowell CA. Acute adolescent menorrhagia. *Am J Obstet Gynecol.* 1981;139:277–280.
Deligeoroglou E. Dysfunctional uterine bleeding. *Ann NY Acad Sci.* 1997;816:158–164.
DeVore GR, Owens O, Kase N. Use of intravenous Premarin in the treatment of dysfunctional uterine bleeding—a double-blind randomized control study. *Obstet Gynecol.* 1982;59:285–291.
Livingstone M, Fraser IS. Mechanisms of abnormal uterine bleeding. *Hum Reprod Update.* 2002;8:60–67.
Munro MG. Dysfunctional uterine bleeding: advances in diagnosis and treatment. *Curr Opin Obstet Gynecol.* 2001;13:475–489.
Reich H, Ribeiro SC, Vidali A. Hysterectomy as treatment for dysfunctional uterine bleeding. *Baillieres Best Pract Res Clin Obstet Gynaecol.* 1999;13:251–269.
Rosenfield RL, Barnes RB. Menstrual disorders in adolescence. *Endocrinol Metab Clin North Am.* 1993;22:491–505.
Shankar M, Lee CA, Sabin CA, Economides DL, Kadir RA. von Willebrand disease in women with menorrhagia: a systematic review. *BJOG.* 2004;111(7):734–740.

# 10 CONTRACEPTION: INTRAUTERINE DEVICE

*Jane L. Davis*

## LEARNING POINT

It is important to select patients that are good candidates for using the intrauterine device (IUD).

## VIGNETTE

A 30-year-old, G3P3, woman presents for a routine gynecologic evaluation. She is currently using a low-dose oral contraceptive, but would possibly like to change to the IUD. She is in a mutually monogamous relationship with her husband. They are uncertain if they wish to have additional children. She denies any history of sexually transmitted diseases.

The patient has regular cycles every 30 days. She has had three-term, normal spontaneous vaginal deliveries. The patient's past medical and surgical histories are negative. The patient does not smoke or use recreational drugs. She is a social drinker.

The physical exam reveals a Caucasian woman. Vital signs reveal a blood pressure of 110/68, pulse of 82/min, respiratory rate of 18/min, and temperature of 98.6°F. Thyroid is nonpalpable, lungs are clear, and heart has regular rate and rhythm, without audible murmurs. Abdomen has normal bowel sounds present, is soft, nontender, without palpable masses. Pelvic exam reveals external genitalia without lesions, vagina is well rugated, cervix with multiparous os, uterus is anteverted and normal size, and adnexa are nontender with no palpable masses. Rectovaginal exam is confirmatory.

### QUESTION 1

*What two IUDs are currently available in United States?*

### ANSWER 1

Copper containing systems (Cu T380A-ParaGard)—Available for use since 1988; approved for 10 years of contraceptive use, probably efficacious for 12 years.

Levonorgestrel-intrauterine system (Mirena)—52 mg levonorgestrel total, releases 20 ug/day; approved for 5 years of contraceptive use, probably efficacious for 7 years.

### QUESTION 2

*How do IUDs prevent pregnancy?*

### ANSWER 2

1. Prefertilization effects (more common with copper containing IUDs)
   a. Interference with sperm transport from the cervix to the fallopian tube: IUDs alter biochemical and cellular composition of cervical mucus, endometrial secretions, and tubal fluid.
   b. Inhibition of sperm capacitation and survival: Copper is detrimental to sperm capacitation and motility. Progesterone released in the endometrial cavity may alter tubal motility and sperm or egg viability in the tube.
2. Postfertilization effects
   a. Endometrial changes that inhibit the process of implantation: Significant increases in macrophages, lymphocytes, and plasma cells have been observed in both histologic sections of the endometrium and endometrial fluid of IUD users. Levonorgestrel-containing IUDs also cause decidualization and suppression of endometrial function.

### QUESTION 3

*Who is the ideal patient for an IUD?*

## ANSWER 3

An IUD is well suited for women who:

1. Are older, parous, nonpregnant, and who desire contraception, but who do not desire permanent sterilization.
2. Are in stable monogamous relationships (both patient and her partner).
3. Have no history of pelvic inflammatory disease (PID).
4. Do not have a history of a prior ectopic pregnancy (EP) (this is a relative contraindication).

## QUESTION 4

*What are the complications of IUD insertion?*

## ANSWER 4

Complications of IUD placement include PID, uterine perforation, cervicitis, vasovagal reaction, expulsion, and pregnancy (see Table 10-1).

## QUESTION 5

*How should you counsel a patient prior to inserting an IUD?*

**TABLE 10-1. IUD Complications of Uterine Insertion**

| COMPLICATION | FREQUENCY | RISK FACTORS |
|---|---|---|
| PID within 20 days | 1/1000 | BV, cervicitis, contamination with insertion |
| Uterine perforation | 1/1000 | Immobile, markedly verted uterus |
| | | Breast-feeding woman |
| | | Inexperienced, unskilled inserter |
| Vasovagal reaction or fainting with insertion | Rare | Stenotic os, pain prior vasovagal reaction |
| Expulsion | | Insertion on menses, immediately postpartum, not high enough in fundus or nulliparous |
| Pregnancy | | Poor placement, expulsion |

SOURCE: Reprinted with permission from: Hatcher RE, Zieman M, Cwiak C, Darney PD, Crenin MD, Stosur HR. *A Pocket Guide to Managing Contraception 2005–2007.* Tiger, Georgia: Bridging the Gap Foundation, 2005.

## ANSWER 5

Prior to inserting an IUD, patients should be counseled regarding the following:

1. Complications of IUD insertion.
2. Pregnancy prevention failure rate of the IUD is approximately 1% per year.
3. Twenty percent of women discontinue using the IUD after 1 year because of bleeding, cramping, or spontaneous expulsion.
4. Partial or complete perforation of the uterine wall occurs in approximately 1/1000–2000 insertions.

## QUESTION 6

*What should be done when patients with an IUD are diagnosed with a pregnancy?*

## ANSWER 6

Evaluate the patient to rule out an EP, since there is an increased likelihood that pregnancies with an IUD in place will be extra-uterine. The risk of an EP, if a pregnancy occurs, is 25% for levonorgestrel-containing IUDs and 3–4% for copper-containing IUDs.

Once an EP has been excluded, if the patient elects to continue the pregnancy, the IUD should be removed as soon as possible if the string can be located (ultrasound guidance may be helpful). If the IUD is removed in the first trimester, the risk of a miscarriage is dependent on where the IUD is located; alternatively, the risk of a second or third trimester fetal loss is not increased. If the IUD remains in place, the patient should be counseled that the risk of first trimester miscarriage, septic abortions (especially in the second trimester), and premature births in the third trimester will increase.

## BIBLIOGRAPHY

Foreman H, et al. Intrauterine device usage and fetal loss. *Obstet Gynecol.* 1981;58:669–677.

Furlong LA. Ectopic pregnancy risk when contraception fails. *J Reprod Med.* 2002;47:881–885.

Hatcher RA, Zieman M, Cwiak C, Darney PD, Crenin MD, Stosur HR. *A Pocket Guide to Managing Contraception,* 2005–2007. Tiger, Georgia GA: Bridging the Gap Foundation; 2005.

Stanford JB, Mikolajczyk RT. Mechanisms of action of intrauterine devices. Update. *ACOG.* February 1992. Technical Bulletin No. 164.

Stanford JB, Mikolajczyk RT. Mechanisms of action of intrauterine devices. Update and estimation of postfertilization effects. *AJOG.* 2002;187:1699–1708.

# 11 CONTRACEPTION: TUBAL STERILIZATION

*Jane L. Davis*

## LEARNING POINT

Proper presterilization counseling is critical to minimize patient regret and dissatisfaction.

## VIGNETTE

A 32-year-old, G4P3013, female presents desiring information regarding sterilization. She is in a mutually monogamous, stable relationship with her husband for 8 years. She has three children who are alive and well, between the ages of 1–7 years. She has tried other methods of contraception, but has had problems with each method including the intrauterine device (IUD) and combination oral contraceptive pills. Both the patient and her husband are certain that they do not want any additional children, and her husband does not wish to have a vasectomy if possible.

The patient has regular cycles every 28–30 days, with menses lasting 3–4 days. Her obstetrical history is significant for three-term pregnancies and three spontaneous vaginal deliveries. The patient's medical and surgical histories are both negative. She does not smoke or use recreational drugs. She is a social drinker.

The physical exam reveals a slender, Caucasian woman. Vital signs: blood pressure 110/70, pulse 80/min, respiratory rate 18/min, temperature 98.6°F. Thyroid nonpalpable, lungs clear, heart regular rate and rhythm; without audible murmurs, abdomen with normal bowel sounds, soft, nontender, no palpable masses. Pelvic exam: external genitalia without lesions, vagina well estrogenized, multiparous cervical os, otherwise normal, uterus anteverted and normal size, adnexa nontender, without palpable masses. Rectovaginal confirms.

## QUESTION 1

*What presterilization counseling/assessment should patients receive?*

## ANSWER 1

1. Counsel regarding alternative methods, including male sterilization.
2. Inform patient that the procedure is permanent.
3. Evaluate patient for risk factors that affect regret of sterilization:
   a. Approximately 6% of sterilized women report regret or request information about sterilization reversal within 5 years of procedure (1–2% of men seek information on vasectomy reversal). Postpartum tubal ligation is associated with increased guilt and regret over interval procedures.
   b. Risk factors that affect regret:
      i. Young age at the time of sterilization regardless of parity or marital status. Women between the ages of 20–24 years at sterilization are twice as likely to experience regret than women between the ages of 30–34 years.
      ii. Marital instability increases the probability of regret.
4. Probability of sterilization failure, including ectopic pregnancy.
5. Potential complications from both the operation and anesthesia (death related to procedure 1–2/100,00 procedures).
6. Discuss potential of "posttubal syndrome," i.e., the onset of irregular menses and dysmenorrhea, reported to occur in 10–15% of patients. However, well-controlled prospective studies have failed to provide convincing evidence that this syndrome exists.
7. Advise patient that sterilization offers no protection against sexually transmitted diseases.

## QUESTION 2

*What are the failure rates of tubal ligations?*

## ANSWER 2

The failure rates of bilateral tubal ligation (BTL) procedures are generally accepted to be less than 1%. However, the findings from the U.S. Collaborative Review of Sterilization (multicenter, prospective cohort study following 10,685 women for 8–14 years who underwent a BTL) indicate that the failure rates are higher than expected with significant differences between methods. Furthermore, the failure persists for years after the procedure and varies by the method used and the age of the patient at the time that the procedure was performed.

The highest failure rates are reported after clip sterilizations (36.5/1000 procedures) and lowest after unipolar coagulation (7.5/1000 procedures) and postpartum salpingectomy (7.5/1000 procedures). Cumulative risk of pregnancy was highest among women sterilized at a young age with bipolar coagulation (54.3/1000 procedures) and clip application (52.1/1000 procedures).

## QUESTION 3

*What are some of the different methods for performing postpartum tubal ligation?*

## ANSWER 3

There are various types of BTL in use today:

1. Pomeroy or Modified Pomeroy Procedure: Ligation/excision of midsegment of tube with absorbable suture (Fig. 11-1).
2. Irving Procedure: Ligation/transection of proximal portion of each tube and implantation of the cut end of the tube into a pocket in the uterine wall (lowest failure rate, but more complicated to perform).
3. Uchida Procedure (also performed as interval procedure): Tube is dissected from mesosalpinx with injection of saline. Mesosalpinx is then incised and the tube is transected. Proximal end of the tube is sutured within the leaves of the broad ligament.
4. Kroener Fimbriectomy: Excise distal tube and fimbriae ligating ends with silk suture (failure rate can be as high as 3%).

## QUESTION 4

*What are the usual regulations for performing sterilizations in state and federaly funded programs?*

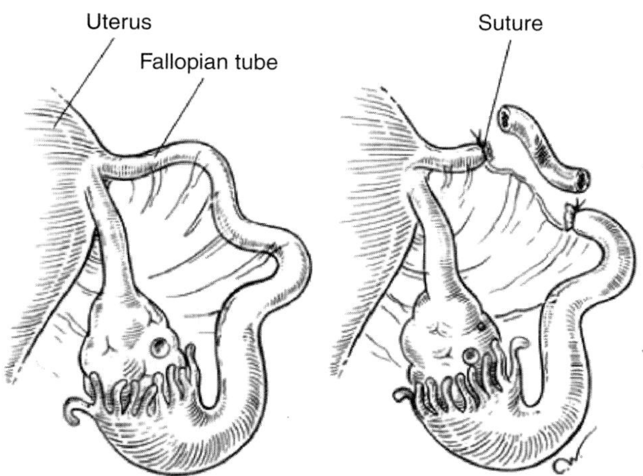


**FIG. 11-1** Pomeroy tubal ligation.

## ANSWER 4

1. Patient must be at least 21 years of age.
2. Patient must be mentally competent.
3. Patient must sign informed consent at least 30 days prior to the procedure (sign prior to or at 36 weeks). *Consent expires after 180 days.*
4. In cases of premature or emergent surgical delivery, the consent must be signed at least 72 hours in advance.

## BIBLIOGRAPHY

ACOG Technical Bulletin No. 222. April 1996.

Hendrix NW et al. Sterilization and its consequences. *Obstet Gynecol Survey*. 1999;54:766–777.

Hillis SD, et al. Poststerilization regret. Findings from the United States collaborative review of sterilization. *Obstet Gynecol*. 1999;93:889.

Peterson HP, et al. The risk of pregnancy after tubal sterilization: findings from the U.S. collaborative review of sterilization. *Am J Obstet Gynecol.* 1996;174:1161–1170.

Wilcox LA, et al. Risk factors for regret after tubal sterilization: 5 years of follow-up in a prospective study. *Fertil Steril.* 1991; 55:927–933.

# 12 CONTRACEPTION: DEPO-PROVERA

*John Kuo*

## LEARNING POINT

Understanding the use, advantages and contraindications of Depo-Provera use for contraception.

## VIGNETTE

A 25-year-old, G1P0010, African-American female presents desiring information regarding alternative contraception methods. She is currently sexually active with her steady boyfriend of 1 year and has been using oral contraceptive pills for contraception. However, she reports that she forgets to take her contraceptive pills on occasion due to her busy schedule and wishes to learn about other forms of contraception. Her past medical history is significant for sickle cell trait and epilepsy controlled on carbamazepine. She denies a personal history of thromboembolism and does not use tobacco or recreational drugs. Her obstetrical history is significant for a first trimester therapeutic termination at age 18. She has regular menses and no history of sexually transmitted diseases.

Physical examination reveals an African-American woman of normal body habitus. Her vital signs are blood pressure 120/80, pulse 70/min, respiratory rate 12/min, temperature 98.6°F. Examination reveals normal thyroid, heart, lung, abdomen, back, pelvic, and extremities.

## QUESTION 1

*What is Depo-Provera?*

## ANSWER 1

Depo-Provera is a contraceptive injection containing medroxyprogesterone acetate. It is formulated as microcrystals, suspended in an aqueous solution. The dosage for contraception is 150 mg given intramuscularly (gluteal or deltoid) every 3 months (11–13 weeks). The typical failure rate is 0.3% during the first year of use. The pregnancy rate is about 1 per 100 women after 5 years of consistent use. Its primary mechanism of action is suppression of gonadotropins, which prevents follicular maturation and ovulation. In addition, the endometrium is altered preventing implantation and the cervical mucus thickens forming a barrier to sperm penetration. The first injection should be administered within the first 5 days of the menstrual cycle, or a backup method is necessary for 2 weeks.

## QUESTION 2

*What are the advantages of Depo-Provera?*

## ANSWER 2

Advantages:

- Easy to use, no daily or coital action required
- Private as use is not detectable
- Highly effective long-acting contraception, with success rates comparable to sterilization, intrauterine device (IUD), and implants
- Free from estrogen-related side-effects
- Reduced menstrual flow and anemia
- Less endometriosis
- Decreased risk of endometrial cancer
- Less ovarian cysts
- Fewer uterine fibroids
- Fewer ectopic pregnancies
- Less pelvic inflammatory disease (PID)
- Inhibits invivo sickling and reduces the frequency and intensity of sickle cell crises
- Raises the seizure threshold (probably due to sedative properties of progestins), making it an excellent choice if taking antiepileptics
- Can be administered immediately after delivery
- Lactation enhanced with negligible concentration in the breast milk and no effects on infant growth and development

## QUESTION 3

*Are there any contraindications to the use of Depo-Provera?*

## ANSWER 3

Absolute contraindications:

- Known or suspected pregnancy
- Unexplained vaginal bleeding
- Known or suspected malignancy of the breast
- Active thrombophlebitis, current or past history of thromboembolic disorders, or cerebral vascular disease
- Significant liver disease
- Previous sex steroid-induced liver adenoma
- Known hypersensitivity to Depo-Provera (medroxyprogesterone acetate or any of its other ingredients)

Relative contraindications

- Severe cardiovascular disease
- Liver disease
- Rapid return to fertility desired
- Difficulty with injections
- Severe depression

## QUESTION 4

*What are the side effects of Depo-Provera?*

## ANSWER 4

Irregular menstrual bleeding occurs in about 70% of users during the first 3 months and it is the reason up to 25% of users discontinue in the first year. Bleeding and spotting decrease over time with 55% of users becoming amenorrheic after 12 months and 68% after 24 months. Depo-Provera has also been associated with a significant loss of bone mineral density in the hip and lumber spine as bone metabolism accommodates to a lower estrogen level. Bone loss is greater with increasing duration of use and this bone loss may not be completely reversible (see Fig. 12-1). It is unknown whether use during adolescence or early adulthood, a critical period of bone accretion, will reduce peak bone mass and increase the risk for osteoporotic fracture later in life.

There is a tendency for women using Depo-Provera to gain weight, which averages 5.4 lb after 1 year and 8.1 lb after 2 years. Because Depo-Provera has a prolonged contraceptive effect, there may be a 6–18 month delay following the last injection before the return of ovulation. In addition, there is no protection against HIV infection or other sexually transmitted diseases. Long-term case-controlled studies of Depo-Provera found slight or no increased overall risk of breast cancer and no overall increased risk of ovarian, liver, or cervical cancer.

Adverse reactions reported by more than 5% of subjects are menstrual irregularities (bleeding or amenorrhea, or both), abdominal pain or discomfort, weight changes, dizziness, headache, asthenia (weakness or fatigue), and nervousness. Decreased libido or anorgasmia, pelvic pain, backache, breast pain, leg cramps, no hair growth or alopecia, depression, bloating, nausea, rash, insomnia, edema, leukorrhea, hot flashes, acne, arthralgia, and vaginitis were reported by 1–5% of subjects.

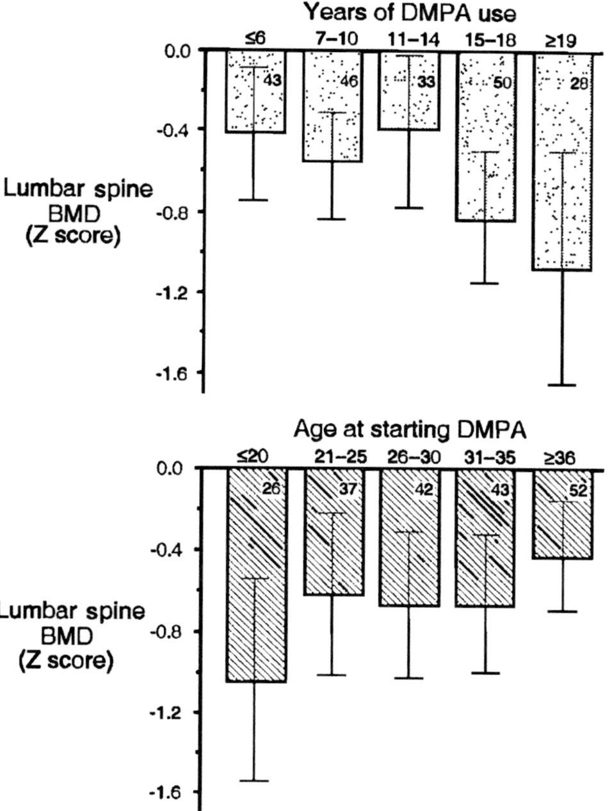


**FIG. 12-1** Mean lumbar spine bone mineral density z score (with 95% confidence intervals) according to number of years use of depot medroxyprogesterone acetate (DMPA) and according to age at starting DMPA.

SOURCE: From Cundy T, Cornish J, Roberts H, et al. Spinal bone density in women using depot medroxyprogesterone contraception. *Obstet Gynecol.* 1998;92:569.

## BIBLIOGRAPHY

Cundy T, Cornish J, Roberts H, et al. Spinal bone density in women using depot medroxyprogesterone contraception. *Obstet Gynecol.* 1998;92:569.

de Abood M, de Castillo Z, Guerrero F, et al. Effect of Depo-Provera or microgynon on the painful crises of sickle cell anemia patients. *Contraception* 1997;56:313.

Depo-Provera Contraceptive Injection package insert by Pharmacia & Upjohn Company, Division of Pfizer Inc, Nov 2004.

Mattson RH, Cramer JA, Caldwell BV, et al. Treatment of seizures with medroxyprogesterone acetate: preliminary report. *Neurology.* 1984;34:1255.

Schwallie PC, Assenzo JR. Contraceptive use—efficacy study utilizing medroxyprogesterone acetate administered as an intramuscular injection once every 90 days. *Fertil Steril.* 1973;24:331.

Skegg DCG, Noonan EA, Paul C, et al. Depot medroxyprogesterone acetate and breast cancer: a pooled analysis from the World Health Organization and New England studies. *JAMA.* 1995;273:799.

Speroff L, Fritz MA. *Clinical Gynecologic Endocrinology and Infertility.* 7th ed. Philadelphia, Lippincott Williams & Wilkins; 2005.

Trussell J, Hatcher RA, Cates W, et al. A guide to interpreting contraceptive efficacy studies. *Obstet Gynecol.* 1990; 76:558.

Westhoff C. Depot-medroxyprogesterone acetate injection (Depo-Provera): a highly effective contraceptive option with proven long-term safety. *Contraception.* 2003;68:75.

WHO: Multinational comparative clinical trial of long-acting injectable contraceptives: norethisterone enanthate given in two dosage regimens and depot-medroxyprogesterone acetate. Final report. *Contraception.* 1983;28:1.

# 13 EMERGENCY CONTRACEPTION

*Susan Sarajari*

## LEARNING POINT

Options and effective use of emergency contraception.

## VIGNETTE

A 24-year-old, G0, presents to your office stating that she had unprotected intercourse yesterday night. She is near midcycle and is worried that she might get pregnant. The last time she had intercourse was 2 months ago and a urine pregnancy test today is negative. The patient has regular menstrual cycles, with menses lasting 4–5 days. She has never been pregnant and has no surgical history. She has no medical problems and is not taking any medications. She does not smoke, use drugs, and only drinks a glass of wine occasionally. The patient has used oral contraceptive pills in the past but has run out and has not seen a physician to renew her prescription. She has heard about emergency contraception from a friend and wants to know whether she would be a candidate for it.

### QUESTION 1

*What is emergency contraception and who is a candidate for emergency contraception?*

### ANSWER 1

Emergency contraception is also known as postcoital contraception and is the administration of drugs to prevent pregnancy in women who have had unprotected intercourse, failure of another contraception method, or were victims of sexual assault. Women of reproductive age who had unprotected intercourse within the previous 72 hours, independent of the time in the menstrual cycle are candidates for emergency contraception. See Table 13-1.

### QUESTION 2

*What is the mechanism of action of emergency contraception?*

### ANSWER 2

There is no single mechanism of action but inhibition or delay of ovulation, regression of corpus luteum, interference with tubal transport, and changes in the endometrium interfering with implantation have all been reported.

Ninety-eight percent of patients will menstruate 21 days after treatment with emergency contraceptives and menses will occur at the expected time in more than 50% of patients. In 90% of women, menses will be of normal duration. If treatment is given during the follicular phase of the cycle, menses may occur 3–7 days earlier than expected. If treatment is given in the luteal phase, menses may be delayed. A pregnancy test should be done if the patient did not start her menses after 21 days.

### QUESTION 3

*How is emergency contraception provided?*

**TABLE 13-1. Potential Indications for Use of Emergency Contraception**

| |
|---|
| Unprotected intercourse (consensual or rape) within the previous 120 hours. |
| Suspected contraceptive failure within the previous 120 hours, including: |
| • Breakage, slippage, or leakage of a male condom |
| • Dislodgment, breakage, or incorrect use of a diaphragm, cervical cap, or female condom |
| • Failure of a spermicide tablet or film to melt before intercourse |
| • Failure to withdraw before ejaculation |
| • Expulsion of an intrauterine device |
| • Missed oral contraceptive pills |
| • Late injection of injectable contraceptive (>2 weeks late for a progestin-only formulation, or >3 days late for a combined estrogen plus progestin formulation) |

SOURCE: Adapted from Grimes, DA, Raymond, EG. Emergency contraception. *Ann Intern Med.* 2002;137:180.

## ANSWER 3

1. Plan B:
   a. Levonorgestrel 0.75 mg given twice 12 hours apart.
   b. May be better tolerated and more effective than the estrogen-progestin regimen.
2. Preven: Four combination tablets, each containing 50 mcg of ethinyl estradiol and 0.25 mg of levonorgestrel. Take two tablets twice 12 hours apart (also known as the Yuzpe regimen). Discontinued production in 2004.
3. Mifepristone (RU-486): An antiprogestin, given as 10 mg in one dose is as effective as levonorgestrel.
4. Copper intrauterine device: The device may still be inserted 5–7 days after unprotected intercourse except in cases of rape or sexually transmitted disease. The advantage of this method is that it provides continuing contraception.
5. Other options: Dosage equivalents using common oral contraceptive pills. See Table 13-2.

## QUESTION 4

*What are the potential side effects and contraindications of emergency contraception?*

## ANSWER 4

1. Nausea and vomiting are the most common side effects. Nausea occurs in 30–66% of patients and emesis in 12–22% of patients. Antiemetics can be taken 1 hour before the first dose of emergency contraception and decrease the incidence of nausea and vomiting. Antiemetics do not seem to be effective if taken after the onset of symptoms. With the progestin-only method, nausea and vomiting occur significantly less.
2. Breast tenderness occurs anywhere from 1% to 47%.
3. Uncommon side effects include irregular bleeding, fatigue, dizziness, headache, and lower abdominal pain.

**TABLE 13-2. Oral Contraceptives That Can be Used for Emergency Contraception in the United States[a]**

| BRAND | COMPANY | PILLS PER DOSE[b] | ETHINYL ESTRADIOL PER DOSE (μG) | LEVONORGESTREL PER DOSE (mg)[c] |
|---|---|---|---|---|
| | | PROGESTIN-ONLY PILLS: TAKE ONE DOSE[b] | | |
| Plan-B | Barr/Duramed | 2 white pills | 0 | 1.5 |
| Ovrette | Wyeth-Ayerst | 40 yellow pills | 0 | 1.5 |
| | | COMBINED PROGESTIN AND ESTROGEN PILLS: TAKE TWO DOSES 12 HOURS APART | | |
| Alesse | Wyeth-Ayerst | 5 pink pills | 100 | 0.50 |
| Aviane | Barr/Duramed | 5 orange pills | 100 | 0.50 |
| Cryselle | Barr/Duramed | 4 white pills | 120 | 0.60 |
| Enpresse | Barr/Duramed | 4 orange pills | 120 | 0.50 |
| Jolessa | Barr/Duramed | 4 pink pills | 120 | 0.60 |
| Lessina | Barr/Duramed | 5 pink pills | 100 | 0.50 |
| Levlen | Berlex | 4 light-orange pills | 120 | 0.60 |
| Levlite | Berlex | 5 pink pills | 100 | 0.50 |
| Levora | Watson | 4 white pills | 120 | 0.60 |
| Lo/Ovral | Wyeth-Ayerst | 4 white pills | 120 | 0.60 |
| Low-Ogestrel | Watson | 4 white pills | 120 | 0.60 |
| Lutera | Watson | 5 white pills | 100 | 0.50 |
| Nordette | Wyeth-Ayerst | 4 light-orange pills | 120 | 0.60 |
| Ogestrel | Watson | 2 white pills | 100 | 0.50 |
| Ovral | Wyeth-Ayerst | 2 white pills | 100 | 0.50 |
| Portia | Barr/Duramed | 4 pink pills | 120 | 0.60 |
| Quasense | Watson | 4 white pills | 120 | 0.60 |
| Seasonale | Barr/Duramed | 4 pink pills | 120 | 0.60 |
| Seasonique | Barr/Duramed | 4 light-blue-green pills | 120 | 0.60 |
| Tri-Levlen | Berlex | 4 yellow pills | 120 | 0.50 |
| Triphasil | Wyeth-Ayerst | 4 yellow pills | 120 | 0.50 |
| Trivora | Watson | 4 pink pills | 120 | 0.50 |

[a] Plan-B is the only dedicated product specifically marketed for emergency contraception. Alesse, Aviane, Cryselle, Enpresse, Jolessa, Lessina, Levlen, Levlite, Levora, Lo/Ovral, Low-Ogestrel, Lutera, Nordette, Ogestrel, Ovral, Portia, Quasense, Seasonale, Seasonique, Tri-Levlen, Triphasil, and Trivora have been declared safe and effective for use as ECPs by the U.S. Food and Drug Administration. Worldwide, about 50 emergency contraceptive products are specifically packaged, labeled, and marketed. For example, Gedeon Richter and HRA Pharma are marketing in many countries the levonorgestrel-only products Postinor-2 and NorLevo, respectively, each consisting of a two-pill strip with each pill containing 0.75 mg levonorgestrel. Levonorgestrel-only ECPs are available either over-the-counter or from a pharmacist without having to see a clinician in 42 countries.

[b] The label for Plan B says to take one pill within 72 hours after unprotected intercourse, and another pill 12 hours later. However, recent research has found that both Plan B pills can be taken at the same time. Research has also shown that that all of the brands listed here are effective when used within 120 hours after unprotected sex.

[c] The progestin in Cryselle, Lo/Ovral, Low-Ogestrel, Ogestrel, Ovral, and Ovrette is norgestrel, which contains two isomers, only one of which (levonorgestrel) is bioactive; the amount of norgestrel in each tablet is twice the amount of levonorgestrel

SOURCE: Reproduced with permission from the American College of Obstetricians and Gynecologists (ACOG Clinical Review).

4. Emergency contraception should not be used in patients with a known or suspected pregnancy, undiagnosed abnormal genital bleeding, or hypersensitivity to any component of the drug.
5. There is neither evidence of increased risk nor evidence of decreased safety among patients who have contraindications to the use of daily oral contraceptives. However, for women with a history of idiopathic thrombosis, the progestin-only regimen may be preferable.
6. There is no evidence of an increased incidence of anomalies with emergency contraception; however, no specific studies have investigated this effect.

## BIBLIOGRAPHY

American College of Obstetricians and Gynecologists. ACOG practice bulletin No. 25. Emergency oral contraception. 2001. *Int J Gynaecol Obstet*. 2002;78(2):191–198.

Zieman M. Emergency contraceptives. In: Rose BD (ed.). *UpToDate*. Waltham, MA:UpToDate;2006. www.Update.com

# 14 ORAL CONTRACEPTION

*Susan Sarajari*

## LEARNING POINT

Proper patient evaluation and selection is critical before prescribing oral contraceptive pills.

## VIGNETTE

A 38-year-old, G3P3003, presents to your office for her annual exam and Pap smear. She has had three vaginal deliveries, does not desire any more children, and wants a prescription for oral contraceptive pills. She has regular periods, which last 3–4 days. She has no surgical history and does not desire surgical sterilization. She has tried the intrauterine device (IUD) before but had increased abdominal cramping and vaginal spotting while the IUD was in place, and it was removed 3 months after insertion. The patient states that she had mildly elevated blood pressure for which she took medication several years ago, but now is no longer on medication. She does not drink alcohol or use drugs but smokes about three cigarettes per day. Her family history is unremarkable except for a father with diabetes. Her physical exam, including the pelvic exam and vital signs are within normal limits, except for a blood pressure of 149/83.

### QUESTION 1

*What is the pharmacology and mechanism of action of oral contraceptive pills?*

### ANSWER 1

1. Combination oral contraceptive pill: Contain both an estrogen component and a progestin component. The estrogen component is usually ethinyl estradiol and the progestin component is usually a 19-nortestosterone derivative, such as norethindrone, norethynodrel, norethindrone acetate, ethynodiol diacetate, lynestrenol, norgestrel, norgestimate, desogestrel, and gestodene. Pills with varying doses of ethinyl estradiol (20, 25, 30, 35 mcg) are available.
   a. Monophasic pills: Contain the same dose of estrogen and progesterone.
   b. Bi/triphasic pills: Contain varying doses of progestin or estrogen. There is no rearly advantage over monophasic pills.
2. Progestin-only pill (mini-pill): Contain no ethinyl estradiol. Progestin is usually norethindrone or norgestrel. Are associated with more breakthrough bleeding and slightly higher failure rates than combination oral contraceptives but provide an option for patients who want a contraceptive pill but need to avoid estrogen.
3. Mechanism of action: Estrogen-induced inhibition of the midcycle LH surge of gonadotropin secretion, therefore preventing ovulation. Other potential estrogenic mechanisms include suppression of gonadotropin secretion during the follicular phase of the cycle, thereby preventing follicular maturation, decrease in ovarian steroid production due to suppression of gonadotropin secretion, and possibly a decreased pituitary responsiveness to gonadotropin-releasing hormone. Progestin-related mechanisms include causing the endometrium to be less suitable for implantation, rendering the cervical mucus less permeable to sperm, and decreasing tubal motility and peristalsis.
3. Efficacy: Theoretical failure rate is 0.1% but actual failure rate is 2–3% (see Table 14-1).

### QUESTION 2

*What are the contraindications to oral contraceptives?*

**TABLE 14-1. Selected Oral Contraceptives**

| DRUG | PROGESTIN, MG* | ESTROGEN† | COST‡ |
|---|---|---|---|
| **Monophasic combinations** | | | |
| Cyclessa 28 (Organon) | Desogestrel (0.1) | Ethinyl estradiol (25) | $32.76 |
| April 28 (Barr) | Desogestrel (0.15) | Ethinyl estradiol (30) | 25.20 |
| Desogen 28 (Organon) | Desogestrel (0.15) | Ethinyl estradiol (30) | 27.72 |
| Ortho-Cept 21 (Ortho-McNeil)[δ] | Desogestrel (0.15) | Ethinyl estradiol (30) | 32.55 |
| Yasmin 28 (Berlex) | Drospirenone (3) | Ethinyl estradiol (30) | 29.40 |
| Demulen 1/35 21 (Pharmacia)[δ] | Ethynodiol diacetate (1) | Ethinyl estradiol (35) | 32.13 |
| Zovia 1/35 21 (Watson)[δ] | Ethynodiol diacetate (1) | Ethinyl estradiol (35) | 23.73 |
| Demulen 1/50 21 (Pharmacia)[δ] | Ethynodiol diacetate (1) | Ethinyl estradiol (50) | 35.70 |
| Zovia 1/50E 21 (Watson)[δ] | Ethynodiol diacetate (1) | Ethinyl estradiol (50) | 25.41 |
| Alesse 21 (Wyeth-Ayerst) | Levonorgestrel (0.1) | Ethinyl estradiol (20) | 31.71 |
| Aviane 21 (Barr)[δ] | Levonorgestrel (0.1) | Ethinyl estradiol (20) | 21.00 |
| Lessina 28 (Barr) | Levonorgestrel (0.1) | Ethinyl estradiol (20) | 29.40 |
| Levlite 28 (Berlex) | Levonorgestrel (0.1) | Ethinyl estradiol (20) | 32.20 |
| Levlen 21 (Berlex)[δ] | Levonorgestrel (0.15) | Ethinyl estradiol (30) | 31.71 |
| Levora 21 (Watson)[δ] | Levonorgestrel (0.15) | Ethinyl estradiol (30) | 25.83 |
| Nordette 21 (Wyeth-Ayerst)[δ] | Levonorgestrel (0.15) | Ethinyl estradiol (30) | 32.13 |
| Ovcon 35 21 (Warner Chilcott)[δ] | Norethindrone (0.4) | Ethinyl estradiol (35) | 31.71 |
| Brevicon 21 (Watson)[δ] | Norethindrone (0.5) | Ethinyl estradiol (35) | 20.37 |
| Modicon 28 (Ortho-McNeil) | Norethindrone (0.5) | Ethinyl estradiol (35) | 34.16 |
| Necon 0.5/35E 21 (Watson)[δ] | Norethindrone (0.5) | Ethinyl estradiol (35) | 19.95 |
| Nortrel 0.5/35 28 (Barr) | Norethindrone (0.5) | Ethinyl estradiol (35) | 27.72 |
| Necon 1/50 21 (Watson)[δ] | Norethindrone (1) | Mestranol (50) | 21.42 |
| Norinyl 1/50 21 (Watson)[δ] | Norethindrone (1) | Mestranol (50) | 15.33 |
| Ortho-Novum 1/50 28 (Ortho-McNeil) | Norethindrone (1) | Mestranol (50) | 32.20 |
| Necon 1/35 21 (Watson)[δ] | Norethindrone (1) | Ethinyl estradiol (35) | 21.42 |
| Norinyl 1/35 21 (Watson)[δ] | Norethindrone (1) | Ethinyl estradiol (35) | 28.14 |
| Nortrel 1/35 21 (Barr)[δ] | Norethindrone (1) | Ethinyl estradiol (35) | 23.31 |
| Ortho-Novum 1/35 21, 28 (Ortho-McNeil) | Norethindrone (1) | Ethinyl estradiol (35) | 31.92 |
| Ovcon 50 28 (Warner Chilcott) | Norethindrone (1) | Ethinyl estradiol (50) | 34.72 |
| Loestrin 1/20 21, 28 (Pfizer) | Norethindrone acetate (1) | Ethinyl estradiol (20) | 32.13 |
| Microgestin 1/20 28 (Watson) | Norethindrone acetate (1) | Ethinyl estradiol (20) | 28.28 |
| Loestrin 1.5/30 21 (Pfizer)[δ] | Norethindrone acetate (1.5) | Ethinyl estradiol (30) | 32.34 |
| Microgestin 1.5/30 28 (Watson) | Norethindrone acetate (1.5) | Ethinyl estradiol (30) | 28.84 |
| Ortho-Cyclen 21 (Ortho-McNeil)[δ] | Norgestimate (0.25) | Ethinyl estradiol (35) | 31.92 |
| Lo/Ovral 21 (Wyeth-Ayerst)[δ] | Norgestrel (0.3) | Ethinyl estradiol (30) | 33.39 |
| Low-Ogestrel 21 (Watson)[δ] | Norgestrel (0.3) | Ethinyl estradiol (30) | 24.99 |
| Ogestrel-28 (Watson) | Norgestrel (0.5) | Ethinyl estradiol (50) | 38.36 |
| Ovral 21 (Wyeth-Ayerst)[δ] | Norgestrel (0.5) | Ethinyl estradiol (50) | 48.51 |
| **Muliphasic combinations** | | | |
| Kariva 28 (Barr) | Desogestrel (0.15) | Ethinyl estradiol (20, 0, 10) | 30.80 |
| Mircette 28 (Organon) | Desogestrel (0.15) | Ethinyl estradiol (20, 0, 10) | 30.52 |
| Tri-Levlen 21 (Berlex)[δ] | Levonorgestrel (0.05, 0.075, 0.125) | Ethinyl estradiol (30, 40, 30) | 28.98 |
| Triphasil 21 (Wyeth-Ayerst)[δ] | Levonorgestrel (0.05, 0.075, 0.125) | Ethinyl estradiol (30, 40, 30) | 30.87 |
| Trivora-28 (Watson) | Levonorgestrel (0.05, 0.075, 0.125) | Ethinyl estradiol (30, 40, 30) | 26.60 |
| Necon 10/11 21 (Watson)[δ] | Norethindrone (0.5, 1) | Ethinyl estradiol (35) | 21.42 |
| Ortho-Novum 10/11 28 (Ortho-McNeil) | Norethindrone (0.5, 1) | Ethinyl estradiol (35) | 34.44 |
| Ortho-Novum 7/7/7 21 (Ortho-McNeil) | Norethindrone (0.5, 0.75, 1) | Ethinyl estradiol (35) | 30.03 |
| Tri-Norinyl 21 (Watson) | Norethindrone (0.5, 1, 0.5) | Ethinyl estradiol (35) | 28.14 |
| Estrostep 28 (Pfizer)[¶] | Norethindrone acetate (1) | Ethinyl estradiol (20, 30, 35) | 32.20 |
| Ortho Tri-Cyclen 21 (Ortho-McNeil)[δ, ¶] | Norgestimate (0.18, 0.215, 0.25) | Ethinyl estradiol (35) | 30.45 |

*(Continued)*

**TABLE 14-1. Selected Oral Contraceptives (*Continued*)**

| DRUG | PROGESTIN, MG* | ESTROGEN† | COST‡ |
|---|---|---|---|
| **Progestin-only pills** | | | |
| Micronor (Ortho-McNeil) | Norethindrone (0.35) | | 38.06 |
| Nor–QD (Watson) | Norethindrone (0.35) | | 31.92 |
| Ovrette (Wyeth-Ayerst) | Norgestrel (0.075) | | 33.63 |

*Different progestins are not equivalent on a milligram basis.
†Ethinyl estradiol and mestranol are not equivalent on a milligram basis; the results of some studies indicate that 30–35 μg of ethinyl estradiol is equivalent to 50 μg of mestranol.
‡Average cost to the patient for 28 days' use, based on data from retail pharmacies nationwide provided by Scott-Levin's Source Prescription Audit (SPA), May 2001 to April 2002.
§Also available in 28-day regimen at slightly different cost.
¶Also FDA-approved.
SOURCE: Reproduced with permission from *The Medical Letter on Drugs and Therapeutics*. Vol. 44 (Issue 1133). New Rochelle, NY. The Medical Letter. 2002. A Nonprofit Publication. www.medicalletter.org

## ANSWER 2

Contraindications to oral contraceptive use are:

- History of an estrogen-dependent tumor
- Previous thromboembolic event or stroke
- Active liver disease
- Pregnancy
- Undiagnosed abnormal uterine bleeding
- Hypertriglyceridemia
- Women over the age of 35 who smoke
- The pros and cons of oral contraceptive use for women with poorly controlled hypertension, women receiving anticonvulsant therapy and women with migraine headaches should be carefully evaluated prior to starting oral contraceptives.

## QUESTION 3

*What are the side effects of oral contraceptives?*

## ANSWER 3

Side effects of oral contraceptives include:

- Early side effects: Nausea, bloating, breast tenderness, and mood changes.
- Breakthrough bleeding: Most common side effect of oral contraceptives, increased with low-dose estrogen pills and progestin-only pills.
- Amenorrhea: Occurs in 5–10% of cycles and is due to the development of an atrophic endometrium. Can be treated by changing to a pill containing a higher dose of estrogen or adding a small dose of estrogen.
- Postpill amenorrhea: No longer common since the availability of low-dose oral contraceptives.
- Drug interactions: Oral contraceptive metabolism is accelerated by any drug that increases microsomal enzyme activity in the liver, such as barbiturates (phenobarbital), rifampin, phenytoin, carbamazepine, and griseofulvin.
- Weight: Weight changes are not consistently found.

## QUESTION 4

*What are the noncontraceptive effects of oral contraceptives?*

## ANSWER 4

Noncontraceptive effects of oral contraceptive pills are a decreased risk or incidence of:

- Dysmenorrhea
- Iron deficiency anemia (reduction in menstrual flow)
- Ectopic pregnancy
- Benign breast disease
- Ovarian cysts (higher dose estrogen pills only)
- Ovarian cancer
- Endometrial cancer (progestin effect)
- Postmenopausal hip fracture

May be useful in the treatment of:

- Acne (pills with low androgenic progestin)
- Hirsutism or Hyperandrogenism (e.g., polycystic ovary syndrome)
- Menorrhagia
- Endometriosis
- Hypothalamic amenorrhea
- Hormone replacement in women with primary hypogonadism

## QUESTION 5

*What are the risks of oral contraceptive use?*

## ANSWER 5

Risks of oral contraceptive use include:

- Carriers of hereditary thrombiphilia mutations (factor V Leiden, prothrombin gene mutation, protein S and protein C deficiencies, antithrombin) and patients with hyperhomocystenemia are at increased risk of cerebral vein thrombosis.
- Increased risk of thrombosis in obese women.
- Increased risk of venous throboembolic disease.
- Small increase in ischemic stroke risk; hemorrhagic stroke risk does not seem to be increased.
- There does not seem to be an increased risk of breast cancer, however data are conflicting.
- Increased risk of cervical cancer.
- Decreased risk of nonhereditary ovarian cancer.
- Decreased risk of endometrial cancer.
- Effect on risk of melanoma is unclear.

## QUESTION 6

*How are oral contraceptive pills administered?*

## ANSWER 6

Pills should be preferably started on the first day of the period to provide maximum protection, however, most pill packs start on the first Sunday after the period. If a patient starts on a Sunday, another form of back-up contraception should be used in the first month, since the first pill pack might not provide the maximum contraceptive effect. Oral contraceptive pills can be given monthly or every 3 months.

## BIBLIOGRAPHY

ACOG Practice Bulletin. Clinical management guidelines for Obstetrician-Gynecologists. The use of hormonal contraception in women with coexisting medical conditions 18, 2001.

Speroff L, Fritz MA. *Clinical Gynecologic Endocrinology and Infertility*. Philadelphia, PA: Lippincott Williams & Wilkins; 2005.

Martin KA, Barbieri RL. Overview of the use of estrogen-progestin contraceptives. In: Rose BD (ed). *UpToDate*. Waltham. MA: UpToDate,2006. www.Uptodate.com

Martin KA, Barbieri RL. Risks and side effects associated with estrogen-progestin contraceptives. In: Rose BD (ed). *UpToDate*. Waltham, MA:UpToDate,2006. www.Uptodate.com

# 15 HIDRADENITIS SUPPURATIVA

*Jane L. Davis*

## LEARNING POINT

Review the treatment options of hidradenitis suppurativa (HS).

## VIGNETTE

A 24-year-old, G0, African-American woman presents with multiple ulcers involving the vulva and perianal area.

The patient has had multiple sexual partners in the past, but has been in a mutually monogamous relationship over the last 2 years. However, recently she has been unable to have sex secondary to dyspareunia due to the perineal ulcerations. The patient's medical and surgical history is negative. Her only medications are a low-dose combination oral contraceptive. She denies substance abuse and socially uses alcohol. The patient smoked one pack of cigarettes per day up until 1 year ago. She currently does not smoke.

The physical exam reveals an African-American female in no acute distress.

Weight 180 lb, height 6 ft 2 in. blood pressure 120/80, pulse 78/min, respiratory rate 18/min, temperature 98.6°F.
Thyroid: nonpabable.
Breasts: no palpable masses.
Lungs: clear.
Heart: regular rate and rhythm, no audible murmurs.
Abdomen: soft, nontender, no palpable masses.
External genitalia: multiple ulcerations with large sinus tracts involving labia majora and perianal area.
Vagina: well rugated, without lesions.
Cervix: nulliparous os, no lesions
Uterus: anteverted, normal size, nontender
Adnexal: no palpable masses. Rectovaginal exam without masses or induration.

The wet mount is negative at follow-up. Cultures for herpes simplex, gonococcus, and chlamydia are negative. Biopsy of one of the lesions revealed only chronic inflammatory changes. Serology for human immunodeficiency virus (HIV), rapid plasma reagin (RPR), hepatitis B surface antigen (HbsAg), and hepatitis C antibody is all negative.

## QUESTION 1

*What is HS including its etiology and epidemiology?*

## ANSWER 1

HS is a chronic, recurrent inflammatory process involving the apocrine glands of the axilla, groin, perineal, and perianal regions. The disorder is characterized by chronically draining wounds and sinus tracts. The etiology remains unclear, but the primary process involves occlusion of either the apocrine or follicular ducts, followed by secondary infection of the apocrine system with extension into the surrounding subcutaneous tissues. HS may progress differently in different individuals. See Table 15-1.

The exact incidence in the general population is unknown secondary to underreporting and misdiagnosis. However, it is estimated to affect 1 in 300 adults, usually presenting after puberty and before the age of 40. HS may be more common in African-American women who have a greater density of apocrine glands. However, perianal disease is twice as common in males as in females.

## QUESTION 2

*What are the predisposing factors for HS?*

## ANSWER 2

Predisposing factors:

1. Obesity (shearing forces on the involved skin)
2. Conditions associated with androgen excess
3. Smoking, although no etiologic relationship demonstrated
4. Family history

**TABLE 15-1. Stages of Hidradenitis Suppurative**

| |
|---|
| STAGE I—Solitary or multiple isolated abscess formation without scarring or sinus tracts |
| STAGE II—Recurrent abscessed, single or multiple widely separated lesions, with sinus tract formation and cicatrization |
| STAGE III—Diffuse or broad involvement across a regional area with multiple interconnected sinus tracts and abscesses |

SOURCE: From www.hs-usa.org, June 2003.

## QUESTION 3

*What is the differential diagnosis for HS?*

## ANSWER 3

The differential diagnosis of HS includes furunculosis, pyoderma, granuloma inguinale, lymphogranuloma venereum, pilonidal disease, inflammatory bowel disease, condyloma accuminata, carcinoma, and immunodeficiency syndromes.

Diagnosis is often difficult to make and biopsy of the affected area may need to be performed. We should note that squamous carcinoma can develop in long-standing cases of HS after an average of 20 years.

## QUESTION 4

*What is the treatment of HS?*

## ANSWER 4

Medical therapy

1. Conservative measures: Initiated first aiming toward relief of pain, and maintaining or improving hygiene to reduce bacterial load (warm baths, hydrotherapy, topical cleansing agents). Patient should be advised to wear loose-fitting clothing and lose weight if they are obese.
2. Topical and systemic antibiotics: Antibiotic therapy should include antistaphylococcal agents for axillary disease and broad spectrum for perineal disease. Both systemic tetracycline and topical clindamycin have been shown to be effective. Chronic administration of antibiotics does not seem to prevent recurrences of HS.
3. Hormonal therapy: A few case reports have suggested that estrogen-progesterone combination therapy may be effective although definitive studies are lacking.
4. Isotretinoin (Accutane): Variable success with this drug has been reported in patients with HS.

Surgical therapy: Various factors will influence the extent of surgery undertaken including the site affected, the extent of the disease, and whether patients present with acute or chronic disease. Specific procedures include:

1. Local incision and drainage: May control acute symptoms, but recurrence is quite common.
2. Unroofing of sinus tracts and marsupialization: Very tedious and time-consuming, but often allows

for best healing and regeneration of epidermis. With more extensive disease, have higher risk of recurrence.

3. Wide excision with skin graft: Reserved for chronic and extensive disease. Excision should be carried out to 1–2 cm beyond visible disease area. Most surgeons agree that wide excision in the perineal area is best managed by allowing wounds to granulate in without skin grafting. However, recovery is quite long and good wound care is crucial.

## BIBLIOGRAPHY


Brown CF, et al. Hidradenitis suppurativa of the anogenital region: response to isotretinoin. *AJOG.* 1988;158:12–15.

Camisa C, et al. Treatment of hidradenitis suppurativa with combination hypothalamic-pituitary-ovarian and adrenal suppression. A case report. *J Reprod Med.* 1989;34: 543–546.

Goldberg JM, et al. Advanced hidradenitis suppurativa presenting with bilateral vulvar masses, *Gynecol Oncol.* 1996;60:494–497.

Manolitsas T, et al. Vulvar squamous cell carcinoma arising in chronic hidradenitis suppurativa. *Gynecol Oncol.* 1999;75: 285–288.

Mitchell KM, Beck DE. Hidradenitis suppurativa. *Surg Clin N Am.* 2002;82:1187–1197.


# 16 MENOPAUSE: OSTEOPOROSIS PREVENTION AND TREATMENT

*John Kuo*

## LEARNING POINT

Understanding osteoporosis risk factors, screening, and treatments.

## VIGNETTE

A 60-year-old, G2P2002, Caucasian female presents for a routine annual examination. She has been postmenopausal for 12 years and has never been on hormone replacement therapy. Her past medical history is significant for hypertension and hypothyroidism. She is currently taking benazepril and levothyroxine. There have not been any recent changes in her medication dosages and the last check of her thyroid function tests were 3 years ago. She denies any abnormal vaginal bleeding or urinary incontinence. However, she does complain of back pain and has noticed a gradual loss of height. She has occasional hot flashes and night sweats, but these are not bothersome. She ambulates with a cane and denies any excessive fatigue. She has smoked about one pack per day of cigarettes for the last 30 years.

Physical examination reveals a thin Caucasian woman who appears her stated age. Her vital signs are blood pressure 136/82, pulse 90/min, respiratory rate 12/min, and temperature 98.6°F. Examination is significant only for moderate kyphosis, mild lumbar tenderness to palpation, and atrophy of her vaginal epithelium.

## QUESTION 1

*What is osteoporosis?*

## ANSWER 1

Osteoporosis is characterized by decreased bone mass, normal ratio of mineral to matrix, and microarchitectural deterioration leading to an increased risk of fractures. Almost all bone mass in the hip and vertebral bodies is accumulated in women by late adolescence. After adolescence, there is only a slight gain in total skeletal mass that ceases around age 30. This is followed by a slow decline in bone density (~0.7% per year) until menopause when bone loss accelerates for 5 years largely due to estrogen deficiency (1–1.5% of total bone mass per year). Approximately 13–18% of U.S. women aged 50 years and older have osteoporosis while another 37–50% have osteopenia. Hip and vertebral fractures are significant sources of morbidity and mortality in women.

## QUESTION 2

*What are the risk factors for osteoporosis?*

## ANSWER 2

Common risk factors for osteoporotic fractures:

- History of prior fragility fracture
- Family history of osteoporosis
- Increasing age
- Caucasian or Asian race
- Low weight and body mass index

- Eating disorder or poor nutrition
- Long-term low calcium, low vitamin D, or low phosphorus intake
- Smoking
- Alcoholism
- Excessive caffeine intake
- Estrogen deficiency (early menopause, surgical menopause, prolonged premenopausal amenorrhea)
- Inadequate physical activity (sedentary, prolonged bedrest, hemiplegia)
- Medical conditions (including Cushing's syndrome, hyperthyroidism, hyperparathyroidism, renal disease, hepatic disease)
- Medications (including heparin, anticonvulsants, thyroxine, corticosteroids)
- Impaired eyesight despite adequate correction
- History of falls
- Dementia

## QUESTION 3

*How is osteoporosis diagnosed?*

## ANSWER 3

The World Health Organization (WHO) has defined osteopenia and osteoporosis on the basis of axial skeleton measurements of bone density to facilitate screening and identifaction of individuals at risk. These definitions apply specifically to T scores derived from the use of dual-energy x-ray absorptiometry (DXA) of the lumbar spine or hip. The Z score is the number of standard deviations from the mean bone mineral density of a reference population of the same sex, race, and age, while the T score is based on the mean peak bone mineral density of a normal, young adult population. The Z score is used for younger women and the T score is used for menopausal women.

The WHO defines osteopenia as a bone mineral density between 1 and 2.5 standard deviations below the young adult mean and osteoporosis as a bone mineral density 2.5 standard deviations or more below the young adult peak mean (see Table 16-1). At the spine and hip, a decrease of 1 standard deviation in bone mass is associated with approximately a twofold increase in fracture risk. The National Osteoporosis Foundation has chosen a T score of −2 for women without risk factors and −1.5 for women with additional risk factors as the threshold for therapeutic intervention. Treatment should also be initiated in postmenopausal women who have experienced a previous fragility or low-impact fracture.

**TABLE 16-1. World Health Organization Definition of Osteoporosis Based on Bone Mineral Density of Total Hip**

| BONE CLASSIFICATION | T SCORE* |
|---|---|
| Normal | Greater than or equal to −1 |
| Osteopenia (low bone mass) | Less than −1, but more than 2.5 |
| Osteoporosis | Less than or equal to −2.5 |

*Number of standard deviations from the mean peak bone mineral density of a normal, young, gender-matched population.
SOURCE: Data from WHO. Assessment of fracture risks and its application to screening for postmenopausal osteoporosis. WHO Technical Report Series 843. Geneva: WHO, 1994.

Bone mineral density should be assessed in postmenopausal women presenting with fractures, who have one or more risk factors for osteoporosis, or who are aged 65 years or older. Bone mineral density testing may also be useful for premenopausal and postmenopausal women with certain medical conditions or take certain drugs associated with an increased risk of osteoporosis. Measurement of bone mineral density may be helpful in deciding about preventive therapy, diagnosing the severity of disease, and accessing the efficacy to current therapy. In untreated postmenopausal women without new risk factors, subsequent screening should not be repeated until 3–5 years. For women receiving therapy, monitoring before 2 years of therapy does not provide clinically useful information and may lead to erroneous assumptions about the effect of therapy.

## QUESTION 4

*What are the available treatment options for osteoporosis?*

## ANSWER 4

Prevention and treatment should always begin with lifestyle modifications. Modifications include adequate dietary intake of calcium and vitamin D, regular weight-bearing and muscle-strengthening exercises, smoking cessation, moderation of alcohol and caffeine consumption, reduction of medication that reduce strength and balance, and initiating fall prevention strategies.

The Women's Health Initiative (WHI) demonstrated a statistically significant reduction of hip and clinical vertebral fractures by 34% in healthy postmenopausal women using 0.625 mg/day of conjugated equine estrogen and 2.5 mg/day of medroxyprogesterone acetate. Other studies have demonstrated improved bone density with doses as low as 0.3 mg/day of conjugated equine estrogen with or without 1.5 mg/day of medroxyprogesterone acetate. Transdermal estrogen has also been found to increase bone mineral density of the spine and hip. Generally, hormone therapy is believed to work best if it is started in the first 5 years after menopause. The WHI indicated an increased risk of cardiovascular events and breast cancer for women taking combined estrogen and progestin therapy. Thus, hormone therapy should be based on an individual's history and risk factors, including the need for treatment of vasomotor symptoms.

Bisphosphonates and selective estrogen receptor modulators (SERMs) are commonly prescribed for prevention and teatment of osteoporosis. Bisphosphonates (i.e., alendronate, risedronate) prevent bone loss by inhibiting bone resorption. These agents increase bone mineral density at both the spine and hip and reduce fractures in women with established osteoporosis at all assessed locations by approximately 30–50%. Because bisphosphonates may cause upper gastrointestinal side effects and has very poor absorption, it is important to take this medication on an empty stomach with plain water and the patient must remain upright for at least 30 minutes without additional food or drink. SERMs (i.e., raloxifene, tibolone, tamoxifen) have estrogenic effects on skeleton bone density and antiestrogenic properties on endometrial and breast tissue. The U.S. Food and Drug Administration has determined that raloxifene is safe and effective for the prevention of osteoporosis. In postmenopausal women, raloxifene significantly increases bone mineral density and reduces vertebral fractures by 35–50% in women with established osteoporosis. Hip fracture reduction has not been demonstrated and the risk of deep vein thrombosis is similar to estrogen.

Salmon calcitonin and human recombinant parathyroid hormone are also available for osteoporosis treatment. Fluoride, thiazides, statins, growth hormone, and phytoestrogens have all been investigated with variable results and are not considered first-line agents for the prevention or treatment of osteoporosis.

## BIBLIOGRAPHY


ACOG Practice Bulletin No. 50. Osteoporosis. January 2004.

Anonymous. Osteoporosis prevention, diagnosis, and therapy. NIH Consensus Statement. 2000;17:(1):1–45.

Anonymous. Osteoporosis: review of the evidence for prevention, diagnosis and treatment and cost-effectiveness analysis. Executive summary. *Osteoporos Int.* 1998;8(Suppl. 4):S3–S6.

Delmas PD, Bjarnason NH, Mitlak BH, et al. Effects of raloxifene on bone mineral density, serum cholesterol concentrations, and uterine endometrium in postmenopausal women. *N Engl J Med.* 1997;337:1641.

Ettinger B, Black DM, Mitlak BH, et al. Reduction of vertebral fracture risk in postmenopausal women with osteoporosis treated with raloxifene: results from a 3-year randomized clinical trial. Multiple Outcomes of Raloxifene evaluation (MORE) investigators [published erratum appears in *JAMA.* 1999;282:2124]. *JAMA.* 1999;282:637.

Looker AC, Wahner HW, Dunn WL, et al. Updated data on proximal femur bone mineral levels of US adults. *Osteoporos Int.* 1998;8:468.

Matkovic V, Jelic T, Wardlaw GM, et al. Timing of peak bone mass in Caucasian females and its implication for the prevention of osteoporosis: inference from a cross-sectional model. *J Clin Invest.* 1994;93:799.

National Osteoporosis Foundation: Physician's guide to prevention and treatment of osteoporosis. Washington, DC: NOF; 2003.

NIH Consensus Development Panel on Osteoporosis Prevention, Diagnosis, and Therapy. Osteoporosis prevention, diagnosis, and therapy. *JAMA.* 2001;285:785.

Rossouw JE, Anderson GL, Prentice RL, et al. Risks and benefits of estrogen plus progestin in healthy postmenopausal women: principal results from the Women's Health Initiative randomized controlled trial. *JAMA.* 2002;288:321.

Sirola J, Kroger H, Honkanen R, et al. Factors affecting bone loss around menopause in women without HRT: a prospective study. *Maturitas.* 2003;45:159.

Speroff L, Fritz MA. *Clinical Gynecologic Endocrinology and Infertility.* 7th ed. Philadelphia, PA: Lippincott Williams & Wilkins; 2005.

World Health Organization: Assessment of fracture risks and its application to screening for postmenopausal osteoporosis. WHO Technical Report Series 843. Geneva: WHO; 1994.


# 17 MENOPAUSE: PERIMENOPAUSE

*Margareta D. Pisarska*

## LEARNING POINT

The "perimenopause" more appropriately called the menopausal transition is a period of variable ovarian function leading to unique symptoms during this time of a woman's life.

## VIGNETTE

A 45-year-old, G4P4004, comes in because her period is 2 weeks late. She states that she is sexually active but uses a condom. She also complains that she has been feeling irritable and is always hot. Occasionally she has to go outside in order to relieve her symptoms.

Gynecologic history: Age on onset of menses at 12 with 28 day cycles and menses lasting for 5 days.
No history of fibroids, ovarian cysts, or sexually transmitted diseases.
Obstetrics history: Four normal spontaneous deliveries without complications.
Medical history and surgical history is negative.
Social history: She does not smoke, drink alcohol, or use illicit drugs. She is not taking any medications and has no allergies to medications. She states that her mother has some type of thyroid condition.
Physical exam reveals a healthy appearing female.
Vital signs: Blood pressure 110/70, pulse 80/min, respiratory rate 18/min, temperature 98.6°F.
Thyroid: Nonpalpable, lungs clear, heart regular rate and rhythm without audible murmurs.
Abdomen: Normal bowel sounds: soft, nontender, no palpable masses.
Pelvic exam: Normal external genitalia, cervix multiparous, no lesions, uterus anteverted normal size, adnexa nontender, no masses bilaterally. Rectovaginal confirms.

Blood work reveals the following: $\beta$ human chorionic gonadotropin (hCG) is negative, follicle-stimulating hormone (FSH) is 25 mIU/mL, and thyroid-stimulating hormone (TSH) is 2 mIU/mL.

## QUESTION 1

*What is the definition of perimenopause?*

## ANSWER 1

"Perimenopause" or "climacteric" should be more appropriately identified as the menopausal transition. The Stages of Reproductive Aging Workshop (STRAW) was held to better define the terms of the menopausal transition and developed a staging system (see Fig. 17-1). The Menopausal transition begins when a woman has variations in her menstrual cycles with increasing FSH and ends with the final menstrual period. The final menstrual period is retrospectively defined after 1 year of amenorrhea. The perimenopause begins at the same time as the menopausal transition and ends 1 year after the final menstrual period. This takes place 2–8 years preceding menopause and continues until 1 year after the final menstrual period. The average transition begins at age 47 and takes about 4 years.

## QUESTION 2

*What are the endocrine changes during the menopausal transition?*

Final Menstrual Period (FMP)

| Stages: | −5 | −4 | −3 | −2 | −1 | 0 | +1 | +2 |
|---|---|---|---|---|---|---|---|---|
| Terminology: | Reproductive | | | Menopausal transition | | Postmenopause | | |
| | Early | Peak | Late | Early | Late* | Early* | | Late |
| | | | | Perimenopause | | | | |
| Duration of stage: | Variable | | | Variable | | ⓐ 1 yr | ⓑ 4 yrs | Until demise |
| Menstrual cycles: | Variable to regular | Regular | | Variable cycle length (>7 days different from normal) | ≥2 Skipped cycles and an interval of amenorrhea (≥60 days) | Amen x 12 mos | None | |
| Endocrine: | Normal FSH | | ↑ FSH | ↑ FSH | | ↑ FSH | | |

↑= Elevated

*Stages most likely to be characterized by vasomotor symptoms

**FIG. 17-1** Stages of the menopausal transition. American Society for Reproductive Medicine, A Practice Committee Report, The Menopausal Transition. 2001;1–5.

## ANSWER 2

FSH increases in the early menopausal transition due to decreased negative feedback to the hypothalamus and pituitary. Inhibin, which is produced in the granulosa cells of the ovary, normally inhibits FSH secretion. Ovarian inhibin decreases with age and this decrease in negative feedback leads to the increase in FSH levels. There are two types of inhibin, inhibin A and inhibin B. Inhibin B in the follicular phase of the cycle appears to be decreased in the early menopausal transition, concomitant with the rise in FSH. The elevated FSH levels may lead to increased estradiol production at times greater than seen in younger women. Ovarian function is unpredictable during this stage. Ovulatory cycles are interspersed with periods of chronic anovulation. There are periods of hypoestrogenism, hyperestrogenism, and inadequate progesterone production.

## QUESTION 3

*What are the symptoms of women in the menopausal transition and how would you treat them?*

## ANSWER 3

Abnormal uterine bleeding commonly occurs in women during this transition as a result of periods of hyperestrogenism and progesterone deficiency due to chronic anovulation. It is important to exclude other causes of abnormal bleeding prior to treatment. Oral contraceptive pills are effective in stabilizing the endometrium. Oral contraceptive pills can be used in women who do not smoke and do not have any other contraindications to use. They are also effective in preventing pregnancy. Although ovarian function is waxing and waning during this period, ovulatory cycles do occur and pregnancy can result. Continuous hormone replacement therapy may be considered in these women and is more likely to be successful in women with at least 6 months of amenorrhea. Depot medroxy-progesterone acetate (DMPA) may also be considered, however, its use is limited secondary to concerns of bone mineral density reductions. Progestin-containing intrauterine devices (IUDs) may help control bleeding and serve as contraception. Although widely used, cyclic and oral medroxyprogesterone was not found to be effective for bleeding.

Hot flashes can occur during this period and symptoms can be resolved either with oral contraceptive pills, or estrogen/progestin combination therapy (HT), or estrogen therapy (ET). In women where estrogen therapy is contraindicated, clonidine, progestins (megestrol acetate, norethindrone, DMPA), and low-dose serotonin reuptake inhibitors, may provide partial relief of hot flashes. Nonpharmaco-logic measures include layering clothing, avoiding caffeine and alcohol, and keeping the ambient temperature a few degrees cooler.

## BIBLIOGRAPHY


American Society for Reproductive Medicine. A Practice Committee Report, The Menopausal Transition. 2001;1–5.

Lethaby A, Irving G, Cameron I. Cyclical progestogens for heavy menstrual bleeding. *Cochrane Database Syst Rev.* 2000; CD00106.

Casper RF. Diagnosis and clinical manifestations of menopause. In: Rose BD (ed.). *UpToDate*. Waltham, MA:UpToDate;2006. www.Uptodate.com

Santoro N, Brown JR, Adel T, Skurnick JH. Characterization of reproductive hormonal dynamics in the perimenopause. *J Clin Endocrinol Metab.* 1996;81:1495–1501.

Sherman BM, Korenman SG. Hormonal characteristics of the human menstrual cycle throughout reproductive life. *J Clin Invest.* 1975;55(4):699–706.


# 18 MENOPAUSE: HORMONE THERAPY COUNSELING

*Margareta D. Pisarska*

## LEARNING POINT

Hormone therapy should be considered in symptomatic menopausal women. However, it is not recommended for prevention.

## VIGNETTE

A 55-year-old, G2P2002, recently heard a report on the risks of hormone therapy. She states she was started on hormone therapy 4 years ago when she was having severe hot flashes and cycle irregularity. She states she was told that the hormones would also help keep her *young*. She feels great on hormone therapy but is concerned about the potential risks.

Gynecologic history: Age at onset of menses at 12 with 28 day cycles and menses lasting for 5 days.

No history of fibroids, ovarian cysts, or sexually transmitted diseases.

Obstetrics history: Two normal spontaneous deliveries without complications.

Medical history and surgical history is negative.

Social history: She does not smoke, drink alcohol, or use illicit drugs. She is taking estrogen for 28 days and a progesterone pill for the first 12 days of the month. She has no allergies to medications. She states that her mother and grandmother both had severe osteoporosis.

Physical exam reveals a healthy appearing thin female.

Vital signs: Blood pressure 110/70, pulse 80/min, respiratory rate 18/min, temperature 98.6°F.

Thyroid: Nonpalpable.

Lungs: Clear.

Heart rate: Regular and rhythm without audible murmurs.

Abdomen: Normal bowel sounds, soft, nontender, no palpable masses.

Pelvic exam: Normal external genitalia, cervix multiparous, no lesions, uterus anteverted normal size, adnexa nontender, no masses bilaterally. Rectovaginal confirms.

## QUESTION 1

*What were the findings from the Women's Health Initiative (WHI)?*

## ANSWER 1

The estrogen and progestin hormone therapy (HT) arm of the WHI which enrolled 16,608 healthy women with a uterus, was designed to explore whether hormone therapy protected against heart disease and osteoporosis. Average age at entry was 63 years. The study was discontinued prematurely after only 5.2 years because the risks for the study group on combined HT outweighed the benefits. Moreover, the risks, although small, were outside of the safety standards set for the study, which led to early termination of the study. Risks included a small but significant increased risk of breast cancer (38 women out of 10,000 women per year compared to 30 women taking placebo), heart attacks (37 women out of 10,000 women per year compared to 30 women taking placebo), strokes (29 women out of 10,000 women per year compared to 21 women taking placebo), and blood clots (34 women out of 10,000 women per year compared to 16 women taking placebo) for the group of women on HT.

However, there were benefits as well. HT users had a lower risk of spine and hip fractures. In the HT group, there was a 24% reduction in total fractures, and a 34% reduction in hip fractures. On average, per year, there were 10 cases of hip fracture per 10,000 women on HT compared to 15 per 10,000 women on placebo. The WHI also reported a reduced risk of colon cancer among HT users, which was down by 37% (or 10 cases of colorectal cancer per 10,000 women per year on HT compared to 16 cases per 10,000 women per year on placebo). However, the greater risks for breast cancer and cardiovascular problems outweighed the benefits for most women.

Another part of the WHI, involving 11,000 healthy postmenopausal women who were using estrogen therapy (ET) alone, was continued but early in 2004, that arm of the study was halted as well. They found that estrogen alone was not protective against cardiovascular disease and there was also an increased risk of stroke and blood clots similar to the estrogen/progestin arm. Women on estrogen had 12 more strokes per year for every 10,000 women than did those who took a placebo (44 on ET vs. 32 on placebo) and an increased risk of blood clots (21 on ET vs. 15 on placebo). In the estrogen-only arm, there was no change in risk of breast cancer compared to the placebo group and there was also a decreased risk of hip fractures.

## QUESTION 2

*Should hormone replacement therapy (HRT) be administered for cardiovascular disease prevention?*

## ANSWER 2

No. Although there have been a number of epidemiological studies that reported a reduced risk of coronary artery disease (CAD) and myocardial infarction (MI), the randomized controlled trials (RCT) did not find that HT or ET were effective for primary or secondary prevention of nonfatal MI and coronary heart disease (CHD) deaths. A summary of these early epidemiological studies appeared in World Health Organization (WHO) Technical Report in 1996 suggesting that HT use reduced the risk of nonfatal MI or CAD death by 44%. Additionally, from the Nurses Health Study, the relative risk of a major coronary event (nonfatal MI or CHD mortality) was lower among current users of HT compared to never-users.

The results of three of the largest randomized controlled trials, (Heart and Estrogen/Progestin Replacement Study [HERS], European Strategic Programme for Research and

Development in Information Technology [ESPRIT], and WHI) found no evidence that HT or ET was effective for primary or secondary prevention of nonfatal MI and CHD deaths. The HERS secondary prevention trial involved 2763 women with CAD who were postmenopausal and who had an intact uterus. These women were randomized to receive either HT or placebo. There was no difference in MI or CHD death between the two groups. The smaller ESPRIT study randomized 1017 postmenopausal women with a recent first MI to placebo or ET for 2 years. The frequency of nonfatal reinfarction or cardiac death did not differ between the two groups. The WHI, which was designed to be a primary prevention trial, did not show any cardiovascular benefit.

## QUESTION 3

*What are some of the benefits of HT and ET?*

## ANSWER 3

Hormone therapy is the most effective medication available for treating hot flushes. Relief from flushes improves sleep and may improve quality of life. Although the WHI did not find an improvement in quality of life for women taking HT, most of the women in the WHI were 10 years older than most women who use hormones to relieve menopausal symptoms, and most of the WHI study participants had no menopausal symptoms while they were enrolled in the study. Estrogen is also effective for symptoms of urogenital atrophy, such as vaginal dryness and sexual discomfort as a result of vaginal dryness. Vaginal route of administration appears to be better for urogenital symptoms. The ACOG task force on hormone therapy recommends using the lowest effective dose for the shortest period of time to relieve symptoms.

RCT uniformly indicate that HT maintains or improves bone mineral density in the spine, proximal femur, and radius although, results have not been as consistent with respect to prevention of clinical fractures. There is epidemiologic evidence and two small RCS that suggest current HT use may prevent clinical fractures. In addition, the WHI study found a significant overall reduction in osteoporotic fractures (hip, vertebral, and other osteoporotic fractures). Approximately 85% of osteoporotic fractures observed in the WHI trial were nonvertebral and nonhip fractures. However, if it is utilized only for the prevention of osteoporosis, other alternatives are available that can help prevent osteoporosis and fractures without the added risks.

For bone health, all peri- and postmenopausal women should consume 1200–1500 mg of calcium per day, a multivitamin containing vitamin D, and engage in regular weight-bearing exercise such as walking, regardless of use of other agents for osteoporosis prevention.

## BIBLIOGRAPHY

ACOG Task Force for Hormone Therapy. American College of Obstetricians and Gynecologists Women's Health Care Physicians. Summary of balancing risks and benefits. *Obstet Gynecol*. 2004;104(Suppl. 4):128S–129S.

Practice Committee of the American Society for Reproductive Medicine. Estrogen and progestogen therapy in postmenopausal women. *Fert Steril*. 2004;81(1):231–241.

# *19* CHRONIC PELVIC PAIN CAUSES

*Ricardo Azziz*

## LEARNING POINT

To understand the definition, prevalence, differential diagnosis, and causes of chronic pelvic pain (CPP).

## VIGNETTE

A 36-year-old, G0, presents to your office complaining of progressive pelvic pain. Pain began some 6 years ago and has waxed and waned, although generally with an increasingly more severe course. While she feels general "soreness" in her pelvis, pain is significantly worse immediately preceding and at the time of menstruation, which requires her to stay at home 2–3 days per month. She has been experiencing increasing dyspareunia, primarily with deep penetration. Although changing coital position helped in the past, this has had less effect recently, and the patient has taken to avoiding intercourse altogether. She denies problems with bowel movements, which are generally once daily, except at the time of her menses when she experiences increased loose stools and painful defecation. She denies difficulty urinating, including polyuria, nocturia, hesitancy, and the feeling of incomplete voiding. She experiences a small amount of pain relief with ibuprofen 600 mg every 6 hours, but denies taking narcotics or other such medications.

On examination, the pelvis feels normal, as does the cervix, with the exception that the left adnexa feels somewhat thickened and is 3/4 + tender. She has no cervical motion tenderness. Cervix appears normal to visualization. You suspect, among other possible diagnoses, that the patient suffers from CPP secondary to endometriosis.

## QUESTION 1

*What is the definition and prevalence of CPP?*

## ANSWER 1

CPP is defined as nonmenstrual pelvic pain of 6 or more months duration that is severe enough to cause functional disability or require medical or surgical treatment. CPP is estimated to have a prevalence of 3.8% in women aged 15–73 years, although a Gallup poll found that 15% of women ages 18–50 years surveyed complained of CPP. CPP is estimated to account for 10% of all referrals to gynecologists, is the indication for 12% of all hysterectomies, and accounts for over 40% of gynecologic diagnostic laparoscopies.

## QUESTION 2

*What are the principal etiologies of CPP? How often is endometriosis found in patients with CPP, and how does this compare with normal?*

## ANSWER 2

Endometriosis, adenomyosis, irritable bowel syndrome (IBS), interstitial cystitis (IC), pelvic adhesions, chronic pelvic inflammatory disease (PID), and degenerating uterine fibroids are the principal etiologies of CPP (Table 19-1). Most reports indicate that endometriosis is

**TABLE 19-1. Diseases/Conditions That May be Associated with Chronic Pelvic Pain in Women**

| GYNECOLOGIC | GASTROINTESTINAL | MUSCULOSKELETAL | UROLOGIC | OTHER |
|---|---|---|---|---|
| **Extrauterine** | | | | |
| Adhesions | Carcinoma of the colon | Chronic coccygeal pain | Bladder neoplasm | Abdominal epilepsy |
| Adnexal cysts | Colitis | Degenerative joint disease | Interstitial cystitis | Abdominal migraine |
| Chronic ectopic pregnancy | Constipation | Disk herniation or rupture | Radiation cystitis | Depression |
| Chlamydial endometritis or salpingitis | Inflammatory bowel disease | Abdominal wall myofascial pain (trigger points) | Chronic urinary tract infection | Bipolar personality disorders |
| Endometriosis | Hernias | Faulty or poor posture | Stone/urolithiasis | Neurologic dysfunction |
| Endosalpingiosis | Diverticular disease | Fibromyositis | Urethral diverticulum | Porphyria |
| Neoplasia of the genital tract | Irritable bowel syndrome | Low back pain | Urethral syndrome | Shingles |
| Ovarian retention syndrome (residual ovary syndrome) | Chronic intermittent bowel obstruction | Compression of lumbar vertebrae | Recurrent, acute cystitis | Familial Mediterranean fever |
| Ovarian remnant syndrome | | Muscular strains and sprains | Urethral caruncle | Sleep disturbances |
| Ovarian dystrophy or ovulatory pain | | Hernias: ventral, inguinal, femoral, Spigelian | Recurrent, acute urethritis | Somatic referral |
| Postoperative peritoneal cysts | | Neuralgia of iliohypogastric, ilioinguinal, and/or genitofemoral nerves | Uninhibited bladder contractions (detrusor dyssynergia) | Abdominal cutaneous nerve entrapment in surgical scar |
| Residual accessory ovary | | Rectus tendon strain | | |
| Subacutte salpingo-oophoritis (chronic PID) | | Pelvic floor myalgia (levator ani spasm) | | |
| Tuberculous salpingitis | | Spondylosis | | |
| Pelvic congestion syndrome | | Piriformis syndrome | | |
| **Uterine** | | | | |
| Adenomyosis | | | | |
| Atypical dysmenorrhea or ovulatory pain | | | | |
| Cervical stenosis | | | | |
| Chronic endometritis | | | | |
| Endometrial or cervical polyps | | | | |
| Intrauterine contraceptive device | | | | |
| Leiomyomata | | | | |
| Symptomatic pelvic relaxation (genital prolapse) | | | | |

SOURCE: Modified with permission from Howard FM. Chronic Pelvic Pain. *Obstet Gynecol.* 2003;101:594–611.

present in 40–80% of patients with CPP, with rates in the general population of between 0.1% and 10%.

## QUESTION 3

*How often is CPP associated with multiple causes?*

## ANSWER 3

Approximately 50% of patients with CPP have multiple concomitant pathologies including endometriosis, IBS, IC, levator ani spasm, and fibromyalgia. For example, one study noted that in a sequential sample of 60 women with IBS and 26 women with inflammatory bowel disease (IBD), CPP was reported in 21 (35.0%) of IBS patients versus 4 (13.8%) of those with IBD ($p < 0.05$). It has also been estimated that approximately 75% of the women seeing a gynecologist for complaints of a variety of CPP syndromes also have symptoms of urgency/frequency or irritative voiding symptoms, suggestive of IC.

## QUESTION 4

*What is IC, and what proportion of patients with CPP have it?*

## ANSWER 4

IC is a clinical syndrome of frequency, urgency, and/or pelvic pain in the absence of any other identifiable pathology, such as urinary tract infection, bladder carcinoma, or cystitis induced by radiation or medication. Patients with IC report various degrees and locations of pain, including lower abdomen, urethra, lower back, and vaginal areas.

It has been estimated that approximately 75% of the women seeing a gynecologist for complaints of a variety of CPP syndromes have symptoms of urgency/frequency or irritative voiding symptoms.

## QUESTION 5

*Are abuse and CPP related?*

## ANSWER 5

Approximately 30–40% of CPP patients report some form of abuse, either physical, psychological, or sexual. The relationship is strongest with sexual abuse prior to age 15–17 years, and generally involving genital penetration (major sexual abuse).

## BIBLIOGRAPHY

Howard FM. Chronic pelvic pain. *Obstet Gynecol.* 2003;101: 594–611.

Jamieson DJ, Steege JF. The prevalence of dysmenorrhea, dyspareunia, pelvic pain, and irritable bowel syndrome in primary care practices. *Obstet Gynecol.* 1996;87:55–58.

Kontoravdis A, Chryssikopoulos A, Hassiakos D, Liapis A, Zourlas PA. The diagnostic value of laparoscopy in 2365 patients with acute and chronic pelvic pain. *Int J Gynaecol Obstet.* 1996;52:243–248.

Lampe A, Doering S, Rumpold G, Solder E, Krismer M, Kantner-Rumplmair W, Schubert C, Sollner W. Chronic pain syndromes and their relation to childhood abuse and stressful life events. *J Psychosom Res.* 2003;54:361–367.

Lampe A, Solder E, Ennemoser A, Schubert C, Rumpold G, Sollner W. Chronic pelvic pain and previous sexual abuse. *Obstet Gynecol.* 2000;96:929–933.

Mathias SD, Kuppermann M, Liberman RF, Lipschutz RC, Steege JF. Chronic pelvic pain: prevalence, health-related quality of life, and economic correlates. *Obstet Gynecol.* 1996;87:321–327.

Parsons CL, Dell J, Stanford EJ, Bullen M, Kahn BS, Willems JJ. The prevalence of interstitial cystitis in gynecologic patients with pelvic pain, as detected by intravesical potassium sensitivity. *Am J Obstet Gynecol.* 2002;187:1395–1400.

Rapkin AJ, Kames LD, Darke LL, Stampler FM, Naliboff BD. History of physical and sexual abuse in women with chronic pelvic pain. *Obstet Gynecol.* 1990;76(1):92–96.

Toomey TC, Hernandez JT, Gittelman DF, Hulka JF. Relationship of sexual and physical abuse to pain and psychological assessment variables in chronic pelvic pain patients. *Pain.* 1993;53:105–109.

van Os-Bossagh P, Pols T, Hop WC, Bohnen AM, Vierhout ME, Drogendijk AC. Voiding symptoms in chronic pelvic pain (CPP). *Eur J Obstet Gynecol Reprod Biol.* 2003;107:185–190.

Walker EA, Gelfand AN, Gelfand MD, Green C, Katon WJ. Chronic pelvic pain and gynecological symptoms in women with irritable bowel syndrome. *J Psychosom Obstet Gynaecol.* 1996;17:39–46.

Walling MK, Reiter RC, O'Hara MW, Milburn AK, Lilly G, Vincent SD. Abuse history and chronic pain in women: I. Prevalences of sexual abuse and physical abuse. *Obstet Gynecol.* 1994;84:193–199.

Whitehead WE, Palsson O, Jones KR. Systematic review of the co-morbidity of irritable bowel syndrome with other disorders: what are the causes and implications? *Gastroenterology.* 2002;122:1140–1156.

Zondervan KT, Yudkin PL, Vessey MP, Dawes MG, Barlow DH, Kennedy SH. Prevalence and incidence in primary care of chronic pelvic pain in women: evidence from a national general practice database. *Br J Obstet Gynaecol.* 1999;106:1149–1155.

Zondervan KT, Yudkin PL, Vessey MP, Jenkinson CP, Dawes MG, Barlow DH, Kennedy SH. Chronic pelvic pain in the community—symptoms, investigations, and diagnoses. *Am J Obstet Gynecol.* 2001;184:1149–1155.

# 20 INTERSTITIAL CYSTITIS

*Cynthia D. Hall*

## LEARNING POINT

Interstitial cystitis (IC) should be contemplated with every patient with pelvic pain, but treatment can be difficult.

## VIGNETTE

A 35-year-old female who complains of pain in the central lower abdomen presents to the office. It began about a year ago and is constant, but gets worse before and during her nocturia menses. She urinates every hour to 1.5 hours during the day, but feels almost a constant pressure to urinate. She does not have urge incontinence. She has superficial and deep dyspareunia, which is burning in quality, and she often feels the need to urinate during coitus. She has been treated with antibiotics four times in the past year for presumed urinary tract infection (UTI), but at least one of the cultures was negative. She gets mild relief on the antibiotics, but only after 7 days or so. She had a diagnostic laparoscopy that was negative. She has been taking oral contraceptive pills (OCPs) with no relief of symptoms.

### QUESTION 1

*What is the differential diagnosis of chronic pelvic pain (CPP)?*

### ANSWER 1

CPP is a major medical problem. In one study, it was found that 14.7% of women have CPP, defined as pain > 3 months in duration. CPP accounts for 10% of referrals to a gynecologist, 40% of laparoscopies, and 18% of hysterectomies. It is responsible for time out of work, and many women are depressed. Patients with CPP consistently score poorly on quality of life questionnaires.

Multiple organ systems can be responsible for CPP, and there may be multiple and overlapping causes in a single patient. The cause for CPP may be undefined in as many as 61% of patients. The primary differential includes:

- Endometriosis
- Adenomyosis
- Pelvic masses
- IC
- Irritable bowel syndrome
- Musculoskeletal pain

See also Table 19-1.

### QUESTION 2

*How is a patient with CPP evaluated?*

### ANSWER 2

The evaluation begins with a good history. The location, onset, and contributing factors of the pain should be noted. Especially important is to see what exacerbates the pain (e.g., constipation, bowel movements, urination, any urinary frequency or urgency, menses, dyspareunia).

Physical examination should include palpation of the abdomen for the presence of rebound or guarding and determining if the pain gets better or worse with valsalva (musculoskeletal pain often will increase with valsalva). A pelvic exam is always indicated. Start with evaluation for vulvar vestibulitis syndrome (VSS), which often coexists with other conditions. Separating the labia with one hand, inspect and touch the area just outside the hymenal ring (the vestibule) with a Q-Tip. With VVS, the patient may experience pain, burning, or discomfort, and there may be areas of erythema. With one finger, palpate individually the levator ani musculature, the urethra, the bladder, the cervix (determining any cervical motion tenderness), and the uterosacral ligaments. Ask about pain with palpation. A bimanual examination is often sufficient to rule out pelvic masses.

### QUESTION 3

*If IC is suspected, how does one confirm the diagnosis?*

### ANSWER 3

To diagnose IC, one must have a high index of suspicion in any patient with CPP. Specific features include suprapubic location, presence of urinary frequency, urgency or nocturia, and bladder or urethral tenderness. The presence of dyspareunia is common and can represent the IC itself, concurrent levator spasm, VVS, or endometriosis. IC and endometriosis occur together in 36–90% of women.

A voiding diary indicating frequent small volume voids is the usual pattern. Some women with IC may urinate as many as 15–20 times per day, with volumes of 100–150 cc (usually 300–400 cc). A UTI should be ruled out by sending a urine sample for culture. Urinalysis is not as sensitive for UTI, but may show hematuria in IC patients.

An abnormal potassium sensitivity test (PST) can support the diagnosis of IC. It tests for abnormal epithelial permeability, one of the theories for the pathogenesis of IC. Begin by asking the patient to void, then inserting a urethral catheter and noting the post void residual. Then fill the bladder with 40 cc of sterile water, and after 5 minutes, have the patient rate her pain and urgency on a scale of 0–5. Empty the bladder and instill a dilute solution of potassium chloride. Repeat the patient's rating of discomfort. An increase of more than 2 points in either pain or urgency is considered a positive test. A positive PST occurs in 70–80% of patients with IC.

Cystoscopy under anesthesia is still considered the gold standard for diagnosis. After distending the bladder to 80 cm of water, the physician empties and then partially refills the bladder. The diagnosis of IC is made by identifying petechial hemorrhages, glomerulations, or, rarely, Hunner's ulcers (Fig. 20-1).

## QUESTION 4

*What are the treatment options for IC?*

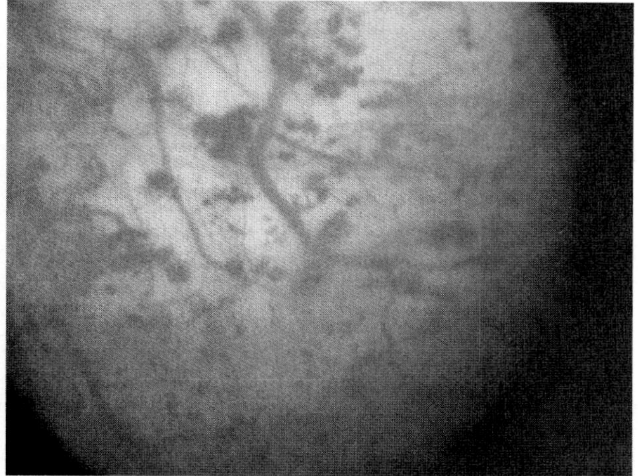

**FIG. 20-1** Cystoscopy after hydrodistention in an IC patient. Both petechial hemorrhages and glomerulations are present.

## ANSWER 4

Unfortunately, not every patient will respond to any one treatment for IC. Therefore it may take some trial and error to find the best treatment for a particular patient. Diet, especially avoiding acidic or spicy foods, alcohol, and caffeine among other things, can be very helpful. Additionally, one usually begins with oral medications, either pentosan polysulfate alone or in combination with amitriptyline or hydroxyzine. Pentosan polysulfate resembles the protective glycosaminoglycan layer of the bladder. Most practitioners will proceed to intravesical treatment if there has not been a response with oral therapy after 3–6 months. Surgical therapy such as the sacral nerve stimulator or cystectomy should be reserved for refractory patients.

Oral therapy:

- Pentosan polysulfate (Elmiron) 100 mg bid
- Amitriptyline (Elavil) 10–50 mg qhs
- Hydroxysine (Atarax or Vistaril) 10–50 mg qhs
- "Prelief" (over the counter) 1–2 tabs with meals
- Other antidepressant or anticonvulsant medications

Intravesical therapy:

- Dimethyl sulfoxide (DMSO)
- Heparin
- Lidocaine
- Hydrocortisone or other steroid
- Sodium bicarbonate

## BIBLIOGRAPHY


Chung MK, Chung RP, Gordon D. Interstitial cystitis and endometriosis in patients with chronic pelvic pain: the "Evil Twins" syndrome. *JSLS.* 2005;9(1):25.

Hanno PM, Buehler J, Wein AJ. Use of amitriptyline in the treatment of interstitial cystitis. *J Urol.* 1989;141:846.

Lifford KL, Barbieri RL. Diagnosis and management of chronic pain. *Urol Clin North Am.* 2002;29(3):637.

Mathias SD, Kuppermann M, Liberman R, et al. Chronic pelvic pain: prevalence, health-related quality of life, and economic correlates. *Obstet Gynecol.* 1996;87:321.

Parsons CL, Dell J, Stanford EJ, et al. The prevalence of interstitial cystitis in gynecologic patients with pelvic pain, as detected by intravesical potassium sensitivity. *Am J Obstet Gynecol.* 2002;187:1395.

Parsons CL, Housley T, Schmidt JD, et al. Treatment of interstitial cystitis with intravesical heparin. *Br J Urol.* 1994;73:504.

Parsons CL, Lilly JD, Stein P. Epithelial dysfunction in nonbacterial cystitis (interstitial cystitis). *J Urol.* 1991;145:732.

Parsons CL, Mulholland SG. Successful therapy of interstitial cystitis with pentosanpolysulfate. *J Urol.* 1987;138:513.

Samraj GP, Kuritzky L, Curry RW. Chronic pelvic pain in women: evaluation and management in primary care. *Compr Ther.* 2005;31(1):28.

# 21 CHRONIC PELVIC PAIN TREATMENTS

*Lee Kao*

## LEARNING POINTS

To understand the definition and prevalence of pelvic pain; etiology and current treatment recommendations for ednometriosis-associated pelvic pain.

## VIGNETTE

This is a 24-year-old, G0, Caucasian female who is self-referred due to a long history of pelvic pain and dyspareunia. The patient was told that she may have pelvic endometriosis by other practitioners and was put on different kinds of medications for the past year or so. Unfortunately, the patient did not experience improvement of her pelvic pain. She has recently married and is experiencing severe dyspareunia along with pelvic pain.

### QUESTION 1

*Define chronic pelvic pain (CPP) and its prevalence.*

### ANSWER 1

One definition of CPP is noncyclic pain of 6 or more months' duration that localizes to the anatomic pelvis, anterior abdominal wall at or below the umbilicus, the lumbosacral back, or the buttocks and is of sufficient severity to cause functional disability or lead to medical care. Pain describes an unpleasant sensory and emotional experience associated with actual or potential tissue damage, and is always subjective. Many patients report pain in the absence of tissue damage or any likely pathophysiologic cause and may have a psychologic basis. If patients regard their experience as pain and report it in the same ways as pain caused by tissue damage, it should be accepted as pain. There is no generally accepted definition of CPP; most have used a minimal duration of 6 months as the major criterion for chronicity. Some temporal characteristics include cyclic (e.g., dysmenorrhea), intermittent (e.g., dyspareunia), or noncyclic pain. "Pelvic" often is assumed to be an adequate description of location, but visceral pelvic pain can be vaguely sensed at the periumbilical area, whereas somatic pelvic pain usually is better localized, as in the sacroiliac joint at the posterior buttocks.

The prevalence of CPP in the general population has not been established, but, available data suggests that it is more common than generally recognized. Approximately 15–20% of women aged 18–50 years suffer from CPP of greater than 1 year's duration.

### QUESTION 2

*What are common causes of CPP?*

### ANSWER 2

It can be helpful to classify CPP into gynecologic and nongynecologic causes, but an obstetrician-gynecologist certainly can diagnose and treat many nongynecologic disorders. For many of the diseases often listed as causes of CPP, only limited evidence or expert opinion supports an etiologic relationship. Potential visceral sources of CPP include the genitourinary (GU) and gastrointestinal (GI) tracts and potential somatic sources include pelvic bones, ligaments, muscles, and fascia. CPP may also result from psychologic disorders or neurologic diseases, either central or peripheral.

Some of the most commonly associated causes are:

1. Physical and sexual abuse: Women with a history of sexual abuse and high somatization scores have been found to be prone to nonsomatic pelvic pain, suggesting a link in-between. Studies have found that 40–50% of women with CPP have a history of abuse, physical or sexual.
2. Pelvic inflammatory disease (PID): Approximately 18–35% of all women with acute PID develop CPP.
3. Endometriosis: Although endometriosis may be a direct cause of CPP, it may also indirectly indicate women who are at increased risk for CPP.
4. Interstitial cystitis (IC): Pelvic pain can be the presenting symptom or chief complaint for IC. It has been estimated that about 38–85% of women presenting with CPP may have IC. Women with known IC are significantly at risk of having CPP.
5. Irritable bowel syndrome (IBS): Irritable bowel syndrome is characterized by a chronic, relapsing pattern of abdominopelvic pain and bowel dysfunction with constipation or diarrhea. It is a common functional bowel disorder of uncertain etiology. It appears

to be associated with CPP most commonly. Symptoms consistent with IBS are found in 50–80% of women with CPP.

6. Obstetric history: Pregnancy and childbirth can cause trauma to the musculoskeletal system and may lead to CPP. Historical risk factors associated with pregnancy and pain include lumbar lordosis, delivery of a large infant, muscle weakness and poor physical conditioning, a difficult delivery, vacuum or forceps delivery, and use of gynecologic stirrups for delivery.
7. Past surgery: A history of abdominopelvic surgery is associated with CPP.
8. Musculoskeletal disorders: Musculoskeletal disorders as causes of or risk factors for CPP have not been widely discussed in gynecologic publications. They may be more important, however, than generally recognized.

## QUESTION 3

*What are the current recommendations for the treatment of CPP?*

## ANSWER 3

Although the etiologic relationships of many of the proposed disorders are not well established, in clinical practice, most of these proposed causes are treated if found in women with CPP. Treatment options according to the level of evidence available are indicated below:

*Based on good and consistent scientific evidence (Level A):*

1. Combined oral contraceptive (OC) should be considered as a treatment option to decrease pain from primary dysmenorrhea.
2. Gonadotropin-releasing hormone agonists are effective in relieving pelvic pain associated with endometriosis and IBS, as well as in women with symptoms consistent with endometriosis who do not have endometriosis. Thus, empiric treatment with GnRH agonists without laparoscopy should be considered as an acceptable approach to treatment.
3. Nonsteroidal antiinflammatory drugs, including cyclooxygenase-2 (COX-2) inhibitors, should be considered for moderate pain and are particularly effective for dysmenorrhea.
4. Progestins in daily, high doses should be considered as an effective treatment of CPP associated with endometriosis or primary dysmenorrhea.
5. Laparoscopic surgical destruction of endometriosis lesions should be considered to decrease pelvic pain associated with endometriosis.
6. Presacral neurectomy may be considered for the treatment of centrally located dysmenorrhea but has limited efficacy for CPP or pain that is not central in its location. Uterine nerve ablation or transection of the uterosacral ligament also can be considered for centrally located dysmenorrhea, but it appears to be less effective than presacral neurectomy. Combining uterine nerve ablation or presacral neurectomy with surgical treatment of endometriosis does not further improve overall pain relief.
7. Adding psychotherapy to medical treatment of CPP appears to improve response over that of medical treatment alone and should be considered in all patients.

*Based on limited or inconsistent scientific evidence (Level B):*

1. Gonadotropin-releasing hormone agonists should be considered as a treatment option for CPP because they have been shown to relieve endometriosis-associated pelvic pain.
2. Surgical adhesiolysis should be considered to decrease pain in women with dense adhesions involving the bowel, but it is unclear if lysis of other types of adhesions is effective.
3. Hysterectomy is an effective treatment for CPP associated with reproductive tract symptoms that results in pain relief in 75–95% of women and should be considered.
4. Sacral nerve stimulation may decrease pain in up to 60% of women with CPP and should be considered as a treatment option.
5. Various physical therapy modalities appear to be helpful in the treatment of CPP and should be considered as a treatment option.
6. Nutritional supplementation with vitamin $B_1$ or magnesium may be recommended to decrease pain of dysmenorrhea.
7. Injection of trigger points of the abdominal wall, vagina, and sacrum with local anesthetic may provide temporary or prolonged relief of CPP and should be considered.
8. Treatment of abdominal trigger points by the application of magnets to the trigger points may be recommended to improve disability and reduce pain.
9. Acupuncture, acupressure, and transcutaneous nerve stimulation therapies should be considered to decrease pain of primary dysmenorrhea.

*Based primarily on consensus and expert opinion (Level C):*

1. A detailed history and physical examination are the basis for differential diagnosis of CPP and should be used to determine appropriate diagnostic studies.
2. Antidepressants may be helpful in the treatment of CPP.

3. Opioid analgesics can be used to provide effective relief of severe pain with a low risk of addiction but do not necessarily improve functional or psychologic status and are not well studied in patients with CPP.

## BIBLIOGRAPHY

ACOG Committee on Practice Bulletins—Gynecology. ACOG Practice Bulletin No. 51. Chronic pelvic pain. *Obstet Gynecol.* 2004;103(3):589–605.

# 22 SEXUAL ASSAULT

*Alison C. Madden*

## LEARNING POINT

Sexual assault is common, and obstetrician-gynecologists must educate themselves on the appropriate care of victims of sexual assault.

## VIGNETTE

A 21-year-old, G1P0010, presents to the emergency room (ER). The patient is quiet and does not make eye contact. The previous evening, she had gone to a college party. The patient doesn't remember leaving the party, and next remembers being awoken by her roommate at 5 A.M. when the roommate came home. The patient was lying in bed partially clothed. She was sore "everywhere" and exhausted, and retreated into the shower. She noted pain upon urination, and bright red blood streaks when wiping. The patient doesn't remember anything after the first few drinks at the party; the roommate suspects date rape. She convinced the patient to be evaluated in the ER.

Her history indicates with menarche at age 13. Last menstrual period (LMP) is 2 weeks prior. She is not on any form of contraception. She denies any sexually transmitted diseases (STDs), and has never had an abnormal pap. She has had 1 first trimester SAb. Her past medical and social histories are both negative. She takes no medications and has no known drug allergies. She is a college student. She denies any illicit drug use, and identifies herself as a "social drinker and smoker."

On physical examination, she is afebrile and her vital signs are stable. The exam is done by a rape crisis nurse. All findings are normal. Survey reveals no bruising. Pelvic exam is done and reveals no cervical motion tenderness, bleeding, or discharge. There are some mild abrasions at the anterior introitus. Wet mount and urine chorionic gonadotrophin is negative.

### QUESTION 1

*What is the incidence of sexual assault, and who is the typical victim?*

### ANSWER 1

Federal statistics include only "forcible rapes" that are reported. Only 10–15% of sexual assaults are reported to police. Therefore, statistics obtained probably grossly under represent the incidence of sexual assault in this country. U.S. Department of Justice statistics indicate an annual incidence of sexual assault of 70 per 100,000 persons in 1987, then increasing to 200 per 100,000 persons in 1994. An American Medical Association report from 1995 indicates 1 in 5 women under the age of 21 will be sexually assaulted.

Sexual assault occurs in all age, race, and socioeconomic groups. There are many misconceptions associated with societal perception of rape. There is no typical victim. Blame is often placed with the victim, whether overtly or implied, despite the fact that the victim is the recipient of a criminal act. Societal preconceptions of the female victims' style of clothing, behavior, past sexual history, and motivations in pressing charges do not hold true. The young and old, and the mentally and physically handicapped, are at higher risk of being victimized.

### QUESTION 2

How does one evaluate a suspected victim of sexual assault?

### ANSWER 2

Ideally a rape evaluation is done by an experienced practioner or some one who specializes in this sort of evaluation. Most ERs have a "sexual assault kit," and many have a nurse or other practioner who is a specialist in these exams. There are also specialized centers for rape evaluations in some cities.

A detailed history and physical is obtained and recorded, using the patient's own words and taking photographs of all physical findings. The history should record all details that the patient can remember, and also include a detailed recent sexual history. Bruises and lacerations are noted. Wood's Lamp is used to see semen. Wet mount is done, and initial STD screens, including *Neisseria* gonorrhoea/*Chlamydia* trachmatis, human immuno deficiency virus (HIV)/Hepatitis B and Syphilis are obtained. Counseling must be made available to deal with the psychologic impact of sexual assault. Fingernail scrapings and combings of pubic hair are done to find traces of assaulter's DNA. Sensitivity to the patient should be foremost in the practioner's mind, as many rape victims have described the thorough assault examination as "another rape."

### QUESTION 3

*Should any treatment be offered?*

### ANSWER 3

Empiric postexposure treatment for STDs is somewhat controversial. The U.S. Centers for Disease Control and Prevention (CDC) recommends empiric antibiotic prophylaxis because many assault victims are lost to follow-up. Empiric therapy includes Ceftriaxone 125 mg IM and Azithromycin 1 g PO × 1 (or Doxycycline 100 mg PO bid × 7d) for (see Chap. 13) and chlamydia. Metronidazole 2 g PO × 1 is recommended for the treatment of bacterial vaginitis or Trichomonas. Also controversial is empiric therapy for Hepatitis B (CDC recommends Hep B Vaccination without Hepatitis B immune globulin (HBIG)) and HIV prophylaxis (300 mg AZT and 150 mg 3TC bid × 4 weeks). All victims of sexual assault should be counseled regarding the availability of emergency contraception regardless of menstruation timing gonorrhea.

### QUESTION 4

*What is the so-called "Date Rape Drug?"*

### ANSWER 4

Gamma-hydroxybutyrate (GHB) is known as the "date rape drug." It has no color or smell, and comes in liquid, powder, and pill form. It usually takes its effect in 10–20 minutes. Victims of date rape who have been slipped this drug "black out" prior to the assault. Effects include the following: drowsiness, dizziness, nausea, vomiting, and changes in blood pressure, trouble breathing, aggressive behavior, impaired judgment, hallucinations, seizures, coma, and death. The closest FDA-approved drug relative is Xyrem, used for treatment of narcolepsy. Another drug available since the 1990s is also known as the "date rape drug": flunitrazepam (Rohypnol), a benzodiazepine. Flunitrazepam initially reduces anxiety, inhibitions, and muscular tension. Higher doses produce anterograde amnesia, lack of muscular control, and loss of consciousness. Onset is in approximately 30 minutes, and effects last 8–12 hours. Both GHB and flunitrazepam have synergistic effects with alcohol and other drugs.

## BIBLIOGRAPHY


ACOG Educational Bulletin. *Sexual Assault*. 1997.

Centers for Disease Control and Prevention. Sexually transmitted diseases treatment guidelines 2002. *Morb Mortal Wkly Rep.* 2002;51 (No RR-6);1.

Centers for Disease Control and Prevention. First line drugs for HIV postexposure prophylaxis. *Morb Mortal Weekly Rep* 47. 1998;(RR-7);1.

Sporer KA, et al. Gamma-hydroxybutyrate serum levels and clinical syndrome after severe overdose. *Ann Emerg Med.* 2003;42:3–8.

Rambow B, Adkinson C, Frost TH, Peterson GF. Female sexual assault: medical and legal implications. *Ann Emerg Med.* 1992;21:727.

Silverman JG, Raj A, Clements K. Dating violence and associated sexual risk and pregnancy among adolescent girls in the United States. *Pediatrics.* 2004;114:220–225.

Weir E. Drug-facilitated date rape. *Can. Med. Assoc. J.* 2001; 165(1):80.

Wilken J, Welch J. Management of people who have been raped. *BMJ.* 2003;326:458–459.


# 23 SYPHILIS

*Alison C. Madden*

## LEARNING POINT

To understand the approach to the diagnosis and management of syphilis.

## VIGNETTE

A 25-year-old healthy, single female presents to her primary care physician's office with complaints of a painless sore near her labia. She states it started as a bump, but now it has developed into an ulcer. She denies any insect bites, ill-contacts, or recent travel. She has no significant past medical or surgical history and does not take any medications except for birth control pills. She has a new male sexual partner and her last sexual encounter was 1 week ago. She denies any history of sexually transmitted diseases and her last pap smear was 3 months ago and was normal. Her exam is remarkable for a 1 cm, slighted elongated nontender ulcerative lesion, with a clear base and an indurated margin on the outer area of her left labia. Another lesion is located on the inside of her labia. The patient also has mild inguinal lymphadenopathy bilaterally.

## QUESTION 1

*What is the incidence and epidemiology of syphilis?*

## ANSWER 1

Cases of syphilis peaked around WWII and declined dramatically thereafter, concomitantly with the availability of penicillin. In the United States, there was a significant resurgence of early syphilis in homosexual males and drug-abusing heterosexuals in the late 1980s, which peaked in the early 1990s, and then steadily declined. However, the rate of primary and secondary syphilis in men increased in 2000 and 2001, while continuing to decline in women. In 2002, the incidence of syphilis was 2.4 cases per 100,000 population and was 3.5 times higher among men than in women.

## QUESTION 2

*What is the natural history of syphilis?*

## ANSWER 2

Syphilis is a chronic, systemic infection caused by the obligate parasite *Treponema pallidum* and characterized by periods of active disease and latency. The disease is acquired by sexual contact and by vertical transmission from mother to fetus. In the early stage of primary syphilis and approximately 10–90 days after exposure, a painless papule appears at the initial inoculation site. Within a few days, the chancre grows in diameter and ulcerates. The ulcer has a clear base with indurated margins. Frequently, there is modest enlargement of regional lymph nodes and usually there are multiple lesions present. Most frequently, the lesions appear in the genital area, however, any part of the body that is exposed can be affected. In the absence of treatment, the chancres will heal spontaneously in 3–6 weeks.

Within a few weeks to months (or even coincident with the primary lesion), a variable systemic illness develops, which is characteristic of the secondary stage of early syphilis. Patients develop low-grade fevers, malaise, sore throat, headache, adenopathy, and a rash. Some patients may even have alopecia or mild hepatitis.

The latency period is divided into two stages and is characterized by historical or serological evidence for syphilis, but no clinical manifestations. Early latency is defined as 1 year from the onset of infection as this is the period when untreated individuals are likely to have infectious relapses. Late latency is defined as the period from 1 to 5 years after the onset of infection.

Tertiary (late) syphilis is characterized by clinical manifestations of the disease in the central nervous system (CNS), cardiovascular system, and skin and bones. The cutaneous and osseous lesions (gummas) have characteristic gross and microscopic appearances and are the most frequent late syphilis manifestation. Neurosyphilis can manifest as gummas, meningitis, tabes dorsalis, paresis, or ophthalmic disease depending upon the anatomical site involved. Cardiovascular syphilis may result in aortic aneurysm, aortic insufficiency, coronary stenosis, and myocarditis.

## QUESTION 3

*How do you diagnose syphilis?*

## ANSWER 3

Since *T. pallidum* cannot be cultured in the lab, the disease must be identified by direct visualization or serology. The most sensitive and specific method for diagnosing primary syphilis is by demonstrating treponemes by darkfield microscopy. Another method is by direct fluorescent antibody testing (DFA-TP).

In most cases, however, syphilis is diagnosed by serological testing. Serological tests include nontreponemal tests and treponemal tests. The nontreponemal tests, the rapid plasma reagin (RPR) test and the Venereal Disease Research Laboratory (VDRL) tests measure the level of antibody to a cardiolipin-cholesterol-lecithin antigen. This reactivity reflects syphilitic activity and disappears with treatment. The treponemal tests are more complex and are used as confirmatory tests. They include the fluorescent treponemal antibody absorption (FTS-ABS) test, the microhemagglutination test for antibodies to

**TABLE 23-1. Treatment of Syphilis**

| | RECOMMENDED REGIMENS | ALTERNATIVE REGIMENS |
|---|---|---|
| Primary, secondary, and early latent | Benzathine penicillin G 2.4 million units IM | • Doxycycline 100 mg PO bid × 2 weeks OR<br>• Tetracycline 500 mg PO qid × 2 weeks OR<br>• Ceftriaxone 1 g IM/IV QD × 8–10 days OR<br>• Azithromycin 2 g PO |
| Late latent or unknown duration | Benzathine penicillin G 2.4 million units IM, given in 3 doses at 1-week intervals | • Doxycycline 100 mg PO bid × 4 weeks OR<br>• Tetracycline 500 mg PO qid × 4 weeks |
| Neurosyphilis | Aqueous crystalline penicillin G 3–4 million units IV q4 hours × 10–12 days | • Procaine penicillin G 2.4 million units IM QD × 10–14 days plus Probenecid 500 mg PO qid × 10–14 days OR<br>• Ceftriaxone 2 g IM/IV QD × 10–14 days |
| **Pregnant women** | | |
| Primary, secondary, and early latent | Benzathine penicillin G 2.4 million units IM | • None |
| Late latent or unknown duration | Benzathine penicillin G 2.4 million units IM, given in 3 doses at 1-week intervals | • None |
| Neurosyphilis | Aqueous crystalline penicillin G 3–4 million units IV q4 hours × 10–12 days | • Procaine penicillin G 2.4 million units IM QD × 10–14 days plus Probenecid 500 mg PO qid × 10–14 days |
| HIV infection | | |
| Primary, secondary, and early latent | Benzathine penicillin G 2.4 million units IM | • Doxycycline 100 mg PO bid × 2 weeks OR<br>• Tetracycline 500 mg PO qid × 2 weeks |
| Late latent or unknown duration | Benzathine penicillin G 2.4 million units IM, given in 3 doses at 1-week intervals | • None |
| Neurosyphilis | Aqueous crystalline penicillin G 3–4 million units IV q4 hours × 10–12 days | • Procaine penicillin G 2.4 million units IM QD × 10–14 days PLUS Probenecid 500 mg PO qid × 10–14 days |

*T. pallidum* (MHA-TP), and the *T. pallidum* particle agglutination assay (TPPA).

The use of a single serological test is usually inadequate because of the potential for false positive results. Thus, the diagnostic algorithm is to screen with a nontreponemal test and if positive, to confirm the diagnosis with a treponemal test.

The Centers for Disease Control currently recommend examination of the cardio-spinal fluid in persons with latent syphilis and in the presence of any of the following: ophthalmic signs or symptoms, evidence of active tertiary syphilis, treatment failure, and HIV infection with latent syphilis or syphilis of unknown duration.

## QUESTION 4

*Who should be routinely screened for syphilis?*

## ANSWER 4

The United States Preventive Service Task Force issued updated guidelines for syphilis screening in 2004. A review of the evidence supports screening all pregnant women and people at higher risk of acquiring syphilis, such as men who have sex with men who engage in high-risk behaviors, commercial sex workers, persons who exchange sex for drugs, and those in adult correctional facilities.

## QUESTION 5

*What is the treatment for syphilis?*

## ANSWER 5

Treatment depends on stage of disease, pregnancy, and HIV status (see Table 23-1). Desensitization protocols are required for penicillin-allergic pregnant women and patients with late latent or unknown stage of syphilis and coexisting HIV.

## BIBLIOGRAPHY

Calonge N. Screening for syphilis infection: recommendation statement. *Ann Fam Med.* 2004;2:362.

Centers for Disease Control and Prevention. Primary and secondary syphilis—United States, 2002. *Morb Mortal Weekly Rep.* 2003;52:1117.

Centers for Disease Control and Prevention. Sexually transmitted diseases treatment guidelines 2002. *Morb Mortal Weekly Rep.* 2002;51(RR–6):1.

Holmes KK, et al. (eds). *Sexually Transmitted Diseases.* New York, NY: McGraw-Hill; 1999:473–509.

Hook EW, Marra CM. Acquired syphilis in adults. *N Engl J Med.* 1992;326:1060.

Rolfs RT, et al. A randomized trial of enhanced therapy for early syphilis in patients with and without human immunodeficiency virus infection. The syphilis and HIV study group. *N Engl J Med.* 1997;337:307.

U.S. Preventive Services Task Force. *Guide to Clinical Preventive Services.* 3rd ed. Available online at http://www.ahrq.gov/clinic/prevnew.htm.

# 24 SALPINGITIS

*Neil S. Silverman*

## LEARNING POINT

To learn diagnostic criteria for pelvic inflammatory disease along with current guidelines for its treatment.

## VIGNETTE

A 19-year-old nulligravid woman presents to the emergency room with a chief complaint of persistent lower abdominal pain for 2 days. Her last menstrual period was 2 weeks ago, and she reports unprotected sexual intercourse on at least two occasions over the past 3 months with a single male partner. She denies being aware of any symptoms of sexually transmitted diseases (STDs) in her partner. She denies any bowel abnormalities, but also reports a lack of appetite due to her pain. She states that she may occasionally feel chilled.

On physical exam, an ill-appearing young woman is seen, rocking to try to be comfortable and holding her lower abdomen. Her temperature is 101.4°F, with a heart rate of 98 and a blood pressure of 100/72. Her lungs are clear to auscultation. On abdominal exam, she has rebound with marked tenderness focally in both lower quadrants. Pelvic exam reveals copious yellowish vaginal discharge which demonstrates sheets of white blood cells microscopically. Bimanual exam is extremely difficult due to the patient's anxiety and discomfort, but marked cervical motion tenderness is elicited, with no masses appreciated. The patient's urine pregnancy test is negative, and her white blood count is 13, 800 with 88% neutrophils and 5% bands.

## QUESTION 1

*What are the diagnostic criteria for pelvic inflammatory disease (PID)?*

## ANSWER 1

Approximately 18.9 million new cases of STDs occurred in 2000, of which 9.1 million were in individuals aged 15–24. In 2002, females aged 15–24 had the highest rates of gonorrhea compared with females in all other age groups. Left undiagnosed and untreated, cervical STDs have high rates of progression to salpingitis and PID, with subsequent risks of tubal infertility.

PID is difficult to diagnose because of the wide variation in signs and symptoms. A clinical diagnosis of symptomatic PID has a positive predictive value for salpingitis of 65–90% in comparison to laparoscopy, which is viewed as a "gold standard," with identification of classic pelvic inflammation and adhesions (Fig. 24-1). Combining two or more clinical findings to define a diagnosis, however, may exclude women who do not have PID at the expense of reducing the number of women with PID who are identified.

Empiric treatment of PID should be initiated in sexually active young women and others at risk for STDs if all the following minimum criteria are present and no other cause(s) for the illness can be identified.

- Lower abdominal tenderness
- Adnexal tenderness, and
- Cervical motion tenderness

Additional criteria may be used to enhance the specificity of the minimum criteria listed above:

- Oral temperature > 101°F (> 38.3°C)
- Abnormal cervical or vaginal discharge
- Elevated erythrocyte sedimentation rate (sed rate)
- Elevated C-reactive protein
- Laboratory documentation of cervical infection with *N. gonorrhoeae* or *C. trachomatis*

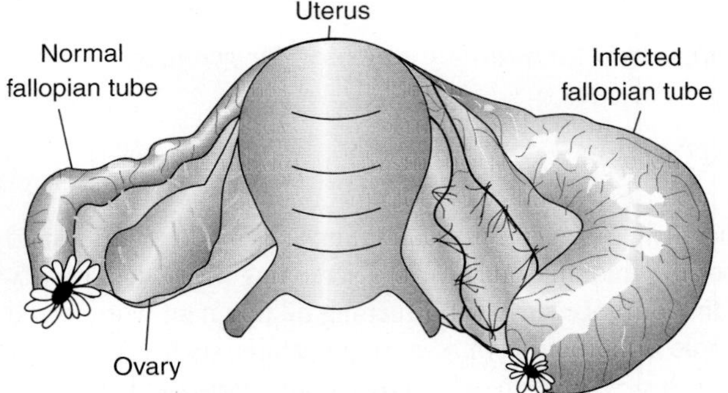


**FIG. 24-1** Acute salpingitis (PID).

## QUESTION 2

*What are the current outpatient and inpatient treatment guidelines for salpingitis and PID?*

## ANSWER 2

Currently, because of high reported resistance rates of gonorrhea to quinolones, oral and parenteral regimens, for PID should not include these agents empirically unless susceptibility testing has been specifically performed prior to initiating therapy. All the regimens below which include a quinolone agent are listed with that critical limitation understood.

Outpatient regimens:

- Ceftriaxone 250 mg IM in a single dose or cefoxitin 2 g IM in a single dose with probenecid 1 g PO administered concurrently, plus doxycycline 100 mg PO twice daily for 14 days with or without (depending on clinical severity) metronidazole 500 mg PO twice daily for 14 days (preferred).
- Ofloxacin 400 mg PO twice daily for 14 days or levofloxacin 500 mg PO once daily for 14 days with or without metronidazole 500 mg PO twice daily for 14 days.

Parenteral regimens:

- Cefotetan 2 g IV q12 hours or cefoxitin 2 g q6 hours plus doxycycline 100 mg IV or PO q12 hours (there is no advantage to the route of administration doxycycline in terms of tissue levels and bioavailability—decisions should be made based on the patient's ability to tolerate oral medications. Doxycycline is extremely irritating to the veins and oral doxycycline should be used as soon as clinically reasonable).
- Gentamicin loading dose IV/IM (2 mg/kg) followed by maintenance dose (1.5 mg/kg) q8 hours or daily gentamicin dosing plus clindamycin IV 900 mg q8 hours.
- Other options: ofloxacin 400 mg IV q12 hours or levofloxacin 500 mg IV daily with metronidazole 500 mg IV q8 hours or ampicillin/sulbactam 3 g IV q6 hours with doxycycline 100 mg IV/PO q12 hours.

Parenteral therapy is stopped 24 hours after a patient improves clinically, with initiation of oral therapy with doxycycline or clindamycin to complete 14 days of therapy. Both drugs are used together for 14 days if a tubo-ovarian abscess was present.

## QUESTION 3

*What are the criteria for hospitalization for the treatment of PID?*

## ANSWER 3

Hospitalization should be considered for the patient with suspected PID when:

- Surgical emergencies such as appendicitis cannot be excluded
- The patient is pregnant
- The patient does not respond clinically to oral antimicrobial therapy (if oral outpatient therapy is tried first, must be able to reevaluate patient by 24 hours to see if she is improving)
- The patient unable to follow or tolerate an outpatient oral antibiotic regimen
- The patient has severe illness, nausea/vomiting, or high fever
- A tubo-ovarian abscess is present.

No clear data exist to suggest that adolescent women empirically do better with hospitalization.

## BIBLIOGRAPHY

Centers for Disease Control and Prevention. Increases in fluoroquinolone-resistant *Neisseria gonorrhoeae* among men who have sex with men—United States, 2003, and revised recommendations for gonorrhea treatment, *Morb Mortal Weekly Rep.* 2004;53:335.

Centers for Disease Control and Prevention: *Sexually Transmitted Disease Surveillance* 2002. Atlanta, GA: CDC; 2003.

Centers for Disease Control and Prevention: Sexually transmitted diseases treatment guidelines 2006. *Morb Mortal Weekly Rep.* 2006;55(RR-11):1.

Sweet RL. Pelvic inflammatory disease: treatment. In Mead PB, Hager WD, Faro S (eds). *Protocols for Infectious Diseases in Obstetrics and Gynecology.* 2nd ed. Malden, MA: Blackwell Science; 2000:400.

Weinstock H, Berman S, Cates W Jr. Sexually transmitted diseases among American youth: incidence and prevalence. *Perspect Sex Reprod Health.* 2004;36:6.

# 25 NONSURGICAL MANAGEMENT OF PELVIC ORGAN PROLAPSE

*Cynthia D. Hall*

## LEARNING POINT

The use of pessaries can be a short- or long-term solution for pelvic organ prolapse (POP).

# VIGNETTE

A 75-year-old, G6P5015, female presents with complaints of fullness in the vaginal area. It is more noticeable and uncomfortable if she has been standing all day and is less noticeable in the morning. She does not complain of urinary or fecal incontinence. Her past medical history is significant for hypertension, obesity, and chronic bronchitis. She has never had any surgery.

Physical exam reveals an obese woman who appears her stated age. There are no palpable abdominal masses. Her introitus is somewhat widened, and, on valsalva, she has a grade 2 cystocele, a grade 2 rectocele, and the cervix descends to the introitus. The anal sphincter feels intact and of normal tone. The uterus feels of normal size, and the adnexa are nonpalpable.

## QUESTION 1

*What is POP and how is it graded?*

## ANSWER 1

POP is a descent of the pelvic organs (bladder, uterus and/or vaginal vault, small bowel, rectum), which is caused by weakening of the pelvic floor support. It is essentially a hernia. POP is extremely common and can seriously hinder a woman's quality of life. Typical symptoms are a feeling of pressure, fullness, or protrusion from the vagina, and lower abdominal or back pain that worsens on standing. Loss of anterior vaginal support often leads to a hypermobile bladder neck with urinary stress incontinence; but kinking of the urethra or trapping of stool in a rectocele may result in difficulty in urination or defecation. It is estimated that 11% of women will undergo prolapse surgery in their lifetimes, and many others either manage their prolapse nonsurgically or live with the problem.

Terms used to describe specific types of female genital prolapse include:

- Cystocele: hernia of the bladder with associated descent of the anterior vaginal segment
- Uterine prolapse: descent of the uterus and cervix
- Vaginal vault prolapse: descent of the vaginal apex (following hysterectomy)
- Rectocele: hernia of the rectum with associated descent of the posterior vaginal segment
- Enterocele: herniation of the small bowel/peritoneum into the vaginal lumen, most commonly presenting following hysterectomy in conjunction with vaginal vault prolapse

However, it is preferable to use the terms anterior, apical, and posterior vaginal prolapse as vaginal topography does not reliably predict which viscera are herniating. One of the most commonly used systems is the Baden-Walker, or "halfway," system for each compartment as follows:

G0: normal position
G1: halfway to hymen
G2: to hymen
G3: halfway past hymen
G4: fully past hymen

Despite the fact that the Baden-Walker system has good intraobserver consistency, it does not describe other factors that are important to describe pelvic floor support. Therefore, in 1997, members of the International Continence Society (ICS) devised another system: the pelvic organ prolapse quantification or POPQ scale (see Figs. 25-1 and 25-2).

## QUESTION 2

*Describe the technique of the pelvic examination in a patient with symptomatic prolapse.*

## ANSWER 2

Start by measuring the urogenital (UG) hiatus and perineal body (PB), then have the patient bear down with the labia separated to see whether anything descends to the introitus. Then with a dissembled speculum, each compartment is evaluated separately. The degree of POP

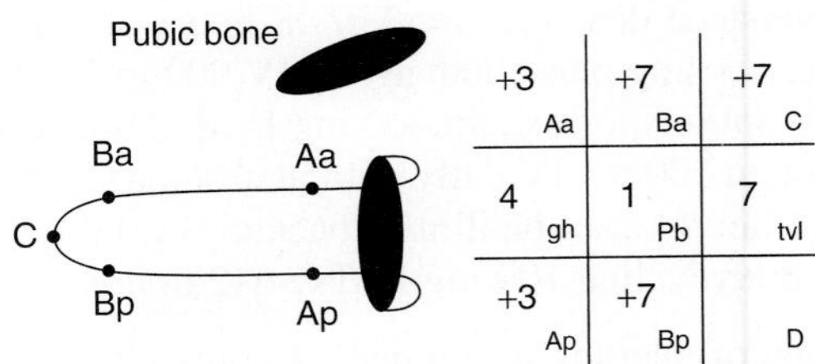


**FIG. 25-1** Three-by-three grid used to express the quantified pelvic organ prolapse (POP-Q) system. Aa = point A of the anterior wall; Ba = point B of the anterior wall; C = cervix or cuff; D = posterior fornix; gh = genital hiatus; pb = perineal body; tvl = total vaginal length; Ap = point A of the posterior wall; Bp = point B of the posterior wall.
SOURCE: Reproduced with permission from Harvey M-A, Versi E. Urogynecology and pelvic floor dysfunction. In: Kistner's Gynecology and Women's Health. 7th ed, Ryan KJ. Berkowitz RS. Barbieri RL, Dunaif A (eds.). St. Louis, Mosby; Elsevier: 1999. Copyright © 1999.

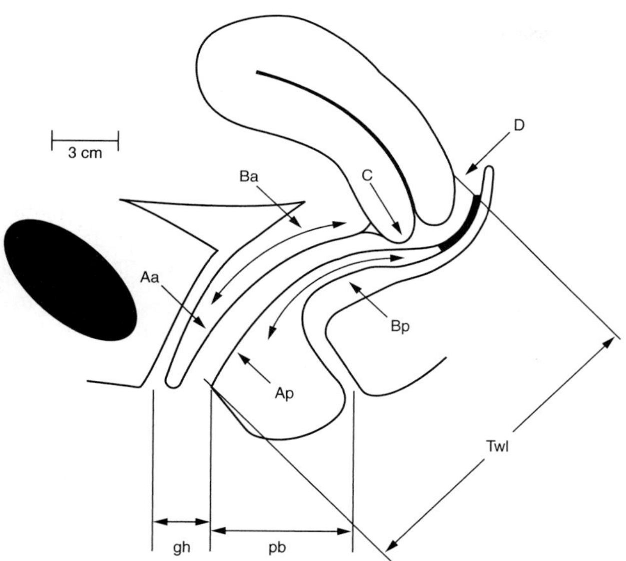


**FIG. 25-2** Pelvic organ support quantitation. Six sites (points Aa, Ba, C, D, Bp, Ap), genital hiatus (gh), perineal body (pb), and total vaginal length (tvl) used for pelvic organ support quantitation. SOURCE: Reproduced with permission from Bump, RC, Mattiasson, A, Bo, K, et al. The standardization of terminology of female pelvic organ prolapse and pelvic floor dysfunction. *Am J Obstet Gynecol* 1996; 175:10. Copyright © 1996 Mosby, Inc.

can vary from day to day and by degree of valsalva and patient position (supine vs. standing), so it is important that the exam corresponds to the patient's history of maximal descent. When in doubt, have the patient return for another examination. In a patient with stress incontinence (SUI), urethra-vesical hypermobility can be quantified by the Q-Tip test, where the lubricated head of a Q-Tip is placed into the urethra to just before the internal sphincter. An angle greater than 30° from the horizontal on straining, measured by the movement of the shaft of the Q-Tip, is considered abnormal, additionally, all patients with prolapse past the introitus should be evaluated for "potential" or "occult" SUI, as prolapse can result in urethral kinking which can mask SUI.

## QUESTION 3

*What are the risk factors for pelvic floor support disorders?*

## ANSWER 3

One of the greatest risk factors for POP is childbirth. Specific factors relating to childbirth, which increase a woman's risk, are multiparity, increased fetal weight, operative vaginal delivery, and prolonged second stage. Childbirth may result in neurologic, muscular, and possibly direct connective tissue damage, which leads to poor pelvic floor support and subsequent prolapse. Genetic predisposition plays a role, but this has been poorly defined. Other risk factors include advanced age, estrogen deficiency, neurogenic dysfunction of the pelvic floor, obesity, previous pelvic surgery, and any condition that chronically increases intraabdominal pressure, such as chronic constipation and pulmonary disease. The majority of patients with clinically significant prolapse will have at least two or more of these factors cumulatively. Over time, these factors contribute to a worsening of the prolapse with age.

## QUESTION 4

*What are non surgical options for treatment?*

## ANSWER 4

Treatment depends upon the anatomic defect and the patient's symptoms, but generally include reassurance, pelvic floor exercises, use of a pessary, or reconstructive surgery. Because POP is a quality of life issue, treatment should be based on symptoms and their impact on patient comfort. It was believed that POP progressed over time. However, this concept has been challenged by the findings of the Women's Health Initiative at UC Davis, which suggested that POP might actually regress in some women over time.

Pelvic floor (Kegel's) exercises can improve symptoms of prolapse, especially in mild to moderate cases. They may also improve urinary and fecal incontinence if present. However, it is important to evaluate a patient's ability to isolate her pelvic muscles. A study of women given written and verbal instructions indicated that only 49% of women could adequately isolate, and consequently control, their pelvic floor musculature. Biofeedback, which gives feedback (verbally or visually) on the effectiveness of muscle isolation, can be used to teach patients these exercises. Regular follow-up also seems to improve compliance.

Pessaries are another option for women with symptomatic prolapse that results in high satisfaction rates for women who choose this option. Pessaries come in all shapes and sizes and can be used even in women with complete procidentia (i.e., grade 4 prolapse of all compartments). Pessaries can often be managed by the patient, inserting and removing the pessary as needed for cleaning or for sexual activity, or can be managed by the practitioner. They should be removed at least once every 3 months and the vagina inspected for any erosions that might occur. Erosions are from direct local irritation and are less common if the vaginal tissue is well estrogenized. Therefore local or systemic hormone replacement is often recommended in conjunction with pessary use.

## BIBLIOGRAPHY

Bump RC, Hurt WG, Fantl JA, et al. Assessment of Kegel pelvic muscle exercise performance after brief verbal instruction. *Am J Obstet Gynecol.* 1991;165(2):322.

Bump RC, Mattiasson A, Bo K, et al. The standardization of terminology of female pelvic organ prolapse and pelvic floor dysfunction. *Am J Obstet Gynecol.* 1996;175(1):10.

Clemons JL, Aguilar VC, Tillinghast TA, et al. Patient satisfaction in prolapse and urinary symptoms in women who were fitted successfully with a pessary for pelvic organ prolapse. *Am J Obstet Gynecol.* 2004;190(4):1025.

Handa VL, Garrett E, Hendrix S, et al. Progression and remission of pelvic organ prolapse: a longitudinal study of menopausal women. *Am J Obstet Gynecol.* 2004;190(1):27.

Karram MM, Bhatia NN. The Q-Tip test: standardization of the technique and its interpretation in women with urinary incontinence. *Obstet Gynecol.* 1988;71:807.

Kobak WH, Rosenberger K, Walters MD. Interobserver variation in the assessment of pelvic organ prolapse. *Int Urogynecol J Pelvic Floor Dysfunct.* 1996:7(3):121.

Olsen AL, Smith VJ, Bergstrom JO, et al. Epidemiology of surgically-managed pelvic organ prolapse and urinary incontinence. *Obstet Gynecol.* 1997;89:501.

Snooks SJ, Swash M, Setchell M, et al. Injury to innervation of pelvic floor sphincter musculature in childbirth. *Lancet.* 1984;2:546.

Swift S, Woodman P, O'Boyle A, Kahn M, Valley M, Bland D, Wang W, Schaffer J. Pelvic Organ Support Study (POSST): the distribution, clinical definition, and epidemiologic condition of pelvic organ support defects. *Am J Obstet Gynecol.* 2005; 192(3):795–806.

# 26 DIAGNOSIS, DIFFERENTIAL, AND TREATMENT OF ANAL INCONTINENCE

*Cynthia D. Hall*

## LEARNING POINT

Anal incontinence has multiple causes, including birth trauma. There are conservative and surgical treatments, depending on the etiology of the incontinence.

## VIGNETTE

A 75-year-old P3 female complains of stress urinary incontinence (SUI) and anal incontinence of solid and liquid stool. The fecal incontinence (FI) began approximately 6 months ago and she had at least 10 episodes of leakage. Sometimes the leakage occurs with fecal urgency, but she also has had hard small stool pass without urgency. She has no symptoms of prolapse but has trouble evacuating the stools when they are hard.

Her past surgical history is significant for a vaginal hysterectomy done for prolapse and an appendectomy. Her medical problems include hypertension and type 2 diabetes mellitus (DM) not requiring insulin for 25 years. She delivered all her children vaginally. The largest infant was 9 lb and was delivered by forceps. She remembers a lot of stitches after that delivery but is unclear whether her rectum had been torn.

On examination, she has a G1 cystocele using the Badan-Walker system (see Chap. 25), and the vagina is short and descends approximately to the ischial spines. She also has a moderate rectocele, and her perineal body is very thin. The external anal sphincter (EAS) feels absent anteriorly and has decreased resting and squeeze tone.

## QUESTION 1

*What are the causes of FI?*

## ANSWER 1

FI is a devastating condition that has enormous social implications. Anal incontinence can be of flatus, liquid, or solid stool. A systematic review estimated the prevalence to be 11–15% of community-dwelling adults. Other data showed a prevalence of 47% of elderly patients in nursing homes. Fecal streaking is equally prevalent in men and women, but women overall have twice the prevalence of major FI.

Overflow FI can occur with fecal impaction. Decreased sphincter pressure can result from either sphincter disruption (obstetrical laceration or other types of trauma such as surgical trauma) or neurologic causes (pudendal nerve damage at vaginal delivery, chronic straining at stool with pudendal nerve stretching, long-standing diabetes, spinal cord injuries, or nerve compression). Decreased functional status and altered mental status can also contribute to FI. Rectovaginal or rectoperineal fistulas can bypass the anal canal and result in FI (see Table 26-1).

## QUESTION 2

*What does one look for on physical examination?*

## ANSWER 2

Overall mental status and mobility should be noted. A targeted neurologic exam should be done. The

**TABLE 26-1.**

| |
|---|
| **Risk factors for neurologic injury:** |
| Longer second stage |
| Larger infants |
| Number of deliveries |
| Prompted pushing as opposed to patient-guided pushing (?) |
| **Risk factors for sphincter laceration:** |
| Midline episiotomy |
| Operative delivery, especially forceps |
| Larger infants |
| Previous sphincter laceration (10–15%) |

bulbocavernosis reflex is elicited by stroking the perianal skin or lightly tapping the clitoris and looking for an anal wink. A thorough pelvic examination should always be performed, looking for lack of support in all compartments and for the presence of a rectocele that could result in fecal trapping and defecatory dysfunction as well as fecal leakage. Look for stool in the vagina and examine the perineal body for a "dovetail" sign (smooth skin anteriorly, gathered posteriorly). The anal sphincter should feel intact on digital examination, and decreased sphincter tone should be ruled out.

## QUESTION 3

*What additional diagnostic tests may be helpful?*

## ANSWER 3

Transanal ultrasound is extremely sensitive and specific in identifying sphincter defects. A 360° probe can visualize the internal anal sphincter (IAS), which is responsible for most of the resting anal tone. The EAS is responsible for most of the volitional squeeze pressure. Ultrasound can also visualize the puborectalis muscle.

Anal manometry measures the anal and rectal pressures. It also gives information about the sensation thresholds of the patient. Anal manometry correlates reasonably well with ultrasound in diagnosing sphincter defects.

Pudendal nerve testing is useful to identify previous neurologic damage. Patients who have neurologic damage in addition to sphincter damage have lower success rates for sphincterplasty.

Defecography is useful for patients with constipation or fecal trapping. A barium paste enema is given. The other pelvic structures such as the bladder, vagina, and small bowel can also be opacified. Films are taken during and after attempted defecation. Defecography can identify anismus (inability to relax the puborectalis and the EAS), or a rectocele, sigmoidocele, or enterocele, or the presence of rectal prolapse or internal intussusception. It can also quantify the amount of barium trapping and the amount of perineal descent, as well as visualize passive leakage of stool through a gaping anus.

## QUESTION 4

*What treatments are available?*

## ANSWER 4

Specific treatment should be sought for the underlying cause in all patients who have diarrhea. Regardless of etiology, formed stool is easier to control than liquid stool. Stool consistency can be improved by supplementing the diet with a bulking agent. Stool frequency can be reduced with antidiarrheal drugs. Anticholinergic agents (such as hyoscyamine) taken before meals may be helpful in patients who tend to have leakage of stools after eating.

Patients who have stool impaction should be disimpacted and treated with a bowel regimen to prevent recurrent impaction. Patients who have incontinence related to mental dysfunction or physical debility may benefit from assistance with a regular defecation program. Limited experience suggests that low doses of the tricyclic antidepressant, amitriptyline, can improve symptoms in patients with idiopathic FI.

Electrical stimulation of the sacral nerve roots can restore continence in patients with structurally intact muscles. The mechanism of action is not entirely clear, but physiology studies in patients with sacral nerve stimulation have shown improvement in resting and squeeze pressures of the anal sphincter as well as improved rectal sensation.

Surgical repair can consist of an end-to-end versus overlapping sphincterplasty (Fig. 26-1). Some studies suggest the overlapping repair is superior when performed remote to obstetrical trauma. Postanal repair imbricating the anal sphincter and levator ani musculature may be useful in the absence of a specific sphincter defect.

## QUESTION 5

*How can we minimize birth injuries and their sequelae?*

## ANSWER 5

Clearly, cesarean section before the onset of labor is protective. However, offering elective primary cesarean sections is controversial and is beyond the scope of this discussion. Multiple cesarean deliveries significantly increase maternal morbidity and mortality.

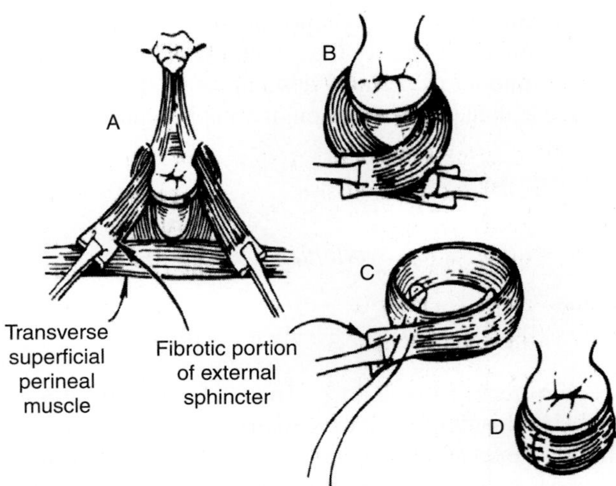


**FIG. 26-1** Overlapping sphincterplasty.

Many of the risk factors for neurologic injury and sphincter disruption are not modifiable. Avoiding midline episiotomy, especially with an operative delivery, is recommended. Cesarean section in patients with a previous third or fourth degree laceration (recurrence risk 10–15%) should at least be considered. Proper identification and repair of obstetric lacerations is essential.

Anal sphincter tears were detected by anal endosonography in 35% of primiparous and 40% of multiparous women in whom symptoms of anal incontinence or fecal urgency were present in 13% and 23%, respectively. However, FI can occur years or even decades after the injury. One series evaluating the outcome of primary repair of third degree obstetric lacerations in 50 women found that 85% had a persistent anal sphincter defect detected by anal endosonography.

Good surgical technique including adequate lighting, anesthesia, and retraction are essential. Often this means transfer to a formal operating room with suction and cautery available. Both the IAS (rubbery layer just underneath the rectal mucosa) and EAS should be repaired. The goal of sphincter repair (either primary or secondary) is reconstruction of a muscular cylinder that is at least 2 cm thick and 3 cm long.

## BIBLIOGRAPHY

Cheetham M, Brazzelli M, Norton C, et al. Drug treatment for faecal incontinence in adults. *Cochrane Database Syst Rev.* 2003;2:CD002116.

Coller JA, Sangwan YP. Fecal incontinence. *Surg Clin N Am.* 1994;74:1377.

Falk PM, Blatchford GJ, Cali RL, et al. Transanal ultrasound and manometry in the evaluation of fecal incontinence. *Dis Colon Rectum.* 1994;37:468.

Jesudason V, Furner S, Nelson R. Fecal incontinence in Wisconsin nursing homes: prevalence and associations. *Dis Colon Rectum.* 1998;41:1226.

Keating JP, Stewart PJ, Eyers AA, et al. Are special investigations of value in the management of patients with fecal incontinence? *Dis Colon Rectum.* 1994;40:896.

MacLeod JH. Management of anal incontinence by biofeedback. *Gastroenterology.* 1987;93:291.

Macmillan AK, Merrie AEH, Marshall RJ, et al. The prevalence of fecal incontinence in community-swelling adults: a systematic review of the literature. *Dis Colon Rectum.* 2004;47:1341.

Malouf AJ, Norton CS, Engel A, et al. Long-term results of overlapping anterior anal-sphincter repair for obstetric trauma. *Lancet.* 2000;355:260.

McKenna DS, Ester JB, Fischer JR. Elective cesarean delivery for women with a previous anal sphincter rupture. *Am J Obstet Gynecol.* 2003;189:1251.

Oberwalder M, Connor J, Wexner SD. Meta-analysis to determine the incidence of obstetric anal sphincter damage. *Br J Surg.* 2003;90:1333.

Rosen HR, Urbarz C, Holzer B, et al. Sacral nerve stimulation as a treatment for fecal incontinence. *Gastroenterology.* 2001;121:536.

Sultan AH, Kamm MA, Bartram CI, et al. Third degree obstetric anal sphincter tears: risk factors and outcome of primary repair. *BMJ.* 1994;308:887.

Sultan AH, Kamm MA, Hudson CN, et al. Anal-sphincter disruption during vaginal delivery. *N Engl J Med.* 1993;329:1905.

# 27 VAGINITIS: RECURRENT CANDIDA

*Alison C. Madden*

## LEARNING POINT

Evaluation and treatment of recurrent candidal vaginal infections.

## VIGNETTE

A 25-year-old woman presents with the chief complaint of recurrent yeast infections. She states that she has had a yeast infection every month for the last year. She had been initially diagnosed with a vaginal yeast infection after a course of antibiotics and was treated with Diflucan prescribed by her doctor. Her symptoms improved for about 2–3 weeks and then returned. At this time she used an over-the-counter yeast treatment, which also worked for only a few weeks. She is sexually active with one male partner. She takes oral acidophilus, which she purchases at a health food store. She takes a low-dose birth control pill. She denies any use of feminine deodorant products or douches. She has no known medical problems and has never had any significant illnesses. Currently she reports having an itchy, white vaginal discharge accompanied by dysuria.

## QUESTION 1

*How can one diagnosis vaginal candidiasis?*

## ANSWER 1

Patients may present with symptoms including pruritis, burning, dysuria, pain, dysparunea, or simply an increased discharge. Exam can reveal thick whitish discharge, erythema, and sometimes excoriations from scratching. The discharge associated with vulvovaginal candidiasis is classically described as thick, cottage cheese-like but it can also be thin and similar to discharges seen with other forms of infectious vaginitis. Vaginal pH is normal in the range of 4.0–4.5. Examination using microscopy with both saline and potascium hydrocloride (KOH) is essential, although 10–50% of the time these may be negative in acute candidial vulvovaginitis. In cases where the diagnosis is in question culture can be obtained, although the lab must be alerted to look for and identify yeasts. On saline preparation, hyphae may be visible and on KOH prep one may see budding yeast. See Fig. 27-1.

Self diagnosis of vulvovaginal candidiasis by patients is quite common with over-the-counter medications frequently used without a definitive diagnosis. Studies have shown that this was accurate at best 35% of the time and often women would treat with over-the-counter yeast infection medications for infections such as bacterial vaginosis or trichomomas.

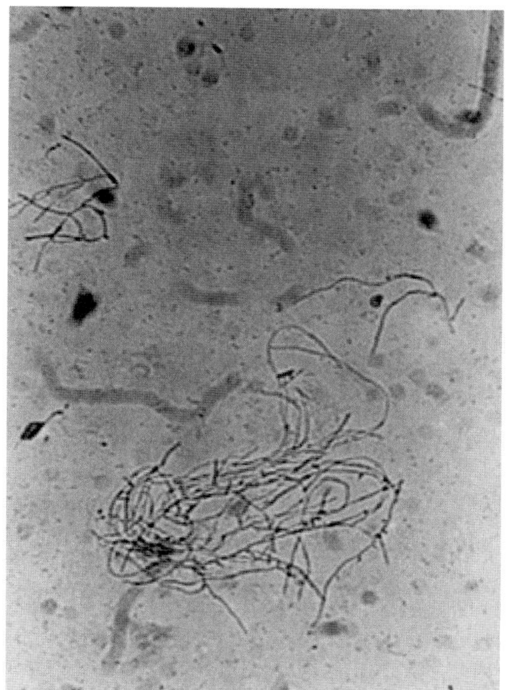

**FIG. 27-1** *Candida albicans vaginitis*. Low-power micrograph of hyphal elements seen on 10 percent KOH examination of a patient with *C. albicans vaginitis*. Courtesy of Jack D Sobel, MD. SOURCE: UpToDate 13.1. Overview of vaginitis.

## QUESTION 2

*What is the differential diagnosis?*

## ANSWER 2

Other conditions which can mimic vulvovaginal candidiasis in symptoms and which may also have a normal pH include allergic or hypersensitivity reactions such as those ocurring with prolonged use of steroid creams or sometimes with over-the-counter antifungal preparations. Vulvar cancer can present with severe prurits and normal appearing discharge and pH. Bacterial vaginosis or trichomonas usually have elevated pH but may also present with similar symptoms.

## QUESTION 3

*What is the treatment?*

## ANSWER 3

Treatment is only indicated for symptomatic patients. Culture and microscopy of asymptomatic women may reveal the presence of candida but does not warrant treatment. Oral and topical antifungal treatments are available and no clear superiority of any formulation has been found. For nonalbicans, candidial infections or recurrent infections, other medications including boric acid have been used with some success. The general recommendation in pregnancy is to use topical formulations for 7 days.

## QUESTION 4

*What about for recurrent vaginal candidiasis?*

## ANSWER 4

Recurrent vulvovaginal candidiasis occurs in approximately 5% of women. It is usually defined as the occurrence of a documented vulvovaginal candidial infection >3 times in a year. It is important to note that self-diagnosis and treatment of recurrent candidial infection often represents misdiagnosis and treatment of other infections. If candidial infections are recurrent, it is important to rule out infection with a resistant form of Candida, although most women will have infections with azole sensitive species—Candida albicans. Risk factors for recurrent infection include HIV infection and diabetes. More controversial, potential risk factors may include oral contraceptives, pregnancy, sexual activity with a partner colonized with Candida, hygiene practices including douching, antibiotic use, and diet.

The use of lactobacillus as a "probiotic" to recolonize the vagina with healthy bacteria has been successful in some small trials. The quality of the lactobacillus products available varies widely and is not regulated. They are only available over the counter and in compounding pharmacies. Boric acid has also been used for the treatment of recurrent vulvovaginal candidal infections.

A recent randomized trial showed a modest benefit to the use of long term suppressive fluconazole for women with recurrent candidial infections.

## BIBLIOGRAPHY

Ferris DG, Dekle C, Litaker MS. Women's use of over-the-counter antifungal medications for gynecologic symptoms. *J Fam Pract.* 1996;42:595.

Ferris DG, Nyirjesy P, Sobel JD, et al. Over-the-counter antifungal drug misuse associated with patient diagnosed vulvovaginal candidiasis (1). *Obstet Gynecol.* 2002;99:419.

National guideline for the management of vulvovaginal candidiasis. Clinical Effectiveness Group (Association of Genitourinary Medicine and the Medical Society for the Study of Venereal Diseases). *Sex Transm Infect.* 1999;75(Suppl. 1):S19.

Reed B. Risk factors for Candida vulvovaginitis. *Obstet Gynecol Survey.* 1992;47(8):551.

Sobel JD, Brooker D, Stein GE, et al. Single oral dose fluconazole compared with conventional clotrimazole topical therapy of Candida vaginitis. *Am J Obstet Gynecol.* 1995;172:1263.

Sobel JD, Chaim W, Nagappan V, et al. Treatment of vaginitis caused by Candida glabarata: use of topical boric acid and flucytosine. *Am J Obstet Gynecol.* 2003;189:1297.

Sobel, JD. Epidemiology and pathogenesis of recurrent vulvovaginal candidiasis. *Am J Obstet Gynecol.* 1985;152:924.

Sobel JD. Bacterial vaginosis In: Rose BD (ed.). *UpToDate.* Waltham, MA:UpToDate;2006. www.Uptodate.com

Sobel JD. Vulvovaginitis: when Candida becomes a problem. *Dematol Clinic.* 1998;16(4):763.

Sobel JD, Wiesenfeld HC, Martens M, et al. Maintenance fluconazole therapy for recurrent vulvovaginal candidiasis. *N Engl J Med.* 2004;351:876–883.

# 28 VAGINITIS: BACTERIAL VAGINOSIS AND TRICHOMONAS

*Alison C. Madden*

## LEARNING POINT

Evaluation and treatment of bacterial vaginosis and trichomonas.

## VIGNETTE

A 31-year-old woman presents complaining of a foul-smelling vaginal discharge for the last 2 weeks accompanied by pelvic pain and cramping. She denies any itching, fevers, or dysuria. She reports recently starting a relationship with one male partner approximately 3 months ago and states she would like to become pregnant in the next year. She denies any history of previous vaginal infections or sexually transmitted disease. She reports using condoms periodically for birth control. On speculum examination, she has an erythematous, cervix and a thin greenish vaginal discharge which has a pH of 5.0. Pelvic exam reveals some mild diffuse tenderness without cervical motion tenderness. There is a noticeable fishy odor with KOH prep. On saline prep multiple clue cells are present and motile trichomands are visible.

## QUESTION 1

*What are the clinical features of bacterial vaginosis and trichomonas?*

## ANSWER 1

Both bacterial vaginosis and trichomonas can present with malodorous discharge but may also be asymptomatic.

Bacterial vaginosis can sometimes present with dysuria and dyspareunia but this is rare. Trichomonas can present with burning, pruruits, pelvic pain, dysuria, and dyspareunia. Bacterial vaginosis and trichomonas tend to produce a thin grey or greenish discharge in contrast to vaginal infections caused by yeast, which tend to be thicker and whitish.

There is large variation, however, and overlap can exist. Many women who self-treat for vulvovaginal candidiasis without resolution of their symptoms have been shown to have bacterial vaginosis or trichomonas. Trichomonas is generally sexually transmitted and bacterial vaginosis is generally not thought to be sexually transmitted. Risk factors for bacterial vaginosis include frequent douching, orogenital sexual relations, and African-American ethnicity. Bacterial vaginosis is referred to as a "vaginosis" rather than a vaginitis as inflammatory reactions tend to be absent with this infection.

## QUESTION 2

*What are the diagnostic criteria for bacterial vaginosis?*

## ANSWER 2

Three of four Amstel criteria are needed for the diagnosis of bacterial vaginosis:

1. Abnormal discharge (grayish-white, homogenous)
2. Vaginal pH >4.5
3. Positive whiff test (fishy odor due to release of amines with 10% KOH)
4. Clue cells on saline wet mount

Cards have been developed by surgical supply companies, which incorporate the amine and pH portion of the test into a bedside test for detection of bacterial vaginosis but the gold standard for diagnosis remains the Amstel criteria including microscopy (see Fig. 28-1 B). The Nugent scoring system is seen in some studies and involves a scoring system based on a gram stain of vaginal discharge. Vaginal culture alone is not useful for establishing the diagnosis as it is often positive in the absence of symptoms. In addition, bacterial vaginosis is thought to be multifactorial and likely due to a decrease in healthy hydrogen peroxide-producing lactobacilli and an increase in multiple potentially pathogenic bacteria including *gardnerella vaginalis*, Mycoplasma, and many others.

## QUESTION 3

*What are the diagnostic criteria for trichomonas?*

## ANSWER 3

*Trichomonas vaginalis* is a flagellated protozoan, which is usually diagnosed by direct visualization of the motile organism on saline wet prep (see Fig. 28-1 D). The physical exam can reveal frothy green discharge, erythema, and punctuate hemorrhages of the cervix. These physical findings may be absent and some women and most men are asymptomatic. Wet mount detection of trichomonas is only about 50–70% sensitive for trichomonas. Other diagnostic tools include a DNA-based probe or monoclonal antibodies, which are about 90% sensitive. Culture can also be performed using diamond's media but not widely available for clinical purposes and is usually reserved for identification of resistant organisms or research studies. Trichomonads are also seen on pap smears but this method also lacks sensitivity.

## QUESTION 4

*What are the treatment options for bacterial vaginosis? What about in pregnancy?*

## ANSWER 4

Treatment options for bacterial vaginosis include oral or vaginal metronidazole, tinidazole, or clindamycin. Multiple doses have been reported for all medications. Cure rates are similar for these medications with significant relapse rates for all treatments. In general, metronidazole or tinidazole may have slightly higher efficacy in longer duration dosages such as 500 mg PO bid × 7 days compared with 2 g single doses and studies have not shown an increased cure rate with oral versus vaginal metronidazole, although this does not target the decidua where bacterial infections may exert their deleterious effect in predisposing to preterm labor. Tinidazole is similar to metronidazole but may be better tolerated due to lower side effects. Clindamycin is equally efficacious to metronidazole for the treatment of bacterial vaginosis in some studies and is the most frequently studied drug for treatment of this disease in pregnancy. The exact relationship of bacterial vaginosis and preterm delivery is controversial as it is the optimal method for screening and treatment of bacterial vaginosis in pregnancy. However, a definite association is present and the general recommendation is to treat bacterial vaginosis in pregnancy with oral medication and monitor for response. Other important parts of a treatment plan for eradicating bacterial vaginosis is personal hygiene modification such as eliminating douching, which has been found to increase the risk for bacterial vaginosis.

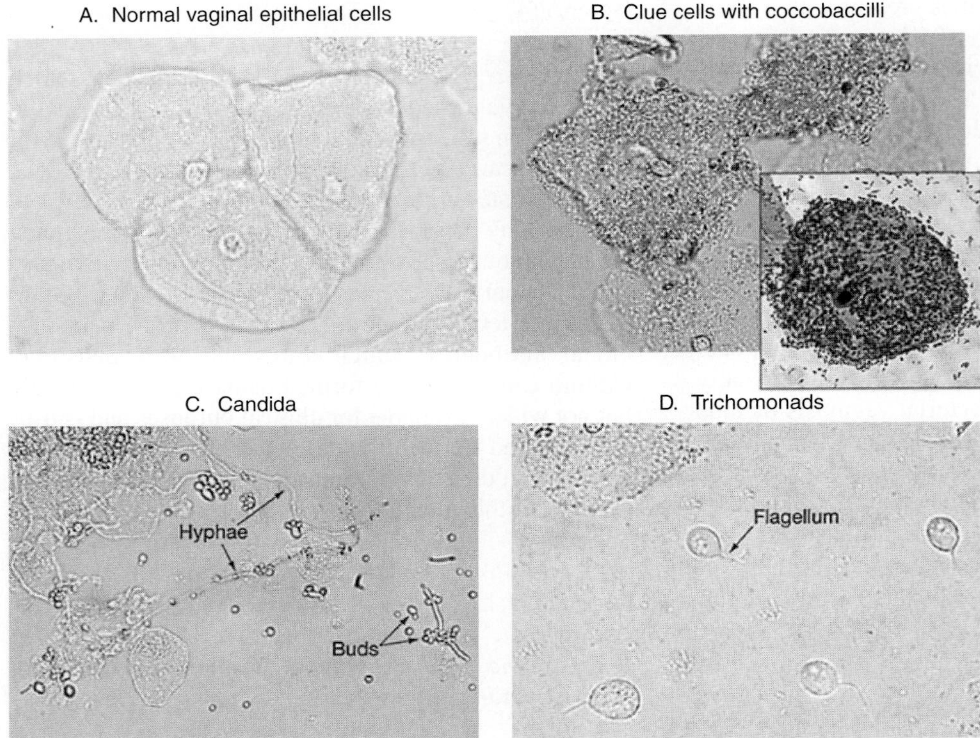


**FIG. 28-1** Microscopic examination of vaginal samples. (A) Normal saline wet mount showing a clump of three normal vaginal epithelial cells (original magnification × 600). Reproduced with permission from William L. Thelmo, MD. (B) Normal saline wet mount showing two clue cells (original magnification × 400). Inset, Gram stain demonstrating how coccobaccilli on the surface of vaginal epithelial cells create the characteristic granular appearance and indistinct borders of clue cells (original magnification × 1000). Reproduced with permission from Lorna Rabe, Magee-Womens Research Institute, Pittsburgh, PA. (C) Normal saline wet mount showing numerous *Candida* hyphae and buds (original magnification × 400). Reproduced with permission from Lorna Rabe. (D) Normal saline wet mount showing four trichomonads. Trichomonads can often be identified easily because of their characteristic jerky motility (original magnification × 600). Reproduced with permission from the Medical Laboratory Evaluation proficiency testing program of the American College of Physicians Services Inc.

SOURCE: From Anderson MR, Klink K, Cohrssen A. Evaluation of vaginal complaints. *JAMA*. 2004;291(11):1368–1379.

## QUESTION 5

*What are the treatment recommendations for trichomonas?*

## ANSWER 5

The first line treatment for nonpregnant patient with trichomonas is a single 2 g dose of metronidazole for both the patient and her partner. There is some controversy regarding the treatment of asymptomatic trichomonas in pregnancy. A randomized study by the National Institute of Child Health and Human Development has shown an increase in preterm birth before 37 weeks for patients with trichomonas treated with metronidazole in pregnancy. This was an unexpected finding and is thought that it might be due to an inflammatory response to the dying trichomonads. The Centers for Disease Control and Prevention (CDC) has stated that metronidazole is safe in all trimesters of pregnancy and can be used in a 2 g single dose for treatment of symptomatic patients. Alternative treatments for nonpregnant patients of symptomatic pregnant patients is metronidazole 500 mg bid for 7 days or tinadazole in same dosages as metronidazole for single or 7-day treatment. Resistant strains of trichomonas are becoming more common. Most are still responsive to higher dose treatment with metronidazole or tinidazole at doses reported as high as 2–4 g a day with combined oral and vaginal formulations. The CDC is available for consultation on these cases and is developing second line treatments, which include topical treatments with paronomycin, nonoxynol-9, and furazolidone.

## BIBLIOGRAPHY

Amsel R, Totten PA, Spiegel CA, et al. Nonspecific vaginitis: diagnostic criteria and microbial and epidemiologic associations. *Am J Med.* 1983;74:14–22.

DeMeo LR, Draper DL, McGregor JA, et al. Evaluation of a deoxyribonucleic acid probe for the detection of Trichomonas vaginalis in vaginal secretions. *Am J Obstet Gynecol.* 1996;174:1339.

Ferris DG, Dekle C, Litaker MS. Women's use of over-the-counter antifungal medications for gynecologic symptoms. *J Fam Pract* 1996;42:595.

Ferris DG, Nyirjesy P, Sobel JD, et al. Over-the-counter antifungal drug misuse associated with patient diagnosed vulvovaginal candidiasis *Obstet Gynecol.* 2002;99:419.

Kiss H, Petricevic L, Husslein P. Prospective randomized controlled trial of an infection screening programme to reduce the rate of preterm delivery. *BMJ.* 2004;329(7462):371.

Klebanoff MA, Carey JC, Hauth JC, et al. Failure of metronidazole to prevent preterm delivery among pregnant women with asymptomatic Trichomonas vaginalis infection. *N Engl J Med.* 2001;345:487–493.

Klebanoff MA, Schwebke JR, Zhang J, et al. Vulvovaginal symptoms in women with bacterial vaginosis. *Obstet Gynecol.* 2004;104:267.

MacDermott RI. Bacterial vaginosis. *Br J Obstet Gynaecol.* 1995;102:92.

Morris M, Nicoll A, Simms I, et al. Bacterial vaginosis: A public health review. *Br J Obstet Gynaecol.* 2001;108:439.

Ness RB, Hillier SL, Richter HE, Soper DE, Stamm C, McGregor J, Bass DC, Sweet RL, Rice P. Douching in relation to bacterial vaginosis, lactobacilli, and facultative bacteria in the vagina. *Obstet Gynecol.* 2002;100(4):765.

Nugent RP, Krohn MA, Hillier SL. Reliability of diagnosing bacterial vaginosis is improved by a standardized method of gram stain interpretation. *J Clin Microbiol.* 1991;29:297–301.

Nyirjesy P, Sobel JD, Weitz MV, et al. Difficult to treat trichomoniasis: results with paronomycin cream. *Clin Infect Dis.* 1998;26:986–988.

Okun N, Gronau KA, Hannah ME. Antibiotics for bacterial vaginosis or Trichomonas vaginalis in pregnancy: a systematic review. *Obstet Gynecol.* 2005;105(4):857–868.

Sobel JD, Nyirjesy P, Brown W. Tinidazole treatment for metronidazole resistant vaginal trichomoniasis. *Clin Infect Dis.* 2001;33:1341–1346.

Soper DE. Trichomonas: under control or undercontrolled? *Am J Obstet Gynecol.* 2004;190:281.

Spence MR, Hollander DH, Smith J, et al. The clinical and laboratory diagnosis of Trichomonas vaginalis infection. *Sex Transm Dis.* 1980;7:168.

Ugwumadu A, Manyonda I, Reid F, et al. Effect of early oral clindamycin on late miscarriage and preterm delivery in asymptomatic women with abnormal vaginal flora and bacterial vaginosis: a randomized controlled trial [see comment]. *Lancet.* 2003;361(9362):983–988.

# 29 VULVAR DIEASE: LICHEN SCLEROSUS

*Andrew John Li*

## LEARNING POINT

Vulvar lesions must be biopsied to exclude malignancy before treatment with topical creams.

## VIGNETTE

A 72-year-old, G0P0, female presents with intermittent vaginal spotting. She also reports a pruritic lesion on her vulva that is white to appearance. She denies any bloody stools or hematuria, and denies fevers, nausea, or anorexia. She denies any bloating or inguinal masses.

The patient's family history is negative for breast, uterine, colon, or ovarian cancer. She denies regular alcohol use but reports a remote history of tobacco use. She is married but was unable to conceive. She denies any history of sexually transmitted diseases or abnormal pap smears.

The physical exam reveals a thin Caucasian female. Vital signs: blood pressure 100/60, pulse 80/minute, respiratory rate 16/minute, temperature 98.6°F. Chest is clear to auscultation; cardiac demonstrates a regular rate and rhythm; abdomen is soft, nondistended, with a tender mass palpable in the left lower quadrant. On pelvic exam, she has normal external female genitalia. On her left labium is a 2 by 4 cm white lesion with excoriations. Her right labia is without lesions. There is no blood in her vagina and her cervical, uterine, adnexal, and rectal exams are within normal limits. A biopsy confirms the diagnosis of lichen sclerosus.

### QUESTION 1

*What are the classic presenting findings associated with lichen sclerosus, and what is the initial management?*

## ANSWER 1

Lichen sclerosis is a chronic inflammatory skin disease that causes substantial discomfort and morbidity, most commonly in adult women, but also in men and children. Any skin site may be affected (and, rarely, the oral mucosa) but lichen sclerosus is most common in the anogenital area. The underlying cause is unknown, but there seems to be a genetic susceptibility and a link with autoimmune mechanisms. The usual symptoms are pruritis, pain, dyspareunia, and burning. Lichen sclerosus characteristically presents with decreased subcutaneous fat such that the vulva is atrophic, with small or absent labia minora, thin labia majora, and sometimes phimosis of the prepuce. The surface is pale with a shiny, crinkled pattern, often with fissures and excoriation. The lesion tends to be symmetrical and often extends to the perineal and perianal areas. The diagnosis is confirmed by biopsy.

## QUESTION 2

*What are the histologic findings associated with lichen sclerosus?*

## ANSWER 2

Criteria to diagnose lichen sclerosus include variable degrees of thinning of the squamous epithelium with progressive loss of the epithelial folds (i.e., the rete ridges). The dermis just beneath the squamous epithelium has a characteristic acellular, homogeneous appearance, and chronic inflammatory cells are found deep to the homogeneous zone. Hyperkeratosis or parakeratosis may be present, but often the keratin layer is normal.

## QUESTION 3

*What is the treatment and management of lichen sclerosus?*

## ANSWER 3

The treatment of choice for anogenital lichen sclerosus is potent topical corticosteroid ointment for a limited time. Approximately 80% patients with lichen sclerosus respond satisfactorily to 0.05% clobetasol. After initial therapy, some patients might only use corticosteroids as needed, while others may require a twice-weekly maintenance therapy. Alternatively, 2% testosterone cream may be used, although it can produce masculinizing side effects and must be continued indefinitely. Surgery may be considered in some women, to relieve effects of scarring or to treat coexisting carcinoma.

## BIBLIOGRAPHY

Bracco GL, Carli P, Sonni L, et al. Clinical and histologic effects of topical treatments of vulval lichen sclerosis: a critical evaluation. *J Reprod Med.* 1993;38:37–40.

Friedrich EG. *Vulvar Disease.* Philadelphia, PA: W.B. Saunders Company; 1983;132–33.

Funaro D. Lichen sclerosus: a review and practical approach. *Dermatol Ther* 2004;17(1):28–37.

Hillard PA. Benign diseases of the female reproductive tract: symptoms and signs. In: Berek JS, Adashi EY, Hillard PA (eds.). *Novak's Gynecology*, 12th ed. Williams & Wilkins; Baltimore, MD: 1988. 388–389.

Powell JJ, Wojnarowska F. Lichen sclerosus. *Lancet.* 1999; 353:1777–1783.

## Section 3

# OFFICE MANAGEMENT: OBSTETRICS

## 30 BREAST-FEEDING AND MASTITIS

*Jane L. Davis*

### LEARNING POINT

There are many advantages and few contraindications to breast-feeding, and mastitis should not be a contraindication for breast-feeding.

### VIGNETTE

A 28-year-old, G1P1, African-American female is 4 weeks postpartum. She has been breast-feeding without difficulty until this morning when she noted feeling flushed with a fever of 102°F and unilateral breast tenderness. The patient denies any additional complaints.

The physical examination reveals a slender African-American female in no acute distress. Vital signs reveal blood pressure 11/68, pulse 80/minute, respiratory rate 18/minute, and temperature 102.2°F. Breast examination reveals the right breast without palpable three masses. The left breast has a firm, indurated area in the right upper, inner quadrant; the breast is erythematous, warm, and tender to palpation throughout, but especially over the area of induration.

#### QUESTION 1

*What are the advantages of and contraindications to breast-feeding?*

#### ANSWER 1

The advantages of breast-feeding include:

1. Human milk is the most appropriate nutrient for human infants.
2. Breast milk provides immunologic protection against infection by providing secretory IgA; breast-fed infants have fewer hospitalizations for infection and fewer problems with allergies later in life.
3. Breast-feeding stimulates more rapid involution of uterus.
4. Breast-feeding can satisfy an infant's nutritional needs for the first 4–6 months at a relatively economical cost.
5. Generally convenient.
6. Encourages natural child spacing.
7. Promotes good maternal-infant bonding.

Contraindications to breast-feeding include:

1. Active herpetic lesion near the breast.
2. Active tuberculosis in mothers who have not yet received adequate treatment for their infection.
3. Primary cytomegalovirus (CMV) infection (during acute phase of the infection).
4. Maternal HIV infection.
5. Maternal varicella infection.
6. When the mother is taking certain drugs (bromocriptine, cocaine, cyclophosphamide, cyclosporine, doxorubicin, ergotamine, lithium, methotrexate, phencydidine pill (PCP), or radioactive iodine; see Table 30-1).
7. In infants with galactosemia.
8. In mothers taking "street drugs."

Note: Mothers who are HBsAg positive may breast-feed provided that their infants have received hepatitis B immune globulin (HBIG) and hepatitis vaccine.

**TABLE 30-1. Medications Contraindicated during Breast-Feeding**

| MEDICATION | REASON |
|---|---|
| Bromocriptine | Suppresses lactation |
| Cocaine | Cocaine intoxication |
| Cyclophosphamide | Possible immune suppression; unknown effect on growth or association with carcinogenesis, neutropenia |
| Cyclosporine | Possible immune suppression; unknown effect on growth or association with carcinogenesis |
| Doxorubicin | Possible immune suppression; unknown effect on growth or association with carcinogenesis |
| Ergotamine | Vomiting, diarrhea, convulsions (at doses used in migraine medications) |
| Lithium | One-third to one-half of the therapeutic blood concentration in infants |
| Methotrexate | Possible immune suppression; unknown effect on growth or association with carcinogenesis, neutropenia |
| Phencyclidine | Potent hallucinogen |
| Phenindione | Anticoagulant; increased prothrombin and partial thromboplastin time in one infant; not used in the United States |
| Radioactive iodine and other radio-labeled elements | Contraindications to breast-feeding for various periods |

SOURCE: Modified with permission from ACOG Educational Bulletin. No. 258. *Breastfeeding: Maternal and Infant Aspects.* 2000.

## QUESTION 2

*What are nonhormonal and hormonal contraceptive methods recommended for use in breast-feeding women?*

## ANSWER 2

Nonhormonal contraceptive methods recommended for use in breast-feeding women include:

1. Exclusive breast-feeding for up to 6 months in mothers meeting lactational amenorrhea criteria, i.e., if baby is fed mother's milk or is given supplement feedings only to a minor extent and the woman has not experienced a postpartum menses. In this setting, breast-feeding provides 98% protection from pregnancy provided intervals between feedings not exceed 4 hours during the day or 6 hours during the night.
2. Prelubricated latex condoms.
3. Copper intrauterine contraceptive devices.
4. Male or female sterilization if permanent contraception is desired.

Hormonal contraceptive methods include:

1. Progestin-only oral contraceptives, prescribed or dispensed at discharge from the hospital to be started 2–3 weeks postpartum (e.g., the first Sunday after the newborn is 2 weeks old).
2. Depot medroxyprogesterone acetate (DMPA) initiated at 6 weeks postpartum. A few studies have shown no adverse effect on the newborn or breast-feeding with starting long-acting progesterone injectables earlier than 6 weeks. However, package inserts for DMPA are more conservative, and this should be discussed first with the patient. Often it is useful to administer DMPA prior to hospital discharge since some patients may have difficulty following up with their postpartum visit.
3. Combined estrogen-progestin contraceptives, provided they are not started before 6 weeks postpartum and only when lactation is well established and the infant's nutritional status well monitored.

## QUESTION 3

*What is mastitis and how is it treated?*

## ANSWER 3

Mastitis occurs in 1–2% of breast-feeding women. Patients present with a tender, reddened area on one breast, often accompanied by chills and fever. The differential diagnosis includes an obstructed milk duct, marked engorgement, and inflammatory breast cancer. Obstructed milk ducts respond to wet compresses and manual massage. Breast engorgement is usually bilateral. Inflammatory breast cancer can be excluded if a prior, recent breast examination was normal.

*Staphococcus aureus* is the most common causative organism, occurring in 40% of cases. Most cases respond to dicloxacillin (500 mg four times daily), hydration, bedrest, and acetominophen. Additionally, the patient should be counseled to empty the affected breast frequently by either breast-feeding or by manually or mechanically expressing the milk. Mastitis per se is not a contraindication to breast-feeding. Breast abscess formation may occur if the treatment of mastitis is delayed.

## BIBLIOGRAPHY

*Breastfeeding: Maternal and Infant Aspects*. ACOG Educational Bulletin. No. 258. 2000.

American Academy of Pediatrics, Committee on Drugs. The transfer of drugs and other chemicals into human milk. *Pediatrics*. 1994;93:137–150.

American Academy of Pediatrics and American College of Obstetricians and Gynecologists. *Guidelines for Perinatal Care*. 4th ed. Washington, DC: American Academy of Pediatrics and American College of Obstetricians and Gynecologists; 1997.

# 31 HYPEREMESIS GRAVIDARUM

*John Williams III*

## LEARNING POINT

Early diagnosis and treatment of nausea and vomiting of pregnancy can prevent escalation of symptoms and need for hospitalization.

## VIGNETTE

A 26-year-old, G2P0010, woman at 10 weeks gestational age presents to her obstetrician's office for her second prenatal visit with a complaint of severe nausea and vomiting. She states that she vomits four to six times per day and she has been unable to keep down solid food or fluids for the past 2 days.

Her obstetric history is significant for an elective termination at 12 weeks in her prior pregnancy. Her medical and surgical histories are noncontributory.

The physical examination reveals a well-developed Caucasian woman. Height is 5 ft/4 in. Weight is 111 lb (loss of 5 lb since her first visit at 7 weeks). Vital signs: Temperature: 98.4°F; blood pressure: 100/60; pulse: 90/min; respirations: 18/min. Mucus membranes appear dry. Skin: poor turgor, no visible lesions. Lungs: clear to auscultation; Heart: regular rhythm, no audible murmurs. Abdomen: normal bowel sounds, soft, nontender, no masses or hepatosplenomegaly. Pelvic examination: normal-appearing external genitalia; Vagina: well rugated, positive Chadwick sign. Uterus: mid position, soft, approximately 10 week's size. Adnexa: nontender without palpable masses. Urinalysis shows 3 + ketones and is negative for glucose.

### QUESTION 1

*What is the spectrum of nausea and vomiting during pregnancy? What is hyperemesis gravidarum?*

### ANSWER 1

Nausea and vomiting affects 70–85% of all pregnancies. Nausea and vomiting may begin as early as 5–6 weeks from the last menstrual period. Symptoms peak in severity by 9 weeks and then begin to subside. Although in 90% of pregnancies symptoms are resolved by 16 weeks, 10–15% of women will continue to have symptoms beyond 20 weeks or for the duration of the pregnancy. Even though nausea and vomiting has historically been referred to as "morning sickness," less than 2% of women experience symptoms solely in the morning. Eighty percent of women experience symptoms throughout the day with peaks between 6 A.M. and 12 P.M. However, the timing of symptoms varies. Overall, no adverse effects are on seen on the pregnancy. There are data that suggest that women with nausea and vomiting of pregnancy have a more favorable outcome than women without.

Hyperemesis gravidarum is the most severe form of nausea and vomiting of pregnancy. It complicates 0.5–1% of all pregnancies and is characterized by persistent vomiting, weight loss exceeding 5% of prepregnancy weight, dehydration, and ketonuria. The etiology has not clearly been defined, but is probably secondary to placental hormones (human chorionic ganadotrophin [hCG] and estradiol).

### QUESTION 2

*What is the basic evaluation for nausea and vomiting of pregnancy?*

## ANSWER 2

A through history, physical, and laboratory examination should be performed.

When did the symptoms begin?

Nausea and vomiting begins prior to 10 weeks. Symptoms of pregnancy beginning after 10 weeks are most likely due to other causes.

Does the patient have a history of preexisting conditions associated with nausea and vomiting such as diabetes mellitus, porphyria, cholelithiasis, or migraines?

Physical findings *not* associated with nausea and vomiting of pregnancy:

Abdominal tenderness other than epigastric discomfort
Fever
Headache (Note: Severe, prolonged nausea and vomiting may cause a thiamine-deficient encephalopathy and associated neurological findings.)
Goiter

Laboratory findings in nausea and vomiting of pregnancy:

Hyperchloremic metabolic alkalosis, which with severe dehydration can progress to acidosis
Elevated liver transaminase (<300 U/I)
Elevated total bilirubin (<4 mg/dL)
Elevated amylase (up to five times greater than normal level)
Decreased TSH (a nonsuppressed TSH suggests that nausea is secondary to something besides pregnancy)
Elevated free thyromine (T4) index

Examination:

Ultrasound
Rule out multiple gestation, gestational trophoblastic disease, and certain anomalies associated with hyperemesis gravidarum (partial mole/triploidy, trisomy 21, and hydrops)

## QUESTION 3

*What are the treatment options for nausea and vomiting of pregnancy and hyperemesis gravidarum?*

## ANSWER 3

Early treatment of nausea and vomiting can prevent escalation of symptoms and need for hospitalization

1. Lifestyle and dietary changes
   - Eating small, frequent meals high in carbohydrate and proteins, and low in fats prevent hypoglycemia and avoid gastric distension, which may trigger vomiting
   - Bland, dry diet-chips and crackers
   - Drinking small amounts of cold, clear, carbonated, or sour liquids
   - Increase resting time
   - Fresh air as needed
   - Avoid offensive smells and food (have patients keep diary)
   - Avoid iron preparations
   - Provide psychological support

The success of any of these is empiric since there is little evidence-based research in this area.

2. Medications:
   - Various algorithms have been developed for more severe symptoms involving IV hydration and medications. An algorithm developed by the Motherisk Program, (Hospital for Sick Children, Toronto, Canada) is shown in Fig. 31-1.

     It is interesting to note that most symptoms will subside within 24–48 hours of starting IV hydration regardless if medications are used. Some feel that correcting dehydration and electrolyte imbalance alone help resolve the symptoms.
   - Ondansetron HCL has been shown to be very safe to use during pregnancy. However, a small, randomized controlled trial in 30 patients found that it offered no benefits over Phenergan. Additionally, it has very little effect on nausea.
   - Vitamin $B_6$ (10–25 mg three to four times daily with or without doxylamine has been shown to be effective.

3. Alternative therapies
   Herbal teas, ginger, acupuncture, acupressure, and hypnosis

## QUESTION 4

*Many pregnant women are reluctant to take medication for nausea and vomiting during pregnancy because of perceived risks of teratogenicity. How should you counsel such a patient regarding the safety of antiemetic drugs in pregnancy?*

## ANSWER 4

It is common for pregnant women and health care providers to overestimate the teratogenic risk of drugs in pregnancy. In the case of nausea and vomiting of pregnancy, the perception of teratogenic risk is unrealistically high, even for medications that have been proven safe. This misperception often leads to underutilization of pharmacologic therapy and termination of otherwise

**Nausea and vomiting of pregnancy: treatment algorithm**[a,b]
**(If no improvement, proceed to next step)**

**Monotherapy:**
Vitamin $B_6$ 10 mg–25 mg, tid or qid

**Add:**
Doxylamine 12.5 mg, tid or qid[c]
Adjust schedule and dose according to severity of patient's symptoms

**Add:**
Promethazine 12.5–25 mg q4h PO/PR
***Or***
Dimenhydrinate 50–100 mg q4–6h PO/PR
(not to exceed 400 mg/d; not to exceed 200 mg/d if patient is also taking doxylamine)

| **No dehydration** | **Dehydration** |
|---|---|
| **Add** any of the following:<br>(presented here in alphabetical order)<br><br>Metoclopramide<br>5–10 mg q8h IM/PO<br>***or***<br>Ondansetron[d]<br>8 mg q12h IM/PO<br>***or***<br>Prochlorperazine<br>5–10 mg q3–4h IM/PO<br>25 mg BID PR<br>***or***<br>Promethazine<br>12.5–25 mg q4h IM/PO/PR | IV fluid replacement[e]<br>IV multivitamin supplementation[f]<br>Dimenhydrinate<br>50 mg (in 50 mL saline/20 min) q4–6h IV<br><br>**Add** any of the following:<br>(presented here in alphabetical order)<br><br>Metoclopramide<br>5–10 mg q8h IV<br>***or***<br>Prochlorperazine<br>2.5–10 mg q3–4h IV<br>***or***<br>Promethazine<br>12.5–25 mg q4h IV<br>**Add:**<br>Methylprednisolone[g]<br>16 mg q8h IV/PO for 3 days. *Taper over 2 weeks to lowest effective dose.* If beneficial, limit total duration of use to 6 weeks.<br>***Or***<br>Ondansetron[d]<br>8 mg, over 15 min q12h IV |

**FIG. 31-1** Treatment algorithm for nausea and vomiting of pregnancy.
[a]This algorithm assumes that other causes of nausea and vomiting have been excluded.
[b]At any step, consider parenteral nutrition, if indicated.
[c]In the United States, doxylamine is available as the active ingredient in Unison Sleep Tabs; one-half of a scored 25 mg table can be used to provide a 12.5 mg dose of doxylamine.
[d]Safety, particularly in the first trimester of pregnancy, not yet determined; has no major effect on nausea.
[e]No study has compared different fluid replacements for nausea and vomiting of pregnancy.
[f]100 mg thiamin IV daily for 2–3 days (followed by IV multivitamins) is recommended for every woman who requires IV hydration and has vomited for more than 3 weeks.
[g]Steroids may increase risk for oral clefts in first 10 weeks of gestation.
SOURCE: Koren G, Levicheck Z. The teratogenicity of drugs for nausea and vomiting of pregnancy: perceived versus true risk. *Am J Obstet Gynecol.* 2002;186:S248–S252.

wanted pregnancies. A meta-analysis by Mazzota and Magee, indicates that doxylamine/pyridoxine, indicates $H_1$ blockers and phenothiazines are both safe and effective for the treatment of nausea and vomiting of pregnancy. Therefore, patients with nausea and vomiting requiring pharmacologic therapy can be reassured that antiemetic drugs pose little to no teratogenic risk.

## BIBLIOGRAPHY


Goodwin TM. Hyperemesis gravidarum. *Clinical Obstet Gynecol.* 1998;41:597–605.

Herbert WN, et al. Nausea and vomiting of pregnancy. APGO Educational Series on Women's Health Issues, Association of Professors of Gynecology and Obstetrics, Washington, DC. 2001.

Koren G, Levicheck Z. The teratogenicity of drugs for nausea and vomiting of pregnancy: perceived versus true risk. *Am J Obstet Gynecol.* 2002;186:S248–S252.

Lacroix R, et al. Nausea & vomiting in pregnancy: a prospective study of its frequency, intensity, and patterns of change. *Am J Obstet Gynecol.* 2000;182:931–937.

Mazzota P, Magee LA. A risk-benefit assessment for pharmacological treatments for nausea and vomiting of pregnancy. *Drugs.* 2000;59:781–800.

Murphy PA. Alternative therapies for nausea and vomiting in pregnancy. *Obstet Gynecol.* 1998;91:149–155.

Nageotte M, et al. Droperidol and diphenhydramine in the management of hyperemesis gravidarum. *Am J Obstet Gynecol.* 1996;174:1801–1806.

Sahakian V, et al. Vitamin $B_6$ is effective therapy for nausea and vomiting of pregnancy: a randomized double-blind placebo-controlled study. *Obstet Gynecol.* 1991;78:33–36.

Sullivan CA, et al. A pilot study of intravenous ondansetron for hyperemesis gravidarum. *Am J Obstet Gynecol.* 1996;174:1565–1568.

Vutyavanich T, et al. Pyridoxine for nausea and vomiting of pregnancy: a randomized, double-blind, placebo controlled trial. *Am J Obstet Gynecol.* 1995;173:881–884.


# INFECTIOUS DISEASES IN PREGNANCY

## 32 SYPHILIS

*Marguerite Lisa Bartholomew*

### LEARNING POINT

Syphilis during pregnancy can cause severe maternal and fetal sequelae if not recognized and treated properly.

## VIGNETTE

A 26-year-old, G1P0020, comes to clinic for abdominal swelling. A singleton 23-week pregnancy is confirmed by limited ultrasound. She denies medical problems and sexually transmitted diseases, but reports that her "throat closed" after taking penicillin a few years ago. For 2 years, she has been using intravenous heroin and exchanged sex for drugs and money on several occasions. A physical examination is unremarkable except for tract marks on her arms. The genital examination is unremarkable. She is referred to a substance abuse treatment center. Blood is drawn with the following findings: HIV negative, hepatitis B surface antigen negative, rapid plasma reagin (RPR) reactive (1:32); all other prenatal labs are unremarkable. A urinalysis is unremarkable. She is called in for a fluorescent treponemal antibody (FTA) titer which is positive and is diagnosed with latent syphilis of unknown duration. A targeted ultrasound indicates normal fetal growth and anatomy. Liver function tests and creatinine are normal.

She is hospitalized for penicillin desensitization. After successful desensitization, she is treated with benzathine penicillin G, 2.4 million units intramuscular (IM) weekly for 3 weeks.

### QUESTION 1

*Describe the stages of syphilis infection and the rates of perinatal transmission.*

### ANSWER 1

Syphilis can be divided into primary, secondary, latent, and tertiary, as follows:

*Primary syphilis* is characterized by a painless genital ulcer (chancre) and inguinal lymphadenopathy.

One-third of patients exposed to early syphilis will acquire the disease. Primary lesions will develop approximately 21 days after exposure, but can present from 10 to 90 days after exposure.

*Secondary syphilis* occurs within a few weeks to several months after the primary lesion, and indicates hematogenous and lymphatic spread of the disease. Symptoms include low-grade fever, malaise, sore throat, headache, adenopathy, and cutaneous or mucosal rash. The characteristic rash on the palms and soles is seen at this time.

*Latent syphilis* is divided in two phases, early latent and late latent. Early latent is defined as occurring less than 1 year after the primary infection; late latent is defined as more than 1 year after the primary infection. Both phases of latent syphilis are asymptomatic. Due to the painless nature of the primary infection, the unlikely event of a documented seroconversion, and unreliable histories, the time interval is often unknown, and patients are often designated as having latent syphilis of unknown duration.

*Tertiary syphilis* is characterized by organ manifestations. Tertiary syphilis occurs in one-third of untreated patients. The most common manifestation is gummatous lesions of the skin, bone, and mucosa. Central nervous system and/or cardiac involvement (aortic aneurysm and/or insufficiency) occur in 25% of patients with the tertiary form.

The incidence of congenital syphilis in 2002 was 11.2/100,000 live births (a 21% decline from 2000). Spirochetes can transfer across the placenta at any time during pregnancy and delivery. Clinical manifestations in the fetus include hydrops, growth restriction, hydrocephalus, skeletal abnormalities, and fetal demise and are not apparent until after 16 weeks gestation when the fetus develops immunocompetence. Between 50% and 100% of untreated pregnant women with primary or secondary disease will vertically transmit it to the fetus, and 50% of these infants will have congenital syphilis. One half of infants with congenital syphilis will be stillborn or deliver prematurely. Early latent syphilis transmission rates are approximately 40%, but only 20% result in a preterm delivery or perinatal mortality. Late latent and tertiary syphilis have a frequency of transmission of 10%, and there is no increase in preterm delivery or perinatal mortality.

## QUESTION 2

*How is syphilis diagnosed during pregnancy?*

## ANSWER 2

The U.S. Centers of Disease Control and Prevention (CDC) recommends that all pregnant women should be screened serologically for syphilis with the RPR test or the Venereal Disease Research Laboratories (VDRL) test early in pregnancy. In populations with a high prevalence of syphilis, or for high-risk patients, serologic screening should also be performed twice during the third trimester (28–32 weeks and at delivery). Any woman delivering a stillborn fetus after 20 weeks of gestation should also be screened. The CDC also recommends that no infant should be discharged from the hospital without knowledge of the result of at least one maternal serologic screen.

The RPR and the VDRL tests are nonspecific antibody tests used for screening. Nonspecific tests can also be used for follow-up of treated disease. If the initial nonspecific screening test is positive, it should be followed with a specific test such as the fluorescent treponemal antibody absorbed (FTA-ABS), the *Treponema-pallidum* immobilization (TPI), or the microhemagglutination-*T-pallidum* (MHA-TP) test. If the specific test is positive, it is diagnostic for syphilis.

In most patients, the nonspecific test (RPR or VDRL) will eventually become nonreactive after treatment; however, it is not unusual for the nonspecific test to remain positive at a low level for life. A fourfold change in the titer level of the nonspecific test is required to document a new infection after treatment or a treatment failure; the RPR or VDRL titer levels correlate with active disease. For most patients, the specific tests will remain positive for life (Fig. 32-1).

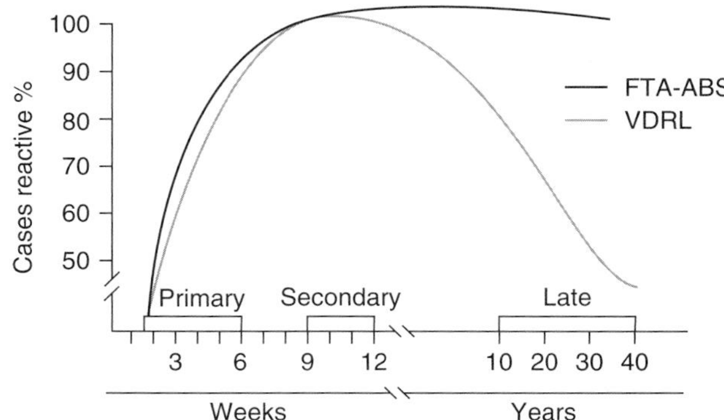


**FIG. 32-1** Time course of antibody development during syphilis. A comparison of the reactivity of the VDRL and FTA-ABS during the course of untreated syphilis. A substantial proportion of persons with primary syphills may not have developed a diagnostic antibody response at the time the chancre of primary syphilis appears.

SOURCE: Courtesy of Hicks CB, MD; modified from the VD Program, Centers for Disease Control, US Public Health Service. ©2005 UptoDate. www.uptodate.com.

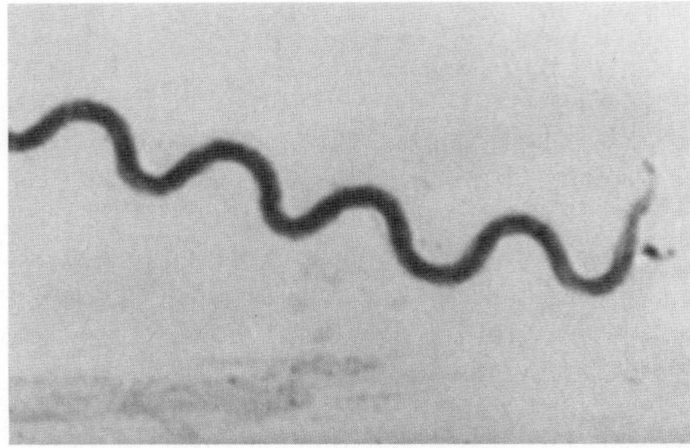

**FIG. 32-2** Darkfield examination of spirochete. Darkfield examination of an exudate from a penile ulcer in a patient with syphilis. When viewed in a fresh specimen, *Treponema pallidum* moves with a characteristic forward and backward motion with rotation around the longitudinal axis.
SOURCE: Adapted with permission from: Hicks CB. In: Rose BD (ed.). UpToDate, Waltham, MA: UptoDate; 2006 www.uptodate. com

**TABLE 32-1. CDC Guidelines for the Treatment of Syphilis in HIV Negative Nonpregnant Adults**

| STAGE | TREATMENT |
|---|---|
| Primary<br>Secondary<br>Early latent | Benzathine penicillin G, 2.4 million units IM<br>In a single dose (1.2 million units in each buttock)<br>Penicillin allergic: Doxycycline 100 mg bid PO or<br>Tetracycline 500 mg PO aid for 14 days |
| Late latent<br>Tertiary<br>Unknown duration | Benzathine penicillin G, 7.2 million units total<br>(2.4 million units IM every week for 3 weeks)<br>Penicillin allergic: Doxycycline 100 mg bid PO or<br>Tetracycline 500 mg PO qid for 14 days for early latent and 30 days for late latent |
| Neurosyphilis | Aqueous crystalline penicillin G, 12–24 million units daily (2–4 million units IV every 4 hours) for 10–14 days or<br>Procaine penicillin G, 2.4 million units IM (plus probenacid 500 mg PO qid) daily for 10–14 days |

When a syphilitic chancre first appears, both the specific and nonspecific tests may be nonreactive. Chancre lesions should be sampled with direct dark field examination for spirochetes, which is 100% diagnostic if spirochetes are seen (Fig. 32-2). Four to six weeks after the chancre appears, 100% of patients with primary syphilis will have positive specific and nonspecific test results.

Regardless of pregnancy status, a cerebrospinal fluid examination is recommended if the following is observed:

1. Neurologic or ophthalmic signs and symptoms
2. Evidence of active tertiary syphilis (aortitis, gumma, iritis, and the like)
3. Treatment failure
4. Concomitant HIV infection with late latent syphilis or syphilis of unknown duration

## QUESTION 3

*How does the treatment of syphilis during pregnancy differ from the treatment of nonpregnant individuals?*

## ANSWER 3

The drug of choice for all stages of syphilis is parenteral benzathine penicillin G. Penicillin is the most efficacious and easily crosses the placenta. Only 1–2% of infants born to adequately treated women will have congenital syphilis. Treatment during pregnancy is the same as that for nonpregnant individuals (Table 32-1) with the following exceptions. Alternative treatments (doxycycline or tetracycline) recommended for nonpregnant penicillin-allergic patients are not acceptable during pregnancy due to the unpredictable placental transfer. Penicillin desensitization is recommended for pregnant penicillin-allergic patients with subsequent penicillin treatment. Skin testing is not necessary if there is a well-described history of anaphylactic symptoms after penicillin. Skin testing is only reliable if major and minor antigens are available, usually found only in tertiary centers. The alternative treatment of neurosyphilis with procaine penicillin G plus oral probenacid is not a good choice for pregnant women due to the need for strict compliance.

## QUESTION 4

*What is the Jarisch-Herxheimer reaction and what are its implications during pregnancy?*

## ANSWER 4

The Jarisch-Herxheimer reaction can occur during treatment of primary, secondary, or early latent syphilis. During pregnancy, this reaction has been reported to occur in 100% of treated primary infections, 60% of treated secondary infections, and none of the treated latent infections. The reaction typically consists of fever, chills, myalgia, headache, hypotension, tachycardia, and transient accentuation of cutaneous lesions. It usually occurs within several hours of treatment and resolves in 24–36 hours.

During the latter half of pregnancy, the reaction can precipitate uterine contractions (67%) and decreased fetal movement (67%) along with the fever (73%). Fetal tachycardia may accompany the maternal fever. Transient late decelerations have been noted in 30%.

The etiology of the reaction is thought to be a result of the cytokine cascade initiated by the immune response to the dying spirochetes' cellular components. There are no prophylactic measures available. Because of this possible reaction, fetal monitoring and ultrasound are recommended before treatment is initiated in those women with viable fetuses who have primary or secondary disease. If the fetal evaluation appears normal, penicillin therapy can be administered on an ambulatory basis. If there are signs of congenital syphilis or fetal compromise, hospitalization for therapy and fetal monitoring is recommended.

## BIBLIOGRAPHY

Centers for Disease Control and Prevention. Sexually transmitted diseases treatment guidelines 2002. *Morb Mortal Wkly Rep.* 2002; 51(No. RR-6):1.

Fiumara NJ, Fleming WL, Downing JG, et al. The incidence of prenatal syphilis at the Boston City Hospital. *N Engl J Med.* 1952;247:48.

Hollier LM, Cox SM. Syphilis. *Semin Perinatol.* 1993;22:323.

Klein VR, Cox SM, Mitchell MD, et al. The Jarisch-Herxheimer reaction complicating syphilotherapy in pregnancy. *Obstet Gynecol.* 1990;75:375.

Sweet RL, Gibbs RS. Sexually transmitted diseases. In: Sweet RL, Gibbs RS (eds.). *Infectious Diseases of the Female Genital Tract.* 4th ed. Philadelphia, PA: Lippincott Williams & Wilkins; 2002:136.

Sweet RL, Gibbs RS. Sexually transmitted diseases. In: Sweet RL, Gibbs RS (eds.). *Infectious Diseases of the Female Genital Tract.* 4th ed. Philadelphia, PA: Lippincott Williams & Wilkins;2002:138.

Sweet RL, Gibbs RS. Sexually transmitted diseases. In: Sweet RL, Gibbs RS (eds.). *Infectious Diseases of the Female Genital Tract.* 4th ed. Philadelphia, PA: Lippincott Williams & Wilkins; 2002:142.

# 33 HERPES SIMPLEX VIRUS

*Marguerite Lisa Bartholomew*

## LEARNING POINT

Standard of care for the management of herpes simplex virus (HSV) in pregnancy has changed in recent years and currently relies on precise history taking and physical examination.

## VIGNETTE

A 25-year-old, G1P0, presents at 38 weeks gestation in active labor. The cervix is 5 cm dilated, 100% effaced, and +1 station. Her contractions are painful, palpably strong, and occur every 3 minutes. The membranes are still intact. She states that she is healthy, but had genital herpes outbreaks every 3–6 months for the past year. Her first known outbreak was 1 year ago, and her last was 1 month ago. She denies prodromal symptoms of genital HSV. She declined to take antiviral prophylaxis in late pregnancy. The genital examination is remarkable for two 5-mm vesicular lesions on the left labia minora, which are painful to the touch (Fig. 33-1). The rest of the perineum and perianal area appear free of lesions. A speculum examination indicates no other lesions visible on the vaginal mucosa or cervix. A primary cesarean delivery is recommended and performed.

### QUESTIONS 1

*What kind of virus is the HSV? Can HSV-1 cause genital lesions and HSV-2 cause oral lesions?*

### ANSWER 1

HSV is a double-stranded DNA virus. It is only transmitted by direct intimate contact, not fomites. Condoms may help reduce risk of transmission but are not fully protective. Following the initial infection, the virus remains dormant in neuronal ganglia (trigeminal and/or lumbosacral) and may reactivate at later times.

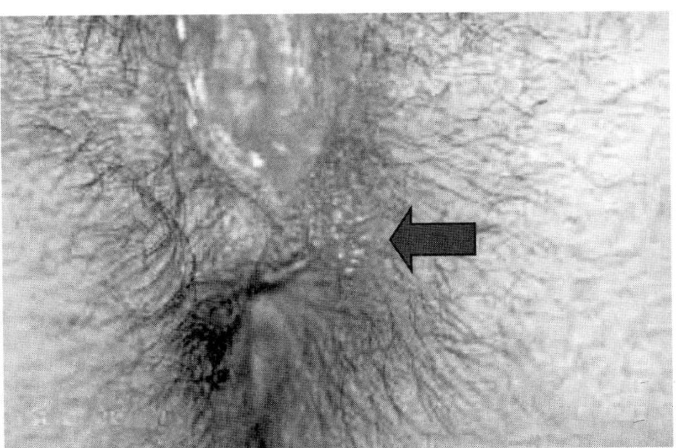

**FIG. 33-1** Vesicular lesions characteristic of genital HSV.

Two strains of the virus have been identified, HSV-1 and HSV-2. The former causes primarily oropharyngeal infection and the latter genital tract infection. However, 30% of new genital cases and 5% of genital recurrences are caused by HSV-1; conversely, 60% of new genital cases and 95% of genital recurrences are caused by HSV-2.

## QUESTION 2

*What is the seroprevalence rate of genital HSV? How many pregnant women acquire overt HSV during pregnancy? What is the incidence of neonatal infection?*

## ANSWER 2

The seroprevalence of genital HSV is about 25% among reproductive aged women in the United States. Approximately 1% of women have an overt herpetic infection during pregnancy. The majority (~80%) of the overt infections are recurrent, while 2% of susceptible women acquire HSV during pregnancy. The majority (~60%) of new infections during pregnancy are asymptomatic.

About 400 cases of neonatal herpes occur annually in the United States, and the estimated incidence of neonatal infection ranges from 1 in 2000 to 15,000 live births.

## QUESTION 3

*Describe the classification system for HSV infection.*

## ANSWER 3

The current classification of HSV infections is described in Table 33-1. Essentially, there are three types: primary, nonprimary but first overt episode, and recurrent.

**TABLE 33-1. Classification of Herpes Simplex Virus Infection**

| CLASSIFICATION | CRITERIA |
|---|---|
| Primary | First clinical infection<br>HSV-1 or HSV-2 isolated with culture or PCR<br>No preexisting antibody |
| Nonprimary, first episode | No history of genital tract infection<br>HSV-1 or HSV isolated with culture or PCR<br>Positive antibody for the other strain of the virus (HSV-1 or HSV-2) causing present infection |
| Recurrent | Prior history of clinical infection<br>Positive antibody for the same strain of virus causing the present infection |

## QUESTION 4

*Does late third trimester antiviral suppression provide any benefits?*

## ANSWER 4

Yes, suppression with a cyclovir (100 qid–400 tid beginning at 36 weeks through delivery) has been shown in many small randomized clinical trials, and in a meta-analysis of 799 subjects, to significantly decrease: (a) the risk of clinical HSV at delivery, (b) the cesarean section rate for the indication of recurrent genital HSV, and (c) HSV viral shedding at delivery. Data are limited with regards to prevention of neonatal herpes, due to the need for very large sample sizes.

## QUESTION 5

*What are the recommendations for care of the pregnant woman with HSV?*

## ANSWER 5

Clinical management of HSV infection has changed dramatically in recent years. For several reasons, surveillance cultures of the genital tract in patients with a history of HSV infection have been ineffective in preventing neonatal HSV infection and are not recommended. First, cultures are not highly sensitive and are costly. Second, correlation between asymptomatic shedding and neonatal infection is poor. Third, culture results are not always readily available at the time a patient is admitted for delivery. Fourth, most children with neonatal HSV infection are actually born to women who do not have a history of prior infection and who, hence, would not be targeted for surveillance cultures. Routine antenatal screening for maternal HSV antibodies is also not cost-effective and cannot be readily utilized for the purposes of planning the labor and delivery.

Accordingly, the following simplified guidelines have now been recommended by the Infectious Diseases Society for Obstetrics and Gynecology and are endorsed by the American College of Obstetricians and Gynecologists.

- At the time of the patient's initial prenatal appointment, she should be questioned about a prior history of HSV infection. If her history is positive, she should be screened for other sexually transmitted diseases such as gonorrhea, chlamydia, syphilis, hepatitis B and C, and HIV. Antiviral therapy is recommended for women with primary or recurrent infections to reduce shedding and enhance healing.

- When the patient ultimately is admitted for term or near term delivery, she should be asked about prodromal symptoms and examined thoroughly for cervical, vaginal, and vulvar lesions. If no prodromal symptoms or overt lesions are present, vaginal delivery should be anticipated. If symptoms or lesions are present, a cesarean delivery should be performed. Cesarean section is indicated even in the presence of ruptured membranes, since operative delivery in this setting significantly decreases the size of the viral inoculum to which the infant is exposed; there is no evidence that there is a particular duration of premature rupture of membranes beyond which the fetus does not benefit from cesarean delivery. Premature rupture of the membranes in the preterm pregnancy necessitates balancing of risks and benefits on a case-by-case basis.
- Mothers with symptomatic infection do not need to be isolated from their infants or other patients. They should wash their hands carefully before handling the infant and shield the baby from any contact with vesicular lesions. Breast-feeding is permissible as long as no skin lesions are present on the breast area.

## BIBLIOGAPHY


Brown ZA, Baker DA. Acyclovir therapy during pregnancy. *Obstet Gynecol.* 1989;73:526.

Brown ZA, Selke S, Zeh J, et al. The acquisition of herpes simplex virus during pregnancy. *N Engl J Med.* 1997;337:509–515.

Fleming DT, McQuillan GM, Robert RE, et al. Herpes simplex virus type 2 in the United States, 1976–1994. *N Engl J Med.* 1997;337(16):1105–1111.

Gabbe SG, Niebyl JR, Simpson JL. *Obstetrics: Normal and Problem Pregnancies*. Philadelphia, PA: Churchill Livingstone; 2003:1318–1320.

ACOG Technical Bulletin No. 102. *Herpes Simplex Virus Infection.* 1987.

ACOG Practice Bulletin No 8. *Management of Herpes in Pregnancy.* 1999.

Sheffield JS, Hollier LM, Lisa M, Hill JB, Stuart GS, Wendel GD. Acyclovir prophylaxis to prevent herpes simplex virus recurrence at delivery: a systematic review. *Obstet Gynecol.* 2005;102(6):1396–1403.

Thung SF, Grobman WA. The cost-effectiveness of routine antenatal screening for maternal herpes simples virus-1 and -2 antibodies. *Am J Obstet Gynecol.* 2005;192(2):483–488.


# 34 HEPATITIS C

*Neil S. Silverman*

## LEARNING POINT

To appreciate the risks of hepatitis C infection for both pregnant and nonpregnant women.

## VIGNETTE

A 43-year-old, G2P0010, woman presents at 8 weeks' gestation for genetic counseling for maternal age, and is interested in exploring the possibility of prenatal diagnosis for aneuploidy. Her social history is significant for a history of intravenous drug use, though she has been sober for over 15 years. Her review of symptoms is negative, and she denies tobacco or alcohol use. Her physical examination is significant for multiple tattoos on both arms, which she acknowledges having obtained when she was younger and "using."

Laboratory values: HIV antibody negative, gonorrhea and chlamydia screens negative, RPR and hepatitis B surface antigen negative. Her hepatitis C virus (HCV) antibody is positive, and her liver function tests are all normal.

### QUESTION 1

*What risk factors are associated with both hepatitis C infection and disease progression? What are the long-term sequelae of infection?*

### ANSWER 1

HCV is an RNA virus that targets both hepatocytes and B-lymphocytes. Primary complications of HCV infection are chronic liver disease-cirrhosis and hepatocellular carcinoma (HCC).

HCV is a world-wide pandemic, with 170 million individuals infected—five times more widespread than HIV (Fig. 34-1). In the United States, 1.8% of the general population is antibody-positive, and 0.8–1.0% of pregnant women in urban populations. There is a higher risk of infection among: intravenous drug users (IVDUs) or those with such a history (80%), individuals with a history of sexually transmitted diseases (6%),

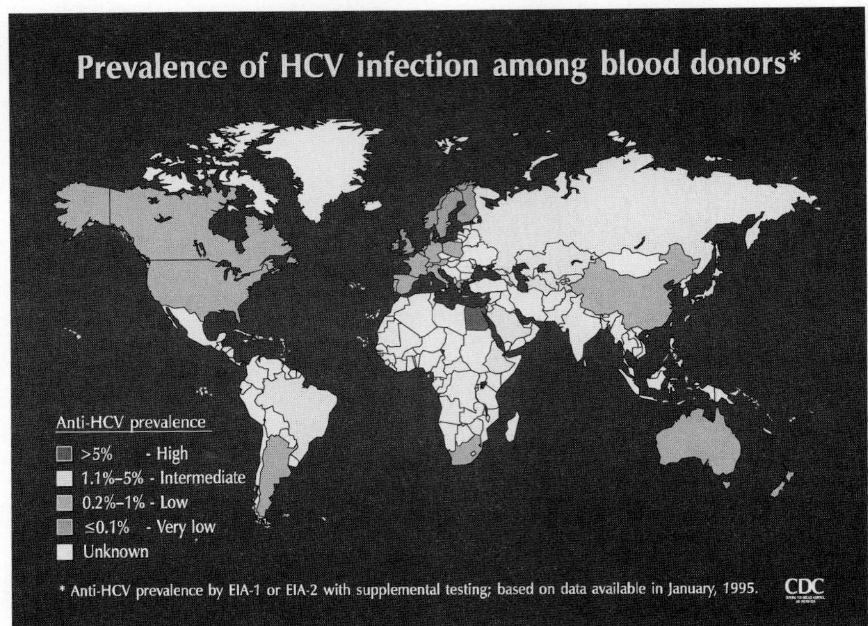


**FIG. 34-1** Worldwide distribution of HCV seropositivity.
SOURCE: Reproduced with permission from Centers for Disease Control and Prevention. Recommendations for prevention and control of hepatitis C virus (HCV) infection and HCV-related chronic disease. *Morb Mortal Wkly Rep.* 1998;47:RR-19.

and those who received blood product transfusions before 1992 (6%). Up to 85% of infected individuals have persistent viremia and never clear the disease (a rate which may be found to be higher as screening tests become more sensitive) (Fig. 34-2).

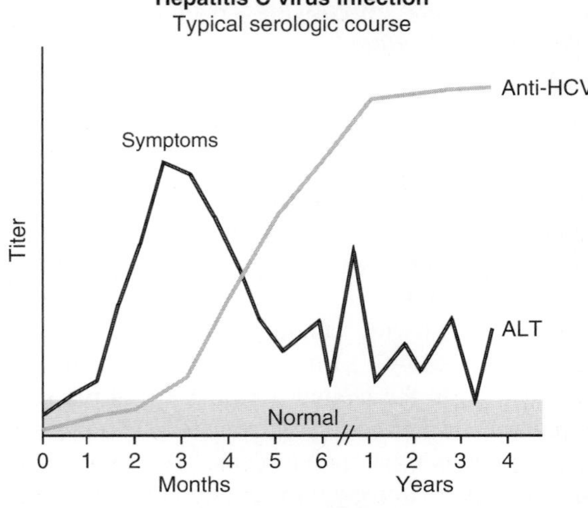


**FIG. 34-2** Serologic picture of hepatitis C infection.

Cirrhosis occurs in 15–20% of those with chronic viremia, with a risk of HCC of 1–4%/year once cirrhosis occurs. There is a higher risk of cirrhosis if the person is also HIV-infected (up to 75% of IVDUs are coinfected): 25% risk at 15 years, compared to 6% if HCV-infected only. Risk factors for cirrhosis/rapid progression (30% of those infected): alcohol, coinfection with HIV or hepatitis B, male age, and older age at the time of infection.

HCV-infected individuals are also at risk for extrahepatic disease, because of lymphocytic involvement. These complications include: mixed essential cryoglobulinemia, non-Hodgkin's lymphoma, and porphyria cutanea tarda.

## QUESTION 2

*What issues are pertinent to HCV infection during pregnancy?*

## ANSWER 2

There is a risk of 7–9% of perinatal (maternal-fetal) transmission, but only among viremic women (if a women is RNA-negative, her risk of perinatal transmission is close to zero). It is not clear if viral load is as critical to transmission as viremia being present at all.

There is currently no role for elective cesarean section to avoid transmission, and breast-feeding is not contraindicated. There does appear to be an increased risk of transmission when fetal scalp leads are used during labor. No role for anti-HCV meds to make mothers non viremic as with HIV, though discussion is ongoing to design clinical trials. Problem with such studies: risk of vertical transmission of HCV is fairly low, so very large trials would be necessary to achieve proper statistical power in such a study; in addition, HCV appears to be a less virulent disease in perinatally acquired cases.

Important testing in pregnancy (or in anyone HCV infected):

1. HIV status—has impact for pregnancy and for long-term maternal health. The risk of vertical HCV transmission is much higher if the mother is also HIV-infected (50%).
2. Ascertain hepatitis B/hepatitis A status if previously uninfected (antibody negative), should vaccinate against both (both vaccines safe during pregnancy, and should be given to high-risk women).
3. Liver function tests (as baseline).
4. HCV-RNA analysis helpful for perinatal transmission counseling—probably helpful only close to the time of delivery (within 2–3 weeks), and useful to the pediatricians following the baby after delivery. Quantitative HCV-RNA is also useful in nonpregnant adults for evaluating the success of anti-HCV therapies when they are given (also to monitor response).

### QUESTION 3

*What other issues need to be discussed with this woman regarding her pregnancy in terms of risks, and does her HCV infection impact at all on her options?*

### ANSWER 3

At her age, she is at increased risk of chromosome abnormalities in her fetus and should be offered genetic counseling and testing. Her overall risk of aneuploidy at age 43 is 1/20 (second-trimester risk), and she would normally be offered either noninvasive screening or invasive diagnostic testing, such as chorionic villus sampling (CVS) or amniocentesis. No data currently exist to state which invasive method is "better" for women with blood-borne infections such as HCV, but amniocentesis is less disruptive to the maternal-fetal interface, especially if traversing the placenta can be avoided, and may be preferable and less risky in terms of procedure-related perinatal viral transmission if definitive genetic testing is requested.

## BIBLIOGRAPHY

Centers for Disease Control and Prevention. Recommendations for prevention and control of hepatitis C virus (HCV) infection and HCV-related chronic disease. *Morb Mortal Wkly Rep.* 1998;47:RR-19.

Hershow RC, Riester KA, Lew J, et al. Increased vertical transmission of human immunodeficiency virus from hepatitis C virus-infected mothers. *J Infect Dis.* 1997;176:414.

Lauer GM, Walker BD. Hepatitis C virus infection. *New Engl J Med.* 2001;345:41.

Leung LT, King SM, Roberts EA. Mother-to-infant transmission of hepatitis C virus. *Hepatology.* 2001;34:223–29.

Silverman NS, Snyder M, Hodinka RL, McGillen P, Knee G. Detection of hepatitis C virus antibodies and specific hepatitis C virus ribonucleic acid sequences in cord bloods from a heterogeneous prenatal population. *Am J Obstet Gynecol.* 1995; 173:1396.

Silverman NS. Hepatitis in pregnancy. In: Sciarra J. (ed.). *Gynecology and Obstetrics.* 2005 ed. Philadelphia, PA; Lippincott, Williams & Wilkins: 2005.

# 35 HUMAN IMMUNODEFICIENCY VIRUS

*Neil S. Silverman*

## LEARNING POINT

To understand the impact on and management of human immunodeficiency virus (HIV) infection during pregnancy.

## VIGNETTE

A 29-year-old, G1P0, women presents for prenatal care at 11 weeks' gestation. This was an unplanned pregnancy; her male partner has a history of heroin abuse and was recently diagnosed with an opportunistic infection related to longstanding (though newly diagnosed) HIV infection. The patient is reluctant to be HIV tested herself but has heard that diagnosis and treatment can be helpful in lowering the risk of newborn infection. She has considered her options and is not interested in pursuing an option of pregnancy termination. Routine prenatal labs are drawn; her HIV ELISA is positive, with a positive confirmatory Western blot.

## QUESTION 1

*What is the risk of vertical (maternal-fetal) transmission of HIV, and what risk factors are associated with increased risks?*

## ANSWER 1

Historically, before the advent and availability of antiretroviral therapy during pregnancy to decrease vertical transmission, the risk of vertical transmission was 25–30% overall, with higher rates quoted for women in developing countries (30–50%) compared to industrialized countries. This difference was thought to be related to access to health care and overall maternal health status in general. In 1994, the National Institutes of Health published the first randomized trial employing retroviral therapy (single-agent zidovudine [AZT]) with the specific intent of reducing the risk of vertical transmission. In this trial, the risk of vertical transmission was significantly lowered from 25% in the placebo group to 8% in the AZT-treated group. Since that time, as antiretroviral treatment has progressed in general for HIV-infected adults, it has also been expanded for the treatment of pregnant women, both to ensure ongoing maternal health and to further decrease the risk of vertical transmission of HIV. Currently, with the use of multiagent highly active antiretroviral therapy (HAART) in pregnancy, the risk of vertical transmission is estimated to be in the range of 1–2%.

The risk of vertical HIV transmission has been reported to increase with: (1) advanced maternal disease (lower CD4 counts, higher HIV-RNA "viral load"), (2) prematurity, (3) breast-feeding, (4) smoking, (5) drug use (both intravenous and inhaled/cocaine). Among all factors, maternal viral load at the time of delivery appears to have the strongest predictive value, and is a critical goal of antiretroviral therapy during pregnancy.

## QUESTION 2

*How important is HIV screening for pregnant women?*

## ANSWER 2

The U.S. Centers for Disease Control and Prevention (CDC) estimates that 40,000 new infection with HIV still occur in the United States every year, including approximately 300 infants per year infected via vertical/perinatal transmission (Fig. 35-1). Early identification and treatment of pregnant women and treatment of newborns in the first hours of life are essential for the prevention of neonatal HIV infection.

Currently, it is recommended that all pregnant women be offered HIV testing. Some states have stronger mandates than others; in California, for example, it is required that all providers delivering care to pregnant women offer HIV testing during their pregnancy. Variations of two different HIV testing strategies are currently being employed in the United States: an "opt-in" approach is a strategy that requires specific informed consent, usually in writing, before HIV testing can be performed, and is the basis for most state laws and regulations in effect today. A number of states and providers, however, are moving to an "opt-out" approach, in which universal HIV testing with patient notification is viewed as a routine component of prenatal care. A pregnant woman is notified that she will be tested for HIV as part of the routine panel of prenatal blood tests unless she declines. The opt-out approach has been associated with higher testing rates than the opt-in approach in a number of studies; rates have approached 85–98% in surveyed areas using this strategy. The CDC recently revised its guidelines to recommend the opt-out approach.

For women who present to labor and delivery with undocumented HIV status, rapid HIV testing can be

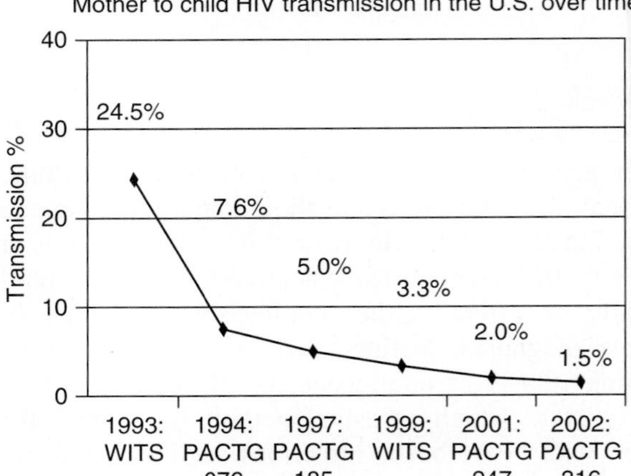


**FIG. 35-1** Historical trends in maternal-fetal HIV transmission.

offered/employed to provide an opportunity to begin prophylaxis of previously undiagnosed infection before delivery. Antiretroviral prophylaxis during labor and prior to delivery has been shown to still have an impact on vertical transmission, though not as large an effect as when begun during pregnancy and continued through delivery. The CDC-sponsored Mother-Infant Rapid Intervention at Delivery (MIRIAD) study group examined the use of a rapid oral HIV test kit in 4849 prenatal patients with unknown HIV status in a multicenter urban-based hospital study. Data from that study showed a sensitivity for the oral test (OraQuick) of 100% and a specificity of 99.9. Turnaround time was 20–40 minutes. As with all screening tests, confirmation needs to be performed with a standard Western blot assay, and the likelihood of a false-positive result is higher in populations with lower prevalences of HIV infection overall.

## QUESTION 3

*What measures can be taken during around the time of delivery to lower the risk of perinatal HIV transmission?*

## ANSWER 3

Maternal treatment during pregnancy with the goal of lowering viral load has been a major advance in lowering the risk of perinatal/neonatal HIV infection, especially since it is estimated that up to one-third of neonatal infections occur in utero, prior to the onset of labor. Ongoing research suggests that later cases of infection occur as the result of fetal exposure to the virus during labor and delivery. At very low maternal viral load levels, however (<1000 copies/mL), the observed incidence of vertical transmission was 0, with a 95% confidence level upper limit of 2%.

In theory, the risk of vertical transmission could be lowered by avoiding vaginal delivery and performing cesareans before the onset of labor and before rupture of membranes. Early studies examining this factor, however, were retrospective, analyzing data from other studies not designed to specifically address route of delivery as a separate risk factor for vertical transmission. Inconsistent results, therefore, were seen in a number of studies, specifically in studies conducted before combined antiretroviral therapy was used routinely, and before maternal viral load testing was a routine component of surveillance. Whether cesarean delivery offers any additional benefit to women on HAART or to women with low or undetectable maternal viral loads is unknown. A recent European multicenter study suggests that it might; however, there was no controlling within centers for how route of delivery was decided for individual patients, which, unfortunately, significantly weakened the power of its conclusions.

Current consensus consists of the following recommendations:

- Women with viral load >1000 copies/mL with or without therapy, should be counseled that elective prelabor cesarean delivery at 38 weeks is recommended to decrease the risk of vertical transmission.
- Data are insufficient to demonstrate a benefit for neonates of women who are durably suppressed on antiretroviral therapy, with viral load <1000 copies/mL.
- Internal scalp leads should not be used during labor.
- Antriretroviral therapy should not be interrupted around the time of delivery, either vaginal or cesarean.

## BIBLIOGRAPHY


ACOG: ACOG Committee Opinion no. 304. Prenatal and perinatal human immunodeficiency virus testing: expanded recommendations. 2004.

ACOG. ACOG Committee Opinion no. 234. Scheduled cesarean delivery and the prevention of vertical transmission of HIV infection. 2000.

Bulterys M, Jamieson DJ, O'Sullivan MJ, et al. Rapid HIV-1 testing during labor: a multicenter study. Mother-Infant Rapid Intervention at Delivery (MIRIAD) Study Group. *JAMA.* 2004;292:219.

Centers for Disease Control and Prevention. Advancing HIV prevention: new strategies for a changing epidemic—United States, 2003. *Morb Mortal Wkly Rep.* 2003;52:329.

Connor EM, Sperling RS, Gelber R, et al. Reduction of maternal-fetal transmission of human immunodeficiency virus type 1 with zidovudine treatment. *N Engl J Med.* 1994;331:1173.

European Collaborative Study. Mother-to-child transmission of HIV infection in the ear of highly active antiretroviral therapy. *Clin Infect Dis.* 2005;40:458.

Garcia PM, Kalish LA, Pitt J, et al. Maternal levels of plasma human immunodeficiency virus type 1 RNA and the risk of perinatal transmission. *N Engl J Med.* 1999;341:385.

Mitchla Z, Sharland M. Current treatment options to prevent perinatal transmission of HIV. *Exp Opin Pharmacother.* 2000;1:239.

Mofenson LM, Lambert JS, Stiehm ER, et al. Risk factors for perinatal transmission of human immunodeficiency virus type 1 on women treated with zidovudine. *N Engl J Med.* 1999;341:385.

Silverman NS, Watts DH, Hitti J, et al. Initial multicenter experience with double nucleoside therapy for human immunodeficiency virus during pregnancy. *Infect Dis Obstet Gynecol.* 1998;6:237.

Wade NA, Birkhead GS, Warren BL, et al. Abbreviated regimens of zidovudine prophylaxis and perinatal transmission of human immunodeficiency virus. *N Engl J Med.* 1998;339:1409.

# 36 PARVOVIRUS

*Neil S. Silverman*

## LEARNING POINT

To learn the risks and potential management options for parvovirus infection during pregnancy.

## VIGNETTE

A 34-year-old, G2P1001, at 26 weeks' gestation receives a note from her 6-year-old child's school that there has been an outbreak of "fifth disease" reported there. Her child has not been ill, nor has she or her husband. She calls her obstetrician distraught, concerned over the potential impact of parvovirus infection for her pregnancy.

### QUESTION 1

*How does parvovirus B19 produce disease or illness?*

### ANSWER 1

Parvovirus B19 is the only known human pathogenic parvovirus, first discovered in 1974 during evaluations of assays for hepatitis B surface antigen as sample no. 19 in panel B of serum samples. *Parvoviridae* (parvo = small) are among the smallest DNA-containing viruses that infect mammalian cells. The virus cannot be easily grown in a lab setting, and humans are the only known host (though other primates have specific erythro viruses of their own). Outbreaks of infection and illness are more common in late winter through early summer.

Parvovirus B19 has erythroid specificity of attack resulting from the virus' cellular receptor, globoside, also known as blood group P antigen. The P antigen is found on erythroid progenitors, erythroblasts, and megakaryocytes. The virus is cytotoxic for these cells. The antigen is also found on endothelial cells, whose infection may help in transplacental transfer as well as in producing the typical rash of "fifth disease." In normal volunteers, B19 infection leads to an acute, self-limited (4–8 days) decrease in red blood cell production and decline in hemoglobin. In patients with normal erythroid turnover, this limited impact does not produce significant anemia, but in patients with high red blood cell turnover due to hemolysis, blood loss, or other factors, the temporary failure of erythropoiesis can precipitate transient aplastic crisis, seem most commonly in patients with underlying hemoglobinopathies. This medical emergency was actually the first clinical illness reported in humans with B19-related disease, in a 1981 series of six Jamaican immigrants in the United Kingdom with sickle cell anemia.

The clinical impact of parvovirus infection is primarily seen in two forms:

- Erythema infectiosum: an exanthematous rash, classically "slapped-cheeks" rash seen 2–5 days after a nonspecific prodrome period following a 7–10 day incubation period. This can then progress to an erythematous maculopapular rash over the trunk and limbs. Rash is seen much more commonly in children with infection than in adults (Fig. 36-1).
- Arthropathy: arthralgia/arthritis that is usually symmetric—seen more commonly in women, often with significant joint swelling, lasting 1–3 weeks. In the absence of a history of rash, this can often be mistaken in women for rheumatoid arthritis. Seen more commonly in adults, though 1/3 of adult infections are asymptomatic.

### QUESTION 2

*How can maternal parvovirus infection impact on pregnancy?*

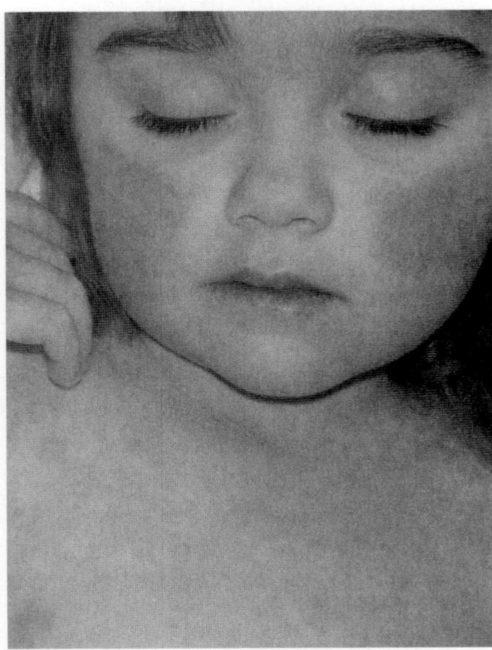

**FIG. 36-1** Typical "slapped-cheek" rash of parvovirus infection.
SOURCE: From U.K. Clinical Virology Network.

## ANSWER 2

Transmission of parvovirus B19 occurs primarily through respiratory secretions/droplet spread and via hand-to-mouth contact. An infected individual is generally infectious 5–10 days after exposure, prior to the onset of rash or symptoms, and is no longer infectious by the time a rash appears.

Seropositivity/existing immunity increases with age, and is approximately 60% in adolescents and adults. The risk of maternal infection in a susceptible woman varies with the level of exposure. The greatest risk is from an infected household member (usually a child), with a 50% risk of seroconversion. The risk of transmission in a child care/classroom setting is lower, ranging from 20–40%.

The risk of fetal morbidity even in the face of documented maternal infection is low, although adverse fetal effects have been described. While transplacental transmission is as high as 33%, rates of fetal loss of 2–9% are based on retrospective series and subject to recall or selection biases. One prospective series followed 52 exposed pregnancies, with confirmation of maternal seroconversion, with none of the pregnancies with loss or ultrasound abnormalities. Some series have attributed up to 18% of cases of nonimmune hydrops to perinatal parvovirus infection. Hydrops may occur as a result of aplastic anemia in the fetus, or from myocarditis or chronic fetal hepatitis resulting from parvovirus infection. Severe effects have been described more commonly when maternal infection occurs from the mid-second trimester to very early third trimester, when there may be more nucleated red blood cells in the fetal circulation proportionally.

## QUESTION 3

*How is parvovirus infection diagnosed, and how is it best managed during pregnancy?*

## ANSWER 3

Parvovirus infection is confirmed serologically through the evolution of positive IgM and IgG antibody fractions. While analysis of fluids such as blood can be performed for parvovirus-specific DNA sequences via polymerase chain reaction (PCR)-based methodologies, the individual is usually no longer viremic by the time a rash appears, triggering suspicion for the infection. Viremia is first present 5–6 days after infection, peaking at 8–9 days. IgM antibody typically appears 10–12 days after infection, with IgG present by 2 weeks. Therefore, acute and convalescent titers (2 weeks apart) can be helpful in an exposed individual without symptoms, though a positive IgM test in a symptomatic adult with an ill child, for example, is also diagnostic.

No treatment is available or recommended for this usually benign and self-limited infection, even in the cases where it may be passed on transplacentally to the fetus, since most infected fetuses clear the infection spontaneously with no long-term sequelae. Overall, with a 33% risk of transplacental transmission, and a maximum 9% risk of fetal impact, there is no more than a 3% risk of significant fetal morbidity in the face of a maternal parvovirus infection during pregnancy. While amniocentesis can and has been used to diagnose fetal infection by detection of parvovirus-specific DNA in amniotic fluid, such invasive testing is neither helpful nor warranted in the absence of fetal ultrasound findings. However, in cases of nonimmune hydrops or with other ultrasound findings suggesting in utero viral infection (e.g., echogenic fetal bowel), amniotic fluid evaluation can help either narrow or exclude a diagnosis of parvovirus infection. Management is otherwise supportive and noninvasive. The maximum window of risk to the fetus after maternal infection appears to be 8–10 weeks. Therefore, most experts recommend a series of fetal ultrasounds and/or nonstress tests during that period, depending on the gestational age. In utero transfusion of infected fetuses with severe anemia resulting in hydrops has been described to surmount the period of acute fetal infection and erythropoietic suppression.

## BIBLIOGRAPHY


ACOG. ACOG Practice Bulletin No. 20. Perinatal viral and parasitic infections. Washington, DC, ACOG, 2000.

Brown KE. Parvovirus B19. In: Mandell GL, Bennett JE, Dolin R (eds.) *Mandell, Douglas, and Bennett's Principles and Practice of Infectious Diseases.* 6th ed. Philadelphia, PA: Elsevier Churchill Livingstone; 2005:1891.

Cartter ML, Farley TA, Rosengren S, et al. Occupational risk factors for infection with parvovirus B19 among pregnant women. *J Infect Dis.* 1991;163:282.

Gillespie SM, Cartter ML, Asch S, et al. Occupational risk of human parvovirus B19 infection for school and day care pesonnel during an outbreak of eryhthema infectiosum. *JAMA.* 1990;281:1099.

Gratacos E, Torres PJ, Vidal J, et al. The incidence of human parvovirus B19 infection during pregnancy and its impact on perinatal outcome. *J Infect Dis.* 1995;171:1360.

Harger JH, Adler SP, Koch WC, Harger GF. Prospective evaluation of 618 pregnant women exposed to parvovirus B19: risks and symptoms. *Obstet Gynecol.* 1998;91:413.

Miller E, Fairley CK, Cohen BJ, Seng C. Immediate and long term outcome of human parvovirus B19 infection in pregnancy. *Br J Obstet Gynecol.* 1998;105:174.

Peters MT, Nicolaides KH. Cordocentesis for the diagnosis and treatment of human fetal parvovirus infection. *Obstet Gynecol.* 1990;75:501.

Rodis JF, Rodner C, Hansen AA, et al. Long-term outcome of children following maternal human parvovirus B19 infection. *Obstet Gynecol.* 1998;91:125.

Torok TJ, Wang QY, Gary GW Jr. Prenatal diagnosis of intrauterine infection with parvovirus B19 by the polymerase chain reaction technique. *Clin Infect Dis.* 1992;14:149.

Yaegashi N, Okamura K, Yajima A, Murai C, Sugamura K. The frequency of human parvovirus B19 infection in nonimmune hydrops fetalis. *J Perinat Med.* 1994;22:159.

# 37 PURIFIED PROTEIN DERIVATIVE TESTING IN PREGNANCY

*Neil S. Silverman*

## LEARNING POINT

To learn diagnostic criteria for tuberculosis, as well as risks and management guidelines during pregnancy.

## VIGNETTE

A 33-year-old nurse presents to her hospital's employee health services for her annual evaluation and screening for communicable diseases. She immigrated to the United States from Panama at age 9, and has been in good health her entire life with so significant medical or surgical problems. She is currently 18 weeks pregnant with her first pregnancy. Her routine tests are all normal, except for a positive purified protein derivative (PPD) at 15-mm induration; her PPD had been negative the previous year. She denies any respiratory symptoms, and her physical examination is normal, including her lung examination. A chest x-ray is performed with abdominal shielding, and shows no evidence of active or old pulmonary disease.

### QUESTION 1

*What are the criteria for a positive PPD, and what risk factors are associated with progression from latent to active disease?*

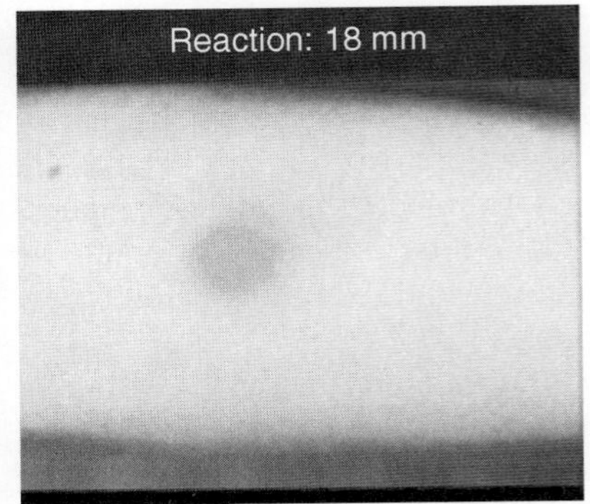


**FIG. 37-1** Positive PPD Result.
SOURCE: From www.vh.org.

### ANSWER 1

A PPD is not contraindicated during pregnancy, since it contains only purified protein, and no actively infectious material. Criteria for a positive test (Fig. 37-1):

1. 5-mm diameter: recent contacts of a person with active tuberculosis (TB), HIV-infected persons, persons with other immunosuppression, persons with chest x-ray findings suggestive of old case of TB
2. 10-mm diameter: recent arrivals from countries where TB rate is high, injection drug users, children <4 years, persons whose medical/social condition puts them at risk for TB exposure or progression, including health-care workers
3. 15-mm diameter: persons with no known risk factors

Infection with HIV is the strongest risk factor known for progression of latent infection with *Mycobacterium tuberculosis* to active disease: 7–10% per year. HIV-infected persons who are newly infected with *M. tuberculosis* have an increased risk of developing active TB disease, often with rapid progression.

### QUESTION 2

*How much of an issue is TB infection among immigrants to the United States, and does previous BCG vaccination impact on TB screening in that population?*

### ANSWER 2

There has been a steady increase in TB cases among foreign-born persons over the past decade (Fig. 37-2). Rates of TB infection are 5–20 times higher in Asia and Latin America than in the United States. The composition of TB cases in the United States reflects those patterns: among immigrants with TB in 1997, 22% were from Mexico, 14% from the Philippines, and 11% from

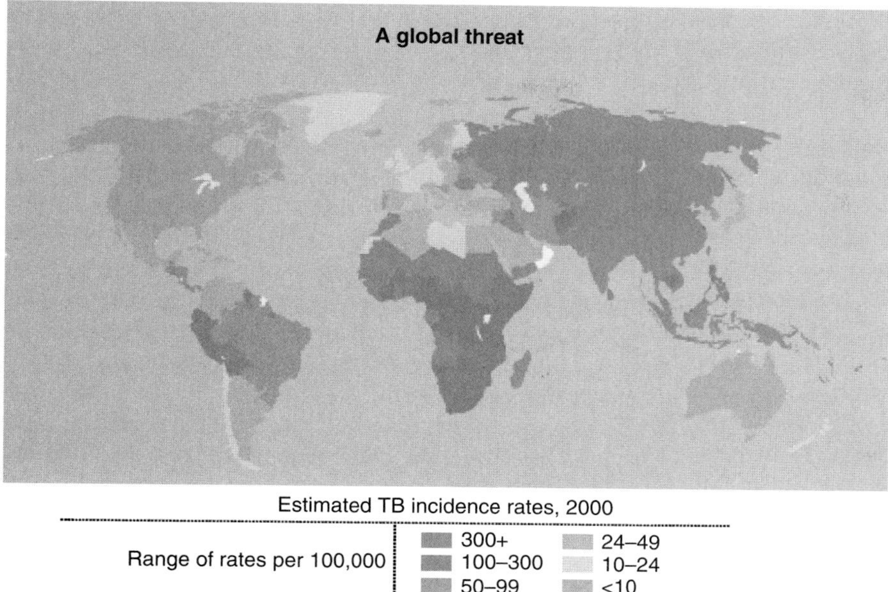


*Source of map*: Global tuberculosis control, WHO report 2000.

**FIG. 37-2** Worldwide prevalence of tuberculosis.
SOURCE: From www.tballiance.org.

Vietnam: 66% of foreign-born persons with TB were reported from California (36% of all national cases, regardless of national origin).

Bacille Caimette Guérin (BCG) vaccine for prevention of TB has been in use since 1921, with >3 billion doses given, though its overall efficacy is still controversial. A meta-analysis in 1994 concluded it was efficacious in reducing the risk of active TB cases and deaths by 50%. This analysis was somewhat limited by the data's ability to predict completely the duration of protection and, in the prospective trials analyzed, to assess specific age groups other than infants.

PPD reactivity caused by BCG vaccination wanes with time and is unlikely to persist >10 years after vaccination in the absence of *M. tuberculosis* exposure and infection. BCG-induced reactivity might be prolonged by giving a PPD/skin test 1 week to 1 year after the initial postvaccine skin test. The presence or size of a post-BCG skin-test reaction does not predict protection. In addition, the size of a skin reaction in a BCG-vaccinated person is not a factor in determining if the reaction is due to TB infection or the previous vaccine. One study showed that a change in the size of a previously noted PPD reaction after a known TB exposure in a vaccinated person was clearly evidence of acute infection, not a vaccine-booster (protective) effect.

PPD testing is *not* contraindicated for individuals previously BCG-vaccinated, with the established size cutoffs staying the same. A diagnosis of active TB should be considered for any BCG-vaccinated person—regardless of skin-test results or HIV status—if they have symptoms suggestive of TB or if they have been recently exposed.

## QUESTION 3

*Should latent TB infection be treated, and can it be treated safely during pregnancy?*

## ANSWER 3

Treatment of latent TB infection is highly effective in preventing active TB infection and progression of disease: efficacy varies with compliance, but ranges 70–90% (98% in a nursing home study). The currently recommended treatment is isoniazid (INH) 300 mg/day for 9 months with 50 mg vitamin B6 daily to prevent peripheral neuropathy. There is no contraindication to its use during pregnancy, and some experts argue that the directly observed period of prenatal care offers an optimal time to initiate INH therapy of latent infection when indicated. The use of an abbreviated regimen of daily rifampin/pyrazinamide (PZA) for 2 months has been investigated for high-risk, low-compliance populations (especially incarcerated HIV-infected individuals), though there is a very high rate of chemical hepatitis with this regimen. Despite earlier concerns, rifampin can be used in pregnancy, though PZA is usually reserved for the treatment of active TB, where multidrug therapy is indicated.

INH hepatitis has been a concern in terms of treatment of latent TB in persons >35 years old. Older studies suggested a risk of hepatotoxicity of 5–20/1000, with a case-fatality a rate of 1–10%. However, those studies included mild liver function test (LFT) elevations in the diagnosis of hepatotoxicity. A 7-year prospective cohort study from a public TB clinic in Seattle studied >11,000 consecutive patients, their definition of hepatotoxicity required: (1) clinical symptoms, (2) LFT elevations five times above normal, and (3) resolution of symptoms after medication was withdrawn. Overall, 11 patients experienced hepatotoxicity, only 1 required hospitalization, and all 11 recovered without sequelae (4 had also been taking acetominophan or other non steroidal anti-inflamatory drugs). The overall rate of hepatotoxicity for those taking preventive therapy was 0.1%, with higher trends among women (8/11) and those >35 years (5/11). They concluded INH prophylaxis could be used more widely in high-risk populations.

## BIBLIOGRAPHY

Centers for Disease Control and Prevention. Recommendations for prevention and control of tuberculosis among foreign-born persons. *Morb Mortal Wkly Rep.* 1998;47:RR-16.

Centers for Disease Control and Prevention. The role of BCG vaccine in the prevention and control of tuberculosis in the US. *Morb Mortal Wkly Rep.* 1996;45:RR-4.

Colditz GA. Efficacy of BCG vaccine in the prevention of tuberculosis. *JAMA* 1994;271:698.

Hamadeh MA, Glassroth J. Tuberculosis and pregnancy. *Chest.* 1992;101:1114.

Horsburgh CR, Feldman S, Ridzon R. Guidelines from the Infectious Diseases Society of America: practice guidelines for the treatment of tuberculosis. *Clin Infect Dis.* 2000;31:633.

Nolan CM. Hepatotoxicity associated with isoniazid preventive therapy. *JAMA.* 1999;281:1014.

Robinson CA, Rose NC. Tuberculosis: current implications and management during pregnancy. *Obstet Gynecol Surv.* 1996;51:115.

# 38 VARICELLA

*Neil S. Silverman*

## LEARNING POINT

To understand the risks of varicella infection during pregnancy for both mother and fetus, along with prevention and treatment guidelines.

## VIGNETTE

A 25-year-old women who recently emigrated from Puerto Rico presents at 25 weeks' gestation with a vesicular rash that erupted asynchronously on her body after an initial period of 36 hours of fever and generalized malaise. The lesions appeared in crops, starting primarily on her trunk and abdomen, with some scattered lesions now on her extremities and face. She is afebrile and denies any respiratory symptoms. Her lungs are clear to auscultation. Some of the lesions have begun to crust over, but some are still vesicular. She lives at home with her boyfriend, who is not ill, and notes that a nephew she cared for 2 weeks ago has developed a rash-like illness.

### QUESTION 1

*What is the natural course of varicella infection?*

### ANSWER 1

Varicella is highly contagious—the attack rate among susceptible contacts is 70–90% after exposure. Humans are the only known reservoir for varicella zoster virus (VZV). Infection is primarily spread through respiratory secretions, with VZV-specific DNA being able to be identified from the nasopharynx of infected individuals. Varicella is primarily a disease of childhood, with 90% of cases occurring in individuals <13 years of age.

The incubation period for the infection is 10–20 days (mean 14 days), with the period of infectivity spanning from 48 hours before the rash appears until all vesicles crust over. Primary infection is defined as chickenpox, characterized by fever, malaise, and a maculopapular pruritic rash that becomes vesicular (Fig. 38-1). After

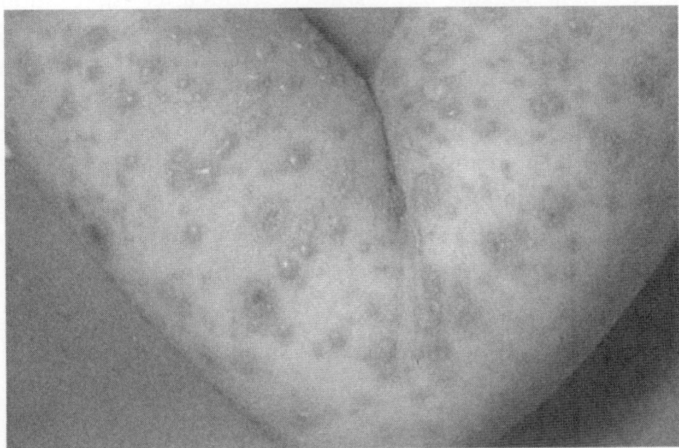

**FIG. 38-1** Varicella rash.
SOURCE: From www.cdphe.state.co.us

primary infection VZV remains dormant in sensory ganglia, like other herpesviruses, and can be reactivated to cause a vesicular erythematous skin rash along a dermatomic distribution, known as herpes zoster. VZV antibody develops within a few days after the onset of infection, and prior VZV infection confers lifelong immunity.

## QUESTION 2

*How common is varicella infection in pregnancy, and how helpful are maternal history and serologic screening in determining risks after exposure?*

## ANSWER 2

Varicella infection is uncommon in pregnancy, occurring in only 0.4–0.7/1000 patients. Approximately 90–95% of reproductive-age women born in North America are VZV-immune, though immunity rates are 80–85% for women born outside the United States, especially in subtropical countries (Central America, Caribbean). Published studies have evaluated the predictive ability of maternal infection status. McGregor et al. serologically tested 37 women with negative or indeterminate histories: 71% of those with negative histories for chickenpox were actually immune, while 90% of those with indeterminate histories were immune. Subsequently, Silverman et al questioned 514 women: 79% gave positive past infection histories, all of whom were varicella immune. Of the 109 women with negative or indeterminate histories, 47% and 94% were serologically immune, respectively. Therefore, when serologic testing is available after a significant exposure of a pregnant woman, testing should be guided by infection history, since at least half of women with no history of infection will be immune. One could also argue for first-trimester serologic testing of all women with *certain* negative histories of chickenpox only. A recent cost-effectiveness study showed that history-targeted screening and postnatal vaccination of nonimmune women could prevent 43% of adult varicella cases, costing $1126 per case prevented, and saving $21.8 million in medical and work-loss costs.

## QUESTION 3

*What concerns are there for mother and fetus in the face of maternal varicella infection?*

## ANSWER 3

In adults, severe complications are more common than in children, particularly pneumonia and encephalitis. Pneumonia is estimated to occur in 1/400 cases of infections in adults, usually occurring 3–5 days into the course of the illness. In a prospective study of male military personnel, x-ray abnormalities were seen in 16% of those with varicella, though only 25% of those had evidence of cough or other clinical symptoms. In pregnant women, morbidity and mortality appear to be higher than among comparable nonpregnant adults. Varicella pneumonia is a risk factor for maternal mortality (Fig. 38-2).

Varicella can be transmitted transplacentally, though the risk of adverse fetal effects appears to be low, no higher than 1–2%, when exposure occurs during the first 20 weeks of pregnancy (probably actually substantially lower due to inherent recall bias in retrospective studies). A congenital varicella syndrome has been described, characterized by skin scarring, chorioretinitis, and microcephaly. While prenatal diagnosis of fetal VZV infection is possible via amniocentesis with VZV-specific-DNA PCR analysis, in the absence of obvious ultrasound findings, such results, if positive, give no information about the severity, if any, of fetal/neonatal disease (unlike cytomegalovirus (CMV), for example, another herpesvirus). Negative results can be reassuring, but positive results don't give much predictive information.

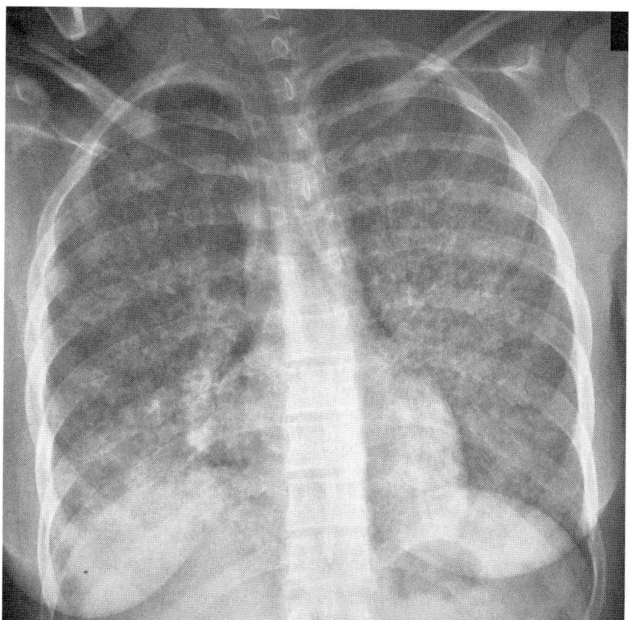

**FIG. 38-2** Varicella pneumonia.
Source: Reproduced with permission from Schwartz DT. *Emergency Radiology: Case Studies.* New York: McGraw-Hill, 2007.

## QUESTION 4

*What treatments are available or recommended to ameliorate maternal or fetal/neonatal illness during pregnancy?*

## ANSWER 4

The American Academy of Pediatrics recommends antiviral treatment for adolescents and adults with primary varicella infection, as well as for other high-risk children. Such treatment ideally is started within 24 hours of onset of illness, and can be: acyclovir 800 mg orally 5 times/day, valacyclovir 1 g orally three times/day or famciclovir 500 mg orally three times/day. Such treatment has been shown to shorten duration of lesion formation, reduce total number of new lesions (by 25%), and diminish constitutional symptoms (in 1/3 of pts). Varicella pneumonia or encephalitis is treated with intravenous acyclovir, with careful inpatient surveillance. Acyclovir has been shown to be safe during pregnancy, even when administered in the first trimester. Valaciclovir is preferable orally: it is the prodrug of acyclovir and 60% more bioavailable than acyclovir. Both valaciclovir and famciclovir appear to be superior to acyclovir for cutaneous healing of varicella lesions. Maternal treatment with these medicationss for maternal illness will have no impact on potential vertical/perinatal transmission.

Perinatally-acquired neonatal varicella is associated with a high death rate when maternal disease develops 5 days before delivery or up to 48 hours postpartum, largely due to both the newborn failing to get protective transplacental antibodies from the mother as well as the immaturity in general of the neonatal immune system. The mortality rate has been reported to be as high as 30%. Varicella zoster immune globulin (VZIG) should be administered to such newborns. VZIG can also be administered to pregnant women known to be seronegative with a significant exposure, but not beyond 72 hours after exposure—this is effective in reducing severity of maternal illness, but does not ameliorate or prevent fetal infection.

## BIBLIOGRAPHY


ACOG. Practice Bulletin No. 20. Perinatal viral and parasitic infections. 2000.

Centers for Disease Control and Prevention. Varicella-related deaths among adults. *Morb Mortal Wkly Rep.* 46:409, 1997.

Centers for Disease Control and Prevention. Varicella-zoster immune globulin for the prevention of chickenpox. *Ann Intern Med.* 1984;100:859.

Enders G, Miller E, Cradock-Watson J, Bolley I, Ridehalgh M. Consequences of varicella and herpes zoster in pregnancy. *Lancet.* 1994;343:1548.

Glantz JC, Mushlin AC. Cost-effectiveness of routine antenatal varicella screening. *Obstet Gynecol.* 1998;91:519.

Kesson AM, Grimwood K, Burgess MA, et al. Acyclovir for the prevention and treatment of varicella zoster in children, adolescents and pregnancy. *J Paediatr Child Health.* 1996;32:211.

McGregor JA, Mark S, Crawford GP, Levin MJ. Varicella zoster antibody testing in the care of pregnanct women exposed to varicella. *Am J Obstet Gynecol.* 1987;87:281.

Ogilvie MM. Antiviral prophylaxis and treatment in chickenpox. A review prepared for the UK Advisory Group on Chickenpox on behalf of the British Society for the Study of Infection. *J Infect.* 1998;36 (suppl. 1):31.

Preblud SR, Orenstein WA, Bart KJ. Varicella: clinical manifestations, epidemiology and health impact. *Pediatr Infect Dis.* 1984;3:505.

Silverman NS, Ewing SH, Todi N, Montgomery O. Maternal varicella history as a predictor of varicella immune status. *J Perinatol.* 1995;27:35.

Smith WJ. Prevention of chickenpox in reproductive-age women. *Obstet Gynecol.* 1998;92:535.

Wallace MR, Bowler WA, Murray NB, Brodine SK, Oldfield EC. 3rd. Treatment of adult varicella with oral acyclovir: a randomized placebo-controlled trial. *Ann Intern Med.* 1992;117:358.


# 39 HEPATITIS B

*Neil S. Silverman*

## LEARNING POINT

To understand risk factors for hepatitis B infection, as well as sequelae of infection both during and outside of pregnancy.

## VIGNETTE

A 28-year-old, G1P0, is seen for initiation of prenatal care for her first pregnancy. She states that she is in excellent health, has no significant chronic complaints, and has a family history significant for a grandmother who died of liver disease. She was born in Taiwan and emigrated to the United States at age 7. Her physical examination is unremarkable. Her prenatal labs are significant for a positive hepatitis B surface antigen (HBsAg) result. On followup visit, additional tests are ordered.

Followup lab results: Aspartate amino transaminase (AST) 18 IU/l (normal <30), alanine amino transferae (ALT) 14 IU/l (normal <30), hepatitis B surface antibody (HBsAb) (–), hepatitis B core antibody (HbcA) (+), hepatitis B core protein antigen (HbeAg) (+), hepatitis B virus antibody (HCV Ab) (–). Her result had been negative.

## QUESTION 1

*What risk factors are associated with hepatitis B virus (HBV) infection, and what are the long-term sequelae of infection?*

## ANSWER 1

Hepatitis B infection is a global public health concern (Fig. 39-1). In the United States, it is responsible for 40–45% of all cases of hepatitis. While the rate of new infections has declined in the United States since 1987 by half, the result of vaccine availability and utilization, over 1 million Americans are chronic HBV carriers. HBV is transmitted by both parenteral (primarily but not exclusively blood-borne) and sexual contact. Vertical transmission from a chronic carrier mother to her newborn is a particularly efficient method and, globally, represents a major reservoir for the perpetuation of the chronic carrier state in endemic populations.

Major risk factors include: (1) Asian, Pacific Islander, or Eskimo descent (immigrant or native), (2) history of acute or chronic liver disease, (3) rejection a blood donor, (4) staff or patient in a dialysis unit, (5) occupational exposure in a medical or dental setting, (6) staff or patient in an institution for the mentally disabled, (7) repeated blood transfusions, (8) household contact with an HBV carrier or dialysis patient, (9) multiple sexually transmitted diseases, (10) tattoos, (11) history of injection or inhalation drug use. Approximately 25% of the regular sexual contacts of infected individuals will themselves become seropositive. Except for individuals whose only risk factor for HBV infection is family ethnicity (usually perinatal transmission), HBV-infected adults are also at risk for and should be tested for HCV and HIV infection.

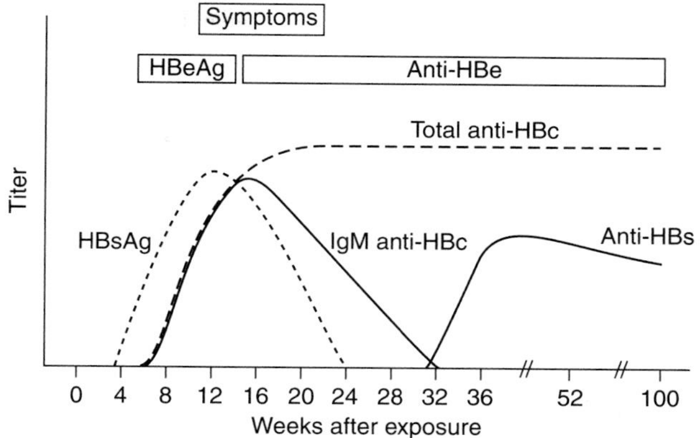


**FIG. 39-2** Serologic picture of acute, resolved Hepatitis B infection.
SOURCE: From Virology Online. http://virology-online.com

Overall mortality associated with HBV infection is 1%. Of those with acute infection (90–95% asymptomatic), 90–95% will clear the infection completely and develop protective neutralizing antibodies (HBsAb), and completely clear the surface antigen, HBsAg. HBsAb and HBsAg for all practical purposes do not exist together serologically (Fig. 39-2). The other 5–10% of patients

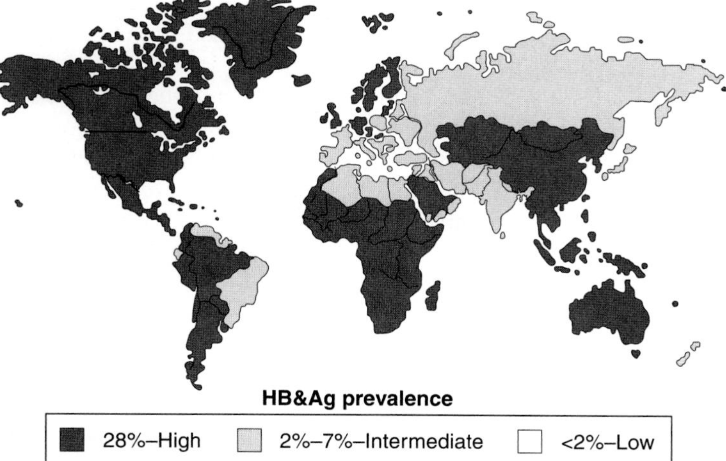


**FIG. 39-1** Global view of HBV endemicity.
SOURCE: From Virology Online. http://virology-online.com

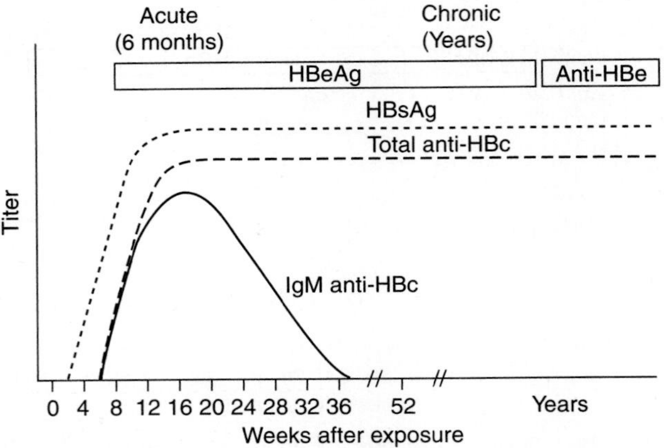


**FIG. 39-3** Serologic picture of chronic Hepatitis B infection. SOURCE: From Virology Online. http://virology-online.com

become chronically infected (chronic carriers) though are still asymptomatic and have normal liver functions tests, but have a lifetime risk of severe liver disease (Fig. 39-3). Twenty five percent will develop chronic active hepatitis, which frequently progresses to cirrhosis. HBV carriers' risk of developing liver cancer is 50–100 times higher than those without HBV infection.

## QUESTION 2

*What pregnancy risks need to be addressed in the face of maternal HBV infection?*

## ANSWER 2

While maternal health will almost certainly not be impacted by her HBV status during the time of her pregnancy, there are significant risks to her newborn if appropriate postdelivery measures are not implemented. Overall, 10–20% of women who are seropositive for HBsAg transmit the virus to their newborns in the absence of appropriate postnatal immunoprophylaxis. If a woman is also seropositive for the e antigen, HBeAg, which is associated with the viral core and represents a state of high viremia and infectivity, the risk of transmission increases to 90%, with 70–90% of those newborns ultimately, becoming chronic carriers.

Between 85–95% of perinatal transmission cases occur as a consequence of intrapartum exposure of the newborn to contaminated blood and secretions. Therefore, knowledge of a woman's serologic HBV status is critical prior to delivery. Testing for HBsAg is now a mandated component of routine prenatal screening (ideally at a woman's initial first trimester presenting visit, but always whenever she first presents for care during a pregnancy). Infants of women who are HBsAg-positive at the time of delivery should receive combined immunoprophylaxis with hepatitis B immune globulin (HBIG) and the first in the series of hepatitis B vaccinations. Both vaccine and HBIG are of no use once an individual is infected. HBIG was the first preventive agent available but offers only transient passive immunity: it prevents vertical transmission as a single agent in 70–75% of cases. The combination of HBIG and HBV vaccine (given within 12 hours of birth, and can be given concomitantly) confers 95% protection against vertical HBV transmission to newborns born to chronic carrier mothers.

## QUESTION 3

*What have been the impacts of prenatal HBV screening and neonatal prophylaxis?*

## ANSWER 3

HBV screening during pregnancy offers an opportunity to offer screening and treatment to other household members. If they are uninfected serologically, then they should be offered HBIG acutely and start their vaccination series. The vaccine series confers 95–97% rates of protection, and, as the first recombinant vaccine developed, has no risks of blood-borne contamination even theoretically possible.

There is clearly a link between chronic HBV infection and both cirrhosis and hepatocellular carcinoma (HCC). In countries where HBV infection has been endemic, implementation of newborn and childhood vaccination programs have decreased both the rate of HBsAg-positivity among children <5 years old (from 10% to 2%) and significantly lowered the rate of childhood HCC. As these children become older, it would be expected that the overall rates of adult complications of chronic HBV infection will also decrease significantly in these endemic areas.

## BIBLIOGRAPHY

Beasley RP, Wang LY, Lee GC, et al. Prevention of perinatally transmitted hepatitis B virus infections with hepatitis B immune globulin and hepatitis B vaccine. *Lancet.* 1983;2:1099.

Centers for Disease Control and Prevention. Hepatitis B virus: a comprehensive strategy for eliminating transmission in the United states through universal childhood vaccination: recommendations of the Immunization Practices Advisory Committee. *Morb Mortal Wkly Rep.* 1991;40 (rr-13):1.

Centers for Disease Control and Prevention. Prevention of perinatal transmission of hepatitis B virus: prenatal screening for all pregnant women for hepatitis B surface antigen. *Morb Mortal Wkly Rep.* 1988;37:341.

Chang MH, et al. Universal hepatitis B vaccination in Taiwan and the incidence of hepatocellular carcinoma in children. *N Engl J Med.* 1997;336:1855.

Hoofnagle JH. Chronic hepatitis B. *N Engl J Med.* 1990;323:337.

Immunization Practices Advisory Committee (ACIP). Protection against viral hepatitis. *Morb Mortal Wkly Rep.* 1990;39 (RR-2):1.

Koziel MJ, Siddiqui A. Hepatitis B virus and hepatitis delta virus, in Mandell GL, Bennett JE, Dolin R (eds.). *Mandell, Douglas, and Bennett's Principles and Practice of Infectious Diseases*, 6th ed. Philadelphia, PA: Elsevier Churchill Livingstone; 2005: 1864.

Lee CL, et al. Hepatitis B vaccination and hepatocellular carcinoma in Taiwan. *Pediatrics.* 1997;99:351.

Silverman NS, Darby MJ, Ronkin SL, Wapner RJ. Hepatitis B prevalence in an unregistered prenatal population: new implications for neonatal therapy. *JAMA.* 1991;268:2852.

# MEDICAL/SURGICAL CONDITIONS ASSOCIATED WITH PREGNANCY

## 40 CHRONIC HYPERTENSION

*Jasvant Adusumalli*

### LEARNING POINT

Evaluation and treatment of chronic hypertension in pregnancy.

### VIGNETTE

A 33-year-old female, G1P0, at 8 weeks gestation, presents to the office for her initial obstetrical visit. She expresses concern because of her history of hypertension. The patient states she had intentionally discontinued her antihypertensive medication approximately 1 month prior to conception, as her family physician had recommended cessation of medication prior to attempting pregnancy. Prior to that time, she had been on antihypertensive medication for approximately 3 years. She underwent a laparoscopic cholecystectomy 2 years ago and currently takes only prenatal vitamins. She denies smoking, alcohol, or drug use, and her family history is significant for hypertension in both parents. Currently, she denies any other complaints with the exception of occasional headaches, which are relieved with acetaminophen. Her vital signs are:

Temperature: 98.6°F
Blood Pressure: 134/82 mm Hg
Pulse: 77 bpm
Respiratory rate: 18 min

### QUESTION 1

*What are the diagnostic criteria for chronic hypertension in pregnancy?*

### ANSWER 1

Approximately 5% of pregnant women are diagnosed with chronic hypertension, which is defined as hypertension present before the 20th week of pregnancy or hypertension present before pregnancy. Specific criteria for the diagnosis of chronic hypertension in pregnancy are as follows. Chronic hypertension in pregnancy can be divided into:

1. Mild hypertension: Systolic blood pressure >140 mm Hg and diastolic blood pressure >90 mm Hg, or
2. Severe hypertension: Systolic blood pressure >180 mm Hg and diastolic blood pressure >110 mm Hg
3. Use of antihypertensive medications before pregnancy, or
4. Onset of hypertension before 20th week of gestation, or Persistence of hypertension beyond the usual postpartum period

## QUESTION 2

*Describe the initial testing involved in chronic hypertension and the maternal and fetal risks associated with chronic hypertension.*

## ANSWER 2

Known risks of hypertensive disease include heart failure, encephalopathy, renal disease, retinopathy, and ischemic heart disease. These risks are independent of pregnancy and consequently monitoring for end-organ involvement should be performed at the initial obstetric visit. A serum creatinine and blood urea nitrogen, hemoglobin, hematocrit, and a 24-hour urine collection for protein and creatinine clearance are useful initial laboratory tests. An opthalmological examination, electrocardiogram, and possibly an echocardiogram, may also be warranted at the initial evaluation to assess the degree of preexisting morbidity.

Chronic hypertension has been associated with an increased risk of the following, depending on whether the patient has mild or severe chronic hypertension:

- Superimposed preeclampsia: 10–25% risk (mild); 50% risk (severe)
- Placental abruption: 0.7–1.5% risk (mild); 5–10% risk (severe)
- Preterm birth <37 weeks: 12–34% risk (mild); 62–70% risk (severe)
- Fetal growth restriction: 8–16% risk (mild); 31–40% risk (severe)

## QUESTION 3

*What type of antepartum assessment and fetal surveillance is recommended in this patient?*

## ANSWER 3

As noted above, pregnancies complicated by chronic hypertension are at greater risk for developing preeclampsia, placental abruption, preterm birth, and growth restriction. The goals of the antepartum assessment should include early detection of preeclampsia and fetal growth restriction. Methods employed in detecting the early development of preeclampsia include more frequent assessments of maternal blood pressure and proteinuria. Evaluation of fetal growth may be performed by the serial measurement of fundal height and sonographic estimation of fetal size. However, currently there is no consensus as to what specific tests should be utilized in the surveillance of pregnancy in patients with chronic hypertension. In addition, there is no consensus on the appropriate timing of the surveillance. Current recommendations include a baseline ultrasound at 16 to 20 weeks gestation and serial ultrasounds every 4 weeks beginning at 28–32 to assess fetal growth. Nonstress testing and a biophysical profile are recommenced when there is suspicion of superimposed preeclampsia or superimposed preeclampsia, biophysical profile, and nonstress testing is controversial.

## QUESTION 4

*What are the therapeutic goals in pregnancies complicated by chronic hypertension and what antihypertensive medications may be utilized?*

## ANSWER 4

In women without end-organ damage, the systolic blood pressure may be maintained as high as 140–150 mm Hg and the diastolic blood pressure may be maintained as high as 90–100 mm Hg. However, in women with evidence of end-organ damage, the blood pressure should be kept lower than 140/90. Treatment of women with uncomplicated mild chronic hypertension has not been shown to improve perinatal outcomes.

There are many antihypertensive medications available, which have all been shown to be effective and safe in pregnancy, including labetalol, nifedipine, hydralazine, and methyldopa. Atenolol has been associated with fetal growth restriction and should not be used in pregnancy. Angiotensin-converting enzyme (ACE) inhibitors and angiotensin receptor antagonists have been associated with fetal and neonatal failure and death and should be discontinued in pregnancy. Thiazide diuretics may be continued, unless there is evidence of uteroplacental compromise. Studies have shown no adverse effects on perinatal outcome when diuretics were taken in pregnancy.

## BIBLIOGRAPHY

ACOG Practice Bulletin No. 29. Chronic Hypertension in Pregnancy. 2001.

Agency for Healthcare Research and Quality. Management of chronic hypertension during pregnancy. Evidence Report/Technology Assessment no. 14. AHRQ Publication No. 00-E011.200.

AHRO Publication No. 00-E011. Rockville, MD: AHRO, 2000.

Anonymous Report of the National High Blood Pressure Education Program Working Group on High Blood Pressure in Pregnancy. *Am J Obstet Gynecol.* 2000;183:S1–S22.

Anonymous the sixth report of the Joint National Committee in prevention, detection, evaluation, and treatment of high blood pressure. *Arch Intern Med.* 1997;157:2413–2446.

Collins R, Yusuf S, Peto R. Overview of randomized trials of diuretics in pregnancy. *Br Med J(Clin Res Ed).* 1985; 290:17.

Ferrer RL, Sibai BM, Mulrow CD, et al. Management of mild chronic hypertension during pregnancy: a review. *Obstet Gynecol.* 2000;96:849–860.

Haddad B, Sibai BM, Chronic hypertension in pregnancy. *Ann Med.* 1999;31: 246–252.

Lydakis C, Lip GY, Beevers M, et al. Atenolol and growth in pregnancies complicated by hypertension. *Am J Hypertens.* 1999;12:541.

Sibai BM. Chronic hypertension in pregnancy. *Obstet Gynecol.* 2002;100:369.

# 41 THYROID DISEASE IN PREGNANCY: HYPERTHYROIDISM

*Marguerite Lisa Bartholomew*

## LEARNING POINT

For optimum pregnancy outcomes, recognition and treatment of hyperthyroid disease is essential.

## VIGNETTE

A 37-year-old, G2P1001, is admitted for severe hyperemesis gravidarum (TH-HEG). Her last period is unknown, and she reports that her menstrual periods are irregular. An ultrasound indicates a singleton intrauterine pregnancy measuring 8 weeks by crown rump length. During her hospital stay, thyroid function tests are drawn with the following results: thyroid-stimulating hormone (TSH) 0.05 μU/mL (normal 1–5.0 μU/mL) and free thyroxine ($T_4$) of 4.0 ng/mL (normal 0.8–2.8 ng/dL). She denies history of goiter, hair loss, and heat intolerance. She lost 10 lbs in the past 4 months and reports occasional anxiety.

Vital signs indicate a blood pressure of 130/70 mm Hg, heart rate of 100 bpm, respiratory rate of 14/min, and temperature of 98.8°F. The physical examination is unremarkable except for a mildly enlarged thyroid without nodules. She is hospitalized three more times for hyperemesis over the ensuing month. The thyroid function tests are repeated 4 weeks after the first set, and the results indicate no significant change, although thyroid-stimulating antibodies are positive. She is diagnosed with hyperthyroidism, with probable Graves' disease. Propylthiouracil (PTU) 100 mg orally three times/day is prescribed. Four weeks later, the TSH is 0.1 μU/mL and the free $T_4$ is 2.5 ng/mL. At 36 weeks gestation, she develops preeclampsia, and labor is induced; she delivers a healthy male infant.

## QUESTION 1

*How do you distinguish between Graves' disease and transient hyperthyroidism of TH-HEG?*

## ANSWER 1

It is difficult to distinguish between Graves' disease and TH-HEG. Moreover, many symptoms of thyroid disease (hyper or hypo) are subtle and are often assumed to be a normal part of pregnancy or neurosis. Certain symptoms of hyperthyroidism (nausea, vomiting, weight loss, tachycardia, tremor, anxiety, and the like) are common to both TH-HEG and Graves' disease.

Diaphoresis, persistent tachycardia unresponsive to hydration, proximal muscle wasting, and severe symptoms are not usually seen in TH-HEG. Symptoms that antedate the pregnancy, goiter, exophthalmos, and TSH receptor antibodies are pathognomonic for Graves' disease and are not seen in TH-HEG. TH-HEG is usually self-limiting, resolving between 14 and 20 weeks gestation and does not require antithyroid medication.

The best way to distinguish between the two is to perform a careful history and physical examination, following serial thyroid function tests, and determining the titers of antithyroid and TSH receptor antibodies. If there is no goiter or exophthalmos, and the symptoms and thyroid function tests spontaneously improve or normalize prior to 20 weeks gestation, Graves' disease is essentially excluded. In both entities, a suppressed TSH lags for a few weeks after normalization of the free $T_4$ levels, whether following spontaneous thyroid hormone normalization (TH-HEG) or normalization after antithyroid treatment (Graves' disease).

## QUESTION 2

*What are the goals for the treatment of hyperthyroidism (Graves' disease) during pregnancy?*

## ANSWER 2

Hyperthyroidism occurs in 1–2/1000 pregnant women, 95% being the result of Graves' disease. Control of hyperthyroidism with medication has been shown to improve perinatal outcomes and is strongly recommended. During pregnancy, the most accurate thyroid function tests are TSH, free $T_4$, and free triiodothyroxine ($T_3$) because they are not affected by changes in thyroglobulin-binding globulin (TBG).

There are two choices for the treatment of Graves' disease, PTU or methimazole. Methimazole is usually reserved only for those patients who will not take PTU because of concern regarding the rare chance of aplasia cutis in some exposed infants. Both drugs are equally effective in controlling thyroid hormone levels and symptoms. Both inhibit $T_4$ formation by thyroid peroxidase-catalyzed iodination of thyroglobulin. PTU has the added benefit of blocking the peripheral conversion of $T_4$ to $T_3$ and is generally less expensive than methimazole. The initial recommended dose of PTU is 100 mg orally three times/day and that of methimazole is 10 mg orally twice/day.

Treatment during pregnancy is designed to balance treatment of the mother with the risk of iatrogenic hypothyroidism and goiter in the fetus, and, as such, the lowest effective dose should be used. With proper monitoring, the risk of fetal hypothyroidism is rare and usually resolves after birth. Thyroid function tests should be checked every 2–4 weeks, and the dose of medication is titrated to keep the free $T_4$ level at the upper limit of the normal range (0.8–2.8 ng/dL). Changes in free $T_4$ will be apparent 2 weeks after a medication change, however, changes in TSH will not be apparent for at least 1 month after medication adjustment and may never normalize during treatment. If the TSH level does normalize, the dose of antithyroid medication should be reduced. Free $T_3$ levels can be followed, but add little clinical benefit once the free $T_4$ level is found to be elevated. If the TSH is suppressed and the free $T_4$ is normal, a free $T_3$ should be obtained to rule out $T_3$ toxicosis syndrome, which may indicate an active thyroid nodule.

Antithyroid medication needs commonly drop in the second and third trimester, and the dose should be adjusted accordingly. Many women with mild disease may be weaned off medications completely prior to delivery, but this is not recommended before 32 weeks due to the high relapse rate. Careful postpartum surveillance is necessary because it is not uncommon for Graves' disease patients to relapse after delivery. Both PTU and methimazole are excreted into breast milk (PTU less than methimazole), but pose little to no risk to the infant. Consequently, the American Academy of Pediatrics considers both drugs compatible with breast-feeding.

Betablockers are rarely needed, but can be used to quell symptoms for the first few weeks in symptomatic patients and are indicated during thyroid storm. Iodine 131 therapy is contraindicated in pregnancy after 10 weeks because it concentrates in the fetal thyroid causing hypothyroidism. Subtotal thyroidectomy is reserved for cases refractory or intolerant to medical therapy.

## QUESTION 3

*What are the complications of untreated or suboptimally treated hyperthyroidism during pregnancy?*

## ANSWER 3

Pregnancy complicated by poorly controlled hyperthyroidism is associated with increased rates of spontaneous abortion, preterm labor, low birth weight, stillbirth, preeclampsia, and maternal heart failure. Thyroid storm crisis occurs in 2% of women who are treated during pregnancy. The risk appears higher in untreated women particularly in association with emergency cesarean delivery and/or infection. In one series, two of seven untreated thyrotoxic women in labor developed thyroid crisis. Pregnant women with uncontrolled hyperthyroidism should undergo antenatal testing. Maintenance of a euthyroid state is protective against the development of thyroid storm.

Fetal hyperthyroidism may occur in women with thyroid-stimulating antibodies, which may cross the placenta and activate the fetal thyroid gland. Antibody levels are independent of the type of maternal treatment, including ablation therapy. Fetal hyperthyroidism occurs in 1–5% of neonates born to women with Graves' disease. The condition usually presents after 24 weeks when fetal antibody levels become significant. Antibody titers are recommended at 28–30 weeks. Levels in excess of three to four times control values are predictive of fetal hyperthyroidism. The effects of the antibodies are mitigated by the maternal use of antithyroid medications.

Symptoms of fetal hyperthyroidism include crainiosynostosis, fetal goiter (extended neck), fetal tachycardia, intrauterine growth restriction, and oligohydramnios. Fetal thyrotoxicosis can be treated with maternal administration of antithyroid medications. The fetal response can be followed clinically or with cordocentesis for determination of fetal TSH levels.

The presentation of Graves' disease in the neonate may be delayed because the stimulating antibodies last longer in the circulation than the antithyroid medications. Transient hypothyroidism may also occur because of antithyroid therapy and/or the concomitant presence of inhibitory antibodies. Pediatricians should be informed regarding the presence of thyroid disease in the mother, the extent of treatment, and the presence or absence of antithyroid autoantibodies.

## QUESTION 4

*Discuss the diagnosis and treatment of thyroid storm during pregnancy.*

## ANSWER 4

Thyroid storm is characterized by an abrupt and severe exacerbation of thyrotoxicosis. The typical findings of thyroid storm are:

1. Fever (temperature >100°F)
2. Maternal palpitations (tachycardia; tachyarrhythmia), fetal tachycardia
3. Hypertension
4. Mental status changes (anxiety, agitation, psychosis)
5. Diaphoresis
6. Weakness, muscle wasting
7. Diarrhea, nausea, vomiting
8. Congestive heart failure
9. Goiter
10. Exophthalmos, lid lag
11. Increased $T_4$ and decreased TSH levels

The goals of therapy are to control the hyperthyroid state by blocking the release of $T_4$ and the peripheral conversion of $T_4$ to $T_3$ and to prevent congestive heart failure. Treatment consists of thionamides, iodide, and beta blockers. Congestive heart failure in the setting of thyroid storm is rapidly reversible when treated with PTU, iodide, and the diuretic furosemide. Initial tests should include free $T_4$, TSH, CBC, electrolytes, liver function tests, glucose, ECG chest x-ray, and urinalysis and culture (see Fig. 41-1). Specific steps are as follows:

*Step 1:* Assess need for intensive care. Provide supportive therapy with intravenous access and hydration, oxygen, and nasogastric tube if patient is unable to swallow. If the fetus is viable, institute fetal monitoring. Do not intervene for fetal indications until the mother is stabilized, as the fetal condition will likely improve.

*Step 2:* Stop peripheral conversion of $T_4$ to $T_3$. Although production of $T_4$ is inhibited by PTU, this is not the immediate goal. Use:

- PTU 1 g by mouth or nasogastric tube followed by 300 mg every 8 hours.
- Hydrocortisone 100 mg IV every 8 hours or Dexamethasone 8 mg orally once per day.

*Step 3:* Inhibit thyroid hormone release from the gland.

- One hour after PTU is started, administer oral Lugols' solution (20–30 drops in a 24-hour period) or sodium iodide (0.5g/12 h) intravenously (IV).

*Step 4:* Control autonomic symptoms using:

- Propranolol 1 mg IV over 5 minutes (may give simultaneously with PTU if needed); titrate to maintain heart rate ≤90 bpm.

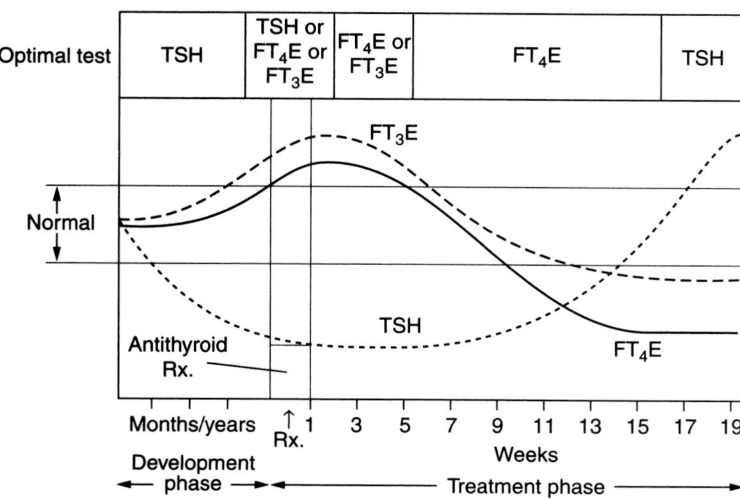


**FIG. 41-1** Optimal tests for hyperthyriodism.

- Cooling blanket and/or acetaminophen to reduce body temperature. However, avoid salicylates because they can displace $T_4$ and $T_3$ from TBG, worsening symptoms.

*Step 5:* Search for sequelae, including:

- Congestive heart failure (consider pulmonary artery catheterization if present)
- Thromboembolism (particularly of the CNS)
- Cardiac arrhythmia

*Step 6:* Identify the inciting factor(s). This is most often an infection (e.g., pyelonephritis). Less common precipitants include preeclampsia, anemia, myocardial infarction, diabetic ketoacidosis (if diabetic), pulmonary embolism, induction of anesthesia, acute surgical emergency, and the onset of labor and delivery.

Iodides and corticosteroids can be discontinued with clinical improvement. PTU should be continued and titrated according to needs. For refractory cases, plasmapheresis and/or subtotal thyroidectomy may be considered.

## BIBLIOGRAPHY

ACOG Practice Bulletin No. 37. Clinical Management Guidelines of Obstetrician-Gynecologists. Thyroid Disease in Pregnancy. 2002.

American Academy of Pediatrics Committee on Drugs. The transfer of drugs and other chemicals into human milk. *Pediatrics*. 2001;108:776.

Bouillon R, Maesens M, Van Assche A, et al. Thyroid function in patients with hyperemesis gravidarum. *Am J Obstet Gynecol*. 1982;143:922.

Clavel S, Madec AM, Bornet H, et al. Anti TSH-receptor antibodies in pregnant patient with autoimmune thyroid disorder. *Br J Obstet Gynecol*. 1990;97:1003.

Davis LE, Lucas MJ, Hankins GDV, et al. Thyrotoxicosis complicating pregnancy. *Am J Obstet Gynecol*. 1988;72:108.

Goodwin TM, Hershman JM. Hyperthyroidism due to inappropriate production of human chorionic gonadotropin. *Clin Obstet Gynecol*. 1997;40:32.

Lowell DE. Thyroid and parathyroid emergencies. In Clark SL, Cotton DD, Hankins GD, Phelan JP (eds.). *Critical Care Obstetrics*, 3rd ed. Malden, MA: Blackwell Science. 1997:540.

Mestman JH. Endocrine diseases in pregnancy In: Gabbe SG, Niebyl JR, Simpson JL (eds.). *Obstetrics: Normal and Problem Pregnancies.* 4th ed. Philadelphia, PA: Churchill Livingstone; 2002:1141–1150.

Pekonen F, Lamberg BA, Ikonen E. Thyrotoxicosis and pregnancy: an analysis of 43 pregnancies in 42 thyrotoxic mothers. *Ann Chir Gynaecol*. 1978;67:1.

Perelman AH. Management of hyperthyroidism and thyroid storm during pregnancy. In: Foley MR, Strong TH (eds.). *Obstetric Intensive Care: A Practical Manual.* Philadelphia, PA: WB, Saunders; 1997:147.

Wing DA, Millar LK, Koonings PP. A comparison of propylthiouracil versus methimazole in the treatment of hyperthyroidism in pregnancy. *Am J Obstet Gynecol*. 1994; 170:90.

# 42 OVARIAN MASSES IN PREGNANCY

*Marguerite Lisa Bartholomew*

## LEARNING POINT

Perinatal outcome for pregnant women with ovarian/adnexal masses includes accurate ultrasound assessment and judicious use of surgery.

## VIGNETTE

A 40-year-old, G2P1001, at 12 weeks gestation, arrives in the emergency room with acute onset of right-sided abdominal pain associated with nausea and vomiting. Upon questioning, she reports that an ovarian cyst was seen during the ultrasound performed the week prior during chorionic villus sampling. She reports carrying a twin pregnancy conceived with in vitro fertilization. Vital signs indicate a blood pressure of 130/80 mm Hg heart rate 100 bpm, respiratory rate 14/min and temperature 98.6°F. The abdominal examination indicates involuntary guarding and tenderness in the lower right abdomen. Pelvic ultrasound indicates a diamniotic dichorionic twin gestation with normal cardiac activity. The right adnexa contains a complex mass measuring 6 cm in maximum diameter; color doppler flow is seen within the mass. The white blood cell count is 10,000 cells/mL, and the hematocrit is 35%. She undergoes a laparoscopy with the findings of a bluish mass comprising the right ovary with obvious torsion. Once untwisted, the normal color returns to the ovary, and a cystectomy is performed without spillage. The final pathology is a mature teratoma with vascular congestion and edema.

### QUESTION 1

*What is the incidence of adnexal masses in pregnancy? What is the most common pathological diagnosis found in adnexal masses removed during pregnancy? How often does torsion occur?*

### ANSWER 1

The incidence of adnexal masses in pregnancy has been estimated to be 1/200 pregnancies, and 1/3000 pregnancies have masses that require exploration. In a study published in 2003 by Sherard and colleagues, 60 masses were found over a 12-year period, equivalent to 15% of pregnancies. The mean time of diagnosis was 12 weeks gestation with mean surgery time of 20 weeks gestation. The average size was 115 mm for malignant masses and 76 mm for benign masses. The pathological diagnoses were as follows: 50% were mature teratomas, 20% were cystadenomas, 13% were functional cysts, and 13% were malignant (63% of these were low malignant potential).

A similar study was published in 2000 by Usui and colleagues from Japan. Over a 17-year period of time, 69 masses were reported. Of these, 47% were mature teratomas, 18% were functional cysts, 12% were mucinous cystadenomas, 9.0% were endometriomas, 6.0% were paraovarian cysts, 4.3% were serous cystadenomas, and 2.8% were malignant. The mean gestational age at surgery was 13 weeks.

Based on retrospective data, the most frequent complication of a benign ovarian cyst during pregnancy is torsion. In a review by Whitecar and colleagues, this complication occurred in 5% of 130 adnexal masses and in 40% of 16 patients with acute pain and peritoneal signs. Several investigators advocate elective exploration and cystectomy in the second trimester for persistent masses greater than 5–6 cm, in order to avoid torsion and undetected malignancy. Others recommend a more conservative approach based on ultrasound findings, with intervention and resection during pregnancy reserved for persistent simple masses greater than 10 cm, persistent complex masses (septae, solid parts, and or papillary projections), or those clinically suspected of torsion.

The diagnosis of ovarian torsion during pregnancy is challenging and remains a clinical assessment. The presence of arterial or venous flow during ultrasound has not been shown to be a reliable method to exclude torsion. Torsion appears to be uncommon after the first trimester, as the mass is usually held in place between the abdominal wall and the growing uterus in the later trimesters. Consequently, the majority of the published reports of ovarian torsion during pregnancy are in the first trimester.

## QUESTION 2

*What are the general ultrasound criteria that distinguish a benign versus a malignant adnexal mass?*

## ANSWER 2

Most importantly, the ultrasound assists in distinguishing an ovarian from an extraovarian mass (i.e., ectopic pregnancy, pedunculated myoma, hydrosalpinx, paraovarian cyst, diverticular abcess, appendiceal abcess, fallopian tube cancer, and the like).

The overall accuracy of the ultrasound diagnosis is good. Reports combining grey scale with doppler have accurately distinguished between a benign and malignant ovarian neoplasm in over 90% of cases. In a retrospective series by Bromley and Benacerraf, ultrasound correctly characterized the type of benign lesion 95% of the time for dermoids, 80% of the time for endometriomas, and 71% of the time for simple cysts (Figs. 42-1 and 42-2). There was one malignancy among the 125 cases which was also correctly diagnosed.

The following ultrasound characteristics distinguish benign from malignant masses:

### Malignant

- Larger than 50 mm
- Complex/solid
- Solid component that is not echogenic
- Thick septations (3 mm or more)
- Nodular or papillary projections
- Color doppler flow in solid component
- Resistive index (RI) on Doppler ultrasonography <0.4 (not diagnostic)
- Ascites

### Benign

- Less than 50 mm
- Simple
- Thin septations
- Solid component very echogenic with shadowing (teratoma)
- (RI)>0.4 (not diagnostic, corpus lutea may have low-resistance doppler indices)

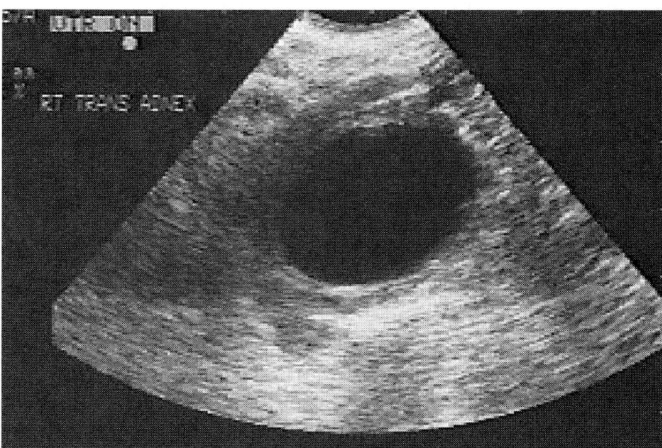


**FIG. 42-1** Ultrasound of simple ovarian cyst.
SOURCE: Image courtesy of Andrew Li, MD.

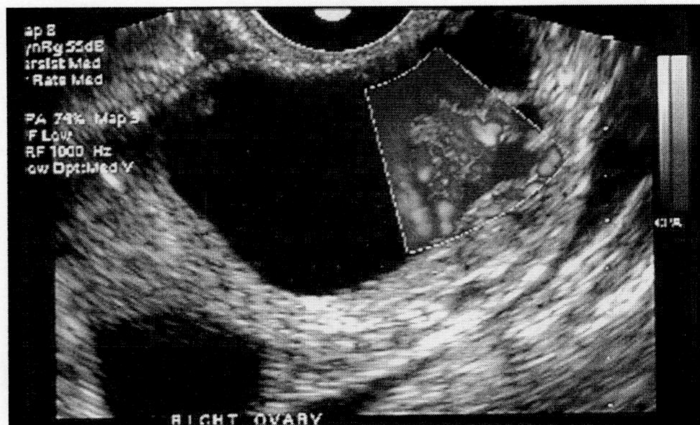


**FIG. 42-2** Ultrasound image of a complex ovarian cyst with presence of central color doppler flow.
SOURCE: Image courtesy of Andrew Li, MD.

## QUESTION 3

*What are the risks to the pregnancy of surgical exploration of an ovarian mass? When is the best time to perform surgery during pregnancy? Has laparoscopy been shown to be safe during pregnancy?*

## ANSWER 3

The risk of spontaneous abortion after surgery is reported to range from 3% to 5%, and the risk of preterm birth is reported to be 9–12%. We should note that these estimates arise from studies where the majority of the surgeries were performed in the second trimester. The perinatal and maternal death rate attributable to the surgical evaluation of adnexal masses in pregnancy is very low.

The best time to perform surgery in order to reduce the risk of a fetal loss is in the early-to-mid second trimester, which has been demonstrated to provide a lower pregnancy loss rate compared with surgery in the first trimester and does not require fetal monitoring. Techniques should be employed to maintain placental perfusion during surgery, including avoidance of long periods of hypotension/hypoxia, left-sided wedge positioning, and avoidance of $CO_2$ over distension during laparoscopy. The intraabdominal pressure during laparoscopy in pregnancy should not exceed 15 mm Hg.

In small series, laparoscopy has been shown to be safe in pregnancy when it is performed by an experienced operator. This technique is controversial, particularly if the surgery is being done to rule out an ovarian malignancy, with concerns regarding tumor spill and delay in definitive surgical therapy noted. In fact, many practitioners would argue that excluding a malignancy would be the only reason to electively operate on a pregnant woman with an ovarian mass.

## BIBLIOGRAPHY

Albayram F, Hamper UM. Ovarian and adnexa torsion: spectrum of sonographic findings with pathologic correlation. *J Ultrasound Med.* 2001;20(10):1083.

Bromley B, Benacerraf B. Adnexal masses during pregnancy: accuracy of sonographic diagnosis and outcome. *J Ultrasound Med.* 1997;16(7):447.

Cunningham FG, Gant NF, Leveno LC, et al. Abnormalities of the reproductive tract. In: *Williams Obstetrics*. 21st ed. New York, NY: McGraw Hill; 2001;930.

Ekerhovd E, Wienerroith H, Staudach A, et al. Preoperative assessment of unilocular adnexal cysts by TV ultrasonography: a comparison between ultrasonographic imaging and histopathologic diagnosis. *Am J Obstet Gynecol.* 2001;184:48.

Fatum M, Rojansky N. Laparoscopic surgery during pregnancy. *Obstet Gynecol Surv.* 2001;56(1):50.

Hess L, Peaceman A, O'Brien W, et al. Adnexal mass occurring with intrauterine pregnancy: report of fifty-four patients requiring laparotomy for definitive management. *Am J Obstet Gynecol.* 1988;158:1029.

Mathevet P, Nessah K, Dargent D, et al. Laparoscopic management of adnexal masses in pregnancy: a case series. *Eur J Obstet Gynecol Reprod Biol.* 2003;108 (2):217.

Sherard GB, Hodson CA, Williams JW, et al. Adnexal masses in pregnancy: a 12-year experience. *Am J Obstet Gynecol.* 2003;189(2):358.

Tekay A, Jouppila P. Validity of pulsatility and resistance indices in classification of adnexal tumors with TV color doppler ultrasound. *Ultrasound in Obstet Gynecol.* 1992;2:338.

Thornton JG, Wells M. Ovarian cysts in pregnancy: does ultrasound make traditional management inappropriate: *Obstet Gynecol.*1987;69:717.

Usui R, Minakami H, Kosuge S, et al. A retrospective survey of clinical, pathologic, and prognostic features or adnexal masses operated on during pregnancy. *J Obstet Gynecol Res.* 2000;26(2):89.

Whitecar P, Turner S, Higby K. Adnexal masses in pregnancy: a review of 130 cases undergoing surgical management. *Am J Obstet Gynecol.* 1999;181:19.

# 43 CHOLESTASIS OF PREGNANCY

*Marguerite Lisa Bartholomew*

## LEARNING POINT

The diagnosis of cholestasis of pregnancy requires attention to symptoms, physical findings, and serum bile acids in order to prevent stillbirth in the late third trimester.

## VIGNETTE

A 30-year-old, G3P2002, at 32 weeks gestation, presents complaining of intense pruritis which began on the palms and soles of her feet and now involves her abdomen. Physical examination indicates excoriations on her abdomen, but no obvious rash or lesions. Her skin and sclera appear nonicteric. A nonstress test is performed and is reassuring. An ultrasound indicates a singleton pregnancy with normal fetal size and amniotic fluid volume. Ursodioxycholic acid 500 mg orally twice/day is prescribed, and serial antepartum testing is ordered (see Table 43-1).

The patient reports an improvement in symptoms with ursodioxycholic acid. An amniocentesis is performed at 36 weeks with mature results. Induction of labor is performed with a successful normal vaginal delivery of a vigorous infant. The pruritis resolves 48 hours after delivery.

### QUESTION 1

*What is cholestasis of pregnancy (ICP), and how is it diagnosed?*

### ANSWER 1

Intrahepatic cholestasis of pregnancy is a rare disorder of unknown etiology that usually occurs after 25 weeks gestation and resolves 48 hours after delivery. The overall prevalence is 1/1000–1/10,000 pregnancies. The highest prevalence has been reported in Scandinavia (2%) and Chile (14%). It is more common in winter and in women with a personal history of ICP, advanced maternal age, and multiple gestations. ICP is the second most common cause of jaundice in pregnancy, after viral hepatitis.

There is no uniform agreement on the criteria for diagnosis. ICP is characterized by pruritis, with or without jaundice. Symptoms are associated with elevated levels (3–100×) of serum bile acids (total, cholic, deoxycolic, chenodeoxycholic acids), alkaline phosphatase (5–10×), transaminases (2–10×), and bilirubin (2–5×), in the absence of other disease processes. The bile acids deposit in the skin causing intense pruritis, although the level of bile acids does not correlate with the intensity of symptoms.

The pruritis occurs first and is followed by the development of jaundice in 1–4 weeks. The pruritis usually starts on the palms and soles and then spreads centrally. Scratching may cause excoriations which should not be mistaken for a rash. There is usually no malaise, nausea, vomiting, abdominal pain, or tenderness. The presentation of ICP contrasts with the pruritic urticarial papules and plaques of pregnancy (PUPPP), which begin centrally, spread peripherally, and manifest skin lesions.

Liver biopsy is not recommended for diagnosis, but usually shows normal hepatocellular architecture. The centrolobular areas may reveal dilated bile canaliculi, bile plugs, and staining without inflammatory cells. These hepatic changes regress after pregnancy.

**TABLE 43-1. Serum Levels of Bile Acids**

| | |
|---|---|
| Total bile acids | 60 μmol/L (normal = 0–10 μmol/L) |
| AST | 100 U/L |
| ALT | 120 U/L |
| Alkaline phosphatase | 300 U/L |
| Total bilirubin | 2.0 mg/dL |

### QUESTION 2

*What are the fetal and maternal risks? What is the recurrence risk?*

### ANSWER 2

There is an increased risk of preterm delivery of approximately 35%, and recent literature indicates that bile acids activate the myometrial oxytocin receptor. Other risks include increased risk of perinatal mortality, intrapartum nonreassuring fetal heart rate patterns (14%), and meconium staining (27%). When untreated, the perinatal mortality ranges from 11% to 20%. When treated, including delivery after lung maturity is documented, perinatal mortality has been reported to be 3.5%. Severity of maternal symptoms is not correlated with fetal prognosis, and antepartum testing has not been shown to be predictive of fetal death. Stillbirths usually occur after 37 weeks. Autopsies of stillborn infants suggest an acute anoxic insult with cardiac and pulmonary petechiae without growth restriction. There is also an association with fetal intracranial hemorrhage.

Maternal risks, aside from significant discomfort, are few. Subclinical steatorrhea and malabsorption of vitamin K (likely exacerbated by cholestyramine treatment) leading to postpartum hemorrhage has been reported. Those women with prior hepatitis C (HCV) are more likely to manifest ICP. In an Italian study, 23% of 56 patients with ICP were positive for HCV or RNA. ICP recurs in 40–60% of subsequent pregnancies. It has been shown to cluster in families and has been linked to at least three cholestais genes (*BSEP, FICI, and MDR3*). Patients with ICP should be advised that estrogen and progesterone-containing contraceptions may cause the condition to recur in the nonpregnant state.

## QUESTION 3

*What are the potential pathophysiological mechanisms underlying ICP?*

## ANSWER 3

A number of different mechanisms have been proposed to explain ICP including:

1. A defect in the biliary excretion of sulfated metabolites, possibly associated with a defect in progesterone metabolism such that ICP women make more sulfated progesterone metabolites. Sulfated progesterones are normally excreted into bile, and both estrogen and progesterone can be converted into cholestatic steroids.
2. Genetic predisposition: A number of potential genetic defects have been suggested, including those of bile salt export pump gene, familial intrahepatic cholestasis 1 gene, and multiple drug resistance 3 genes.
3. Inability of the fetus to remove bile acids from maternal circulation. Bile acid transporters have been found on both sides of the trophoblast.
4. Maternal liver damage causing defects in P450 system, since the P450 system mitigates the effects of cholestasis.
5. Increased opioidergic tone, which results in increased sensitivity to pruritis. Serum from cholestasis patients injected into medullary dorsal horn of monkeys induced scratching behavior, reversible by naloxone, and serum from noncholestasis patients did not induce scratching.
6. Selenium deficiency: An increased incidence of ICP has been observed in seleniumin-deficient Chilean patients. Selenium levels decrease in pregnancy, particularly in winter months.

## QUESTION 4

*Describe treatment options.*

## ANSWER 4

1. Delivery is the ultimate treatment. Fetal lung maturity testing should be performed at 36–37 weeks, and delivery is strongly recommended if mature.
2. Ursodeoxycholic acid (UCDA) is a naturally occurring hydrophillic bile acid that replaces other more hydrophobic and cytotoxic bile acids. It stimulates biliary excretion of steroids with sulfate groups and has been found to improve symptoms, decrease bile acids, and possibly improve fetal outcome. Accumulation in the amniotic fluid and cord blood appears to be very low even when high doses of UDCA (1.5 to 2.0 g/d) have been used. Given the absence of maternal and fetal toxicity, the use of UDCA in ICP is warranted, particularly in patients with severe cholestasis. The optimal dose has yet to be determined, although starting doses of 300–500 mg twice a day are described (14–16 mg/kg/d).
3. S-adenyslmethionine (SAMe) is required as a precursor to transsulfuration (potentiates antioxidants) in the liver and reverses estrogen-induced impairment of bile secretion. The combination of SAMe with UCDA has been found to be more effective than either alone.
4. Cholestyramine: 8–16 g/d in three to four divided doses. Binds excess bile salts in the intestine, thereby inhibiting absorption and increasing excretion. However, it also inhibits absorption of vitamin K and other medications, and some practitioners recommend checking PT and INR weekly and treating with vitamin K as needed. Can also cause bloating and constipation. May take 2 weeks to become effective. Overall, cholestyramine is no longer considered first line therapy for ICP.
5. Corticosteroids such as dexamethasone, 12 mg q day × 6 days, demonstrate benefit in the reduction of symptoms bile acids counts. Also suppresses fetal placental estrogen production.

Oral antipruritic medications, such as benadryl, treats only pruritis and have no effect on suppression of bile acids. Topical antipruritic medications and steroids are generally ineffective.

## BIBLIOGRAPHY

Gabbe SG, Niebyl JR, Simpson JL. *Obstetrics: Normal and Problem Pregnancies.* Philadelphia, PA: Churchill Livingstone; 2003:1218–1220.

Germain AM, et al. Bile acids increase response and expression of human myometrial oxytocin receptor. *Am J Obstet Gynecol.* 2003;189:577–582.

Hirvioja ML, Tuimala R, Vuori J. The treatment of intrahepatic cholestasis or pregnancy by dexamethasone. *Br J Obstet Gynecol.* 1992;99:109–111.

Mazzella G, Rizzo N, Azzaroli F, et al. Ursodeoxycholic acid administration in patients with cholestasis of pregnancy: effects on primary bile acids in babies and mothers. *Hepatology.* 2001;33:504–508.

Mullally B, Hansen W. Intrahepatic cholestasis of pregnancy: review of the literature. *Obstet Gynecol Surv*. 2002;57:47–52.

Nicastri PL, et al. A randomized placebo-controlled trial of ursodeoxycholic acid and S-adenosylmethionine in the treatment of intrahepatic cholestasis or pregnancy. *Br J Obstet Gyn*. 1998;105:1205.

Palma J, Reyes H, Ribalta J, et al. Effects of ursodeoxycholic acid in patients with intrahepatic cholestasis or pregnancy. *Hepatology*. 1992;15:1043–1047.

Paternoster DM, et al. Intra-hepatic cholestasis of pregnancy in hepatitis C virus infection. *Acta Obstet Gynecol Scand*. 2002; 81:99–103.

Reid R, et al. Fetal complications of obstetric cholestasis. *Br Med J*. 1976;1:870–872.

Savander M, et al. Genetic evidence of heterogeneity in intrahepatic cholestasis of pregnancy. *Gut*. 2003;52:1025–1029.

# 44 ADNEXAL MASSES DURING PREGNANCY

*Ilana Cass*

## LEARNING POINT

To understand the appropriate evaluation of an adnexal mass in pregnancy.

## VIGNETTE

A 24-year-old, G1P0, has been followed for an adnexal mass, first noted on ultrasound at 10 weeks gestational age. The mass is still present on follow up ultrasound at 14 weeks gestational age, 7 cm × 6 cm, complex with a single septae. The other ovary is normal in appearance, and there is no reported pelvic fluid. She has mild intermittent pain without any clear precipitating factors. She has no associated bowel symptoms, and has some expected urinary frequency. She has no significant past medical or gynecologic history and no prior surgeries. She denies any family history of cancer.

Physical examination reveals a gravid woman in no apparent distress. Vitals signs: pulse 68, BP 90/50. Head, eyes, ears, nose, and throat examination reveals no adenopathy, chest is clear to auscultation, cardiac examination shows regular rate and rhythm, abdominal examination is consistent with a 16-week gravid uterus. She has no evidence of any ascites; there is slight tenderness to deep palpation in the left lower quadrant without or inguinal adenopathy. Pelvic examination reveals a gravid uterus, cervix is closed with a palpable, slightly tender, mobile mass approximately 6 cm on bimanual examination on the left, with no masses in the rectovaginal septum.

## QUESTION 1

*What is the incidence of ovarian tumors in pregnancy? What are the most common ovarian neoplasms encountered in pregnancy?*

## ANSWER 1

Approximately 1 in 500 pregnancies.

1. Functional cysts—follicular or corpus luteum cysts are the most common ovarian mass in pregnancy
2. Dermoid cysts
3. Serous cystadenoma

## QUESTION 2

*What are some of the risks associated with the management of an ovarian mass in pregnancy, and what is the management of an ovarian mass in pregnancy?*

## ANSWER 2

Risks include: malignancy (2–5%), torsion (10–15%), cyst rupture/hemorrhage with attendant risks of infection, preterm labor or spontaneous abortion, and obstruction of delivery. Management is based on patient symptoms and ultrasound characteristics. Patients with acute pain have a much higher incidence of complications including fetal loss rates of 11–20%, oophorectomy as opposed to cystectomy, larger masses and cyst rupture. Patients without acute pain whose masses persist into the second trimester and are larger than 6–8 cm, rapidly enlarging or complex generally require surgical intervention. Tumor markers are notoriously not helpful as they may be elevated secondary to pregnancy alone.

## QUESTION 3

*When is the optimal time for surgical intervention and why?*

### ANSWER 3

Ideally between 12–16 weeks because functional cysts should have resolved by this point, the reduced incidence of spontaneous abortions at this gestation and because the placenta has completely taken over hormonal support of the pregnancy from the corpus luteum by 12 weeks.

### QUESTION 4

*At which gestational ages is there the highest risk of ovarian torsion, and why?*

### ANSWER 4

The risk of torsin is highest prior to 16 weeks, as the uterus is rising out of the pelvis and during the puerperium, as the uterus involutes.

## BIBLIOGRAPHY

Morrow CP, Curtin JP (eds.). Cancer in pregnancy. Chapter 14. In: *Synopsis of Gynecologic Oncology.* 5th ed. Philadelphia, PA: Churchill Livingstone; 1998;353–367.

Hess LW, et al. Adnexal mass occurring with intrauterine pregnancy: report of 54 pts requiring laparotomy for definitive management. *Am J Obstet Gynecol.* 1988;158:5.

Struyk AP, et al. Ovarian tumors in pregnancy. *Acta Obstet Gynecol Scand.* 1984;63:421.

Wang PH, et al. Ovarian tumors complicating pregnancy, emergency and elective surgery. *J Reprod Med.* 1999;44:279–287.

# 45 PREGNANCY AFTER BREAST CANCER

*Ilana Cass*

## LEARNING POINT

To understand the risks and clinical recommendations for women regarding conception following a diagnosis of breast cancer.

## VIGNETTE

A 38-year-old, G1P1, has been followed in your office for 4 years. She was diagnosed with a ductal carcinoma-in-situ breast cancer 1 year ago. She was treated with lumpectomy with a complete excision and negative margins followed by radiation therapy. She and her husband now come to see you regarding the possibility of having another child. She has been followed by her medical oncologist, who reports that she is in clinical remission.

She has no significant past medical or gynecologic history. She conceived spontaneously at age 34 and had an uncomplicated vaginal delivery at term. She denies any family history of cancer, but reports a maternal history of cardiovascular disease.

The physical examination reveals a well-nourished woman in no apparent distress. Vitals signs: pulse 68/min, BP 110/60 mm Hg. Head, eyes, ears, nose, and throat examination reveals no adenopathy, chest is clear to auscultation, cardiac examination shows regular rate and rhythm. Breast examination reveals a well-healed scar of the left breast. Abdominal examination is normal without any masses or inguinal adenopathy, pelvic examination reveals normal anatomy with a mobile uterus, normal size.

### QUESTION 1

*What are some of the concerns regarding pregnancy after a diagnosis of breast cancer?*

### ANSWER 1

Foremost is the concern that pregnancy, with elevated estrogen levels, may adversely affect the patient's breast cancer course given the existing epidemiological, laboratory, and clinical data that show the impact of hormones on breast cancer. Reproductive history is an established risk factor assessment tool (GAIL model) for breast cancer. Laboratory data suggests that estrogen is important in the initiation and promotion of breast cancer growth in vitro. Most compelling is the data showing a greater than 50% reduction in breast cancer risk among women who have had oophorectomy by age 35 compared to controls. Finally, hormonal manipulation, including oophorectomy, had been successfully used as an adjunctive therapy for breast cancer patients in the past. Another concern is the risk of spontaneous abortion or teratogenesis induced by chemotherapy in women with a history of breast cancer. Available studies have found similar rates of miscarriage among women with a history of breast cancer, ranging from 10% to 24%. No increased teratogenic effects have been seen among infants born to women who have been treated with chemotherapy after breast cancer, although most of the data includes women who waited a minimum of 6 months to conceive after the completion of chemotherapy.

## QUESTION 2

*How does subsequent pregnancy affect mortality in breast cancer survivors? What is one of the potential biases that may affect these results?*

## ANSWER 2

Subsequent pregnancy does not seem to worsen survival in matched case-control studies. However, studies are small, and may be affected by the "healthy mother effect." Women who become pregnant after breast cancer diagnosis may be more likely to be free of disease at the time of pregnancy than similar breast cancer patients who do not have subsequent pregnancy. Studies have tried to control for this by choosing control women who had disease-free intervals identical to the interval between diagnosis and pregnancy, and by analyzing only women with good prognosis disease, and have all found the same results.

## QUESTION 3

*What is the dominant estrogen of pregnancy? Is it a weaker or stronger estrogen than estradiol?*

## ANSWER 3

Estriol, a weaker estrogen than estradiol.

## QUESTION 4

*Are women with a history of breast cancer able to breast-feed?*

## ANSWER 4

Many women who have undergone lumpectomy and radiation will be able to breast-feed but will often have less milk production from the irradiated side and may be more prone to mastitis on that side. Breast-feeding from the contra lateral breast is not affected and is safe.

## BIBLIOGRAPHY


Clarke MJ. Ovarian ablation in breast cancer, 1896–1998: milestones along the hierarchy of evidence from case report to Cochrane review. *BMJ.* 1998;317(7167):1246–1248.

Gail MH, Brinton LA, Byar DP, Corle DK, Green SB, Schairer C, Mulvihill JJ. Projecting individualized probabilities of developing breast cancer for white females who are being examined annually. *JNCI.* 1989;81:1879–1886.

Gelber S, Goldhirsch A, Castiglione-Gertsch M, Marini G, et al. Effect of pregnancy on overall survival after the diagnosis of early-stage breast cancer. *JCO.* 2001;19(6):1671–1675.

Higgins S, Haffty BG. Pregnancy and lactation after breast-conserving therapy for early stage breast cancer. *Cancer.* 1994; 73(8):2175–2180.

Kroman N, Jensen MB, Melbye M, Wohlfahrt J, Mouridsen HT. Should women be advised against pregnancy after breast-cancer treatment? *Lancet.* 1997;350:319–322.

Mueller BA, Simon MS, Deapen D, Kaimineni A, Malone KE, Daling JR. Childbearing and survival after breast carcinoma in young women. *Cancer.* 2003;98(6):1131–1140.

Surbone A, Petrek JA. Childbearing issues in breast cancer survivors. *Cancer.* 1997;79(7):1271–1278.


# 46 ASTHMA

*Jane L. Davis*

## LEARNING POINT

Since asthma has been reported to affect approximately 4–8% of pregnant women in the United States, it is important to know how it impacts upon a pregnancy.

## VIGNETTE

A 26-year-old Caucasian, G1P0, presents for her initial prenatal visit at 6 weeks gestational age. Her past medical history is significant for asthma since 6 years of age. The patient's internist currently treats her with an inhaled beta agonist, and recently also added an aerosolized steroid. The patient's symptoms seem to worsen when she develops upper respiratory infections. The patient received an influenza immunization 4 months ago.

The physical examination reveals a Caucasian woman in no acute distress. Vital signs: blood pressure

118/70, pulse 80/min, respiratory rate 18/min, temperature 98.6°F. Thyroid: nonpalpable; breasts: no palpable masses; lungs: without wheezes or rhonchi; heart: regular rate and rhythm without any murmur; abdomen: soft, nontender; pelvic: normal external genitalia, vagina well estrogenized, cervix nulliparous uterus anteverted, 6-week size, adnexa negative.

## QUESTION 1

*What are the pulmonary physiologic changes that occur during pregnancy?*

## ANSWER 1

Pregnancy is associated with changes in lung volume (Table 46-1) such that: (1) there is a 40% increase in tidal volume (the amount of air moved in one normal respiratory cycle), (2) a 20–50% increase in minute ventilation (volume of air moved per minute), and (3) a decrease in residual volume (the volume of air that remains in the lung at the end of a maximal expiration). These changes are mediated mainly by progesterone, which acts as a respiratory stimulant. During pregnancy arterial blood gases reflect a compensated respiratory alkalosis.

## QUESTION 2

*What effect does pregnancy have on asthma and what effect does asthma have on pregnancy?*

## ANSWER 2

Approximately one-third of asthmatic patients will improve, one-third will worsen, and one-third will remain the same during pregnancy. The clinical course of asthma during pregnancy may be predicted by the course during the first trimester, and most patients have the same pattern of response with repeated pregnancies.

Although data have been conflicting, the largest and most recent studies suggest that maternal asthma increases the risk of perinatal mortality, preeclampsia, preterm birth, and low birth weight infants. More severe asthma has been associated with increased risks.

## QUESTION 3

*Outline the treatment of asthma during pregnancy.*

**TABLE 46-1. Normal Pulmonary Values in Pregnant and Nonpregnant Women**

| TERM | DEFINITION | VALUES . NONPREGNANT | VALUES PREGNANCY | CLINICAL SIGNIFICANCE IN PREGNANCY |
|---|---|---|---|---|
| Tidal volume | The amount of air moved in one normal respiratory cycle | 450 mL | 600 mL (increases up to 40%) | |
| Respiratory rate | Number of respirations per minute | 16/min | Changes very little | |
| Minute ventilation | The volume of air moved per minute; product of respiratory rate and tidal volume | 7.2 L | 9.6 L (increases up to 40% because of the increase in tidal volume) | Increases oxygen available for the fetus |
| Forced expiratory volume in 1 second | | Approx. 80–85% of the vital capacity | Unchanged | Valuable to measure because there is no change due to pregnancy |
| Peak expiratory flow rate | | | Unchanged | Valuable to measure because there is no change due to pregnancy |
| Forced vital capacity | The maximum amount of air that can be moved from maximum inspiration to maximum expiration | 3.5 L | Unchanged | If over 1 L, pregnancy is usually well tolerated |
| Residual volume | The amount of air that remains in the lung at the end of a maximal expiration | 1000 mL | Decreases by around 200 mL to around 800 mL | Improves gas transfer from alveoli to blood |

SOURCE: Data from ACOG Technical Bulletin 224.

## ANSWER 3

The goals in treating asthma during pregnancy are: (1) reduction in the number of attacks, (2) prevention of severe attacks, and (3) assurance of adequate maternal and fetal oxygenation.

1. Treatment of chronic asthma
   a. Inhaled beta agonists (albuterol): Bronchodilators are the mainstay of therapy; can be used on an as needed or scheduled basis. Side effects include cardiac arrhythmias and tachyphylaxis.
   b. Inhaled glucocorticoids (budesonide is the preferred inhaled corticosteroid): Additional therapy used with inhaled beta agonists in patients with more severe asthma. Main side effect is oral candidiasis. Fewer side effects than with oral steroids.
   c. Cromolyn: Anti-inflammatory agent, which prevents mast cell degranulation. No longer a recommended treatment. Currently, preferred treatment is either medium-dose inhaled corticosteroids or a combination of inhaled corticosteroids with long-acting inhaled beta2-agonist.
   d. Aminophylline: Seldom used anymore. Increases cAMP (which causes bronchodilatation) by inhibiting phosphodiesterase.

Of note, all patients with asthma should receive influenza vaccine each year. This vaccine is safe to use during pregnancy since it is a killed vaccine.

2. Treatment of acute asthma
   a. 30–40% concentration of humidified $O_2$
   b. IV hydration
   c. Inhaled beta agonists (albuterol), which is preferred or subcutaneous terbutaline (0.25 mg).
   d. Systemic steroids (Methylprednisolone 100 mg q 6–8 hours or hydrocortisone 100 mg q 4 hours until asthma resolved followed with oral prednisone, which is tapered over 7–14 days). Note: if patient has been receiving oral steroids throughout pregnancy, she will need *stress* doses when in labor (hydrocortisone 100 mg q 4–6 hours in labor and for 24 hours postpartum).

3. Pulmonary function testing.

Pulmonary function testing is now used routinely in the management of chronic and acute asthma. Sequential measurement of the forced expiratory volume in 1 second ($FEV_1$) is the single best measure reflecting severity. An $FEV_1$ less than 1 L, or less than 20% of predicted, correlates with severe disease, defined as hypoxia, poor response to therapy, and a high relapse rate. The peak expiratory flow rate (PEFR) correlates well with the $FEV_1$, and can be measured reliably with inexpensive portable meters. Notably, PEFR does not change over the course of pregnancy in normal women. Consequently, some investigators advocate the use of PEFR home monitoring to adjust medications and determine management. However, some studies also indicate that optimization of asthma control by adjustment of medications may be conducted by either self-adjustment with the aid of a written action plan or by regular medical review, and those individualized written action plans based on PEFR appear to be equivalent to action plans based on symptoms.

## BIBLIOGRAPHY


Asthma and Pregnancy Report. NAEPP Report of the Working Group on Asthma and Pregnancy: Management of Asthma During Pregnancy: Recommendations for Pharmacologic Treatment. NIH Publication No 93-3279. Bethesda, MD: U.S. Department of Health and Human Services; National Institutes of Health; National Heart, Lung, and Blood Institute, Update 2004.

Asthma and Pregnancy Report. NAEPP Report of the Working Group on Asthma and Pregnancy: Recommendations for Pharmacologic Treatment. U.S. Department of Health and Human Services, Update 2004.

Clark SL. Asthma in pregnancy. *Obstet Gynecol.* 1993;82: 1036–1040.

Kallen B, Rydhstroem H, Aberg A. Asthma during pregnancy-a population based study. *Eur J Epidemiol.* 2000;16(2):167–171.

Lemanske RF, Busse WW. Asthma. *JAMA.* 1997;278:1855–1873.

Mabie WC. Asthma in pregnancy. *Clin Obstet Gynecolo.* 1996; 39:56–69.

ACOG Technical Bulletin No. 224. Pulmonary Disease in Pregnancy. 1996.

Schatz M, Zeiger RS, Hoffman CP, Harden K, Forsythe A, Chilingar L, Saunders B, Porreco R, Sperling W, Kagnoff M. Perinatal outcome in the pregnancies of asthmatic women: a prospective controlled analysis. *Am J Resp Crit Care Med.* 1995;151:1170.


# 47 DEPRESSION AND POSTPARTUM PSYCHOLOGICAL REACTIONS

*Jane L. Davis*

## LEARNING POINT

Women who have a history of psychiatric illness prior to pregnancy are at a greater risk of developing a more significant psychological reaction in the postpartum period.

## VIGNETTE

A 36-year-old, G1P1, presents for her 6-week postpartum visit following the delivery of a healthy, term female infant via a normal spontaneous delivery. The patient's husband, who has accompanied her on this visit, states that he has been quite concerned about his wife's behavior. Despite her initial happiness of becoming a mother, the patient appears to be indifferent to her infant. She initially breast-fed, but lost interest in it, and stopped after 2 weeks. She spends most of the day in bed, and allows the nanny to care for her daughter. She is unable to sleep during the night and has lost all of her pregnancy weight along with an additional 10 pounds. She has a 10-year history of depression, including a failed suicide attempt as an adolescent. She was under the care of a psychiatrist prior to this pregnancy and was treated with medication, however, she discontinued treatment prior to conception. Her past medical history is otherwise negative.

### QUESTION 1

*Describe the psychological reactions experienced by women in the postpartum period?*

### ANSWER 1

The psychological reactions experienced by women in the postpartum period includes maternity or postpartum "blues," postpartum nonpsychotic depression, and postpartum psychotic depression. The incidence, definition, etiology, and treatments are detailed as follows:

**Maternity or postpartum blues** (incidence 50–70% of pregnancies)

*Definition:* "Blues" may be a misnomer since these women are predominately happy. This is basically a transient state of emotional lability, anxiety, restlessness, and irritation appearing on any day within the first week postpartum, usually resolving by postpartum day 10. There are no obstetric, social, economic correlates. Since symptoms may vary from one patient to another and since study criteria have also varied, the reported incidence may vary.

*Risk factors/etiology:* Unknown, although two potential mechanisms have been suggested: (1) The abrupt hormonal withdrawal occurring postpartum; the absolute levels of estrogen and progesterone are unrelated, but the greater the change in hormone levels between pregnancy and postpartum, the greater the likelihood of developing symptoms. (2) Activation of a biological mechanism underlying mammalian mother-infant attachment behavior and regulated primarily by oxytocin. Table 47-1 lists factors that may increase the risk of postpartum blues.

*Treatment:* Because syndrome is transient, no specific therapy is indicated other than family support. Since some symptoms may be secondary to sleep deprivation, increased rest may be advised.

**Postpartum nonpsychotic depression** (incidence: 10–20%; the incidence may be higher since it often goes undiagnosed either because of poor screening techniques or mothers' reluctance to admit symptoms)

*Definition:* Only defined officially in the psychiatric nomenclature in 1994 in the *Diagnostic and Statistical Manual of Mental Disorders, 4th ed,* which describes a true depressive disorder specific to the postpartum period. Its onset is usually within 6 weeks postpartum and may last 3–14 months. Prognosis for recovery is good although 50% recur with subsequent pregnancies. In addition to classical signs and symptoms of depression (feelings of inadequacy, sleep and appetite disturbances, and impaired concentration) patients may manifest indifference to family and infant. Patients often are obsessed with thoughts of killing their infants. However, they rarely act on these unless they become psychotic (see later on).

*Risk factors/etiology:* Risk factors include a history of major depression (30% of patients with history will develop), prior postpartum depression (25% risk of recurrence), premenstrual dysphoric disorder, lack of social support, maternal age <20 years, single motherhood, and possibly low socioeconomic status. A hormonal imbalance has not been implicated unless there is a genetic predispostion. It is less common in cultures where there is strong social support of new mothers. It is not related to a woman's educational

**TABLE 47-1. Factors that May Cause "Postpartum Blues"**

| |
|---|
| The emotional letdown that follows the excitement and the fears that most women experience during pregnancy and delivery. |
| The discomforts of the early puerperium. |
| Fatigue from loss of sleep during labor and postpartum. |
| Anxiety over the capability to care for the infant after leaving the hospital. |
| Fears of becoming less attractive. |

SOURCE: Cunningham GF, Leveno KJ, Bloom SL, Hauth JC, Gilstrap LG, Wenstrom. KD. (ed.) *Williams Obstetrics.* 22nd ed. McGraw-Hill; 2005. 705.

level, gender of baby, mode of delivery, or whether the pregnancy was planned or not. Table 47-2 lists additional risk factors for nonpsychotic postpartum depression.

*Diagnosis:* An adequate history and assessment of patient's risk factors is generally sufficient. Some investigators feel that many more patients (up to 35%) would be diagnosed if adequate screening methods (Edinburgh postnatal depression scale) were implemened, and recommend assessment sooner than the 6-week postpartum visit.

*Treatment:* Treatment includes antidepressive medications. Patients should be counseled that nonpsychotic postpartum depression may be a precursor of recurrent depression in the mother. Emotional, behavioral, cognitive, and interpersonal problems in the child may develop if not treated properly.

**Postpartum psychotic depression** (incidence 0.14–0.26%)

*Definition*: Psychosis manifested by delusions, hallucinations, or both occurring 3 weeks postpartum whether for the first time or as part of a recurrent illness. There is often more disorientation and mood lability than seen in nonpostpartum psychosis. Patients with this condition can appear normal, and then acutely become profoundly depressed and psychotic. Women with postpartum psychotic depression are more likely to harm their infants and themselves. Therefore, this is considered a true psychiatric emergency.

**TABLE 47-2. Characteristics of Antenatal Patients that May Increase the Risk for Major Postpartum Depression**

| |
|---|
| Under 20 years of age |
| Unmarried |
| Medically indigent |
| Comes from a family of six or more children |
| Separation for one or both parents in childhood or adolescence |
| Received poor parental support and attention in childhood |
| Limited parental support in adulthood |
| Poor relationship with husband or boyfriend |
| Economic difficulties with housing or income |
| Dissatisfied with amount of education |
| Evidence of emotional problem, past or present |
| Low self-esteem |

Posner NA, Unterman RR, Williams KN. Postpartum depression: the obstetrician's concerns. *Recent Advances in Postpartum Psychiatric Disorders.* In Wood DG (ed.). Washington DC: American Psychiatric Press, Inc; 1985:69.

*Risk factors/etiology:* Postpartum psychotic depression is usually a manifestation of a bipolar disorder. Since a depressive episode can occur during the course of an underlying bipolar disorder, all patients with postpartum depression should be screened with the following questions:

"Have you ever had four continuous days when you were feeling so good, high, excited, or hyper that other people felt you were not your normal self?" and "Have you experienced 4 continuous days when you were so irritable that you found yourself shouting at people or starting fights?"

## QUESTION 2

*What is the differential diagnosis of postpartum psychological reactions?*

## ANSWER 2

The differential diagnosis of postpartum psychological reactions include:

1. Medical conditions such as thyroiditis, hypothyroidism, and B12 deficiency.
2. Substance abuse including the use of lysergic acid diethylamide (LSD), phencydidine (PCP) and methylenedioxy methanphetamine (MDHA or "ecstasy")

## QUESTION 3

*What is the recommended treatment for nonpsychotic and psychotic postpartum depression?*

## ANSWER 3

Antidepressant medication is the mainstay of treatment for nonpsychotic and psychotic postpartum depression with selective serotonin reuptake inhibitors (SSRIs) more commonly used than tricyclic antidepressants since they are more efficacious in women and have fewer side effects; 50–65% of women treated experience improvement in symptoms. Very low concentrations of SSRIs are found in breast milk (citalopram and fluoxetine have the highest concentration in breast milk). Occasionally sleep disturbances, crying, watery stools, and vomiting in infants exposed to SSRIs from breast milk are observed.

Psychotherapy alone without medication may also be efficacious in 45–60% of patients. For postpartum depression without psychosis, patients also benefit from support groups, couples therapy, parenting coaching, and the like.

### QUESTION 4

*Is there a role for prophylactic treatment of women who are at risk for developing postpartum depression?*

### ANSWER 4

Prophylactic treatment of women who are at risk for developing postpartum depression is very controversial. One study has suggested that prophylactic therapy for the patient who has had a prior history of depression may decrease the incidence of postpartum depression. The same medication that the patient previously responded to should be used. However, other investigators feel that only observation is indicated.

## BIBLIOGRAPHY

Evins GG, et al. Postpartum depression: a comparison of screening and routine clinical evaluation. *AJOG.* 2000; 182: 1080–1082.

Josefsson A, et al. Obstetric, somatic, and demographic risk factors for postpartum depressive symptoms. *Obstet Gynecol.* 2002; 99:223–228.

Lamberg L: Safety of antidepressant use in pregnant and nursing women. *JAMA.* 1999;282:222–223.

Miller LJ. Postpartum depression. *JAMA.* 2002;287:762–765.

Supta S, et al. SSRIs in pregnancy and lactation. *Obstet/Gynecol. Survey.* 1999;53:733–736.

Wisner KL, et al. Postpartum depression. *NEJM.* 2002; 347:194–199.

Wisner KL, et al. Prevention of recurrent postpartum depression: a randomized clinical trial. *J Clin Psychiatry.* 2001;62:82–86.

# 48 SEIZURE DISORDERS

*Jane L. Davis*

## LEARNING POINT

Seizure disorders can significantly impact on pregnancy and family planning.

## VIGNETTE

A 28-year-old, G0, Hispanic female presents to her gynecologist for a routine evaluation. The patient has a history of generalized seizures since sustaining head trauma in an automobile accident 10 years ago. Phenytoin adequately controls her seizures. Although, the patient is not currently interested in becoming pregnant, she recently married and is interested in having children eventually. She has heard that phenytoin is a potent teratogen and is interested in what she can do to prevent birth defects in her child. Additionally, she is interested in learning what form of contraception would be most effective for her to use at this time.

The patient has regular cycles every 28–30 days, with menses lasting 3–4 days. The patient's medical and surgical histories are negative except for her history of a seizure disorder. She does not smoke or use recreational drugs and is a social drinker.

The physical examination reveals a slender, Hispanic woman. Vital signs: blood pressure 116/70. Pulse: 80/min, respiratory rate 18/min, temperature 98.6°F. Thyroid: nonpalpable; lungs: clear; heart: regular rate and rhythm; without audible murmurs. Abdomen with normal bowel sounds, soft, nontender, no palpable masses. Pelvic examination: external genitalia without lesions, vagina well estrogenized, nulliparous cervical os, uterus anteverted and normal size, adnexa nontender and without palpable masses. Rectovaginal confirms.

### QUESTION 1

*What are the maternal and fetal effects of anticonvulsants?*

### ANSWER 1

1. Vitamin deficiencies
    a. Folate deficiency: All anticonvulsants interfere with folate metabolism and patients can develop macrocytic anemia. Folate deficiency has been suggested as an etiology for the increased risk of neural tube defects observed in patients on certain anticonvulsants (valproic acid and carbamazepine). Although recent data disputes this, most suggest placing these patients on preconception folate supplementation (4 mg/d). Increasing folate ingestion may increase hepatic microsomal enzymatic function and thus clearance of anticonvulsant medications. Therefore, anticonvulsant levels should be checked more frequently after beginning folate administration.

b. Vitamin D deficiency: Phenytoin, phenobarbital, and primidone may increase metabolism of vitamin D, which can potentially cause neonatal hypocalcemia. Patients should be reminded to take prenatal vitamins that contain adequate amounts of vitamin D (5 mg or 200 1U per day.
c. Vitamin K deficiency: Neonatal hemorrhage secondary to deficiency in vitamin K-dependent clotting factors (II, VII, IX, X) is observed occasionally in patients taking phenobarbital, phenytoin, and primidone.

2. Fetal effect: Cardiac, craniofacial, neural tube defects (see above), and minor abnormalities of the digits malformations may be two to three times the risk in the general population and can be found with all anticonvulsants. The etiology of these malformations has been disputed, i.e., are they secondary to the medications (e.g., folic acid deficiency or other entity, as stated earlier) or are they caused by genetic abnormalities that are part of the mother's seizure disorder (e.g., deficiency of the detoxifying enzyme epoxide hydroxylase)? Children of mothers with idiopathic epilepsy have a four times greater risk of developing epilepsy. Risk may be equivalent if father has epilepsy, but some investigators observe that the risk is less.

## QUESTION 2

*What is the suggested preconception counseling in a patient with a seizure disorder?*

## ANSWER 2

Generally patients can be counseled that most women with seizure disorders do well during pregnancy, and have a minimal, but increased, risk of having a child with congenital malformations (as stated earlier).

1. Women with frequent seizures (especially tonic-clonic) should avoid pregnancy until their seizures are under improved control.
2. If the patient has been seizure free for 2–5 years, with the consultation of a neurologist, consider slowly tapering the patient off her anticonvulsive medication over a 1–3-month period. Approximately 50% of patients will relapse over this period and will need to be restarted on their medications.
3. Preconception folate supplementation (4 mg/d through the first trimester).

## QUESTION 3

*What method of postpartum contraception can be recommended to a patient with a seizure disorder?*

## ANSWER 3

Although all methods of contraception are available to patients with seizure disorders, certain medications (carbamazepine, phenobarbital, phenytoin, felbamate, vigabatrin, and topiramate) decrease the effectiveness of combined, and progesterone-only oral hormonal contraceptives pills (OCPs) by enhancing hepatic metabolism and clearance of steroid hormones. One option is for patients to use condoms with OCPs or to use a higher dose OCP (although efficacy of using an OCP with 50 ug mestranol in this setting has not yet been confirmed). This decreased efficacy has not been seen with depot medroxyprogesterone acetate since the progestogen dose received is usually more than adequate. Additionally, this effect is not seen in patients on valproic acid and, possibly, not in patients on gabapentin, lamotrigine, or tiagabine (Table 48-1).

## BIBLIOGRAPHY

ACOG Practice Bulletin No. 18. The use of hormonal contraception in women with coexisting medical conditions. 2000.

ACOG Technical Bulletin No. 231. Seizure disorders in pregnancy. 1996.

Gabbe SG, et al. *Obstetrics: Normal and Problem Pregnancies.* 4th ed. New York: Churchill Livingstone: 2002.

Holmes LB, et al. The teratogenicity of anticonvulsant drugs. *N Engl J Med.* 2001;344:1132–1138.

Pschirrer ER, Mong M. Seizure disorders in pregnancy. *Obstet Gynecol Clin North Am.* 2001;28:601–611.

Yerby MS. The use of anticonvulsants during pregnancy. Semin Perinatol. 2001:25:153–158.

**TABLE 48-1. Interaction of Anticonvulsants and Combination Oral Contraceptives**

| |
|---|
| Anticonvulsants that decrease steroid levels in women taking combination oral contraceptives |
| Barbiturates (including phenobarbital and primidone) |
| Phenytoin |
| Carbamazepine |
| Felbamate |
| Topiramate |
| Vigabatrin |
| Anticonvulsants that do not appear to decrease steroid levels in women taking combination oral contraceptives |
| Valproic acid |
| Gabapentin* |
| Lamotrigine* |
| Tiagabine* |

*Pharmacokinetic study used anticonvulsant dose lower than that used in clinical practice.

SOURCE: From ACOG Practice Bulletin No. 73. The use of hormonal contraception in women with coexisting medical conditions. 2006.

# 49 APPENDICITIS

*Kimberly D. Gregory*

## LEARNING POINT

Diagnostic work up, differential diagnosis of acute abdominal pain during pregnancy, and management of appendicitis in pregnancy

## VIGNETTE

Ms. Jones is a 24-year-old, G5P0, female at 23 weeks gestation who presents complain of nausea, vomiting, and right lower quadrant pain for the past 24 hours. She denies fever, chills, or genitourinary tract symptoms. She has a history of a previous surgery for removal of multiple myomas. A complete blood count (CBC) was obtained which revealed a hematocrit of 39%, and a white cell count (WBC) of 16,000 cells/mm$^3$. Fetal heart rate was noted to be 150 bpm, and uterine irritability was noted on the tocodynameter. The patient denies vaginal bleeding, or ruptured membranes.

### QUESTION 1

*What is the differential diagnosis for pregnant patients presenting with an acute abdomen?*

### ANSWER 1

The differential diagnosis of acute abdomen in pregnancy is the same as for nonpregnant patients including all organs found in the pelvis and can be conceptualized as obstetric, gynecologic, gastrointestinal, or genitourinary etiologies (see Table 49-1). While acute appendicitis probably occurs less often in pregnancy than in nonpregnant, age-matched controls, it is the most common nonobstetric cause of acute abdominal pain occurring in approximately 1/1500 deliveries. It is more common in the sencond trimester, and can be difficult to diagnose.

### QUESTION 2

*What are some reasons that often make it more difficult to diagnose appendicitis during pregnancy?*

### ANSWER 2

Multiple factors contribute to the difficulty in diagnosing appendicitis in pregnancy. For example:

1. Symptoms of anorexia, nausea, and vomiting that often accompany appendicitis, are commonly found during a normal pregnancy.
2. As the uterus enlarges, the appendix moves upward and outward so that pain and tenderness may not be prominent in the right lower quadrant.
3. Some degree of leukocytosis is the rule during normal pregnancy.
4. During pregnancy other disorders can be confused with appendicitis such as pyelonephritis, renal colic, and abruption.
5. Pregnant women (especially late in pregnancy) with appendicitis may not have symptoms considered "typical" or classic for appendicitis (see comment later on).
6. Reluctance to image pregnant women or to perform surgery on pregnant women due to perceived fetal and maternal risks

While displacement of the appendix with uterine enlargement is a "classic" obstetrical pearl, recent studies suggest that right lower quadrant pain is still by far the leading presenting symptom in all three trimesters, and that the appendix can be found in its normal location 80–90% of the time, suggesting that McBurneys point is the accurate site for incision for both gravid and nongravid women.

**TABLE 49-1. Differential Diagnosis of Acute Abdomen in Pregnancy**

| OBSTETRIC CONDITIONS | GYNECOLOGIC CONDITIONS | GASTROINTESTINAL CONDITIONS | GENITOURINARY CONDITIONS |
|---|---|---|---|
| Abruption | Adnexal torsion | Gall bladder disease | Pyelonephritis |
| Chorioamnionitis | Ectopic pregnancy | Pancreatitis | Renal colic |
| Labor | Salpingitis | Inflammatory bowel disease | |
| Endometritis | Degenerating myoma | Adhesions (bowel obstruction) from prior surgery | |

## QUESTION 3

*What new techniques are available for the diagnosis and treatment of appendicitis?*

## ANSWER 3

Historically, appendicitis was a clinical diagnosis based on serial observations and examinations. Today, imaging techniques are available that can aid in the diagnosis and/or development of a differential diagnosis. Ultrasound, a helical computerized tomography (CT), and magnetic reasonic imaging (MRI) (with or without contrast) have all been used to evaluate the appendix and to confirm or refute the diagnosis. Fetal exposure to diagnostic x-rays is low (< 300 mrads); well below that which is considered dangerous during pregnancy (5 rads).

As with nonpregnant patients, the mainstay for surgical management of appendicitis is laparoscopy. Studies have demonstrated the safety of laparoscopy for all three trimesters; albeit most studies report on the use of endoscopy up through the second trimester.

## BIBLIOGRAPHY


Affleck DG, Handrahan DL, Egger MJ, et al. The laparoscopic management of appendicitis and cholelithiasis during pregnancy. *Am J Surg.* 1999;178:523–529.

Andersen B, Nielsen TF. Appendicitis in pregnancy: diagnosis, management, and complications. *Act Obstet Gynecol Scand.* 1999;78:758–762.

Al-Fozan H, Tulandi T. Safety and risks of laparoscopy in pregnancy. *Curr Opin Obstet Gynecol.* 2002;14:375–379.

Birchard KR, Brown MA, Hayslo WB, et al. MRI of acute abdominal and pelvic pain in pregnant patients. *AMR.* 2005;184;452–458.

Castro MA, Shipp TD, Castro EE, et al. The use of helical computed tomography in pregnancy for the diagnosis of acute appendicitis. *Am J Obstet Gynecol.* 2001;184:954–957.

Cobben LP, Groot I, Haans L, et al. MRI for clinically suspected appendicitis during pregnancy. *AJR.* 2004;183:671–675.

Hodjat H, Kazerooni T. Location of the appendix in the gravid patient: a re-evaluation of the established concept. *Int J Gynecol Obstet.* 2003;81:245–247.

Mazze RI, Kallen B. Appendectomy during pregnancy: a Swedish registry study of 778 cases. *Obstet Gynecol.* 1991;77:835.

Mourad J, Elliott JP, Erickson L, et al. Appendicitis in pregnancy: new information that contradicts long held clinical beliefs. *Am J Obstet Gynecol.* 2000;185:1027–1029.

Oto A, Ernest RD, Shah R, et al. Right lower quadrant pain and suspected appendicitis in pregnant women: evaluation with MR imaging—initial experience. *Radiology.* 2005; 234:445–451.

Popkin CA, Lopez PP, Cohn SM, et al. The incision of choice for pregnant women with appendicitis is through McBUrney's point. *Am J Surg.* 2002;183:20–22.

Rizzo AG. Laparoscopic surgery in pregnancy: long term follow up. *J Laparoendo & Adv Surg Techniques Journal abbrev.* 2003;13:11–15.

Rollins MD, Chan KJ, Price RR. Laparoscopy for appendicitis and cholelithiasis during pregnancy: a new standard of care. *Surg Endosc.* 2004;18:237–241.

Scott LD, Abu-Hamda E. Gastrointestinal disease in pregnancy. In Creasy RK, Resnik R (eds.): *Maternal Fetal Medicine.* 5th ed. Philadephia, PA: Saunders, 2004;1109.

Sharp HT. Gastrointestinal surgical conditions during pregnancy. *Clin Obstet Gynecol.* 1994;37:306.

Sivanesaratnam V. The acute abdomen and the obstetrician. *Best Prac & Research in Clin Obstet Gynecol.* 2000;14: 89–102.


# 50 CARDIAC DISEASE IN PREGNANCY

*John Williams III*

## LEARNING POINT

To understand the prevalence, etiology, and effects of maternal cardiac disease in pregnancy.

## VIGNETTE

A 28-year-old, G2P0010, woman at 10 weeks gestational age presents to her obstetrician's office for her first prenatal visit. She gives a history of being born with a congenital heart defect for which she underwent surgical correction at age 2. She remembers being told that her heart defect was tetralogy of Fallot and that the lesion was completely corrected by her surgery. She states that she has some shortness of breath with moderate exertion. Otherwise, she has no symptoms. She would like to know how the pregnancy will affect her underlying heart condition and what her chances are for having a successful pregnancy and a healthy baby.

## QUESTION 1

*What percentage of pregnancies are complicated by maternal cardiac disease? What are the most common etiologies of maternal cardiac disease?*

## ANSWER 1

Approximately 1% of pregnancies in the United States are complicated by maternal cardiovascular disease. The most common etiology is congenital heart disease (CHD). At one time rheumatic heart disease was common. With improved living conditions and antibiotic treatment for streptococcal infections, the incidence of rheumatic fever has decreased substantially. CHD can be categorized into three different functional groups:

1. Left-to-right shunts resulting in volume overload atrial septal defect [ASD], ventricular septal defect [VSD] patent ductus arteriosus (PDA), and the like).
2. Right-to-left shunts resulting in cyanosis (tetralogy of Fallot, Eisenmenger's).
3. Pressure overload (aortic stenosis, coarctation of aorta, idiopathic hypertrophic subaortic stenosis or IHSS, pulmonary hypertension from release of vena caval obstruction and sustained uterine contractions.

## QUESTION 2

*What are the physiologic changes of pregnancy that affect cardiac function?*

## ANSWER 2

1. A 50% increase in intravascular volume occurs by the early to mid third trimester. In patients with myocardial dysfunction, valvular lesions, or ischemic heart disease, volume overload is poorly tolerated and may lead to congestive heart failure or worsening ischemia.
2. Decreased systemic vascular resistance (SVR). This is important in patients with right to left shunts which will be aggravated by decreasing SVR during pregnancy.
3. Pregnancy is a hypercoagulable state. This increases the need for anticoagulation in patients at risk for arterial thrombosis i.e., those with (prosthetic valves and atrial fibrillation).
4. Marked fluctuations in cardiac output, particularly during labor and delivery. Cardiac output can increase by as much as 50% by the late second stage. Potential for dramatic volume shifts occurs during delivery due to postpartum hemorrhage and as a result of "auto transfusion."

## QUESTION 3

*How should women with cardiac disease be counseled about the risks of pregnancy? What are the systems used for classification of risk for women with cardiac disease in pregnancy?*

## ANSWER 3

Counseling the pregnancy cardiac patient about her prognosis for successful pregnancy is somewhat complex. This is because there is no clinically applicable method of measuring the functional capacity of the heart. The New York Heart Association (NYHA) classification based on the patient's history of past and present disability is a useful index for predicting the response to pregnancy (Table 50-1).

Patients in NYHA classes I and II generally do well in pregnancy. Patients in NYHA classes III and IV have increased risk for complications and maternal death. Recently, the NYHA classification has been replaced by a more complex descriptive system based on etiologic, anatomic, and physiologic features (Clark, 1997).

**Group I**. *Minimal risk of complications* (<1% risk for maternal mortality): ASD, VSD, PDA, pulmonic/tricuspid disease, corrected tetralogy of Fallot, bioprosthetic valve, and Mitral stenosis (MS) (NYHA Class I and II). Marfans syndrome with normal aorta.

**Group II**. *Moderate risk of complications* (5–15% risk of maternal mortality): MS with atrial fibrillation or NYHA Class III or IV, artificial valve, aortic stenosis (AS) coarctation of aorta (uncomplicated), uncorrected tetralogy of Fallot, prior myocardial infection

**Group III**. *Major risk of complications or death* (>25% risk of maternal mortality): pulmonary hypertension, coarctation of aorta (complicated), Marfan's syndrome with dilated aorta.

## QUESTION 4

*How should patients with cardiac disease in pregnancy be managed? What are the indications for cesarean section in pregnant patients with cardiac disease?*

**TABLE 50-1. NYHA Classification of Cardiac Disease**

| | |
|---|---|
| Class I. | No limitation of physical activity |
| Class II. | Slight limitation of physical activity. Comfortable at rest but symptoms with ordinary activity |
| Class III. | Marked limitation of physical activity. Comfortable at rest but symptoms with less than ordinary activity |
| Class IV. | Severe limitation of activity. May have symptoms at rest |

## ANSWER 4

1. Optimal management requires a thorough assessment of anatomical and functional capacity of the heart and analysis of how the physiologic changes of a pregnancy will impact cardiac function. Antepartum, patients should receive meticulous prenatal care with judicious use of bed rest for patients in groups II and III. Intrapartum, management includes laboring in left lateral position, epidural anesthesia (except in cases with severe AS and IHSS where hypotension may result in sudden death), administration of $O_2$, and endocarditis prophylaxis.
2. Vaginal delivery is the preferred approach with use of epidural analgesia for effective pain control (except as noted above) and shortening of the second stage with forceps or vacuum extraction. Cesarean section should be reserved for obstetric indications.

## QUESTION 5

*How should this patient be counseled regarding her risk for offspring with congenital heart defects?*

## ANSWER 5

Women with CHD should be advised that they are at increased risk to have a child with congenital heart defects. The risk for CHD in a first degree relative (child, sibling) of an individual with CHD is 2–3%. Patients with CHD should be offered a fetal echocardiogram at 18–22 weeks' gestational age.

## BIBLIOGRAPHY


Burrow GN, Duffy TP (eds.). *Medical Complications During Pregnancy.* 5th ed. Philadelphia, PA: WB Saunders; 1999; 116–122.

Clark SL, et al (eds.). *Critical Care Obstetrics.* 3rd ed. Blackwell Scientific.1997;290–313.

Lupton M, et al. Cardiac disease in pregnancy. *Curr Opin Obstet Gynecol.* 2002;14:137–143.

Meijer JM, Pieper PG, Drenthen W, et al. Pregnancy, fertility, and recurrence risk in corrected tetralogy of Fallot. *Heart.* 2005;91:801–805.

Reimold SC, Rutherford JD. Valvular heart disease in pregnancy. *N Engl J Med.* 2003;349:52–59.

Zuber M, Gautschi N, Oechslin E, et al. Outcome of pregnancy in women with congenital shunt lesions. *Heart.* 1999; 81:271–275.

# Section 4

# OBSTETRICS

## 51 ABNORMAL LABOR

*Calvin J. Hobel*

### LEARNING POINT

Plotting the Friedman's labor curve can help characterize abnormal labor and the identification of the type of abnormal labor can help understand the pathophysiology of abnormal labor.

### VIGNETTE

The patient is a 30-year-old, G1PO, at 40 6/7 weeks gestation who is admitted to the labor and delivery suite at 3 P.M. in the afternoon with symptoms of early labor and premature rupture of the membranes at 10 A.M. She began to have contractions at 12 noon. Her pregnancy was uncomplicated. An early ultrasound at 12 weeks confirmed her gestational age and a repeat ultrasound at 36 weeks indicated that fetal growth was normal. She had a group B beta streptococcus screen at 36 weeks which was negative.

*Physical examination:* The patient's vital signs are normal. Leopold's maneuver indicates that the presentation was vertex, the lie longitudinal and with the fetal back on the right side. The fetal weight is estimated to be 71/2 lb. This is consistent with the fetal measurements by her ultrasound at 36 weeks. The fetal heart tracing shows a baseline heart rate of 155 bpm with fetal heart rate accelerations that suggest that the fetus has a reactive tracing. Vaginal examination shows that the membranes were ruptured and her cervix is 80% affected and the presenting part is at −1 station with a cervical dilation of 3 cm. The pelvic architecture (pelvimetry) is assessed clinically and the inlet, midpelvis (intraspinous) and the posterior aspect of the pelvis (curvature of sacrum and sacrospinous notch), and the outlet intertuberous distance appear normal.

*Labor course:* During the next 2 hours, the patient begins to experience considerable pain with contractions and she receives epidural anesthesia. Over the next 51/2 hours (8:30 P.M.), she progresses to 6 cm cervical dilation and–2 station. From this point on, her progress is slow and by 9:30 P.M. she progresses to 7 cm and +1 station and the strength of her contraction is felt to be inadequate. Internal monitoring of uterine contractions and fetal heart rate is initiated. At this point, the patient developes clinical amnionitis with a maternal temperature of 101.4°F and fetal tachycardia of 170 bpm. She is started on ampicillin and tobramycin. The uterine activity is noted to be hypotonic (Montevideo units <200) and her labor is augmented with oxytocin. Vaginal examination indicates that the position of the fetal head is right occiput anterior with good flexion (normal). For this patient we have superimposed the normal Friedman labor curve (see Fig. 51-1) according to when this patient was admitted into labor. Her progress remains slow and the vertex was still at a zero station after 20 hours of labor.

### QUESTION 1

*We have plotted out her labor course on the attached Friedman labor curve (Fig. 51-1), which shows the normal latent phase. What type of abnormal labor did she have?*

### ANSWER 1

By plotting her labor progress you can see that she has progressed shortly into active phase of labor, producing

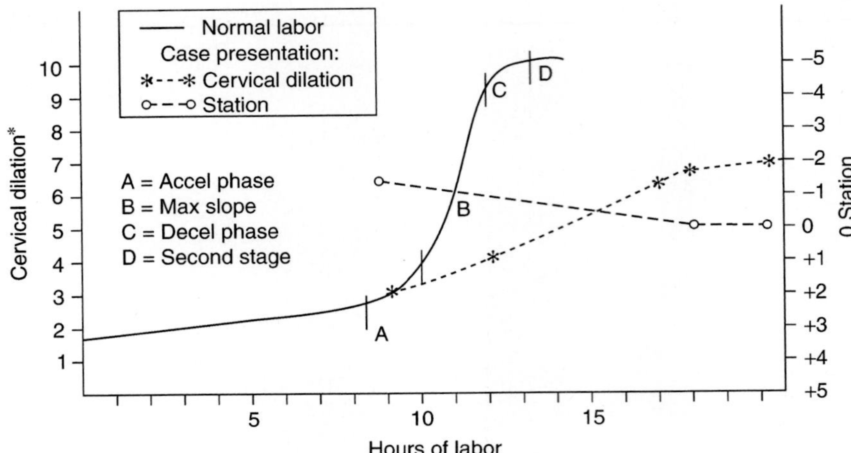


**FIG. 51-1** Friedman's curve of case presentation. *- - *(cervical dilation) superimposed on normal curve (—), o- - o denotes descent (station) of case presentation.

a curve characteristic of *protracted active phase* (<1.2 cm/h) of labor for a woman having her first pregnancy.

## QUESTION 2

*What are the potential etiologies (causes) for this type of abnormal labor?*

## ANSWER 2

1. Abnormalities of expulsion forces: This may be a cause in this patient; however, she was augmented with oxytocin
2. Abnormalities of position of the fetus or abnormality of fetal head: These are unlikely because of normal ultrasound at 36 weeks and normal position 7 A.M.
3. Abnormalities of maternal bony pelvis: This is unlikely because pelvimetry assessment was felt to be normal
4. Abnormal physiology: It is possible that in the presence of amnionitis labor can become abnormal. However, frequently abnormal labor can be due to a combination of factors.

## QUESTION 3

*Define the three stages of labor and provide the upper limits of normal (in hours) for a primigravida and multigravida.*

## ANSWER 3

1. Latent phase of labor begins when a woman perceives regular continuity (usually every 3 minutes with discomfort) as defined onset of labor. The latent phase ends somewhere between 3–5 cm dilation:
   - Nullipara/primigravida = 20 hours (limit)
   - Parous women = 14 hours (limit)
2. Active phase begins when there is a more rapid rate of cervix dilation generally at 3–4 cm:
   - Nulltipara rate 1.2 cm/h
   - Multiparas 1.5 cm/h
3. Second stage of labor begins when the cervical dilation is complete and ends with fetal expulsion:
   - Multipara (limit) equals 2 hours and extended to 3 hours when regional anesthesia is used
   - Multipara (limit) equals 1 hour and extends to hours when regional anesthesia is used

## QUESTION 4

*Define the four times of abnormal labor and consider the etiology for each one.*

## ANSWER 4

1. Prolonged latent phase. The latest phase becomes prolonged when the duration exceeds the limit (stated in answer 3).
   - Etiology may indicate to excessive sedation or conduction anesthesia, unripe cervix, or premature rupture of the membranes at term.

2. Protracted active phase of labor occurs when there is a slow rate of cervical dilation:
   - Less than 1.2 cm in multiparas
   - Less than 1.5 cm in multiparas
   - Etiology may be poor uterine function secondary to infection and/or epidural anesthesia.
3. Arrest of cervical dilation in the active phase of labor is defined as 2 hours without cervical dilation:
   - Most common etiology is cephalopelvic disproportion; however, is not uncommon to have arrest of cervical dilation occurring in patients with a protracted active phase (as in the case presented).
4. Arrest of descent is defined as 1 hour without fetal descent:
   - Most often this occurs in cases of cephalopelvic disproportion. It is not uncommon to observe poor flexion of fetal head and/or arrest in the occiput transverse position.

## BIBLIOGRAPHY


Alexander JM, McIntire DML, Leveno KJ. Chorioamnionbitis and the prognosis for term infants. *Obstet Gynecol.* 1999;94: 274–278.

Cohen WR, Acker DB, Friedman EA. *Management of Labor.* 2nd ed. New York, NY: Aspen Publications; 1989:1–53.

Friedman EA. The graphic analysis of labor. *Am J Obstet Gynecol.* 1954;68:1568–1575.

Satin AJ, Malberry M, Leveno KJ, Sherman ML, Kline DM. Chorio-amnionitis: a harbinger of dystocia, *Obstet Gynecol.* 1992;79:913–915.


# 52 ABRUPTION

*Kimberly D. Gregory*

## LEARNING POINT

To understand and indentify the risk factors for abruption.

## VIGNETTE

A 24-year-old, G3P2, female at 30 weeks gestation with a twin gestation presents after a motor vehicle accident (MVA). She was the passenger and was rear-ended while at a stop light. The approaching car was traveling at approximately 20 miles per hour. She is complaining of abdominal pain, and the tocodynameter reveals occasional contractions with marked uterine irritability. The fetal heart rate is 140 bpm, and reactive. The patient complains of back pain, and vaginal spotting. She denies ruptured membranes. She gives a history of a prior preterm delivery at 34 weeks due to vaginal bleeding. She denies smoking, alcohol, or drug use. On examination, her vital signs are stable. The uterus is soft, nontender, with palpable contractions every 5–7 minutes. An ultrasound is performed and the fetuses are noted to be vertex/breech, diamniotic, dichorionic and size consistent with dates. There is no apparent placental separation noted on ultrasound. The patient's hematocrit is 38%.

### QUESTION 1

*What are the risk factors associated with abruption?*

### ANSWER 1

An abruptio placentae is a separation of a normally implanted placenta prior to birth. Many factors have been associated with abruption. Conditions such as blunt trauma, uterine or umbilical cord anomaly (short cord, myomas at the site of implantation), rupture of membranes with sudden decompression of the uterus, premature rupture of membranes (PROM), multiple gestation, maternal hypertension (both chronic and pregnancy induced) have been associated with abruption, and in fact hypertension is one of the most common risk factors present in approximately 50% of cases. Other reported risk factors include maternal age, parity, inheritable thrombophilias, elevated maternal serum alpha-fetoprotoein (AFP), cigarette smoking, and cocaine use. This patient has several risk factors (blunt trauma after MVA, twin gestation, uterine irritability, vaginal spotting, and a history of prior abruption).

### QUESTION 2

*How would you treat this woman? Is she a candidate for tocolysis?*

### ANSWER 2

Treatment of suspected abruption should be individualized based on maternal status (amount of bleeding, vital signs), fetal status (fetal heart rate, ultrasound documentation of placental hemorrhage/location), ruptured membranes, and gestational age. A term fetus should be delivered. In an otherwise stable mother, a preterm gestation with a fetus who has a normal fetal heart rate tracing can be managed expectantly and/or treated with tocolytics. Although most abruptions present with evidence of vaginal bleeding, approximately 20% can be occult, with retroplacental bleeding that is not externalized; hence, the mother should be monitored closely, and followed with serial hematocrits. Some clinicians favor following fibrinogen levels and coagulation factors as well. Ultrasound is not very sensitive with regard to diagnosing abruptions, especially acutely. Glantz and Parnell reported a sensitivity of 28%, specificity of 99%, PPV 82%, NPV 59% using current day sonographic technology. Since the largest contribution to neonatal mortality and morbidity associated with this diagnosis is due to prematurity, investigators have used expectant management, and judicious use of tocolytics and antenatal corticosteroids to maximize neonatal outcomes.

## QUESTION 3

*How would you counsel this patient regarding recurrence risk of abruption? Does her risk increase with a prior cesarean?*

## ANSWER 3

Depending on the etiology, the risk of recurrence has been reported to be 5.5–16.6%, as much as a tenfold increased risk with subsequent pregnancy. After two consecutive abruptions, the risk of a third increases to 25%. A cesarean delivery in the preceding pregnancy increases the risk of abruption.

## BIBLIOGRAPHY

Ananth CV, et al. Effect of maternal age and parity on the risk of uteroplacental bleeding disorders in prengnacy. *Obstet Gynecol.* 1996;88:511.

Anath CV, et al. Placental abruption and its association with hypertension and prolonged rupture of membrane: a methodologic review and meta-analysis. *Obstet Gynecol.* 1996; 88:309.

Benedetti TJ. Obstetric hemorrhage. In: Gabbe SG, Niebyl JR, Simpson JL (eds.). *Obstetrics Normal and Problem Pregnancies*, 4th ed. *Maternal Fetal Medicine*. 5th ed. Philadephia, PA: Churchill Livingstone; 2002:503.

Glantz C, Purnell L. Clinical utility of sonography in the diagnosis and treatment of placental abruption. *J Ultrasound Med.* 2002;21(8):837–840.

Hladky K, Yankowitz J, Hansen WF. Placental abruption. *Obstet Gynecol Surv.* 2002(57):299–305.

Lydon-Rochelle M, Holt VL, Easterling TR, Martin DP. First-birth cesarean and placental abruption or previa at second birth. *Obst Gynecl.* 2001;97(5, Pt. 1):765–769.

Towers CV, Pircon RA, Heppard M. Is tocolysis safe in the management of third trimester bleeding. *Am J Obstet Gynecol.* 1999;180:1572–1578.

# 53 ANESTHESIA COMPLICATIONS

*Marguerite Lisa Bartholomew*

## LEARNING POINT

Methods, physiology, and complications of obstetrical regional anesthesia.

## VIGNETTE

A 36-year-old, G1P0, is admitted in active labor at 37 weeks gestation. She is healthy and denies medical problems. Her blood pressure is 120/70 mm Hg and heart rate is 80 bpm. The cervical examination is 5 cm dilated, 100% effaced, and 0 station. Contractions are occurring every 2–3 minutes. The fetal heart rate tracing is reassuring. Epidural anesthesia is provided upon request. Five minutes after placement of the epidural, fetal bradycardia is noted down to 80 bpm. The patient's blood pressure is 80/40 mm Hg and she complains of dizziness. She is turned to the left lateral decubitus position, administered a bolus of 250 cc of IV lactated Ringers solution, and receives 5 mg of ephedrine. After 5 minutes, the deceleration spontaneously recovers and maternal blood pressure is 128/76 mm Hg. Seven hours later, she vaginally delivers a vigorous male infant. On postpartum day one, she develops a severe headache that is exacerbated by sitting upright. An epidural blood patch is placed with resolution of the headache.

## QUESTION 1

*What are the pain pathways associated with the first and second stage of labor?*

## ANSWER 1

Pain during the first stage of labor results primarily from uterine contractions and cervical dilation. Painful sensations travel from the uterus via sympathetic nerves and enter the spinal cord at thoracic levels 10, 11, and 12.

Pain during the second stage of labor results primarily from distention of the pelvic floor, vagina, and perineum. The sensory fibers of sacral nerves 2, 3, and 4 (pudendal nerve) transmit painful impulses to the spinal cord.

## QUESTION 2

*What are the anatomic layers that must be traversed to get to the epidural space to effect epidural anesthesia, and at what level is the needle inserted? What is the coaxial technique?*

## ANSWER 2

The anatomic layers that the epidural traverses to reach the epidural space are (in order, from out to in): skin, subcutaneous tissue, interspinous ligament, ligamentum flavum, and epidural space (Fig. 53-1). The subarachnoid space is deep to the epidural space. The epidural needle and catheter are usually inserted at approximately L4 (L2– 4). The lumbar technique allows preservation of sensory and motor function of the perineum and lower extremities with lower doses of local anesthetic. Higher doses of local anesthetic can be used to remove perineal sensation; however, motor function may also be removed.

The coaxial technique allows medication to be placed in the epidural space and the subarachnoic space (spinal effect). The spinal infiltration is performed with a very small needle pushed through the usual epidural needle. The coaxial technique is favored because it has rapid onset, uses very small doses of medication, allows ambulation, and has fewer side effects (very low risk of high spinal and same risk of spinal headache as epidural) than the usual lumbar epidural.

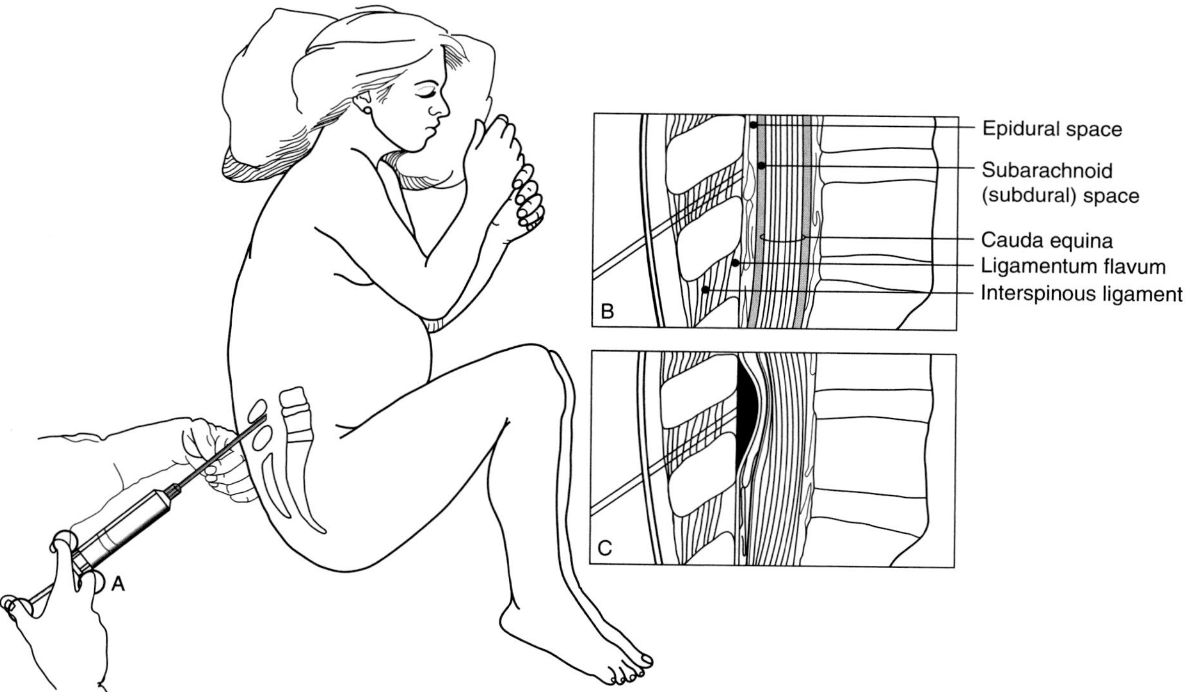


**FIG. 53-1** Technique of lumbar epidural puncture.

SOURCE: Reprinted with permission from Hawkins JL, Chestnut DH, Gibbs CP. Obstetric anesthesia. In: Gabbe S, Niebyl JR, Simpson JL (eds.). *Obstetrics: Normal and Problem Pregnancies.* 4th ed. Philadelphia, PA: Churchill Livingstone; 2002:431–472.

## QUESTION 3

*What are the complications of regional anesthesia in obstetrics? How are they avoided and treated?*

## ANSWER 3

Complications of regional anesthesia in obstetrical patients include:

1. *Death:* Total anesthesia related death occurs in 1.7/1,000,000 live births. Epidural related death occurs in 1.9/1,000,000 live births, and the death rate due to general anesthesia during c-section is 32/1,000,000.
2. *Hypotension:* Occurs after 10% of epidural blocks during labor because of sympathetic blockade and subsequent lower extremity vasodilatation with venous pooling. Venous return decreases with subsequent decreased cardiac output and hypotension. Sympathectomy occurs as a result of the local anesthetic component. Fetal heart rate decelerations may occur and are reversible. The risk of hypotension is reduced by prior IV hydration and uterine displacement. Hypotension is treated with uterine displacement, trendelenburg, IV hydration, and vasopressors. Ephedrine is drug of choice because of its alpha and beta agonist actions and because it is less likely to cause decreased uteroplacental perfusion. Patients with preeclampsia are very sensitive to the hypotensive effects of regional anesthesia (spinal more than epidural); in the setting or preeclampsia, aggressive prophylaxis and slow administration is recommended.
3. *Local anesthesia toxicity:* The incidence of systemic local anesthetic toxicity after lumbar epidural is 0.01%. Central nervous system (CNS) effects are usually first and include excitation, bizarre behavior, ringing in the ears, disorientation, and convulsions, which are usually self-limited. Convulsion due to local anesthetic toxicity was the most common damaging obstetric anesthesia event in a review of closed claims (83% had CNS injury or maternal or neonatal death). Cardiovascular effects may occur after convulsions and include hypertension and tachycardia. Toxicity occurs when the local anesthetic is injected into a vessel or when the dose is miscalculated. The maximum recommended dose of lidocaine is 4 mg/kg without epinephrine and 7 mg/kg with epinephrine. One mL of 1% lidocaine contains 10 mg of lidocaine (not 1 mg). For a 70 kg person, the dose is then about 28 cc without epinephrine and 50 cc with epinephrine. Bupivacaine 0.75% is no longer recommended for use in obstetric patients due to the possibility of prolonged cardiotoxicity. If used, bupivacaine should be given in dilute forms (0.5%) and administered very slowly. Prevention includes using a test dose before the therapeutic dose, careful calculation of doses, and careful placement to avoid vessels. Treatment is limited to supportive care, including oxygen, hydration, cardiovascular support, intubation, anticonvulsants for prolonged convulsions, and delivery if pregnancy impedes resuscitation.
4. *Allergic reaction:* Allergy to local anesthetics is very rare. Allergy to the ester types (chlorprocaine, procaine, tetracaine) is more common than allergy to the amide types (lidocaine, bupivacaine, proivacaine). Side effects from the concomitant epinephrine (palpitations, nausea, and the like) can be mistaken for allergy by patients. Symptoms of rash, hives, or dyspnea should be treated as allergy. Patients with history of allergy can use a local anesthetic from the other group or use narcotics as an alternative.
5. *High or total spinal:* This is defined as a level of anesthesia that rises to the level of the phrenic nerve/diaphragm (C3–5) nerve roots (Fig. 53-2). The incidence of high spinal anesthesia after epidural is less than 0.03%; after a spinal, the risk is 0.2%. Earlier in the process, accessory muscle paralysis will result in apprehension and anxiety. Dyspnea should always be taken seriously. Numbness of hands and fingers indicates a C6–8 level block, numbness of the lower arm C6, and upper arm C5. Numbness at the neck and shoulder, or respiratory arrest, indicates a C2–4 block. Prevention includes careful calculation of doses, avoiding unintentional subarachnoid injection, and careful positioning after spinal administration (spinal anesthesia is affected by patient position, more than epidural). Treatment includes cardiovascular supportive care with oxygen and early intubation. A high index of suspicion for ensuing symptoms is important.
6. *Neurologic injury:* Nerve injury occurs in 0.06% of spinals and 0.02% of epidurals. Reports of paralysis and back pain in the past were found to be related to preservatives in the formulations (sodium bisulfite and EDTA); modern formulations do not contain preservatives. Epidural hematomas are exceedingly rare, but can cause permanent paralysis if not recognized promptly and decompressed emergently. Coagulopathy is a contraindication to epidural or spinal anesthesia.
7. *Chronic back pain:* Chronic back pain is not caused by epidural anesthesia. The incidence of back pain after childbirth is 44% at 2 months and 49% at 18 months, with or without epidural.
8. *Spinal headache:* Caused by a punctured dura that continues to leak cerebrospinal fluid (wet tap). The incidence is 1–3% and is dependent on the experience of the operator. If a wet tap occurs, headache occurs

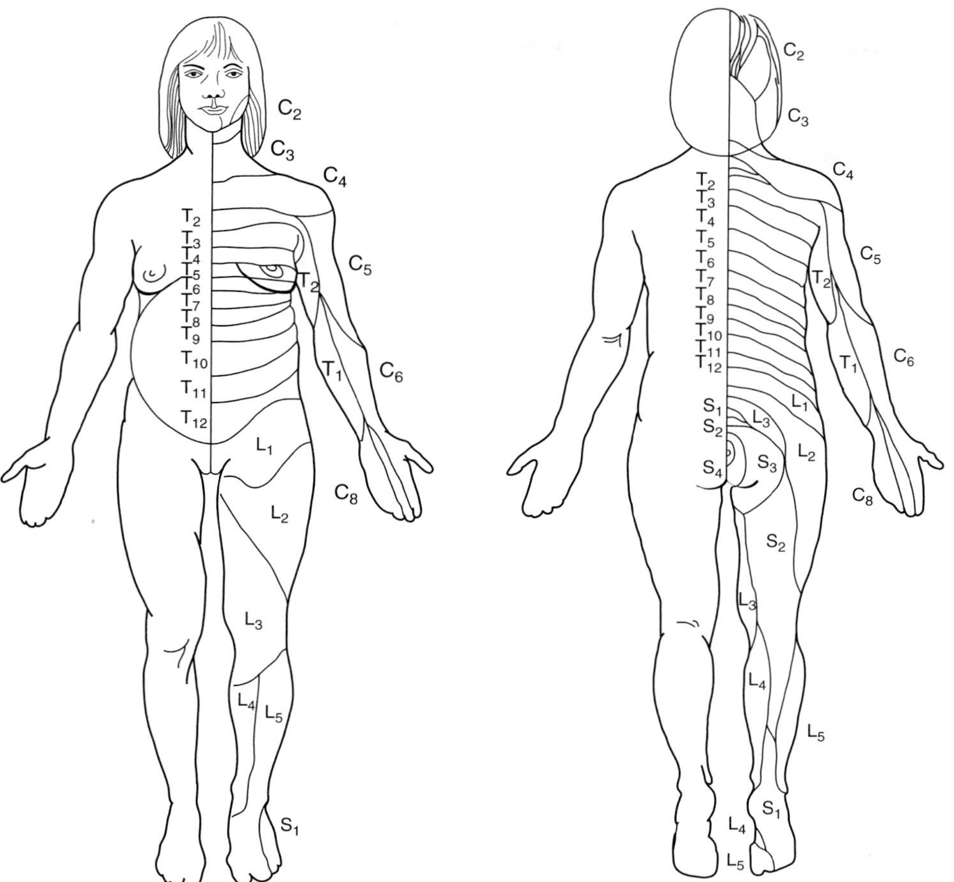


**FIG. 53-2** Dermatome chart.
SOURCE: Reprinted with permission from: Hawkins JL, Chestnut DH, Gibbs CP. Obstetric anesthesia. In: Gabbe S, Niebyl JR, Simpson JL (eds.). *Obstetrics: Normal and Problem Pregnancies.* 4th ed. Philadelphia, PA: Churchill Livingstone; 2002:431–472.

in 70% of patients. There is less risk with spinal than epidural because smaller needles are used in spinals. There is no prevention except for good technique. Treatment includes supine positioning, oral analgesics, caffeine, and hydration. A blood patch can be used if conservative treatment is ineffective; 15 cc of the patients own blood is placed into the epidural space. There is a +95% cure rate with blood patch placement, and prophylactic blood patches have been found to be preventative in some series.

9. *Slower progress of labor:* There is great controversy about progress of labor and mode of delivery in the presence of epidural. Several randomized prospective studies have shown an increased risk of cesarean delivery while others observed no increased risk. The increased risk is found mostly in those patients who receive an epidural early in labor. It is almost impossible to do a randomized controlled trial because of the large crossover rate. Prolonged labor (by 40–90 minutes), increased need for oxytocin (twofold increase), and increased rate of operative vaginal delivery (RR 1.9) have been demonstrated in these patients in prospective studies and meta-analyses. The ACOG Task Force on cesarean delivery rates (2000) recommended that "when feasible the administration of epidural anesthesia in nulliparous woman should be delayed until cervical dilation reaches 4–5 cm and other forms of analgesia be used until that time." However, an ACOG practice bulletin (July 2002) states, "In the absence of a contraindication, maternal request is a sufficient medical indication for pain relief in labor."

## BIBLIOGRAPHY


ACOG Practice Bulletin No. 36. Obstetric Analgesia and Anesthesia 2002.

Breen TW, et al: Factors associated with back pain after childbirth. *Anesthesiology.* 1994;81:29.

Groves PA, et al. Natural history of postpartum back pain and its relationship with epidural anesthesia. *Anesthesiology.* 1994;81:A1167.

Hawkins JL, Chestnut DH, Gibbs CP. Obstetric anesthesia. In: Gabbe S, Niebyl JR, Simpson JL (eds.).: *Obstetrics: Normal and Problem Pregnancies*. 4th ed. Philadelphia, PA: Churchill Livingstone; 2002:431–472.

Thorp JA, et al. Epidural analgesia and cesarean section for dystocia. *Am J Perinatol.* 1991;8:402–410.

Traynor JD, et al. Is the management of epidural analgesia associated with an increased risk of cesarean delivery? *Am J Obstet Gynecol.* 2000;182:1058–1062.

# 54 CHORIOAMNIONITIS

*Kevin R. Justus*

## LEARNING POINT

The diagnosis of chorioamnionitis is associated with significant morbidity.

## VIGNETTE

A 34-year-old woman, G1P0, comes to labor and delivery at 30 weeks of gestation complaining of pelvic pressure and occasional contractions. Her pregnancy was dated by a first trimester ultrasound, which was consistent with her first day of last menstrual period. Physical examination of the cervix demonstrates what appears to be a dilated external cervical os of 2 cm of dilation. Cervical cultures are obtained and a saline wet prep is performed and is negative for bacterial vaginosis. A fetal fibronectin screen is done and returns positive. A detailed ultrasound is performed and reveals a normally growing fetus, with no apparent anomalies. The amniotic fluid index was 13 cm/$H_2O$. The transvaginal ultrasound revealed a cervical length of 1.2 cm with a 1.5 × 2.0 cm "V" shaped funnel. No dynamic changes were noted. Therapy with magnesium sulfate and corticosteroids was initiated. When contractions persisted, amniocentesis was performed to evaluate for intra-amniotic infection.

### QUESTION 1

*What are the risk factors for chorioamnionitis?*

### ANSWER 1

Chorioamnionitis is an intrauterine infection of the fetal membranes and amniotic fluid. It is classically seen in premature rupture of membranes, however, it may occur in preterm premature rupture of membranes. Most cases occur in 90% of deliveries at term, and of those term infants approximately 5% will be affected. The risk factors are mainly those of complicated or prolonged labor. Low parity, prolonged duration of membrane rupture, prolonged duration of labor, larger number of vaginal examinations, and duration of internal fetal monitoring have all been associated with the development of chorioamnionitis.

### QUESTION 2

*What are the histological findings in chorioamnionitis and its significance?*

### ANSWER 2

Chorioamnionitis refers to both the clinical and subclinical syndromes of intrauterine infection and the cellular and molecular processes that accompany these infections including the presence of mononuclear cells and polymorphonuclear leukocytes within the chorion. One of the most consistent observations that occur in preterm birth is the increased likelihood of histological chorioamnionitis. Most cases of histological chorioamnionitis are caused by infection (see Fig. 54-1).

### QUESTION 3

*What findings on amniocentesis fluid would support a diagnosis of intra-amnionitc infection?*

### ANSWER 3

Test that are currently done and available at a clinical lab would include measurement of amniotic fluid glucose concentration (<14 mg/dL in intrauterine infections), quantitative measures of white blood cell count (>50 cells/$mm^3$), gram stain for the presence of bacteria, interleukin-6 (IL-6) concentration (>11.30 ng/mL), and amniotic fluid culture.

### QUESTION 4

*What is the relationship of chorioamnionitis and cerebral palsy?*

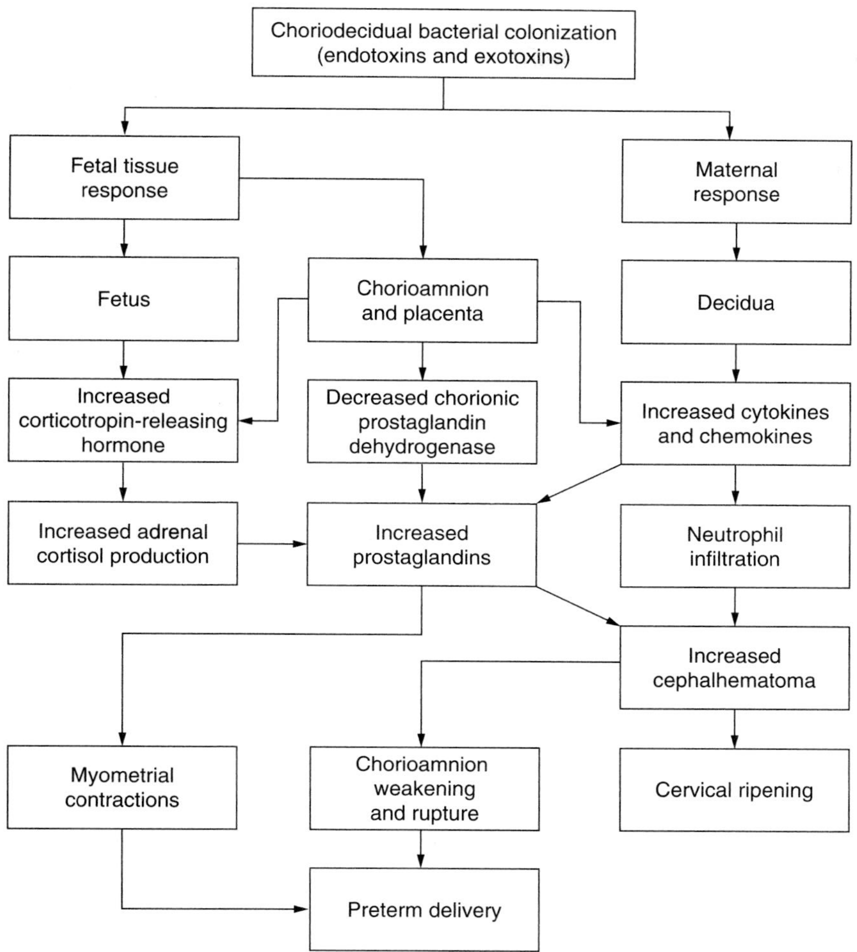


**FIG. 54-1** Potential pathways from choriodecidual bacterial colonization to preterm delivery.

## ANSWER 4

A number of studies now link chorioamnionitis to the development of cerebral palsy. It appears that the earlier the chorioamnionitis occurs in gestation, the greater the association with cerebral palsy. Among term infants, chorioamnionitis increases the background risk of cerebral palsy from 3/1000 to 8/1000 live births. In a number of studies, intrauterine infection has been associated with fetal intracranial hemorrhage and periventricular leukomalacia, a precursor of cerebral palsy.

## BIBLIOGRAPHY


Alexander JM, McIntire DM, Leveno KJ. Chorioamnionitis and the prognosis for term infants. *Obstet Gynecol.* 1999;94: 274–278.

Benirschke K, Kaufmann P. *Pathology of the Human Placenta.* New York, NY: Springer-Verlag; 2000.

Goldenberg RL, Hauth JC, Andrews WW. Intrauterine infection and preterm delivery. *N Engl J Med.* 2000;342:1500.

Hillier SL, Marlius J, Krohn M. A case controlled study of chorioamnionitis infection and histologic chorioamnionitis. *N Engl J Med.* 1988;3198:972–978.

Odibo AO, Rodis JF, Sanders MM, Borgida AF, Wilson F, Egan JF, Campbell WA. Relationship of amniotic fluid markers of intra-amniotic infection with histopathology in cases of preterm labor with intact membranes. *J Perinatol.* 1999; 19:407–412.

Rouse D, Landon M, Leveno K, et al. The maternal fetal medicine units cesarean registry: chorioamnionitis at term and its duration-relationship to outcomes, *Am J Obstet Gynecol.* 2004;1:211–216.

Soper DE, Mayhall CG, Froggatt JW. Characterization and control of intra-amniotic infection in an urban teaching hospital. *Am J Obstet Gynecol.* 1996;175:304–310.

Wu YW, Colford JM Jr. Chorioamnionitits as a risk factor for cerebral palsy: a meta-analysis. *JAMA*. 2000;294:1417.

Wu YW, Escobar G, Grether J, Croen L, Greene J, Newman T. Chorioamnionitis and cerebral palsy in term and near term infants. *JAMA*. 2003;290:2677–2684.

Yoon BH, Romero R, Kim CJ, Jun JK, Gomez R, Choi JH. Amniotic fluid interleukin-6: a sensitive test for antenatal diagnosis of acute inflammatory lesions of preterm placenta and prediction of perinatal morbidity. *Am J Obstet Gynecol*. 1995;172:960–970.

Yoon BH, Romero R, Park JS, Kim SH, Choi JH, Han TR. Fetal exposure to an intra-amniotic inflammation and the development of cerebral palsy at the age of three years. *Am J Obstet Gynecol*. 2000;182:675.

# 55 DIABETIC KETOACIDOSIS IN PREGNANCY

*Marguerite Lisa Bartholomew*

## LEARNING POINT

Diabetic ketoacidosis (DKA) is a medical emergency that should be reversed rapidly to avoid complications for mother and fetus.

## VIGNETTE

A 27-year-old, G2P01-0-1, at 33 weeks gestation, is hospitalized after being seen at her obstetrician's office. She reports malaise, chills, nausea and vomiting, and back pain for 2 days. She has a history of pregestational diabetes diagnosed when she was 5 years old. She has been on an insulin pump for 6 years with satisfactory control. She denies retinopathy and neuropathy. In the first trimester, a 24-hour urine indicated a creatinine clearance of 100 cc/min and 500 mg protein/24 h.

Initial evaluation reveals a temperature of 38.5°C, pulse of 110 bpm, respiratory rate of 30 breaths/min, and blood pressure of 100/60. The fetal heart rate tracing indicates a baseline of 160 bpm, minimal variability, and occasional late decelerations coinciding with occasional contractions. The lungs are clear, and the abdomen is nontender. There is costovertebral angle tenderness on the left. The urine appears cloudy with positive white cells, +1 protein, and +2 ketones on dipstick.

Other laboratory findings include:

1. Hematocrit of 34%
2. Glucose of 270 mg/dL
3. Sodium of 130 mg/dL
4. Potassium of 5.0 mmol/L
5. Chloride of 106 mmol/L
6. Bicarbonate of 11 mmol/L
7. Anion gap (AG) of 19
8. Blood urea nitrogen of 23 mg/dL
9. Creatinine of 1.0 mg/dL
10. Positive serum acetone
11. Blood gas of pH 7.2, $PO_2$ 98%, $PCO_2$ 30%

She is diagnosed with pyelonephritis and DKA. Intravenous (IV) fluids are started including IV insulin, ampicillin, and gentamycin. She is transferred to the obstetrical intensive care unit (ICU) and the fetus is monitored continuously.

### QUESTION 1

*Describe the pathophysiology of DKA and how pregnancy affects its development.*

### ANSWER 1

DKA is a life-threatening complication of diabetes mellitus caused by severe insulin deficiency. The maternal mortality in treated cases is 1% although fetal mortality has been reported to exceed 50%. DKA is a condition characterized by metabolic acidosis, dehydration, and hyperglycemia.

The pathophysiology of DKA is depicted in Fig. 55-1. Without insulin, glucose cannot be transported into the cells of many tissues (e.g., muscle and fat). In response, hormones are produced to promote glucose production inside the cell (i.e., glucagon, cortisol, and catecholamines). As a result, gluconeogenesis and lipolysis increases so that there is a substrate for cellular energy production. The products of lipolysis include ketones (acetone, acetoacetate, and beta-hydroxybutyrate), which are alternative sources of nutrition and energy for the cell.

Unfortunately, ketones are also moderately strong acids that cause a fall in blood pH. In an attempt to normalize the pH by decreasing serum $CO_2$ hyperventilation (or kussmaul breathing) ensues, thereby resulting in a compensatory respiratory alkalosis. Serum bicarbonate ($HCO_3^-$) levels drop as buffers are consumed and the AG increases accordingly (every 1 meq increase in AG = 1 mm/L drop in $HCO_3^-$). Simultaneously, hyperglycemia resulting from the heightened gluconeogenesis causes glycosuria and osmotic diuresis, which results in further water and electrolyte loss.

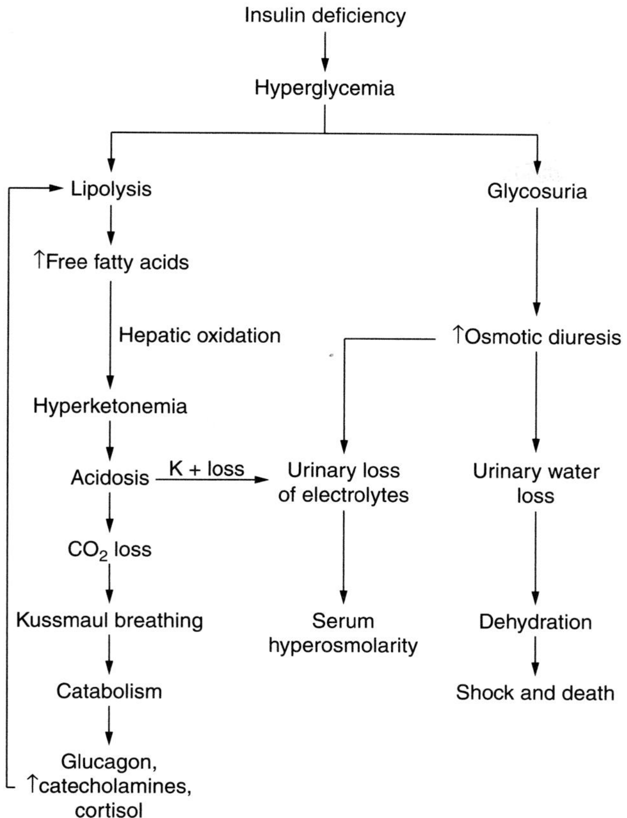


**FIG. 55-1** Physiology of events in diabetic ketoacidosis (DKA). SOURCE: Modified with permission from Foley M. Diabetic ketoacidosis in pregnancy. In: Foley M, Strong T (eds.). *Obstetric Intensive Care: A Practical Guide.* Philadelphia, PA: WB Saunders. 1997:161.

Pregnancy is a state of relative insulin resistance with an increased tendency toward ketosis. These physiologic changes create a lower threshold for the development of DKA in the pregnant patient. DKA has been observed in pregnant patients with plasma glucose levels as low as 180 mg/dL. Furthermore, there is no correlation between the severity of the hyperglycemia and the severity of ketoacidosis in DKA, regardless of the presence or not.

## QUESTION 2

*Outline the acute treatment of DKA during pregnancy.*

## ANSWER 2

The acute treatment of DKA involves four strategies: (a) correction of hypovolemia, (b) insulin therapy, (c) electrolyte correction (most importantly potassium), and (d) identification and treatment of the inciting event. The most common inciting event is infection. Other causes include decreased insulin intake, surgery, trauma, myocardial ischemia, and use of certain medications (e.g., beta-mimetic agents, corticosteroids, and the like). Specific steps should include:

1. Placement of IV line and Foley catheter. Assessment of patient and fetus with physical examination, fetal monitoring, fluid input and output, and laboratory testing (complete blood count, electrolytes, calcium, magnesium, phosphate, $HCO_3^-$, AG, blood gas, serum acetone). A detailed flow sheet should be created, and transfer to intensive care should be considered.
2. Begin IV fluids as soon as possible. Estimate volume deficit to be 100 mL/kg (7–10 L). Start with normal saline and replace 1000 cc in first hour; 500–1000 mL/h for the next 2–4 hours, and then 250 mL/h until patient is 75% replaced. Attempt to get to 75% replacement within 24 hours and 100% replacement within 48 hours. Monitor the electrolytes and fluid balance; if serum sodium increases above 150 mEq/L, switch to 0.45 normal saline.
3. Begin insulin drip. Note tissues that become more resistant to insulin in an acidotic environment. Give an IV bolus of 10–20 units (or 0.2–0.4 units/kg) of regular insulin followed by an infusion of 2–10 units/h (or 0.1 units/kg/h). Monitor serum glucose every hour. If serum glucose is not decreased by 20% within the first 2 hours, double the infusion rate. The decrease in glucose level should not exceed 75/h to avoid rapid changes in serum osmolarity which can precipitate cerebral edema. Begin IV Dantrose 5% in normal saline when the plasma glucose reaches 250 mg/dL. Continue IV insulin until $HCO_3^-$ and AG are normalized ($HCO_3^-$ 18–31 mEq/L and AG <12). After patient is on a regular diet, start subcutaneous insulin before insulin drip is discontinued to avoid rebound hyperglycemia.
4. Follow electrolytes every 2–4 hours. Total body potassium ($K^+$) is depleted by about 5–10 mEq/kg despite the initial hyperkalemia caused by a relative lack of insulin. Insulin therapy, will push $K^+$ into cells thereby, treating the high K in the serum. Do not replace K until the serum level falls to below 5 mEq/L, then give 30–40 mEq/L to replace total body stores.
5. Follow levels of phosphate (usually low in serum) and sodium (total body stores low). Replace phosphate judiciously because rapid replacement may cause hypocalcemia. Potassium phosphate should be considered for potassium replacement if phosphate is <2.0 mg/dL. Sodium is typically replaced when using normal saline. Expect chloride to increase with volume therapy (increased clearance increases

chloride reabsorption in kidneys) and infusion of chloride solutions.

6. The use of sodium bicarbonate (44 mEq in 1 liter 0.45 normal saline) is controversial. It has not been shown to be helpful in the treatment of DKA during pregnancy, although it is recommended if the pH is <7.1 to protect the fetus from acidosis. The goal is not to overcorrect the pH, but to maintain some degree of metabolic acidosis to improve oxygen delivery to the fetus, as oxygen-hemoglobin affinity is increased with alkalosis. Rapid correction of acidosis with bicarbonate can cause hyperosmolarity, hypotension, reduced cardiac output, and increased serum lactate levels.

## QUESTION 3

*What is the endpoint for the treatment of DKA?*

## ANSWER 3

The hallmark of DKA is the combination of hyperglycemia and low serum bicarbonate, typically described as an $HCO_3^-$ of less than 20 mEq/L in the nonpregnant patient; however, the normal $HCO_3^-$ level in pregnancy is between 18–21 mEq/L. The increase in ketoacids should produce an elevated AG; however this is variable, and can be normal in DKA. The renal excretion of ketones is accompanied by an increase in chloride reabsorbtion in the renal tubules, and the resulting hyperchloremia may limit the AG.

The most accurate indicator of resolving DKA is the AG and $HCO_3^-$ levels, used together and not individually. During therapy with insulin and IV fluids, the high AG will begin to decrease while the serum $HCO_3^-$ will remain low because of the dilutional effect of the IV fluids, resulting in a normal AG acidosis or a hyperchloremic metabolic acidosis. The hyperchloremia is due to the chloride load in the IV fluids and the increased renal reabsorbtion of chloride. The pH and the $HCO_3^-$ may not change immediately despite the fact that the DKA is resolving, hence, giving the false impression that the ketoacids are not being cleared.

The best endpoint is the ratio of the AG excess to bicarbonate ($HCO_3^-$) deficit because it takes into account the shift in the pattern of acidosis. The ratio approaches 1.0 with pure organic acidosis and will decrease during therapy of DKA as the expected hyperchloremic metabolic acidosis develops. This ratio is calculated as:

$$\text{AG excess}/HCO_3^- \text{ deficit} = (\text{AG} - 12)/(24 - HCO_3^-)$$

## QUESTION 4

*Why is the fetus at risk for death during DKA, and when is delivery recommended?*

## ANSWER 4

The fetus is at an increased risk of sudden fetal death due to reduced fetal oxygenation stemming from: (a) placental hypoperfusion as a result of maternal hypovolemia, (b) fetal fluid and electrolyte imbalances, and (c) an increased fetal acid load. Correction of the DKA rapidly reverses the untoward fetal effects. Urgent delivery is not recommended for the indication of DKA alone, and delivery during DKA should be reserved only for those fetuses that continue to have nonreasuring testing despite correction of the maternal metabolic state.

## BIBLIOGRAPHY

Foley M. Diabetic ketoacidosis in pregnancy. In: Foley M, Strong T (eds.). *Obstetric Intensive Care: A Practical Guide*. Philadelphia, PA: Saunders; 1997:158.

Landon, MB, Patrick M, Catalano PM, Gabbe SG. Diabetes mellitus In: Gabbe S, Niebyl JR, Simpson JL (eds.). *Obstetrics: Normal and Problem Pregnancies.* 4th ed. Philadelphia, PA: Churchill Livingstone; 2002:1101.

Marino P. The organic acidoses. In: Marino P (ed.). *The ICU Book.* 2nd ed. Philadelphia, PA: Lea & Febiger; 1998:604.

# 56 ACUTE FATTY LIVER OF PREGNANCY

*Jasvant Adusumalli*

## LEARNING POINT

Etiology, evaluation, and treatment of acute fatty liver of pregnancy (AFLP).

## VIGNETTE

A 36-year-old female, G1P0, at 34 4/7 weeks with twin gestation, presents to the labor and delivery unit with a four day history of nausea, vomiting, and epigastric pain. She also states that she has not eaten in 2 days, and her skin and eyes appear to have changed color slightly. Her prenatal course until now has been uneventful. Blood pressure readings and prenatal laboratory studies have all been in the normal range. She had chorionic villus sampling performed at 12 weeks, and the karyotypes are both normal 46, XY. Her past medical history and surgical history are noncontributory. She takes only prenatal vitamins and denies smoking, alcohol, or drug use. Family history is significant for hypertension in both parents.

The physical examination reveals:

Temperature: 98.6°F, BP: 131/81, pulse: 87 bpm, rate: 18/min
General: no acute distress, but general malaise noted
Head, ears, eyes, nose, and throat scleral icterus
Cardiovascular: regular rate and rhythm, normal $S_1$ and $S_2$
Respiratory: lungs clear to auscultation
Abdomen: slight right upper quadrant tenderness upon palpation, no rebound or guarding, normal bowel sounds
Extremities: no cyanosis, clubbing, or edema
Cervix: closed, long, high
Tocometer: no contractions
Fetal monitoring: twin A: 140s bpm, reactive
twin B: 140s bpm, reactive
Ultrasound: reveals breech/breech presentation and no other abnormalities.

## QUESTION 1

*What are the most common symptoms observed in AFLP?*

## ANSWER 1

Acute fatty liver of pregnancy occurs in about 1 in 10,000 deliveries and most commonly occurs in the third trimester. It is characterized by microvesicular fatty infiltration of hepatocytes, and is more frequent in pregnancies with male fetuses or multiple gestations. Over half of the patients with AFLP develop preeclampsia. Severely affected patients may develop fulminant hepatic failure, encephalopathy, hypoglycemia, and renal failure. The most common symptoms of AFLP include:

- Nausea
- Vomiting
- Epigastric pain
- Headache
- Jaundice
- Anorexia
- Central nervous system disturbances

## QUESTION 2

*What laboratory values are seen in AFLP?*

## ANSWER 2

Serum transaminases are moderately elevated although the AST and ALT are generally less than 1000 IU per L, prothrombin time and partial thromboplastin time are prolonged, fibrinogen is decreased, glucose may be decreased, and bilirubin is elevated. In contrast to viral hepatitis, serum transaminases are lower, and platelet counts may be mildly decreased (100,000 to 150,000/mm$^3$), although higher than values seen in the hemolysis, elevated liver, low platelet (HELLP) syndrome (Table 56-1).

**TABLE 56-1. Laboratory Findings in 62 Women with Acute Fatty Liver of Pregnancy**

| | | LABORATORY VALUES—MEAN ±1 SD (RANGE) | | | | |
|---|---|---|---|---|---|---|
| SERIES | PATIENTS | PLASMA FIBRINOGEN (mg/dL) | FIBRIN SPLIT PRODUCTS (μG/mL) | PLATELETS ($10^3$/μL) | CREATININE (mg/dL) | AST (U/L) |
| Usta et al (1994) | 14 | 139 ± 79<br>(37–110) | ND | 126 ± 96 | 2.4 ± 1.0<br>(1.1–3.6) | 1067 ± 1098<br>(200–3670) |
| Castro et al (1996a) | 28 | 125<br>(32–446) | ND | 113<br>(11–186) | 2.5<br>(1.1–5.2) | 210<br>(45–1200) |
| Parkland Hospital | 20 | 134<br>(35–380) | 50<br>(16–256) | 131<br>(9–300) | 2.2<br>(0.9–4.3) | 430<br>(53–1160) |

AST = aspartate aminotransferase; ND = not done.
SOURCE: Adapted with permission from Cunningham FG, et al. *Williams Obstetrics*. 21st ed. New York: McGraw-Hill; 2001:567–618.

## QUESTION 3

*What genetic finding has been linked to the development of AFLP?*

## ANSWER 3

Inherited long-chain 3-hydroxyacyl CoA dehydrogenase deficiency (LCHAD) has been associated with the development of AFLP. This enzyme is important in mitochondrial beta-oxidation of fatty acids, and its deficiency leads to the accumulation of long-chain 3-hydroxyacyl metabolites produced by the fetus or placenta. These metabolites are toxic to the liver and may be the cause of liver dysfunction in many cases. In addition, LCHAD in the neonate has been associated with dilated cardiomyopathy, progressive neuromyopathy, and nonketotic hypoglycemia, and therefore it is important to exclude LCHAD in both mother and infant.

## QUESTION 4

*What is the treatment of AFLP?*

## ANSWER 4

The first course of action is maternal stabilization, including:

- Reversal of coagulopathy by the administration of packed red cells, cryoprecipitate, fresh frozen plasma, or platelets, as needed.
- Glucose infusion.
- Lactulose administration, if ammonia levels are elevated.
- Careful monitoring of fluid status and renal function.

Following maternal stabilization, the treatment of AFLP is prompt delivery.

## BIBLIOGRAPHY

Cunningham FG, et al. *Williams Obstetrics*. 21st ed. New York: McGraw-Hill; 2001:567–618.

Davidson KM, et al. Acute fatty liver of pregnancy in triplet gestation. *Obstet Gynecol.* 1998;91:806.

Hunt CM, Sharara AI. Liver disease in pregnancy. *Am Fam Physician.* 1999;59:(4):829.

McGehee WG, Ouzounian JG, Shaw KJ, et al. Disseminated intravascular coagulation and antithrombin III depression in acute fatty liver of pregnancy. *Am J Obstet Gynecol.* 1996;174:211.

Riely, CA. Acute fatty liver of pregnancy. *Semin Liver Dis.* 1987; 7:47.

Sims H, Brackett J, Powell C, et al. The molecular basis of pediatric long chain 3-hydroxyacyl-CoA dehydrogenase deficiency associated with maternal acute fatty liver of pregnancy. *Proc Natl Acad Sci USA.* 1995;92:841.

Treem WR, Rinaldo P, Hale DE, et al. Acute fatty liver of pregnancy and long-chain 3-hydroxyacyl-coenzyme A dehydrogenase deficiency. *Hepatology.* 1994;19:339.

Usta I, Barton J, Amon E, et al. Acute fatty liver of pregnancy: an experience in the diagnosis and management of fourteen cases. *Am J Obstet Gynecol.* 1994;171:1342.

# 57 FETAL HEART RATE PATTERNS

*Kimberly D. Gregory*

## LEARNING POINT

Definitions, interpretation, and management of fetal heart rate tracings.

## VIGNETTE

A 28-year-old, G1P0, female at 39 weeks gestation presents with spontaneous rupture of membranes, and is 2 cm dilated, 100% effaced, 0 station. She is accompanied by her husband and doula (labor coach). She has informed the labor and delivery nurse about her birth plan and specified that she does not want to be strapped to the bed and electronically monitored continuously throughout her labor, she does not want an IV, she wants to be able to walk around, and eat and drink during her labor, and does not want an epidural. An initial fetal heart rate tracing was obtained, and the fetal heart rate was 140 bpm, and the nurse documented that it was reassuring.

## QUESTION 1

*Should you honor your patient's request regarding continuous fetal heart rate monitoring?*

## ANSWER 1

Multiple studies have demonstrated that intermittent auscultation of the fetal heart rate is equivalent to continuous

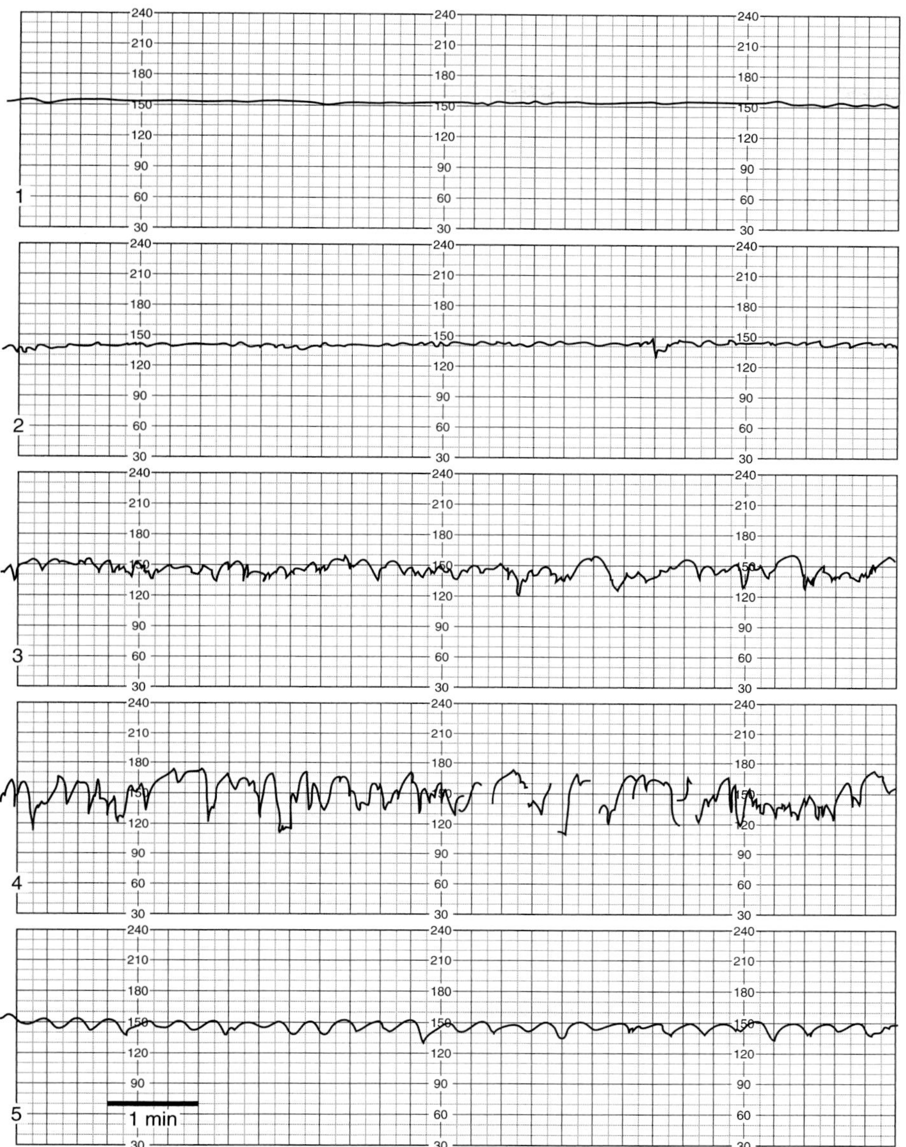


**FIG. 57-1** Fetal heart rate patterns.

SOURCE: (1) Absent variability. No change in amplitude from beat to beat; (2) Minimal variability. Less than or equal to 5 beats per minute (bpm) change in amplitude; (3) Moderate variability. Change in amplitude varies >5 <25 bpm; (4) Marked variability. Change in amplitude >25 bpm; (5) Sinusoidal pattern. Can not interpret variability. The pattern is a smooth sine wave with regular frequency (2–5 cycles per minute), and fixed amplitude (5–15 bpm).

electronic monitoring in assessing fetal status. Intermittent auscultation should be performed at specific intervals, in a nursing environment that allows 1:1 nurse-to-patient ratios. For low-risk patients, the fetal heart rate should be evaluated every 30 minutes in the active phase, and every 15 minutes in the second stage of labor. For high-risk patients, the fetal heart rate should be evaluated every 15 minutes during the active phase of labor, and every 5 minutes during the second stage of labor. If your nursing unit can accommodate 1:1 nurse-to-patient ratio, this patient is low risk, and meets the criteria for intermittent auscultation. The patients should be informed that the status of the baby will need to be assessed and documented at specified intervals.

## QUESTION 2

*What is the definition of a reassuring fetal heart rate tracing?*

## ANSWER 2

A normal heart rate (120–160 bpm, at term) with normal heart rate variability (variation of 3–5 bpm), or moderate variability (6–25 bpm), and the *absence* of patterns are defined as nonreassuring. The presence of fetal heart rate accelerations ≥15 bpm persisting for at least 15 seconds is also considered reassuring.

Other alterations of fetal heart rate exists. Fetal bradycardia is defined as fetal heart rate <110 bpm; fetal tachycardia is defined as fetal heart rate >160 bpm. Periodic fetal heart rate patterns or alterations in the fetal heart rate that occur in association with uterine contractions are as follows:

1. Early decelerations: the onset, nadir, and return to baseline coincide with the beginning, peak, and ending of the uterine contraction
2. Late decelerations: the onset, nadir, and return to baseline occur approximately 30 seconds after the beginning, peak, and ending of the uterine contraction
3. Variable decelerations: abrupt decrease in the fetal heart rate from baseline, the onset, nadir, and duration of the fetal heart rate deceleration varies with successive contractions. Variable decelerations are further quantified as mild, moderate, or severe. Mild variable decelerations are a decrease from baseline of at least 15 bpm for at least 15 seconds. Moderate variable decelerations are a decrease from baseline of 70–80 bpm for greater than 60 seconds or <70 bpm for 30–60 seconds. Severe variable decelerations are when the deceleration is less than 70 bpm for >60 seconds

Variable decelerations are common during labor. They are considered nonreassuring if they become persistent, progressively deeper and/or longer in duration, develop a slow return to baseline.

## QUESTION 3

*What treatment options are available to correct nonreassuring fetal heart rate patterns?*

## ANSWER 3

Attempt should be made to identify the etiology of the fetal heart rate changes, and correct the primary problem if identified. For example, maternal supine position can result in decreased uterine blood flow and placental perfusion resulting in fetal heart rate decelerations that can be alleviated by changing the mother's position; preferably the left lateral recumbent position, albeit any position change (or side) may be sufficient. Maternal hypotension (associated with position, epidural block, or progressive dehydration during labor) can also cause fetal heart rate changes, and can be improved with hydration (and/or fluid boluses as appropriate). Uterine hyperstimulation can lead to fetal heart rate changes due to inadequate fetal oxygenation between contractions. Oxytocin can be decreased or turned off in this setting. Likewise, a tocolytic could be administered if the setting of a prolonged tetanic contraction associated with fetal bradycardia. Amnioinfusion can be used to correct variable decelerations associated with oligohydramnios. In the face of continued nonreassuring fetal heart rate patterns, fetal scalp stimulation or fetal scalp sampling should be attempted. A positive response to fetal scalp stimulation (acceleration 15 bpm lasting 15 seconds) or normal scalp pH indicates the absence of acidosis and labor can continue. If patterns remain nonreassuring, and/or acidosis is present, the patient should be delivered as quickly as possible.

## BIBLIOGRAPHY

ACOG Technical Bulletin No. 207, July 1995. Fetal heart rate patterns: monitoring, interpretation, and management. *Am Col Obstet Gynecol*. 2005. Compendium of Selected Publications. 2004;182–189.

Clark SL, Gimovsky ML, Miller FC. The scalp stimulation test: a clinical alternative to fetal scalp blood sampling. *Am J Obstet Gynecol.* 1984;48:274–277.

Parer JT, Nageotte MP. Intrapartum fetal surveillance. In: Creasy RK, Resnik R (eds.). *Maternal Fetal Medicine*. 5th ed. Philadephia, PA: WB Saunders; 2004:403.

Smith CV, Nguyen HN, Phelan JP, Paul RH. Intrapartum assessment of fetal well-being: a comparison of fetal acoustic stimulation with acid-base determinations. *Am J Obstet Gynecol.* 1986;155:726–728.

# 58 HELLP SYNDROME

*Kimberly D. Gregory*

## LEARNING POINT

Definitions, interpretation, and management of HELLP syndrome.

## VIGNETTE

A 18-year-old, G1P0, African American female at 29 weeks gestation presents with vague complaints of nausea and midepigastric pain. She has not eaten for the past 24 hours. She states she has been constipated throughout her pregnancy. Her last bowel movement was 2 days ago. She is passing flatus. She is afebrile, BP is 130/80, pulse rate 88 bpm. She states the fetus is active, denies uterine contractions, vaginal bleeding, or ruptured membranes. She denies headache, blurred vision, acute change in weight or generalized swelling. On examination, her abdomen is soft, nondistended. She has 2+ midepigastric and right upper quadrant tenderness, trace lower extremity edema, but otherwise, her examination is unremarkable. Laboratory analysis revealed a hematocrit of 30, with platelet count of 95,000. Liver function tests returned with AST of 85, ALT 90, normal lipase, amylase, and lactate dehydrogenase (LDH). Urine protein was traced positive.

### QUESTION 1

*What is the differential diagnosis and how would you proceed to confirm the diagnosis?*

### ANSWER 1

Pertinent findings include nausea, midepigastric, and right upper quadrant pain and tenderness, with elevated liver function tests. Need to evaluate for gall stone disease. The borderline low platelets could be consistent with gestational thrombocytopenia, idiopathic thrombocytopenia, or evolving HELLP syndrome. Comparison with early laboratory tests for baseline hemoglobin, hematocrit, and platelet values would be helpful. Evaluation of a peripheral smear for evidence is essential; however, it can be indirectly inferred by falling hematocrit, increasing LDH, low serum haptoglobin, or evidence of bleeding diathesis. A right upper quadrant ultrasound would be beneficial to rule out cholelithiasis.

Alternatively, serial observation and laboratory evaluation for evolving HELLP syndrome would also be reasonable if this was the leading diagnosis. HELLP syndrome is an acronym for hemolysis, elevated liver enzymes, and low platelets. It is frequently a diagnosis of exclusion, as it can mimic many other diseases (e.g., viral hepatitis, systemic lupus, idiopathic thrombocytopenia purpura [ITP]). It is widely considered to be a variant of preeclampsia and does not necessarily require hypertension and/or proteinuria to confirm the diagnosis. Likewise, there is no formal consensus about the diagnostic criteria for this condition, and is largely considered a diagnosis of exclusion. Nonetheless, it is an important diagnosis to make since treatment and maternal and neonatal prognosis is ultimately tied to the decision for delivery.

### QUESTION 2

*What are the maternal and neonatal risks associated with HELLP syndrome?*

### ANSWER 2

Maternal mortality has been reported to be as high as 24%. Most deaths appear to be associated with delays in diagnosis. Maternal morbidities include cerebral hemorrhage, disseminated intravascular coagulation (DIC), pulmonary edema, acute respiratory distress syndrome (ARDS), renal failure, or hepatic hemorrhage, or hematoma. Pregnancy complications include preterm delivery, abruption, postpartum hemorrhage, and fetal demise. Perinatal mortality rate is also high with reports ranging from 10–37%. Most neonatal mortality and morbidity can be directly attributed to complications of prematurity. Table 58-1 lists rates of neonatal complications observed among patients with HELLP syndrome.

### QUESTION 3

*When and how should this patient be delivered?*

### ANSWER 3

Once the diagnosis of HELLP syndrome is made, the patient should be delivered to optimize maternal safety. Unfortunately, HELLP syndrome can occur late in the second or early in the third trimester and some investigators have argued for temporization to allow administration

**TABLE 58-1. Neonatal Complications Associated with Maternal HELLP Syndrome**

| CONDITION | INCIDENCE (%) |
|---|---|
| Stillbirth | 10 |
| Early neonatal death | 10 |
| Small for gestational age | 44 |
| RDS | 43 |
| Hyperbilirubinemia | 45 |
| Asphyxia | 22 |
| PDA | 16 |
| Neonatal thrombocytopenia | 34 |
| Hypoglycemia | 16 |

of antenatal corticosteroids to improve neonatal outcome. Long-term expectant management before 32 weeks should only be attempted at tertiary care centers and/or under experimental trials. Incidental observations of patients given corticosteroids to improve fetal outcome led to case reports of transient improvements in maternal laboratory values. Subsequently, there were several experimental trials regarding the role of high-dose steroids to treat HELLP syndrome.

A recent meta-analysis reviewed five studies, involving 170 patients (three trials were conducted antepartum and two postpartum). There were no significant differences in the primary outcomes of maternal mortality and morbidity. With regard to the specified secondary maternal outcomes, there was a tendency for a greater platelet count increase over 48 hours, increased mean interval to delivery time in hours, increased mean birthweight, and decreased maternal length of stay for women who received dexamethasone. There were no significant differences in perinatal mortality or morbidity due to respiratory distress syndrome, need for ventilatory support, intracerebral hemorrhage, necrotizing enterocolitis, or 5-minute Apgar less than seven. The authors concluded that there was insufficient evidence to determine whether adjunctive steroid use in HELLP syndrome decreases maternal and perinatal mortality, major maternal and perinatal morbidity. At best, it appears that risk benefit ratio favors attempting treatment for fetal indications, and close observation of maternal indices during this time period. A full course of antenatal steroids (48 hours) may not always be feasible based on worsening maternal status and/or clinical judgment.

The route of delivery should be based on obstetric indications irrespective of gestational age. Appropriate attention to blood pressure control, blood product administration, and magnesium sulfate administration for seizure prophylaxis, should continue postpartum until the HELLP syndrome has resolved. This time course can sometimes extend >72 hours postdelivery.

## BIBLIOGRAPHY

Baxter JK, Weinstein L. HELLP syndrome: The state of the art. *Obstet Gynecol Surv*. 2004;59:838–845.

Eeltink CM, van Lingen RA, Aarnoudse JG, et al. Maternal haemolysis, elevated liver enzymes and low platelets syndrome: specific problems in the newborn. *Eur J Pediatr.* 1993;152:160–163.

Matchaba P, Moodley J. Corticosteroids for HELLP syndrome in pregnancy. *Cochrane Database Syst Rev*. 2006;3.

Sibai BM. Diagnosis, controversies, and management of the syndrome of hemolysis, elevated liver enzymes, and low platelet count. *Obstet Gynecol.* 2004;103:981–991.

# 59 POSTPARTUM HEMORRHAGE

*John Williams III*

## LEARNING POINT

To understand the incidence, differential diagnosis, and management of postpartum hemorrhage.

## VIGNETTE

A 32-year-old, G4P2012, woman has just delivered a 3850 gm male infant at 39 weeks gestation. Her progress in the first stage of labor was slow requiring oxytocin augmentation. During the second stage, she pushed for 2 and one-half hours following which the infant was delivered with low forceps over a median episiotomy. The third stage of labor lasted approximately 30 minutes. The placenta appeared to be intact. Immediately following delivery of the placenta, heavy bleeding with passage of large clots was noted. Bimanual examination revealed a soft, boggy uterus that was unresponsive to massage.

### QUESTION 1

*What is the definition of postpartum hemorrhage, and how often does it occur following a vaginal delivery versus a cesarean delivery?*

### ANSWER 1

Hemorrhage is often a subjective observation, but it is based upon blood loss in excess of the average, which has been described as 500 mL for vaginal delivery and 1000 mL for cesarean section. Hemorrhage occurs in approximately 3.9% of spontaneous vaginal deliveries and 6.4% in cesarean deliveries. However, blood loss is underestimated, 30–50% of the time.

### QUESTION 2

*What is the differential diagnosis of postpartum vaginal bleeding, and what are some of the measures used to control bleeding?*

## ANSWER 2

Postpartum bleeding can be caused by vaginal or cervical laceration, retained products of conception, uterine rupture, uterine atony, uterine inversion, and subsequent disseminated intravascular coagulopathy (DIC). Primary management includes (1) maintenance of intravascular volume with crystalloid fluids and blood component therapy. (2) Aggressive measures to diagnose and treat causative factors including: manual exploration of the uterus and possible curettage for retained products, uterine massage, intravenous oxytocin or intramuscular methylergonovine (Methergine), prostaglandin F analogues (Prostin), suturing of lacerations, vaginal packing, and surgical therapy including: incision and drainage of hematomas, uterine artery ligation, hypogastric artery ligation, uterine compression suture (i.e., B-Lynch, see Fig. 59-1), hysterectomy, and selective arterial embolization.

## QUESTION 3

*Describe the method, rationale, and success rates of uterine devascularization procedures including uterine and hypogastric artery ligation.*

## ANSWER 3

Uterine artery ligation: the ascending branches of the uterine artery are ligated at the level of the vesicouterine peritoneal reflection in order to reduce uterine perfusion. Success rates vary depending on the indication from 80–100%, however, many of these cases may have been elective and most studies are older when more women were taken back to the operating room for bleeding, which now would have been controlled with pharmacological agents. Hypogastric artery ligation involves ligating the anterior division distal to the posterior division take-off, with major complications being tearing the hypogastric vein or sacrificing the posterior division with subsequent gluteal muscle ischemia. Success rates vary between 40–100%. The rationale came from hemodynamic studies, which described that hypogastric artery ligation reduced pelvic blood flow by 49% and pulse pressure beyond the ligation by 85% creating a venous pressure system to provide hemostasis. Uterine compression sutures such as the B-Lynch suture (see Fig. 59-1) have been reported to be highly successful in case reports when other methods have failed and retains future reproductive potential.

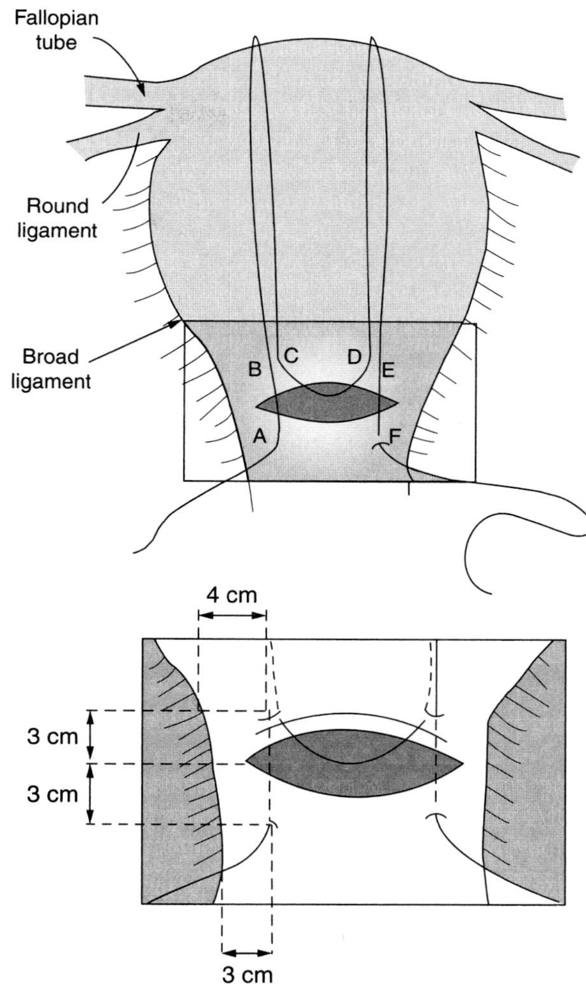


**FIG. 59-1** Anterior uterine wall with B-Lynch suture in place and an enlarged drawing (box) of lower uterine segment with B-Lynch suture in plac.

SOURCE: Reprinted with permission from Ferguson JE II, Bourgeois FJ, Underwood PB, Jr. B-Lynch suture for postpartum hemorrhage. *Obstet Gynecol.* 2000;95:1020–1022.

## QUESTION 4

*What is the role for uterine artery embolization in treatment of postpartum hemorrhage? What is the most common major complication of pelvic artery embolization?*

## ANSWER 4

Selective angiography and embolization have been shown to be effective in controlling vaginal bleeding when other methods have been unsuccessful. The procedure involves the insertion of an intravascular catheter under fluoroscopic guidance into the femoral artery and advancing cephalad into the distal aorta. Angiography is performed to identify the site of bleeding. Once the bleeding site is identified, embolization is carried out using Gelfoam particles or another suitable agent. This procedure should only be done by experienced personnel and in centers where the appropriate equipment is available. The most common major complication of pelvic artery embolization is ischemia and resultant nerve damage. If both branches of the internal iliac artery are embolized, this can interrupt the blood supply of the sciatic and femoral nerves leading to paresis of the lower extremities.

## BIBLIOGRAPHY

ACOG Technical Bulletin No. 243. 1998.

B-Lynch C, Coker A, Lawal AH. The B-Lynch surgical techniques for the control of massive post partum haemorrhage: an alternative to hysterectomy? Five cases reported. *Br J Obstet Gynecol.* 1997;104(3):372–375

Burchell RC. Internal iliac artery ligation: hemodynamics. *Obstet Gynecol.* 1964;24:737–739.

Frisoli G, Leo MV, Sama JC. Postpartum hemorrhage. In: Iffy L, Apuzzio JJ, Vintzileos AM (eds.). *Operative Obstetrics.* 2nd ed. New York, NY: McGraw-Hill;1992.

Gilbert W, Moore T, Resnick R, et al. Angiographic embolization in the management of hemorrhagic complications of pregnancy. *Am J Obstet Gynecol.* 1992;166:493–497.

Hare WSC, Holland CJ. Paresis following internal iliac artery embolization. *Radiology.* 1983;146:47–51.

Vedantham S, Goodwin S, et al. Uterine artery emboliztion. *Am J Obstet Gynecol.* 1997;176:938–948.

# 60 NONIMMUNE HYDROPS

*Kimberly D. Gregory*

## LEARNING POINT

Differential diagnosis of fetal hydrops.

## VIGNETTE

A 33-year-old, G1P0, female presents at 20 weeks for initial prenatal care and is sent for ultrasound to confirm dates. The ultrasound was consistent with dates but the sonologist reported evidence of a pericardial effusion, fetal ascites, scalp edema, and polyhydramnios.

### QUESTION 1

*What is hydrops and how is it diagnosed?*

### ANSWER 1

Hydrops fetalis is a term used to describe generalized edema of the fetus and typically requires evidence of fluid in at least two body cavities. Most cases are diagnosed incidentally on ultrasound (approximately 60%). Other common reasons for referral include polyhydramnios, size greater than dates, fetal tachycardia, decreased fetal movement, antepartum hemorrhage, and maternal preeclampsia. The incidence of nonimmune hydrops at delivery ranges from 1/1500 to 1/3500.

### QUESTION 2

*What is the differential diagnosis of hydrops fetalis?*

### ANSWER 2

Hydrops fetalis can be divided into those related to isoimmunization or nonimmune hydrops. Most isoimmune hydrops is associated with a red blood cell (RBC) antigen (e.g., Rh alloimmunization). This is readily diagnosed by identifying antibodies to an RBC antigen in the maternal serum (indirect Coombs' test). Nonimmune hydrops is more common than isoimmune hydrops, and the differential diagnosis is extremely heterogeneous and is best viewed by systems (see Table 60-1).

### QUESTION 3

*What is the diagnostic workup and overall prognosis for nonimmune hydrops?*

### ANSWER 3

The diagnostic workup for nonimmune hydrops includes the following:

- Maternal CBC with indices including possibly hemoglobin electropheresis

**TABLE 60-1. Differential Diagnosis of Nonimmune Hydrops**

| SYSTEM | EXAMPLE | PREVALENCE (%) |
|---|---|---|
| **Cardiovascular** | | 19 |
| | Malformation | |
| | Arrhytmias | |
| | High output failure syndromes | |
| | Cardiomyopathy | |
| **Pulmonary** | | 10 |
| | Congenital cystic adenomatoid malformation, diaphragmatic hernia, pulmonary sequestration | |
| **Gastrointestinal/genitourinary** | | 10 |
| | Midgut volvulus, malrotation, duplication, prune belly syndrome, congenital nephrosis | |
| **Hematologic** | | 8 |
| | Alpha thalassemia, fetomaternal hemorrhage, G-6-PD deficiency | |
| **Infections** | | 3 |
| | TORCH (toxoplasmosis, CMV, rubella, herpes) Parvovirus, syphilis | |
| **Twins** | | 4 |
| | Twin-to-twin transfusion syndrome, acardiac twin | |
| **Chromosomal** | | 10 |
| | 45×, trisomy 21, 18, 12, triploidy | |
| **Miscellaneous** | | 13 |
| | Skeletal dysplasias (dwarfs), neuromuscular disorders, metabolic syndromes | |
| **Idiopathic** | | 18 |

- Antibody screen
- Kleihauer-Betke stain
- Maternal titers for parvovirus rapid plasma realign (RPR), cytomegolovirus (CMV), toxoplasmosis
- Antibody screen
- Complete fetal ultrasound, including fetal echocardiography, fetal dopplers
- Amniocentesis for fetal karyotype, detection of infectious agents polymerase chain reaction (PCR) based changes.

Overall, the prognosis for nonimmune hydrops is extremely poor. Approximately 70–90% of fetuses die in the perinatal period. In general, the prognosis is related to the underlying problem producing the hydrops. Best prognosis occurs among fetuses with a correctable cardiac arrhythmia, or a potentially treatable fetal anemia. Recent advances in predicting degree of fetal anemia, and ability to transfuse RBCs in this setting have lead to improved outcomes in this particular setting (e.g., fetal parvovirus infection).

## BIBLIOGRAPHY

Bruner JP, et al. Sonography of nonimmune hydrops fetalis. In: Fleischer AC, et al, (eds.). *Sonography in Obstetrics and Gynecology.* 5th ed. New York, NY: McGraw-Hill;1996:564–581.

Sahakian V, Weiner CP, et al. Intrauterine transfusion treatment of nonimmune hydrops fetalis secondary to human parvovirus B19 infection. *Am J Obstet Gynecol.* 1991;164:1090.

Thorp JA, et al. Nonimmune hydrops caused by massive fetomaternal hemorrhage and treated by intravascular transfusion. *Am J Perinatol.* 1992;9:22.

Wilkins I. Nonimmune hydrops. In: Creasy RK, Resnik R (eds.). *Maternal Fetal Medicine.* 5th ed. Philadephia, PA: WB Saunders; 2004:563.

# 61 INCOMPETENT CERVIX/CERCLAGE

*Calvin J. Hobel*

## LEARNING POINT

The classic definition of incompetent cervix is defined as painless cervical dilatation without bleeding in the second trimester of pregnancy with prolapse or ballooning of the membranes followed by delivery of an immature fetus. Often women present with history and physical findings which make it difficult to distinguish true incompetent cervix from other causes of early loss. The following case will illustrate these issues and help the reader develop a focused evidence-based approach to the management of patients with this condition, the cause of which is most likely multifactorial.

## VIGNETTE

A 23-year-old patient presents herself as a new patient for her first prenatal visit at 15 weeks with the following history. She had two elective terminations for her first two pregnancies, both at approximately 10 weeks performed by dilatation and curettage. Her next pregnancy at age 21 ended in the delivery of a very low birth weight infant at 23 weeks after preterm premature rupture of the membranes (PPROM). The patient's physician at that time said she may have an incompetent cervix and she may need a cervical cerclage during her next pregnancy. As part of your workup, you request the medical records from her prior physician and you note that at the time of admission for her prior pregnancy she had oligohydramnios (secondary to PPROM) and normal temperature and a WBC of 7000 cells/mm$^3$, but went into spontaneous labor within 2 days. The infant was born alive at an appropriate birth weight, but expired within 1 hour. The placental pathology showed chorioamnionitis.

For the current pregnancy, the physical examination indicated that this patient had a normal body mass index and no abnormal findings on physical examination. The vaginal examination visually suggested that the cervix appeared normal. The pH of the vaginal secretions was acidic; a sample of vaginal secretions was obtained for a wet mount to assess for bacterial vaginosis and trichomoniasis. The wet mount was normal. A pelvic examination suggested the cervix to be somewhat short and the uterine size was appropriate for gestational age. Because of the concern for her risk of incompetent cervix, the physician performed a vaginal ultrasound and the cervix was 2.8 cm in length.

### QUESTION 1

*Evidence-based medicine requires that one must begin with a proper understanding of the classification of a disease so that one can appropriately categorize the types of patients with an incompetent cervix. What are the three categories of patients with cervical insufficiency and to what category does this patient belong?*

### ANSWER 1

1. There are women with classic historical features of cervical insufficiency who have had two or more second-trimester pregnancy losses without bleeding or clear signs of labor preceding the loss (note that some definitions require two serial losses before calling it classic cervical insufficiency). This type of patient would be a candidate for an elective cerclage.
2. There are those women who present with some shortening of the cervix and funneling. These patients usually have an urgent cerclage.
3. There are those women with clear signs of cervical dilation of 2 cm or more and significant effacement but no evidence of regular painful uterine contractions and may have prolapse of the membranes. These patients require an emergency cerclage.

### QUESTION 2

*What maternal factors are associated with a decreased likelihood of delivery after 28 weeks after the cerclage is paced?*

### ANSWER 2

1. Many studies have used univeriate statistical techniques that have not allowed an assessment of maternal factors that independently predict health outcomes of patients with cerclages. For example, the study by Terkildsen and colleagues demonstrated counterintuitively that the use of tocolytics medications and operator-assisted reduction of prolapsing membranes are associated with decreased success of emergent cerclage. However, these interventions did not attain significance in multivariate analysis after controlling for physical examination findings. They did observe that nulliparity, the presence of membranes prolapsing beyond the external cervical os, and gestational age less than 22 weeks were associated with a decreased chance of delivery at or after 28 weeks after emergent cerclage. Unfortunately, these investigations did not assess the presence or absence of prior spontaneous and therapeutic terminations on the risk of delivery. This would be important in view of the data published by Lumley showing

that the risk of preterm delivery was greater depending on the number of prior spontaneous and therapeutic abortions.
2. Recently, cervical length (short cervix) has been assessed as a risk factor for urgent cerclage placement. Recent randomized clinical trials have reported conflicting results and do not definitively support the placement of a cerclage.
3. Once a cerclage is placed, vaginal fetal fibronectin may be a predictor of the risk of spontaneous preterm delivery. A recent study by Roman et al. suggested that fetal fibronectin assessments may be valuable in identifying women at greater risk. Unfortunately these investigators did not evaluate for the concurrent presence of ascending infection as a possible associated risk factor.
4. Vaginal/cervical ascending infection is a well-known cause of early preterm labor. Many of the documented infections are asymptomatic and may be associated with cervical change without labor. To be certain that infection is not a contributing factor to the cause of the prior loss (as in above case), and a factor in the current pregnancy, the clinician is obligated to assess for the presence of pathogens and treat these prior to placing a cerclage. However, an evidence-based review found no evidence to suggest the routine use of antibiotics, although the incidence of chorioamnionitis as a final outcome ranged from 9% to 37% in the studies reviewed.

## QUESTION 3

*In general what data supports the effectiveness of an elective cerclage, an urgent cerclage, and an emergency cerclage?*

## ANSWER 3

1. In a large prospective randomized trial of approximately 1300 women with nonclassical histories of cervical incompetence, those women randomized to receive an elective cerclage had a significant benefit for delivering after 33 weeks.
2. For patients with shortened cervix, a systematic review of the literature and meta-analysis recently reported that the available evidence does not support the use of elective cerclage for a sonographically detected short cervix.
3. For an emergency cerclage, there are data to suggest that certain techniques, such as amniocentesis and reducing the membranes with a Foley catheter may improve the success of an emergency cerclage. A recent study by Satsaris and colleagues showed that when the cervix was dilated 4 cm or less, pregnancy was prolonged an average of 31 days and if the cervix was dilated greater than 4 cm, the median duration was only 9 days.

## QUESTION 4

*What are the success rates for a patient reaching 33 weeks for placing a cerclage for each of the types of conditions listed in question 1?*

## ANSWER 4

1. Elective cerclage = 87%
2. Urgent cerclage = 56%
3. Emergency cerclage = 43%

## BIBILOGRAPHY


Althuisius SM, Dekker GA, Hummel P. Bekedam DJ. van Geijn HP. Final results of the Cervical Incompetence Prevention Randomized Cerclage Trial (CIPRACT): therapeutic cerclage with bed rest versus bed rest alone. *Am J Obstet Gynecol.* 2001;185(5):1106–1112.

Belej-Rak T, Okun N, Windrim R, Ross S, Hannah ME. Effectiveness of cervical cerclage for a sonographically shortened cervix: a systematic review and meta-analysis. *Am J Obstet Gynecol.* 2003;189(6):1679–1687.

Chasen ST, Silverman NS. Mid-trimester emergent cerclage: a ten year single institution review. *J Perinatol.* 1998; 18(5): 338–342.

Harger JH. Cerclage and cervical insufficiency: an evidence based analysis. *Obstet Gynecol.* 2002;100:1313–1327.

Iams JD, Goldenberg RL, Meis PJ, Mercer BM, Moawad A, Das A, Thom E, McNellis D, Copper RL, Johnson F, Roberts JM. The length of the cervix and the risk of spontaneous premature delivery. National Institute of Child Health and Human Development Maternal Fetal Medicine Unit Network. *N Eng J Med.* 1996;334(9):567–572.

Locatelli A, Vergani P, Bellini P, et al. Amnioreduction in emergency cerclage with prolapsed membranes: comparison of two methods for reducing the membranes. *Am J Perinatol.* 1999;16:73–77.

Lumley J. The association between prior spontaneous abortion, prior induced abortion and preterm birth in first singleton birth. *Prenat Neonat Med.* 1998;3:21–24.

MacNaughton MC, Chalmers IG, Dubowitz V, et al. Final report of the Medical Research Council/Royal College of Obstetricians and Gynaecologists Multicentre Randomized Trial of Cervical Cerclage. *Br J Obstet Gynaecol.* 1993;100: 516–523.

Mays JK, Figueroa R, Sha J, Khakoo H, Kaminsky S, Tejani N. Amniocentesis for selection before rescue cerclage. *Obstet Gynecol.* 2000;95:652–655.

Roman AS, Rebarber A, Sfakianaki AK, Mulholland J, Saltzman D, Paidas MJ, Minior V, Lockwood CJ. Vaginal fetal fibronectin as a predictor of spontaneous preterm delivery in the patient with cervical cerclage. *Am J Obstet Gyecol.* 2003;189:1368–1373.

Rust OA, Atlas RO, Reed J, et al. Revisiting the short cervix detected by transvaginal ultrasound in the second trimester: why cerclage may not help. *Am J Obstet Gynecol.* 2001;185: 1098–1105.

Satsaris V, Senat MV, Gervaise A, Fernanedez H. Balloon replacement of fetal membranes to facilitate emergency cervical/ cerclage. *Obstet Gynecol.* 2001;98:243–246.

Terkildsen MFC, Parilla BV, Kumar P, Grobman WA. Factors associated with success of emergent second-trimester cerclage. *Obstet Gynecol.* 2003;101:565–569.

To MS, Alfirevic Z, Health VCF, et al. Cervical cerclage for prevention of peterm delivery in women with short cervix: randomised controlled trial. *Lancet.* 2004;363:1849–1853.

# 62 INDUCTION OF LABOR AND CERVICAL RIPENING

*Jane L. Davis*

## LEARNING POINT

Proper knowledge of methods of induction of labor and cervical ripening are important to ensure a safer and successful delivery.

## VIGNETTE

A 27-year-old, G1P0, is currently 42 weeks gestation by excellent dating criteria. Although she has had normal antepartum surveillance, she has recently noticed a decrease in fetal movement. She is concerned about this, and questions her obstetrician about induction of her labor. Her prenatal course has been unremarkable. Her past medical history and past surgical history have been negative. Her cervix is 2–3 cm dilated, 50% effaced, and presenting parts rs at –2 station. The cervix is midposition and soft.

## QUESTION 1

*What are indications and contraindications to cervical ripening/induction? What are the rates of induction, and have they changed over time?*

## ANSWER 1

Indications:

- Postterm pregnancy
- Preeclampsia/eclampsia
- Premature rupture of the membranes (PROM) at term or after confirmation of fetal lung maturity in preterm gestation
- Chorioamnionitis
- Suspected fetal jeopardy
- Maternal medical problems (e.g., diabetes)
- Fetal demise
- Logistical factors (e.g., risk of rapid labor, distance from the hospital, psychosocial indications)

Contraindications:

- Placenta previa/vasa previa
- Transverse fetal lie
- Prolapsed umbilical cord
- Prior transfundal uterine incision

Using natality data from the National Center for Health Statistics, Zhang and colleagues reported that between 1989 and 1998, the rate of labor induction increased gradually from 9.0% to 19.4% for all births. The rates varied widely between and within many states (e.g., in 1998, induction rates in Hawaii were 10.9% vs. 41.6% in Wisconsin vs. a range of 6.5–53.2% in counties of New York).

## QUESTION 2

*What are the methods used for cervical and labour ripening?*

## ANSWER 2

Methods of cervical ripening include:

1. Mechanical cervical dilators such as laminaria and Foley catheters. These methods have increased risk of infection.
2. Pharmacologic ripening agents such as prostaglandins (PGE2) and prostaglandin analogs (PGE1 analog-misoprostol), oxytocin, and progesterone antagonists (mifepristone-RU486).

**TABLE 62-1. Bishop Scoring System**

| SCORE | DILATATION (CM) | EFFACEMENT (%) | STATION (−3 TO +3) | CONSISTENCY | POSITION OF CX |
|---|---|---|---|---|---|
| 0 | Closed | 0–30 | −3 | Firm | Posterior |
| 1 | 1–2 | 40–50 | −2 | Medium | Midposition |
| 2 | 3–4 | 60–70 | −1, 0 | Soft | Anterior |
| 3 | 5–6 | 80 | +1, +2 | – | – |

SOURCE: Modified from Bishop EH. Pelvic scoring for elective induction. *Obstet Gynecol* 1964;24:267.

3. Marked "stripping" of membranes.

Methods of induction of labor include:

1. Oxytocin
2. Membrane stripping
3. Amniotomy.

## QUESTION 3

*What criteria are used to assess fetal maturity prior to performing an elective induction?*

## ANSWER 3

If one of the following is met, fetal maturity may be assumed and amniocentesis need not be performed prior to an elective induction:

1. Fetal heart tones have been documented for 20 weeks by nonelectronic fetoscope or for 30 weeks by Doppler.
2. Thirty-six weeks have passed since a positive serum or urine pregnancy test was performed.
3. Ultrasound measurement of the crown-rump length, obtained at 6–11 weeks, supports a gestational age of 39 weeks.
4. Ultrasound at 12–20 weeks confirms a gestational age of 39 weeks determined by clinical history and physical examination.

## QUESTION 4

*What is the Bishop score and what are its five components?*

## ANSWER 4

Bishop designed a scoring system for multiparous patients who were to undergo elective induction in which 0–3 points are given for each of five factors (Table 62-1). When the cervical score exceeded 8, the likelihood of a successful induction was good. Over time, this scoring system has also been applied to primigravid patients.

If the cervix is favorable, cesarean section rates are not necessarily higher if elective induction is undertaken. However, cesarean sections are more common with inductions in primigravid patients in the presence of an unfavorable cervix.

## BIBLIOGRAPHY


ACOG Educational Bulletin No. 230. ACOG. Assessment of Fetal Lung Maturity. 1996.

ACOG Practice Bulletin No. 10. ACOG. Induction of Labor. 1999.

Bishop EH, et al. Pelvic scoring for elective induction. *Obstet Gynecol.* 1964;24:266–268.

Dublin S, et al. Maternal and neonatal outcomes after induction of labor without an identified indication. *Am J Obstet Gynecol.* 2000;183:986–994.

Kaufman KE, et al. Elective induction: an analysis of economic and health consequences. *Am J Obstet Gynecol.* 2002; 187:858–863.

Rayburn WF. Preinduction cervical ripening: basis and methods of current practice. *Obstet Gynecol Survey.* 2002;57:683–692.

Yeast JD, et al. Induction of labor and the relationship to cesarean delivery: a review of 7001 consecutive inductions. *Am J Obstet Gynecol.* 1999;180:628–633.

Zhang J, et al. US national trends in labor induction 1989–1998. *J Reprod Med.* 2002;47:120–124.


# 63 INTRAUTERINE GROWTH RESTRICTION

*Jane L. Davis*

## LEARNING POINT

To learn the definition, diagnosis, and management of intrauterine growth restriction (IUGR).

# VIGNETTE

A 29-year-old, G1P0, female trial attorney has an intrauterine pregnancy at 32 weeks. At her most recent prenatal visit, her obstetrician had measured her uterine fundal height to be 27 cm. An ultrasound revealed fetal head and femur measurements compatible with 32 weeks, but the fetal abdominal circumference was compatible with 26 weeks. The ultrasound estimated fetal weight is less than the 10% for 32 weeks. Both the amniotic fluid index and Doppler velocimetry of the umbilical arteries were within normal limits. A diagnosis of IUGR was entertained.

Although the patient stopped smoking at the beginning of her pregnancy, she recently has been involved in preparing for a difficult trial, and has subsequently resumed smoking one pack of cigarettes each day. Additionally, she has been putting in 14 hour days, driving great distances in order to obtain depositions for her client.

## QUESTION 1

*What is the standard definition of IUGR?*

## ANSWER 1

IUGR is a term used to describe a fetus whose estimated weight appears to be less than expected, usually less than the 10th percentile. IUGR includes normal fetuses at the lower end of the growth spectrum as well as those with specific clinical conditions in which the fetus fails to achieve its inherent growth potential because of extrinsic influences such as maternal smoking or medical conditions or intrinsic genetic defects. Etiologic risk factors for IUGR can be divided into maternal, fetal, and placental (Table 63-1).

**TABLE 63-1. Risk Factor for IUGR**

| |
|---|
| **Maternal risk factors** |
| Hypertension |
| Renal disease |
| Restrictive lung disease |
| Diabetes with underlying vascular disease |
| Cyanotic heart disease |
| Antiphospholipid syndrome |
| Collagen vascular disease |
| Hemoglobinopathies |
| Smoking and substance abuse |
| Severe malnutrition |
| **Fetal risk factors** |
| Multiple gestation |
| Infections |
| Genetic disorders |
| Exposure to teratogens |
| **Primary placental disease** |

## QUESTION 2

*How is IUGR diagnosed antenatally?*

## ANSWER 2

The two steps involved in the antenatal diagnosis of IUGR involve first identification of risk factors and secondly the use of ultrasound to assess fetal size and growth. When necessary, prenatal diagnosis for fetal karyotype and in utero fetal infection may also be required.

The standard measurements of fetal abdominal circumference, head circumference, biparietal diameter, and femur length are obtained. These measurements can be converted into a fetal weight using published formulas and tables. An abdominal circumference within the normal range reliably excludes growth restriction with a false negative rate of less than 10%. A small abdominal circumference or fetal weight estimate less than the 10% suggests the possibility of growth restriction, with the likelihood increasing as the percentile rank decreases. Serial ultrasound measurements are helpful in assessing the progression and/or severity of the restricted growth. Additionally, since IUGR is often associated with aneuploidy and structural abnormalities, a thorough ultrasound assessment for fetal structural abnormalities should be performed.

Oligohydramnios is often found in significant IUGR, and is found in 77–83% of IUGR-affected fetuses. However, amniotic fluid volume may also be normal in pregnancies affected by IUGR.

Although Doppler velocimetry of the umbilical arteries is not useful for diagnosing IUGR, it can be used to follow pregnancies affected by IUGR. Doppler velocimetry has been shown useful in reducing interventions and improving fetal outcomes in pregnancies affected by IUGR.

## QUESTION 3

*What is the fetal morbidity and mortality found in IUGR?*

## ANSWER 3

Perinatal morbidity and mortality is significantly increased in IUGR, especially with weights less than the third percentile. In labor up to 50% of IUGR fetuses exhibit abnormal fetal hear rate tracings. Neonatal complications include polycythemia, hyperbilirubinemia, hypoglycemia, hypothermia, and apneic episodes.

## BIBLIOGRAPHY

ACOG Practice Bulletin Number 12. Intrauterine Growth Restriction. 2000.

Hadlock FP, Deter RL, Harrist RB, Park SK. Estimating fetal age: computer-assisted analysis of multiple fetal growth parameters. *Radiology.* 1984;152:497–501.

Low JA. The current status of maternal and fetal blood flow velocimetry. *Am J Obstet Gynecol.* 1991;164:1049–1063.

McInttire DD, Bloom SL, Casey BM, Leveno KJ. Birthweight in relation to morbidity and mortaligy among newborn infants. *N Eng J Med.* 1999;340:1234–1238.

Phillipson EH, Sokol RJ, Williams T. Oligohydramnios: clinical associations and predictive value for intrauterine growth retardation. *Am J Obstet and Gynecol.* 1983;146:271–278.

Warsof SL, Cooper DJ, Little D, Campbells. Routine ultrasound screen for antenatal detection of intrauterine growth restriction. *Obstet Gynecol.* 1986;67:33–39.

# *64* MECONIUM

*Kimberly D. Gregory*

## LEARNING POINT

Prevalence of meconium passage and the risks of meconium aspiration syndrome (MAS).

## VIGNETTE

A 33-year-old, G2P1, female presents with spontaneous rupture of membranes with thick meconium noted. Her cervical examination is 5 cm dilated, 100% effaced at 0 station. The patient is concerned that her baby has had its first bowel movement inside her uterus.

## QUESTION 1

*What is the incidence of meconium passage?*

## ANSWER 1

Meconium passage in the third trimester is fairly common and has been reported in 2–11% of pregnancies when evaluated using amnioscopy or serial, weekly amniocenteses. During labor, meconium passage is more common with advanced gestational age, such that the rate is approximately 7–22% at term, but approaches 40–50% postterm (see Table 64-1).

## QUESTION 2

*How common is MAS?*

## ANSWER 2

Meconium below the vocal cords and/or in the lungs (meconium aspiration) occurs in approximately 20–60% of infants exposed to meconium amniotic fluid; however, MAS (hypoxia, pulmonary hypertension, and persistent fetal circulation) occurs in approximately 2–8% of exposed infants. Severity of MAS is related to duration of exposure, thickness of amniotic fluid, and associated intrapartum events such as oligohydramnios, abnormal fetal heart rate tracings, hypoxia, and acidemia.

## QUESTION 3

*Is the consistency of meconium important in predicting risk or outcome for MAS?*

## ANSWER 3

The consistency of meconium is variable and is described as light or thin versus dark or thick. There are

**TABLE 64-1. Incidence of Meconium Passage, Meconium Aspiration, and Meconium Aspiration Syndrome**

| MECONIUM PASSAGE | MECONIUM ASPIRATION | MECONIUM ASPIRATION SYNDROME |
|---|---|---|
| 2–50% | 20–60% | 2–8% |

no standardized, reliable ways to measure meconium consistency. Studies have not been able to show a consistent relationship to thick meconium and adverse outcomes in the presence of normal fetal heart rate tracings; however, thick meconium in the presence of abnormal fetal heart rate tracings has been associated with increased risk for MAS.

### QUESTION 4

*Can MAS be prevented?*

### ANSWER 4

In the presence of thick meconium, amnioinfusion during labor has been found to decrease the rate of meconium below the umbilical cords by 84% and several meta-analyses have demonstrated a reduction in MAS. After delivery, there should be DeLee suction of the oropharynx on the perineum and selective use of endotracheal intubation and suctioning for infants who are depressed at delivery.

## BIBLIOGRAPHY

Glantz, JC, Woods JR. Significance of amniotic fluid meconium. In: Creasy RK, Resnik R (eds.). *Maternal Fetal Medicine*. 5th ed. Philadelphia, PA: W.B. Saunders; 2004:441–450.

Hofmeyr GJ. Amnioinfusion for meconium stained liquor in labor. *Cochrane Database Syst Rev.* 2006;3.

Kattwinkel J, Denson S, Zaichkin J, American Heart Association American Academy of Pediatrics Committee on Fetus and Newborn, American Academy of Pediatrics, Niermeyer S. (eds.) *Textbook of Neonatal Resuscitation*. 4th ed. American Academy of Pediatrics Elk Grove Village, I11:2000.

Katz VL, Bowes WA. Meconium aspiration syndrome: reflections on a murky subject. *Am J Obstet Gynecol.* 1992;166:171.

# 65 OPERATIVE VAGINAL DELIVERY

*Kevin R. Justus*

## LEARNING POINT

Vacuum- and forceps-assisted deliveries are two options available when an instrument is needed to facilitate a vaginal birth.

## VIGNETTE

A 29-year-old G4P3003 at 38 weeks of gestation was admitted in active labor to Labor and Delivery. The patient's cervix was examined and was found to be 6 cm, 90% effaced and at −2 station with a bulging bag of membranes present. The estimated fetal weight on Leopold's maneuver was found to be 7 lb. The patient's prenatal history was uncomplicated. Her prior obstetrical history was significant for three terms spontaneous vaginal deliveries with the following weights 7 lb, 7 lb 3 oz, and 7 lb 6 oz, respectively.

The fetal heart tracing was reactive in the 140s with no decelerations. She received regional anesthesia for pain control. She spontaneously ruptured her membranes and the amniotic fluid was clear. The patient was reexamined 2 hours later and was found to be 10 cm, 100% effaced and at +1 station. The position was noted to be right occiput anterior (ROA) with no synclitism present. The mother felt no urgency to push so she was instructed by the nurse to labor down.

You received a call stat to the delivery room to review the fetal heart tracing. Fetal heart tracing was in the 70s for 6 minutes. Her cervical examination was 10 cm, 100% effaced, at +3 station and the position was ROA. The patient attempted to push with good maternal efforts but minimal progress was noted and you decided to perform an operative vaginal delivery.

### QUESTION 1

*What are the indications for an operative vaginal delivery?*

### ANSWER 1

No indication for operative vaginal delivery is absolute. However, the following indications apply when the fetal head is engaged and the cervix is fully dilated:

1. A prolonged second stage in a nulliparous woman with lack of continuing progress for 3 hours with regional anesthesia or 2 hours without regional anesthesia. In a multiparous woman, lack of continuing progress for 2 hours with regional anesthesia, or 1 hour without regional anesthesia.
2. A fetal indication for a nonreassuring fetal heart rate tracing.
3. Maternal indications include disease states that impair the ability to push or conditions that may be worsened by prolonged voluntary pushing efforts such as neurological disorders associated with weakness, certain pulmonary diseases, and maternal cardiac disease.

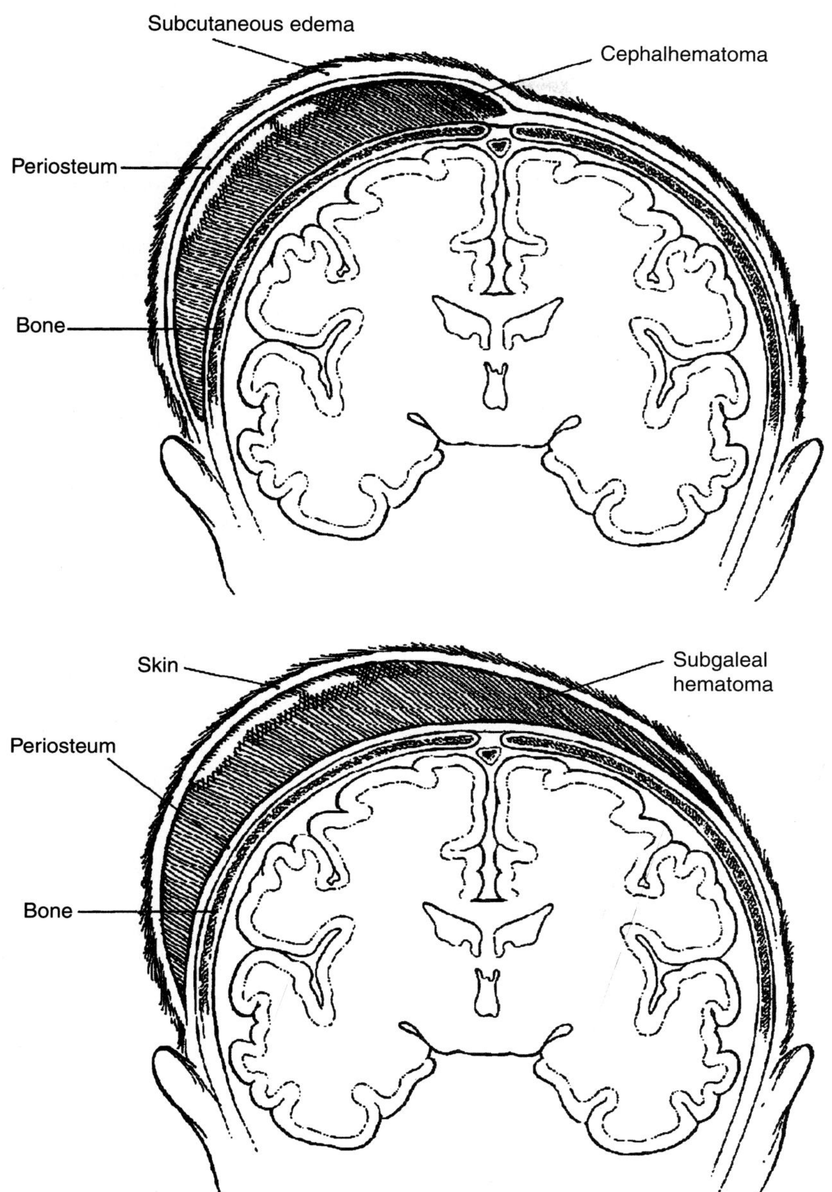


**FIG. 65-1** Cephalhematoma formation.

## QUESTION 2

*What are the criteria for determining what meets classification for a low operative vaginal delivery?*

## ANSWER 2

In 1988, ACOG issued a classification for defining what meets criteria for an outlet, low, and mid forceps delivery. The station of the fetal head in the maternal pelvis was estimated in centimeters. Station referred to the level of the leading bony point of the fetal head at or below the level of the maternal ischial spines. To define engagement, the biparietal diameter had to pass through the pelvic inlet, and that the leading point of the bony edge of the fetal head was at the level of the ischial spines. The fetal head was classified as +5 cm when crowning.

1. Leading point of the fetal skull is at station greater or equal to +2 cm and not on the pelvic floor.
2. Rotation less than 45° or the rotation was greater than 45° and placed the sagittal suture in the midline.

Far more critical than technical proficiency is the knowledge of when operative delivery is used and when it should not be used.

## QUESTION 3

*What are the maternal and fetal risk associated with instrument assisted deliveries?*

## ANSWER 3

Concern for maternal and fetal injury is one of the major reasons for the decline in operative vaginal deliveries. Lacerations of the vagina and cervix are quite common maternal morbidities. Several studies have demonstrated that forcep deliveries have been associated with a greater risk of third and fourth degree rectal lacerations. Vacuum deliveries have been associated with a greater risk of anterior vault and periurethral lacerations. Cephalhematomas (a transient form of scalp trauma caused by bleeding due to rupture of a diploic or emissary vein beneath the periosteum) occur more commonly with the vacuum. A more serious morbidity of the vacuum is the subgaleal hematoma caused by rupture of the diploic vessels in the loose subaponeurotic tissues of the scalp (see Fig. 65-1). This loosely applied connective tissue in the subgaleal space creates the potential for massive bleeding extending from the orbits to the nape of the neck. Bleeding into this space in not limited by the suture lines like it is in cephalhematoma. This is an infrequent but potentially fetal risk that is often associated with vacuum extraction.

## QUESTION 4

*Does the success rate of vacuum and forceps for occiput anterior and occiput posterior vaginal deliveries in low and outlet deliveries differ?*

## QUESTION 4

Forceps are more likely to be successful than vacuum in both occiput anterior and posterior positions in low positions whereas there is no difference with outlet position. However, the use of forceps was associated with a greater risk of rectal sphincter injury than the use of vacuum. The long-term risks of significant perineal injury and the association with fetal incontinence are very important and need to be taken into account when examining the maternal pelvis to determine whether or not an adequate pelvis is present to conduct an operative vaginal delivery.

## BIBLIOGRAPHY

ACOG Practice Bulletin, No 17. Operative Vaginal Delivery. 2000.

ACOG Technical Bulleting, No 152. Operative Vaginal Delivery. 1991.

Damron D, Capeless E. Operative vaginal delivery: a comparison of forceps and vacuum for success rate and risk of rectal sphincter injury. *Am J Obst Gynecol.* 2004;191:907–910.

Damron DP, Capeless EL. Operative vaginal delivery: a comparison of forceps and vacuum for success rate and risk of rectal sphincter injury. *Am J Obstet Gynecol.* 2004;191:907–910.

Demissie K, Rhoads GG, Smulian JC, Balasubramanian BA, Gandhi K, Joseph KS, Kramer M. Operative vaginal delivery and neonatal and infant adverse outcomes: population based retrospective analysis. *BMJ.* 2004;329:24–29.

Gei AF, Belfort MA. Forceps-assisted vaginal delivery. *Obstet Gynecol Clin North Am.* 1999;26:345–370.

Hankins G, Clark S, Cunningham G, Gilstrap L. *Operative Obstetrics.* 2nd ed. Norwalk Connecticut, CT: Appleton & Lange; 2000:180.

Hankins G, Gary DV, Rowe T. Operative vaginal delivery-year 2000. *Am J Obstet Gynecol.* 1996;175:275–282.

Johnson J, Figueroa R, Garry D, Elimian A, Maulik D. Maternal and neonatal effects of forceps and vacuum assisted deliveries. *Obstet Gynecol.* 2004;103:513–518.

ACOG Practice Bulletin, Number 17. Operative vaginal delivery. 2000.

Uchil D, Arulkumaran S. Neonatal subgaleal hemorrhage and its relationship to delivery by vacuum extraction. *Obstet Gynecol Survey.* 2003;10:687–693.

# 66 PLACENTA ACCRETA

*Ilana Cass*

## LEARNING POINT

To understand the ultrasonographic, clinical, and histologic features of placenta accreta, and to recognize the risk factors that lead to abnormal placentation.

## VIGNETTE

A 36-year-old, G5P4, presents with vaginal bleeding at 29 weeks gestational age. The bleeding began without any clear precipitating event and she denies any cramps or pain. She describes the bleeding as heavy for greater than 2 hours despite resting in bed at home. She has had an uneventful pregnancy with regular prenatal visits. An ultrasound performed for anatomy reveals that she has a small gestational age fetus and a complete placenta previa. Her past obstetric history is significant for four prior uncomplicated cesarean-sections at term, following a prior myomectomy at age 21. She has no significant medical history, does not smoke or use any alcohol.

The physical examination reveals a gravid female. Vitals signs: pulse rate 90 bpm, BP 90/60 mm Hg, and afebrile. Chest is clear to auscultation, cardiac examination shows regular rate and rhythm, abdominal examination shows a gravid abdomen with a well-healed pfannenstiel scar. Her fundal height is consistent with a 26-week gestation. Fetal heart tones are auscultated at a normal rate of 140 bpm. She is admitted and during her hospitalization she is given a course of antenatal steroids. A follow-up ultrasound confirms a placenta previa, and is suggestive of a possible placenta accreta.

The patient was discharged home, and followed closely. At 34 weeks gestation, she again develops vaginal bleeding, is hospitalized, and another ultrasound confirms a placenta previa and is suspicious for a placenta accreta. Her bleeding stops with bed rest and after consultation with maternal-fetal medicine and gynecologic oncology, the decision is made to perform an amniocentesis and once fetal lung maturity is documented, deliver her via cesarean-section.

## QUESTION 1

*What is the histological distinction between placenta accreta, increta, and percreta? What are some of the associated ultrasonographic abnormalities suggestive of placenta accreta?*

## ANSWER 1

Placental implantation with abnormally firm adherence to the uterine wall resulting from partial or total absence of the decidua basalis and imperfect development of the fibrinoid (Nitabuch) layer with villi attached to the myometrium (accreta), invading the myometrium (increta) or penetrating through the myometrium (percreta).

Sonographically, the absence or thinning <1 mm of the normal hypoechoic myometrial zone in the anterior lower segment is suggestive of an abnormally adherent placenta. Some also suggest that lacunar vascular spaces within the placental parenchyma, which persist until delivery has been associated with placenta accreta. Thinning or irregularity of the hyperechoic interface between the uterus and bladder wall is also suspicious.

## QUESTION 2

*What is the incidence of placenta accreta? What are the risk factors for placenta accreta/increta/percreta?*

## ANSWER 2

The incidence of placenta accreta ranges from 0.1 to 2.3 per 1000 births, although the incidence varies depending on the definition of placenta accreta that is used. Some studies have included any patient with an adherent placenta that does not spontaneously separate after 2 minutes or those patients who have any retained fragments of placenta within the uterus in a patient with intrapartum or postpartum bleeding. Other studies mandate histological confirmation of the placenta accreta requiring tissue confirmation of the diagnosis.

Risk factors for placenta accreta are any circumstance where placental adherence is defective: placenta previa, uterine scarring, proportionally related to the number of prior cesarean sections, multiparity, past history of uterine curettage.

Approximately one-third of cases of placenta accrete are associated with placenta previa. The risk of placenta accreta increases linearly with placenta previa and the number of prior cesarean sections (see Table 66-1).

## QUESTION 3

*What are some of the complications arising from a placenta accreta/increta/percreta?*

## ANSWER 3

Significant maternal and fetal morbidity have been reported. Hemorrhage, mortality 7–20%, uterine wall rupture, bladder invasion necessitating bladder resection, hysterectomy in 70–80% cases, disseminated intravascular coagulation, surgical reexploration, and uterine inversion. Fetal complications are related to the attendant risks of premature delivery, although a recent study also reported a higher risk of small for gestational age fetuses

**TABLE 66-1.**

| CONDITION | RISK OF ACCRETA |
|---|---|
| Unscarred uterus with placenta previa | 5% |
| One prior cesarean section with placenta previa | 24% |
| More than four cesarean section with placenta previa | 67% |

SOURCE: Clark SL, Koonings SP, Phelan JP. *Obst Gynecol.* 1985;66.

among women with a placenta accrete suggesting that the abnormal placental may affect fetal perfusion.

## BIBLIOGRAPHY


Clark S, Koonings PP, Phelan JP. Placenta previa/accreta and prior cesarean section. *Obstet Gynecol.* 1985;66(1):89–92.

Cunningham FG, MacDonald PC. Abnormalities of the third stage of labor. *Williams Obstetrics.* 19th ed. Stamford, Conn: Appleton & Lange. 1993;620–22.

Gielchinsky Y, Mankuta D, Rojansky N, Laufer N, Gielchinsky I, Ezra Y. Perinatal outcome of pregnancies complicated by placenta accreta. *Obstet Gynecol.* 2004;104(3):527–530.

Guy G. Ultrasonographic evaluation of uteroplacental blood flow patterns of abnormally located and adherent placentas. *Am J Obstet Gynecol.* 1990;163:723–727.

Hudon L, Belfort MA, Broome DR. Diagnosis and management of placenta percreta: a review. *Obstet Gynecol Survey.* 1998:53(8):509–517.

Levine D, Hulka CA, Ludmir J, Li W, Edelman RR. Placenta accreta: evaluation with color Doppler US, power Doppler US, and MR imaging. *Radiology.* 1997;205(3):773–776.

Price F. Placenta previa percreta involving the bladder: a report of 2 cases and review of the literature. *Obstet Gynecol.* 1991;78:509–511.

Silver L, et al. Placenta previa precreta with bladder involvement: new considerations and review of the literature. *Ultrasound Obstet Gynecol.* 1997;9:151–158.


# 67 PLACENTA PREVIA

*Kimberly D. Gregory*

## LEARNING POINT

Definition, risk factors, and management of placenta previa.

## VIGNETTE

A 24-year-old, G2P1, female presents at 20 weeks gestation who presents complaining of vaginal bleeding. She denies contractions, ruptured membranes. Past medical history is significant for a prior term delivery. She had a cesarean delivery for breech presentation. Fetal heart rate was noted to be 150 bpm. A transabdominal ultrasound was performed that noted an anterior low-lying placenta.

### QUESTION 1

*What is the definition and incidence rate of placenta previa?*

### ANSWER 1

Placenta previa is the implantation of the placenta over the cervical os. The incidence rate is approximately 1 in 200 live births. There are three types of placenta previa: (1) total previa where the cervical os is completely covered by the placenta; (2) partial previa where the cervix extends and covers part of the os; (3) marginal previa where the placental edge extends up to but does not cover the cervical os. The incidence rate of placenta previa depends on the gestational age that the patient is being evaluated and the amount of the placenta that covers the os. Between 18 and 25 weeks, low-lying placentas and/or placenta previa has been described in 12–25% of routine ultrasounds. Total placenta previa will persist in approximately 25% of cases, and partial or marginal previa will persist in less than 3% of cases. More objective measurement of the amount of placenta covering the os indicates that if the placenta is within 15 mm of the os, 20% of these will persist as placenta previa at term, whereas if the placenta edge extended to 25 mm, 40% of patients will have placenta previa at term. Placenta previa is most commonly recognized via transabdominal ultrasonography, and accuracy rates approach 90–95%. False positive results can be due to bladder distension. The examination should be repeated after bladder emptying to confirm the diagnosis. Using transvaginal sonography, the reported accuracy rates are approximately 98%.

### QUESTION 2

*What are the more common risk factors for placenta previa?*

### ANSWER 2

There are multiple risk factors for cesarean delivery (see Table 67-1). Previous cesarean delivery is the leading risk factor, and is dose dependent; the more cesareans, the higher the risk (incidence is 1% with one prior cesarean, increases to approximately 10% with four

**TABLE 67-1. Risk Factors for Placenta Previa**

| |
|---|
| Previous cesarean delivery |
| Prior placenta previa |
| Advanced maternal age |
| Ethnicity |
| Multiparity |
| Multiple prior abortions |
| Cigarette smoking |
| Cocaine use |

prior cesareans. Hence, there is concern about the rising rate of cesarean deliveries, since they will likely be accompanied by increased rates of abnormal placentation (both previa and abruption). Smoking has had inconsistent findings in recent epidemiologic-based studies. One population-based prospective cohort study from Nova Scotia confirmed a strong association of cigarette smoking with abruption (relative risk [RR] 2.05, 95% confidence interval [CI] 1.75–2.40) and a weak association with placenta previa (RR 1.36, 95% CI 1.04–1.79)

## QUESTION 3

*What is an appropriate management scheme for a woman with known previa after experiencing an episode of vaginal bleeding?*

## ANSWER 3

Most patients experiencing an episode of vaginal bleeding after viability should be admitted and observed from 24 to 72 hours. Patients who are Rh negative should receive Rhogam. Kleihauer-Betke testing may be of value in patients with bleeding who are Rh negative because of the small risk of fetal hemorrhage. After normal baseline values are obtained there is no need to repeat clotting studies in patient who are not having a bleeding diathesis. If the patient is stable, without further bleeding, one can consider outpatient therapy. One prospective randomized control trial and several retrospective reports have demonstrated safety and cost-effectiveness of outpatient management in candidates with <4 episodes of vaginal bleeding, demonstrated compliance, live proximal to the hospital, have a telephone, and have access to transportation (see Table 67-2).

Patients with persistent bleeding may experience uterine contractions and are candidates for tocolysis, antenatal corticosteroids, and maternal transfusions to maintain maternal hematocrit >30%. Patients receiving

**TABLE 67-2. Summary Outline of Management of Patients with Placenta Previa**

| **Management** |
|---|
| 1. At term → deliver |
| 2. Remote from term (24–36 weeks): |
| **Expectant management** |
| a. Replace maternal blood loss to maintain hematocrit above 30% |
| b. Rhogam to all women who are Rh negative and not sensitized; follow with Kleihauer-Betke with repeated episodes of vaginal bleeding |
| c. Once course of antenatal corticosteroids between 24–34 weeks if actively bleeding and at risk for preterm delivery |
| d. Bedrest (inpatient vs outpatient) |
| e. Amniocentesis at 34–36 weeks, scheduled cesarean delivery if lung maturity confirmed |

tocolysis need to be monitored carefully, but studies suggest pregnancy prolongation by up to 14 days, without significant maternal side effects. Amniocentesis for fetal lung maturity should be performed in stable hospitalized patients. If the gestational age is >34 weeks in the presence of recurrent and/or active bleeding, the patient should be delivered.

## QUESTION 4

*What are the more common complications associated with placenta previa?*

## ANSWER 4

Maternal:

- Anterpartum vaginal bleeding
- Five percent of symptomatic patients will require urgent delivery
- Sixty percent of symptomatic patients who stabilize will have recurrent bleeding episodes
- Abnormal placenta invasion (accreta, increta, percreta)
- Postpartum vaginal bleeding
- Blood transfusion
- Hysterectomy

Fetal:

- Preterm delivery
- Low birth weight
- Stillbirth

## BIBLIOGRAPHY

Ananth CV, Smulian JC, Vintzileos AM. The association of placenta previa with history of cesarean delivery and abortion: a meta-analysis. *Am J Obstet Gynecol.* 1997;177(5):1071–1078.

Benedetti TJ. Obstetric hemorrhage. In: Gabbe SG, Niebyl JR, Simpson JL (eds.). *Obstetrics Normal and Problem Pregnancies.* 4th ed. *Maternal Fetal Medicine.* 5th ed. Philadephia, PA: Churchill Livingstone; 2002:503.

Besinger RE, Moniak CW, Paskiewicz LS, Fisher SG, Tomich PG. The effect of tocolytic use in the management of symptomatic placenta previa. *Am J Obstet Gynecol.* 995;172(16): 1770–1778.

Cunningham FG, Gant NF, Leveno KJ,Gilstrap LC, Hauth JC, Wenstrom KD et al (eds.). Obstetrical Hemorrhage. Chapter 25. In: *Williams Obstetrics.* 21st ed. New York, NY: McGraw-Hill; 2006:619–670.

Droste S, Keil K. Expectant management of placenta previa: cost-benefit analysis of outpatient treatment. *Am J Obstet Gynecol.* 1994;170:1254–1257.

Faiz AS, Ananth CV. Etiology and risk factors for placenta previa: an overview and meta-analysis of observational studies. *J Matern Fetal Neonatal Med.* 2003;13(3):175–190.

Mouer JR. Placenta previa: antepartum conservative management, inpatient versus outpatient. *Am J Obstet Gynecol.* 1994; 170:1683–1685.

Smith RS, Lauria MR, Comstock CH, et al. Transvaginal ultrasonography for all placentas that appear to be low-lying or over the internal os. *Ultrasound Obstet Gynecol.* 1997;9:22–24.

Wing DA, et al. Usefulness of coagulation studies and blood banking in patients with symptomatic placenta previa. *Am J Perinatol.* 1997;14(10): 601–604.

Wing DA, Paul RH, Millar LK. Management of the symptomatic placenta previa: a randomized, controlled trial of inpatient versus outpatient expectant management. *Am J Obstet Gynecol.* 1996;175:806–811.

# 68 PREECLAMPSIA, ECLAMPSIA, AND HELLP SYNDROME

*Marguerite Lisa Bartholomew*

## LEARNING POINT

Definitions, recurrence risk, and complications of hypertensive disorders of pregnancy.

## VIGNETTE

A 19-year-old, G1P0, at 39 weeks gestation, complains of headache, nausea, and vomiting. She denies any medical problems prior to pregnancy. She denies scotomata or right upper quadrant pain. Her blood pressure is 165/112 mm Hg. Urine dipstick indicates +3 proteinuria. The nonstress test is reassuring. Ultrasound indicates an estimated fetal weight at less than the 10th percentile with low normal amniotic fluid volume.

Physical examination indicates lungs clear to auscultation, mild right upper quadrant tenderness, significant facial, and pedal edema. Neurological examination is unremarkable except for brisk patellar reflexes. The cervical is 2 cm dilated, 100% effaced, and at +1 station.

Laboratory values are as follows:

| | |
|---|---|
| Hematocrit | 40% |
| Platelet count | 90,000 |
| AST | 124 mg/dL |
| LDH | 300 mg/dL |

Magnesium sulfate seizure prophylaxis is begun. After pitocin induction, she delivers a 2300 g female with Apgars of 8 at 1 minute and 9 at 5 minutes. Magnesium sulfate is discontinued 24 hours after delivery.

## QUESTION 1

*What are the five types of hypertensive disorders seen in pregnancy? Briefly define.*

## ANSWER 1

The working group of the National High Blood Pressure Education Program (2000) proposed a standardized classification system to avoid nonuniform and confusing terminology that has long been a problem in obstetrics (note that BP = blood pressure, SBP = systolic blood pressure, and DBP = diastolic blood pressure):

- Gestational hypertension (formerly known as pregnancy-induced hypertension [PIH] or transient hypertension)
  1. BP ≥140/90 mm Hg on two occasions 4 hours apart without proteinuria for the first time during pregnancy or in the first 24 hours postpartum.
  2. A 30/15 mm Hg increase over baseline, BP is no longer diagnostic, but these patients warrant further observation.
  3. Resolves by 12 weeks postpartum.
  4. The acronym "PIH" should not be used unless referring specifically to gestational hypertension alone.
  5. Severe range BP is defined as ≥160/110 mm Hg. DBP >120 is associated with loss of cerebral arteriolar auto regulation, and hypertensive encephalopathy may occur when the DBP reaches or exceeds 130–150 mm Hg.

- Preeclampsia
  1. Gestational hypertension plus proteinuria (more than 300 mg/24 h, or 30 mg/dL, (i.e., +1 on urinalysis, on two separate occasions 4 hours apart on random specimens) or gestational hypertension with or without proteinuria in association with persistent central nervous system symptoms, epigastric pain, nausea and vomiting, fetal growth restriction, new onset creatinine elevation, hemolysis, thrombocytopenia (< 100,000/mm$^3$), or elevated AST or ALT.
  2. A 24-hour urine collection for proteinuria is diagnostic and the preferred method if possible.
  3. Generally occurs after 20 weeks gestation unless associated with molar pregnancy or a fetus with alpha thallasemia major (Bart Hb).
  4. Edema occurs in too many women with normal pregnancies to be discriminatory and has been abandoned as a marker in this and other classification schemes. However, despite this statement, centralized edema or rapid weekly weight gain is part of the pathophysiology of the disease and should not be dismissed even if peripheral edema is no longer considered diagnostic.
  5. The Working Group does not specifically distinguish mild from severe preeclampsia (Table 68-1), although The American College of Obstetricians and Gynecologists (ACOG) does recognize this entity (Table 68-2).
- Eclampsia

  Preeclampsia plus seizure, not attributable to other causes.
- Preeclampsia superimposed on chronic hypertension
  1. Hypertension without proteinuria documented before 20 weeks gestation, with new onset proteinuria (+1 on two occasions, 4 hours apart on random specimens, or 300 mg/24 h).
  2. Hypertension and proteinuria documented before 20 weeks with any of the following:
     a. Sudden increase in proteinuria
     b. Sudden increase in BP that was previously well controlled (not due to noncompliance with medications)

**TABLE 68-1. Criteria for Diagnosis of Preeclampsia**

NATIONAL HIGH BLOOD PRESSURE EDUCATION PROGRAM WORKING GROUP 2000

- Blood pressure of 140 mm Hg systolic or higher, or 90 mm Hg or higher diastotic that occurs after 20 weeks of gestation in a woman with previously normal blood pressure.
- Proteinuria, defined as urinary excretion of 300 mg protein or higher, in a 24-hour specimen.

SOURCE: Data from report of the National High Blood Pressure Education Program Working Group Report on High Blood Pressure in Pregnancy. *Am J Obstet Gynecol.* 2000;183:S1–S22.

**TABLE 68-2. Diagnosis of Severe Preeclampsia**

Preeclampsia is considered severe if one or more of the following criteria is present:

- Blood pressure of 160 mm Hg systolic, or higher, or 110 mm Hg diastolic or higher, on two occasions at least 6 hours apart while the patient is on bedrest.
- Proteinuria of 5 g or higher in a 25-hour specimen or 3+ or greater on two random urine samples collected at least 4 hours apart.
- Oliguria of less than 500 mL in 24 hours
- Cerebral or visual disturbances
- Pulmonary edema or cyanosis
- Epigastric or right upper-quadrant pain
- Impaired liver function (>2 times upper limit of normal)*
- Thrombocytopenia (< 100,000/mm$^3$)*
- Fetal growth restriction

*Liver function and platelet thresholds not specified by ACOG, but are the thresholds commonly used by experts: Schiff E, Freidman SA, Sibai BM. Conservative management of severe preeclampsia remote from term. *Obstet Gynecol.* 1994;84:626–630.

SOURCE: Adapted with permission from Diagnosis and Management of Preeclampsia and Eclampsia. ACOG Practice Bulletin No. 33. American College of Obstetricians and Gynecologists. *Obstet Gynecol.* 2002;99: 159–167.

     c. Thrombocytopenia (< 100,000/mm$^3$) or
     d. Elevated AST or ALT.

- Chronic hypertension
  1. Hypertension (≥ 140/90 mm Hg) that is present and observable before pregnancy or diagnosed before the 20th week of gestation or
  2. Hypertension diagnosed for the first time during pregnancy, which does not resolve postpartum.

## QUESTION 2

*On postpartum day 2, this patient asks you if there is anything that can be done to prevent the recurrence of preeclampsia in a subsequent pregnancy. What would you tell her?*

## ANSWER 2

The incidence of preeclampsia is about 5%, and the risk of recurrent preeclampsia after a first severe episode is 12–25%. The recurrence risk after mild disease in the first pregnancy is not as well known. Surveillance during the next pregnancy to identify the condition as early as possible is the best option.

Overall, attempts to prevent preeclampsia have been disappointing, despite the many modalities investigated (antihypertensives, calcium, low-dose aspirin, magnesium, zinc, fish oil, vitamins C and E, and so on). There are at least 15 randomized trials of antihypertensives and diuretics showing no benefit. Randomized trials with limited sample size of magnesium, zinc, and fish oil have also not been shown to prevent preeclampsia.

There are six randomized placebo controlled trials using calcium. Calcium was shown to be of benefit in reducing preeclampsia in three studies evaluating only high-risk women (positive roll over test or increased sensitivity to angiotensin II). However, the largest randomized trial of calcium supplementation in healthy nulliparas sponsored by the National Institutes of Health Care (NIH) (2295 pts in each group) demonstrated no benefit. Calcium supplementation (600–2000 mg) may be of some benefit in particularly high-risk women. A diet that provides 1000 mg of elemental calcium per day is recommended for all women (pregnant or not), and the U.S. Food and Drug Administration (FDA) cites 2500 mg as the upper limit for daily calcium intake.

There appears to be no benefit to low-dose aspirin. Studies that have shown a reduction in preeclampsia did not show a difference in pregnancy outcome. Of the eight randomized placebo controlled trials published since 1993 in different populations around the world (totaling 27,000 women), seven demonstrated no reduction in preeclampsia incidence with prophylactic low-dose aspirin, and the reduction shown in the remaining trial was not statistically significant. In a NIH funded study 2539 women at high risk for preeclampsia (i.e., having pregestational diabetes, chronic hypertension, multifetal gestation, or preeclampsia in a previous pregnancy) were randomized to low-dose aspirin, no benefit was observed over placebo.

Recently, preeclampsia has been linked to increased oxidative stress. One randomized trial suggested the benefits of vitamins C and E supplementation to prevent preeclampsia in high-risk women. Although encouraging, such therapy needs confirmation in larger numbers before recommending it as a preventative measure.

## QUESTION 3

*What percentage of women with preeclampsia will develop the HELLP syndrome and what are the top three serious maternal complications that may occur as a result?*

## ANSWER 3

The reported incidence of the HELLP syndrome in preeclampsia ranges from 2% to 12%, reflecting differences in diagnostic criteria. The syndrome is more common in Caucasian patients and is more likely to be present when preeclampsia occurs remote from term. HELLP syndrome may present with a variety of unusual signs and symptoms, therefore a reasonable index of suspicion, regardless of BP level, is necessary to make the diagnosis. Normal BP does not rule out HELLP syndrome. Serious maternal complications of HELLP syndrome include disseminated intravascular coagulation (DIC) (20%), abruption (16%), acute renal failure (8%), pulmonary edema (6%), intracerebral hemorrhage (1.5%), cerebral edema/eclampsia (1–9%), retinal detachment (1%), laryngeal edema (1%), retinal detachment (1%), subcapsular liver hematoma (1%), acute respiratory distress syndrome (ARDS) (1%), and death (1%).

## BIBLIOGRAPHY

ACOG Practice Bulletin. No. 33. Diagnosis and Management of Preeclampsia and Eclampsia. 2002.

Audibert F, et al. Clinical utility of strict diagnostic criteria for the HELLP syndrome. *Am J Obstet Gynecol.* 1996;175:460.

Chappell LC, Seed PT, Briley AL, et al. Effects of antioxidants on the occurrence of preeclampsia in women at increased risk: a randomized trial. *Lancet.* 1999;354:810–816.

Sibai BM. Hypertension. In: Gabbe SG, Niebyl JR, Simpson JL, (eds.). *Obstetrics: Normal and Problem Pregnancies.* 4th ed. New York: Churchill Livingstone; 2002:945–947.

Report of the National High Blood Pressure Education Program Working Group on High Blood Pressure in Pregnancy. *Am J Obstet Gynecol.* 183(1);2000:S1–S22.

Sabai BM, et al. Maternal morbidity and mortality in 442 pregnancies with hemolysis, elevated liver enzymes, and low platelets. *Am J Obstet Gynecol.* 169;1000:1993.

Sibai BM. Prevention of preeclampsia: a big disappointment. *Am J Obstet Gynecol.* 1998;179(5):1275–1278.

# 69 OBESITY AND BARIATRIC SURGERY

*Kimberly D. Gregory*

## LEARNING POINT

Definition of obesity, criteria for bariatric surgery, procedure options, and impact of procedures on pregnancy outcome.

## VIGNETTE

A 32-year-old, nulligravid, female presents to you for preconception counseling regarding pregnancy after bariatric surgery. She states that she had the procedure

3 years ago, has lost 120 lb, and currently weighs 160 lb. She is recently married, has regular periods, but is concerned about deliberate weight gain, and nutritional requirements associated with pregnancy.

## QUESTION 1

*What is the definition of obesity?*

## ANSWER 1

The criteria for obesity varies by age, race, and height, hence most researchers have advocated for the use of the basal metabolic index (BMI = $kg/m^2$ or weight/height$^2$) as a standardized measure of obesity. This index provides a good measure for body mass and body fat. Overweight is BMI 25–29 $kg/m^2$ and obesity is considered >30 $kg/m^2$, and morbid obesity is defined as greater than 40 $kg/m^2$ or a BMI of >35 $kg/m^2$ with obesity comorbidity.

## QUESTION 2

*What are the treatment options for obesity, and how does obesity impact pregnancy?*

## ANSWER 2

Diet, exercise, behavioral therapy, pharmacologic agents, and surgery have all been used to treat obesity with various success rates. Ideally, some combination of diet, exercise, and behavioral therapy is preferred, with a goal of 10 weight loss in order to see demonstrated health benefits from loss. An NIH consensus development conference concluded that bariatric surgery is the only effective treatment for morbid obesity. Current procedure options include (1) gastric bypass, which involves complete partitioning of the stomach with anastomosis of the proximal gastric segment to a jejunal loop; and, (2) gastric banding, which involves partial partitioning at the proximal gastric segment with placement of gastric outlet opening of a fixed diameter. Both methods create an upper gastric pouch that reduces gastric luminal capacity and causes early satiety and/or malabsorbtion (see Figs. 69-1 and 69-2). In experienced hands, both procedures can be done laparoscopically.

Maternal obesity is associated with adverse pregnancy outcome. Studies have demonstrated increased rates of hypertensive disease (chronic hypertension and

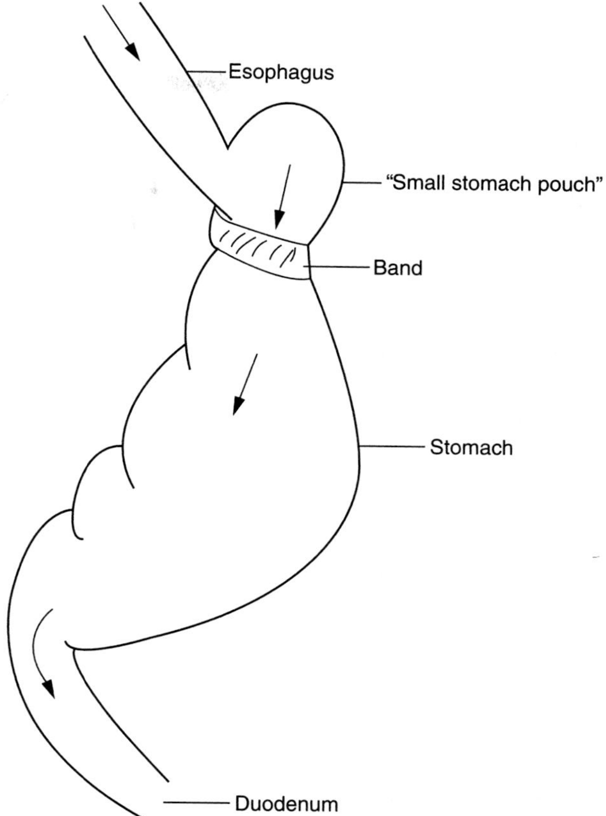


**FIG. 69-1** Gastric banding.

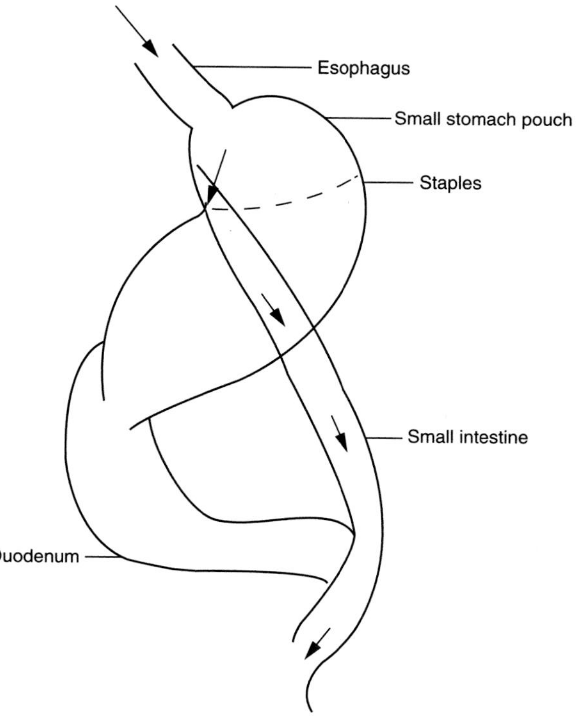


**FIG. 69-2** Gastric bypass.

preeclampsia), diabetes (pregestational and gestational), cesarean section, infections, increased rates of venous thromboembolic disease, and respiratory complications. Fetal and newborn consequences of maternal obesity include increased risk for neural tube defects, fetal mortality, and preterm delivery. Maternal obesity also increases the risk of delivering a large for gestational age or macrosomic neonate, who is at increased risk of subsequent childhood obesity and its associated morbidity. Both maternal and neonatal adverse outcomes are associated with increased costs.

### QUESTION 3

*If the patient gets pregnant, is she at increased risk for pregnancy-related complications due to prior bariatric surgery?*

### ANSWER 3

In a population-based study from Israel, women with prior bariatric surgery were at increased risk for previous cesarean delivery, fertility treatments, premature rupture of membranes, labor induction, and fetal macrosomia. Additionally, these women may be at increased risk of anemia due to iron, folate, and vitamin $B_{12}$ deficiencies. They do not appear to be at increased risk for adverse perinatal outcome.

### QUESTION 4

*What are the long term risks and benefits of bariatric surgery?*

### ANSWER 4

Approximately 60% of patients achieve approximately 60% weight loss after the first year and maintain this weight loss through 5 years. Health benefits include improved quality of life as measured by the SF 36 questionnaire, improved glucose tolerance and reversal of diabetes, hypertension, hyperlipidemia, and overall cardiovascular risk, as well as improvement in sleep apnea. Complications include procedure related mortality (approximately 0.3%), failure (procedure and operator dependent), wound complications (15%), venous thromboembolism, anastomotic leak (1% each).

Long term complications include the following:

- Dumping syndrome: postprandial sweating, weakness, hypoglycemia
- Nutritional defects (e.g., iron, vitamin $B_{12}$, calcium, fat soluble vitamins, folate deficiency, and hyperhomocystinemia)
- Gastroesophageal reflux
- Osteoporosis or metabolic disease
- Gallstones
- Gastrogastric fistula
- Excess skin
- Neurologic complications

## BIBLIOGRAPHY

Berger JR. The neurological compliations of bariatric surgery. *Arch Neurol.* 2004;61:1185–1189.

Castro LC, Avina RL. Maternal obesity and pregnancy outcomes. *Curr Opin Obstet Gynecol.* 2002; 14(6):601–606.

Galtier-Dereure F, Boegner C, Bringer J. Obesity and pregnancy: complications and cost. *Am J Clin Nutr.* 2000;71(Suppl. 5): 1242S–1248S.

Orzano AJ, Scott JG. Diagnosis and treatment of obesity in adults: an applied evidence-based review. *J Am Board Fam Pract.* 2004;17(5):359–369.

Persutti JR, Gorman SR, Swain JM. Primary care perspective on bariatric surgery. *Mayo Clin Proc.* 2004;79:1158–1166.

Rand C, Macgregor A. Medical care and pregnancy outcome after gastric bypass surgery for obesity. *South Med J.* 1989;82:1319–1320.

Sheiner E, Levy A, Silverberg D, Mens TS, Levy L, Katz M, Mazor M. Pregnancy after bariatric surgery is not associated with adverse perinatal outcome. *Am J Obstet Gynecol.* 2004:190:1335–1340.

# 70 SHOULDER DYSTOCIA

*Kimberly D. Gregory*

## LEARNING POINT

Risk factors, complications, and management of shoulder dystocia.

## VIGNETTE

A 22-year-old, G4P3, female at 39 weeks gestation is 10-cm dilated, completely effaced, and at 0 station for the past 2 hours. The baby's estimated fetal weight by an ultrasound performed 2 days ago is 4100 g. Her history is remarkable for a shoulder dystocia in a previous pregnancy. That child weighed 8 lb 5 oz. She has had two subsequent uncomplicated vaginal deliveries. Her largest infant weighed 9 lb. The patient weighs 250 lb, had an abnormal glucose tolerance test (GTT), followed by a normal 3-hour oral glucose tolerance test (OGTT).

## QUESTION 1

*What is the definition of shoulder dystocia and why does it occur?*

## ANSWER 1

Shoulder dystocia is most often defined as delivery that requires additional obstetric maneuvers following gentle downward traction of the fetal head to affect delivery of the shoulders. Shoulder dystocia is caused by impaction of the anterior fetal shoulder behind the maternal pubic symphysis, and can also occur from impaction of the posterior fetal shoulder on the sacral promontory. Since the diagnosis of shoulder dystocia does have a subjective component, it may be either underdiagnosed or overdiagnosed. The reported incidence is 0.6–1.4%.

## QUESTION 2

*Can shoulder dystocia be accurately predicted?*

## ANSWER 2

Shoulder dystocia is most often unpredictable and unpreventable. However, there are some factors that may increase the risk of shoulder dystocia (see Table 70-1). This patient has several risk factors including, multiparity, maternal obesity, previous history of macrosomic infant, previous history of shoulder dystocia (recurrence risk can be as high as 16%), and prolonged second stage. Additionally, although her 3-hour OGTT was normal, she had an elevated glucose tolerance test. While multiple risk factors have been identified, their predictive value is not high enough to be consistently useful in a clinical setting, and primarily serve to heighten clinical awareness to the potential. Several studies have shown that due to the inaccuracy of third trimester ultrasound, elective inductions for macrosomia are not indicated, and may increase the risk for cesarean delivery. Elective cesarean delivery may be considered for ultrasound estimated fetal weight of 5000 g in a nondiabetic and 4500 g in a diabetic.

**TABLE 70-1. Risk Factors for Shoulder Dystocia**

| |
|---|
| Fetal macrosomia |
| Maternal diabetes |
| Maternal obesity |
| Multiparity |
| Postterm pregnancy |
| Previous history of macrosomic infant |
| Previous history of shoulder dystocia |
| Labor induction |
| Epidural anesthesia |
| Operative vaginal delivery |
| Prolonged second stage of labor |

## QUESTION 3

*How should a shoulder dystocia be managed?*

## ANSWER 3

The success in managing shoulder dystocia depends on anticipation and preparation:

1. Patient should be in a delivery room
2. Refrain from pulling on the fetal head
3. Refrain from continued maternal pushing and from giving fundal pressure
4. McRoberts maneuver—hyperflexion of maternal legs on the maternal abdomen. This results in flattening the lumber spine and ventral rotation of the maternal pelvis and symphysis (increases posterior outlet)
5. Suprapubic pressure to disimpact the anterior shoulder
6. Wood's screw maneuver causing rotation of the anterior or posterior shoulder obliquely†
7. Delivery of the posterior arm by flexing the posterior arm at the elbow and sweeping the arm anteriorly over the chest†
8. Deliberate fracture of the fetal clavicle diminishes rigidity and size of shoulder girdle†
9. Zavanelli maneuver*—replacement of the fetal head into the uterus, followed by cesarean delivery
10. Symphysiotomy* (sharp dissection of symphysis and displacement of urethra); rarely reported in the United States

## QUESTION 4

*What the potential maternal and neonatal complications that can occur from shoulder dystocia?*

†Performing a proctoepisiotomy may help with providing more room so that this procedure can be accomplished, but generally does not directly help in managing shoulder dystocia.

*Should be performed unless conventional methods have first been tried.

## ANSWER 4

In a series describing the outcome of 236 shoulder dystocia cases, the maternal complications included postpartum hemorrhage (11%) and fourth degree lacerations (3.8%). Neonatal complications include: brachial plexus injuries, fractures of the clavicle and humerus, hypoxic ischemic encephalopathy, and death. Brachial plexus injuries following shoulder dystocias vary from 4% to 40%. Brachial plexus injuries have been described in the absence of documented shoulder dystocia, and approximately 4% occur after cesarean delivery. Most cases of brachial plexus injury resolve without permanent disability. Fewer than 10% of all cases of shoulder dystocia result in permanent injury.

## BIBLIOGRAPHY

ACOG Practice Bulletin No. 40. 2002.

Beall M, et al. A randomized controlled trial of prophylactic maneuvers to reduce head to body delivery time in patients at high risk for shoulder dystocia. *Obstet Gynecol.* 2003;102:31–35.

Gabbe S, et al. *Obstetrics: Normal and Problem Pregnancies*. 4th ed: 2001.

Gherman RB, et al. Brachial plexus palsy: an in utero injury? *Am J Obstet Gynecol.* 1999;180:1303–1307.

Gherman RB, et al. The McRoberts' maneuver for the alleviation of shoulder dystocia: how successful is it? *Am J Obstet Gynecol.* 1997;176:656–661.

Gilbert WM, et al. Associated factors in 1611 cases of brachial plexus injury. *Obstet Gynecol.* 1999;93:536–540.

Poggi SH, et al. Prioritizing posterior arm delivery during severe shoulder dystocia. *Obstet Gynecol.* 2003;101:1068–1072.

Robinson H, et al. Is maternal obesity a predictor of shoulder dystocia? *Obstet Gynecol.* 2003;101:24–27.

Rouse DJ, et al. The effectiveness and costs of elective cesarean delivery for fetal macrosomia diagnosed by ultrasound. *JAMA.* 1996;276:1480–1486.

Sandberg EC. The Zavanelli maneuver: 12 years of recorded experience. *Obstet Gynecol.* 1999;93:312–317.

# 71 TRAUMA DURING PREGNANCY

*Margurite Lisa Bartholomew*

## LEARNING POINT

Physical trauma complicates one out of 12 pregnancies. Accurate patient education and appropriate obstetrical care are critical to the management of this common problem.

## VIGNETTE

A 23-year-old, G1P0, is brought in by ambulance after being involved in a motor vehicle accident. She is 34 weeks pregnant with regular prenatal care. The paramedics describe that she was a belted driver alone in the car trying to make a left turn when she was hit on the right side by another car going approximately 25 mph. There was no loss of consciousness, head trauma, or direct abdominal trauma. The seatbelt engaged properly, and the airbags deployed. She denies vaginal bleeding, leaking from the vagina, or painful contractions. She reports that her abdomen is sore, but that the fetus is moving well. She denies neck pain and neurological symptoms.

The woman is tearful but alert and oriented. Her vital signs indicate a blood pressure of 120/70, heart rate of 85, respiratory rate of 14, and temperature of 99.9°F. She is wearing a c-spine collar. Her examination is unremarkable except that her abdomen shows some mild bruising over the inguinal/upper thigh area and between her breasts. The abdomen and fundus are nontender without guarding or rebound.

The fetal heart rate monitor reveals a reactive tracing at 150 bpm. There are no decelerations. Irregular contractions are noted every 15–20 minutes (3–4/h) and are palpably mild. Speculum examination indicates no bleeding or pooling. The cervical examination is closed, 50% effaced, and at 0 station. The cervical spine film is normal and the collar is removed. Her blood type is A positive. She is observed and monitored for 6 hours. She is discharged home with analgesics and a kick count chart. A follow-up visit with her obstetrician is scheduled in 24 hours.

## QUESTION 1

*What are the recommendations for monitoring pregnant women (>22–24 weeks gestation) who have sustained trauma?*

## ANSWER 1

The tradition has been to provide fetal/uterine monitoring for 24 hours after trauma, with the reasoning being that most placental abruptions will manifest within that time period of the traumatic event. However, studies indicate that shorter periods of monitoring are an option for selected patients, and the most recent ACOG educational bulletin published in 1998 states the following:

"Because abruption usually becomes apparent shortly after injury, monitoring should be initiated as soon as the woman is stabilized. Recommended minimum time of posttrauma monitoring includes 4 hour and 2–6 hours. None of these times have been validated by large prospective studies. Monitoring should be continued and further evaluation carried out if uterine contractions, a nonreassuring fetal heart rate pattern, vaginal bleeding, uterine tenderness, serious maternal injury, or rupture of membranes is present. If these findings are not present, the patient may be discharged or transferred."

The monitoring periods quoted above were derived from studies where the definitions of contractions were very specific. This is important because normal pregnancies without placental abruption may have regular contractions, particularly in the third trimester.

Pearlman and associates reported no abruptions if uterine contractions were less often than every 10 minutes (6/h) within 4 hours after trauma was sustained. Twenty percent of women who had more frequent contractions had an associated placental abruption. Goodwin and Breen studied noncatastrophic trauma and observed that 11% of those women with three contractions in 20 minutes, uterine tenderness, or vaginal bleeding experienced pregnancy complications related to the trauma. Fifty five percent of the complications were placental abruptions. Alternatively, only 0.9% of women without these signs had pregnancy complications related to the trauma.

In summary, in the absence of significant maternal injury or obstetrical findings (≥6–9 contractions/h, vaginal bleeding, ruptured membranes, or nonreassuring fetal testing), 4–6 hours of monitoring is generally sufficient. Direct abdominal trauma is not a prerequisite for abruption as shearing forces can incite abruption without direct trauma. In addition, the use of x-rays, CT scans, open peritoneal lavage, and surgery should not be withheld from a trauma patient simply because she is pregnant.

## QUESTION 2

*What are the complications that are encountered after trauma in pregnancy?*

## ANSWER 2

Each case should be individually assessed for placental abruption, uterine rupture, fetal-maternal hemorrhage, and fetal injury. The indicators of placental abruption were discussed in part in Answer 1 and include uterine contractions, tetanic contractions, uterine tenderness, vaginal bleeding, nonreassuring fetal heart rate patterns, fetal death, and coagulopathy. Uterine rupture, clinically significant fetal-maternal hemorrhage, and fetal injury are rare and are not usually encountered unless there is severe trauma. Small (less than 15 cc) fetal-maternal hemorrhages are seen commonly after trauma. Many experts discourage the routine use of the Kleihauer-Betke test after trauma because it has not been shown to be clinically more effective in predicting adverse outcome than the usual fetal and uterine monitoring. Significant fetal hemorrhages are more commonly detected by changes in the fetal heart rate monitoring. However, the Kleihauer-Betke test may be reserved for severe trauma cases and for those women who are Rh negative (to determine the appropriate Rhogam dose).

## QUESTION 3

*What are the most common types of trauma observed in pregnancy?*

## ANSWER 3

The three main types of trauma during pregnancy are blunt trauma, penetrating trauma, and thermal injury. Blunt trauma is subdivided into physical abuse, sexual assault, auto accidents, and falls. Penetrating trauma includes knife and gunshot wounds related to assault, suicide, or abortion attempts. Thermal injury includes burns and electric shock.

*Physical/sexual abuse*: It is estimated that up to 25% of women have been physically or sexually abused during the pregnancy, while, according to an ACOG fellows survey, only 40% of obstetricians routinely screen for abuse at the first prenatal visit. Risk factors for physical abuse in pregnancy include social instability (young age, few support systems, undereducation, unemployment, and the like), an unhealthy lifestyle (substance abuse, poor nutrition, and the like), and physical health problems (medical or psychiatric problems, use of prescription medications, and the like).

There is a tendency for physical abuse to increase during pregnancy and in the first few postpartum months. Care and planning must be undertaken before a woman is encouraged to leave her abuser particularly during pregnancy. Separation from the abuser is the time at which a woman is most likely to be seriously injured or killed. In a review of sexual assaults in Dallas, Texas over 6 years, 2% of the women were pregnant. Another study reported that 8% of pregnant adolescents had been sexually assaulted. Almost 50% identified a family member as the perpetrator.

*Motor vehicle accidents*: Automobile accidents are the most common cause of death in young females and are the most common cause of traumatic fetal deaths. Seatbelts are recommended for all pregnant women. Seatbelt use during pregnancy protects both mother and fetus. In studies using "pregnant" crash test dummies, proper use of three point seat belts significantly reduces force transmission to the pregnant uterus (Fig. 71-1). The lap belt should be worn snugly under the uterus and across the pubic symphysis and anterior superior iliac spines. The shoulder belt should be placed snugly between the breasts. The belt should never be placed over the dome of the uterus. Prenatal seat belt education has been shown to be effective in improving compliance and proper use.

*Penetrating Trauma*: During pregnancy, the incidence of major organ injury is less common when compared to nonpregnant victims. The fetus (66%) is more likely than the mother (20%) to be seriously injured after a knife or gunshot wound. The mortality for pregnant women after a gunshot is 3.9%, compared to a 12.5% mortality in nonpregnant patients. Although unpredictable, wounds presenting in the upper abdomen or back are more likely to cause maternal visceral injury. Wounds in the front lower abdomen are more likely to cause fetal injury.

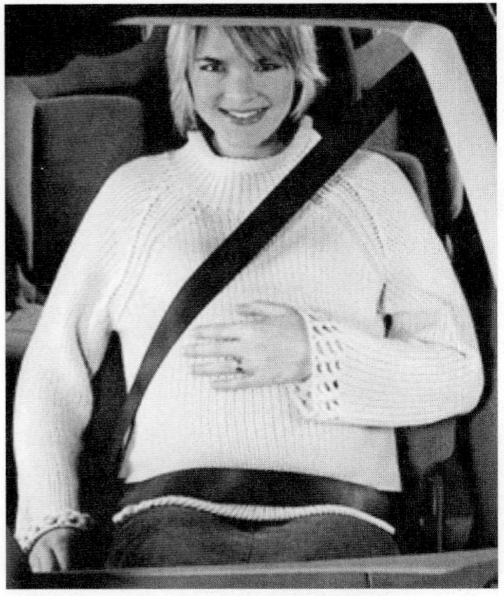

**FIG. 71-1** Proper use of a seatbelt during pregnancy.
SOURCE: From www.baby-marketing.co.uk/automotive/

## QUESTION 4

*What are the guidelines for performing cardiopulmonary resuscitation (CPR) and perimortem cesarean delivery?*

## ANSWER 4

Shock and cardiac arrest are potential complications of trauma during pregnancy. In general, delivering the baby improves the success of maternal CPR. A team approach is necessary for optimal outcomes. Ideally, there are at least nine staff: a code team leader, an airway person, a chest compression person, a vascular access person, a drug administration person, an event recorder, a physician to perform a cesarean delivery, and a neonatologist/ pediatrician.

In nonpregnant individuals CPR results in a cardiac output of only 30% of normal, while CPR performed in the second half of pregnancy is ineffectual unless the uterus is displaced off the vena cava and aorta. The best position is a left tilt using a wedge under the right hip or by tilting the table. Tilting the table makes chest compressions very difficult, therefore the wedge is the preferred method. Outside of maternal positioning and delivery (if necessary), the method of CPR and advanced cardiac life support (ACLS) are usually the same for pregnant and nonpregnant persons.

The longer the fetus is exposed to maternal cardiac arrest, the higher the risk of neurological damage. CPR should be continued throughout the cesarean delivery. The goal is to deliver the baby within 5 minutes of maternal cardiac arrest for optimum fetal outcome. If CPR is successful within 4 minutes in restoring maternal cardiovascular stability, then delivery can be postponed. ACOG recommends cesarean delivery at or before 5 minutes for pregnancies in the third trimester complicated by maternal cardiac arrest. This recommendation is based on the data depicted in Table 71-1.

**TABLE 71-1. Prevalence of Neurologically Intact Infants by Time from Cardiac Arrest to Delivery**

| TIME FROM CARDIAC ARREST TO DELIVERY (MINUTES) | NEUROLOGICALLY INTACT INFANTS (%) |
|---|---|
| 0–5 | 98 |
| 6–15 | 83 |
| 16–25 | 33 |
| 26–35 | 25 |
| 36+ | 0 |

SOURCE: Reprinted from Clark SL, Cotton DB, Hankins GDV, Phelan JP. *Critical Care Obstetrics*. 3rd ed. Boston, MA: Blackwell Science; 1997:691.

Perimortem cesarean delivery *before* 24 weeks gestation would be for maternal benefit only. If at all possible, the patient herself or the family of the critically ill woman should be encouraged to give their input about perimortem cesarean delivery after they have been given accurate gestational age specific information about morbidity and mortality of the mother and future infant.

## BIBLIOGRAPHY

ACOG Educational Bulletin No. 251. Obstetric Aspects of Trauma Management. 1998.

Bajo TM. Cardiopulmonary resuscitation of the pregnant woman. In: Foley MR, Strong TH (eds.). *Obstetric Intensive Care: A Practical Manual*. Philadelphia, PA: WB Saunders; 1997:231.

Clark SL, Cotton DB, Hankins GDV, Phelan JP. *Critical Care Obstetrics*. 3rd ed. Boston, MA: Blackwell Science; 1997:691.

Cuningham FG, Gant NF, Leveno KJ, et al. Critical care and trauma. In: *Williams Obstetrics*. 21st ed. New York, NY: McGraw Hill; 2001:1171.

Goodwin TM, Breen MT. Pregnancy outcome and fetomaternal hemorrhage after noncatastrophic trauma. *Am J Obstet Gynecol*. 1990;162:665.

Katz VL, Dotter DJ, Droegemueller W. Perimortem cesarean delivery. *Obstet Gynecol*. 1986;68:571.

Pearlman MD, Tintinalli JE, Lorenz RP. A prospective controlled study of outcome after trauma during pregnancy. *Am J Obstet Gynecol*. 1990;162:1502.

Shah AJ, Kilcline BA. Trauma in pregnancy. *Emerg Med Clin N Am*. 2003;21:615.

Towery R, English TP, Wisner D. Evaluation of pregnant women after blunt injury. *J Trauma*. 1993;35:731.

# 72 UTERINE INVERSION

*Calvin J. Hobel*

## LEARNING POINT

The risk for uterine inversion is difficult to predict. The immediate identification of this *obstetrical emergency* is important because of maternal hemorrhage and shock. Immediate treatment is vital to reduce the risk of maternal morbidity or mortality.

## VIGNETTE

A 32-year-old, G4P3, at 40 weeks gestation was admitted in active labor with intact membranes. She received prenatal care beginning at 14 weeks and she did not have or develop any medical problems. Her prenatal laboratory work was normal and she had a fetal anatomic survey ultrasound at 18 weeks. The ultrasound revealed a normal-appearing male infant and the placenta was noted to be anterior-fungal location. She had a total of nine prenatal visits and her glucose screen at 28 weeks was reported as normal.

At the time of admission, the physical examination showed that she was 4 cm dilated with intact membranes and the fetal heart tracing was reactive with a normal baseline. Because of moderate pain with labor, the patient received epidural anesthesia. Membranes were ruptured at 6 cm and the fluid was noted to be clear. Her labor progressed rapidly and within 3 hours she spontaneously delivered a 3406 gm male infant with an Apgar score of 9 at 1 minute and 10 at 5 minutes. With minimal traction the placenta was not expelled so the attendant decided to wait 10 minutes and with fundal pressure and traction the placenta delivered, but it remained adherent to something within the vagina forming a rather large mass (attendant had never experienced this situation), but with minimal pealing the placenta detached followed by moderate bleeding from a large raw-appearing surface. The attendant immediately called for assistance recognizing this must be an inverted uterus. An experienced obstetrician arrived along with an anesthesiologist and the diagnosis of uterine inversion was made. The patient was in shock (BP = 60/30 mm Hg and heart rate = 140 bpm) and bleeding moderately. The patient already had an indwelling 18-gauge intravenous catheter.

### QUESTION 1

*What are the immediate steps to be taken in the management of uterine inversion (1–3)?*

### ANSWER 1

1. Immediately call for help, including an anesthesiologist.
2. Have an attendant immediately apply oxygen by facemask.
3. Immediately give a liter of lactated Ringer's solution.
4. If the diagnosis of uterine inversion is obvious, pressure on the exposed inverted uterus will decrease the hemorrhage and often the blood pressure will improve.
5. Since the patient has had an epidural, the uterus may be reduced easily by applying firm pressure (fist or the three middle fingers) at the apex (mid) of the exposed surface and pushing the uterus back into the vagina.

6. If the above attempts fail to reduce the inverted uterus, pharmacologic measures must be considered.
7. Meanwhile the anesthesiologist will continue resuscitation efforts with supporting the blood pressure with Phenylephrine and volume expansion.

## QUESTION 2

*What is the incidence, maternal risk, and classification of uterine inversion?*

## ANSWER 2

The incidence is 1 in 2000 deliveries, but the range can be from 1/2000 to 1 in several hundred thousand. It is important to note that uterine inversion can occur in gynecologic case as well as with the delivery of the placenta.

The maternal risk can be high. Delay in diagnosis results in the need for blood transfusion and prolonged hypotension if the cause is not recognized. Maternal mortality has been reported to be as high as 15%.

The classification of uterine inversion is:

1. Incomplete inversion (No. 2 in Fig. 72-1): The uterine fundus lies within the endometrial cavity without extending beyond the external os. This state could also be considered an subacute inversion.
2. Complete inversion (No. 3 in Fig. 72-1): The inverted fundus extends beyond the external os and is within the vaginal canal.
3. Prolapsed inversion (No. 4 in Fig. 72-1): The inverted uterine fundus extends beyond the vaginal intrtoitus.

## QUESTION 3

*What is the incidence and etiology of uterine inversion?*

## ANSWER 3

The etiology is uncertain but the following factors in order of the frequency of their association (natural vs. operator) are:

Natural causes:

1. Fundal location of placenta
2. Placenta accreta
3. Rapid emptying of the uterus
4. Short umbilical cord
5. The use of oxytocin and magnesium sulfate

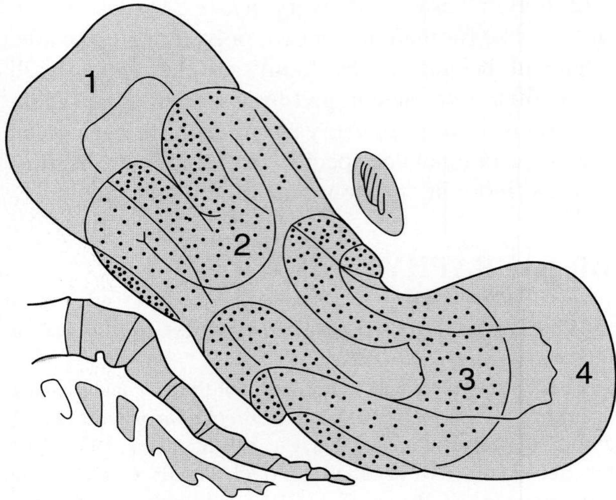


**FIG. 72-1** Progressive degrees of uterine inversion.
SOURCE: Adapted from Cunningham FG, Gant NF, Leveno KJ, Gilstrap LC, Hauth JC, and Wenstrom KD. *Obstetrical Hemorrhage*. Chapter 25. *Williams Obstetrics*. 21st ed. New York, NY: McGraw-Hill;2001.

6. Anomalies of the uterus
7. Prolonged distention as with multiple gestations and polyhydramios

Operator associated causes:

1. Excessive traction on the umbilical cord
2. Excessive fundal pressure

## QUESTION 4

*What are the methods for treating uterine inversion?*

## ANSWER 4

1. Manual correction of the inversion through the vagina is known as the Johnson maneuver, which consists of pushing the inverted fundus through the cervical ring with pressure using the middle three fingers on the inverted fundus directed toward the umbilicus. Oxytocic agents should be withheld until the uterus is replaced. If this fails then uterine relaxants must be used to relax the cervix and lower uterine segment.
2. Several intravenous drugs have been used to relax the uterus. These are magnesium sulfate, terbutaline, and nitroglycerin. Recently, a sublingual nitroglycerin spray in 0.4 mg/metered doses is easy and safe to use. Usually no more than three doses are required. The choice drug is nitroglycerin because it is very quick in action and its primary effect is to reduce hypertonus or spasm and it does not eliminate the basal

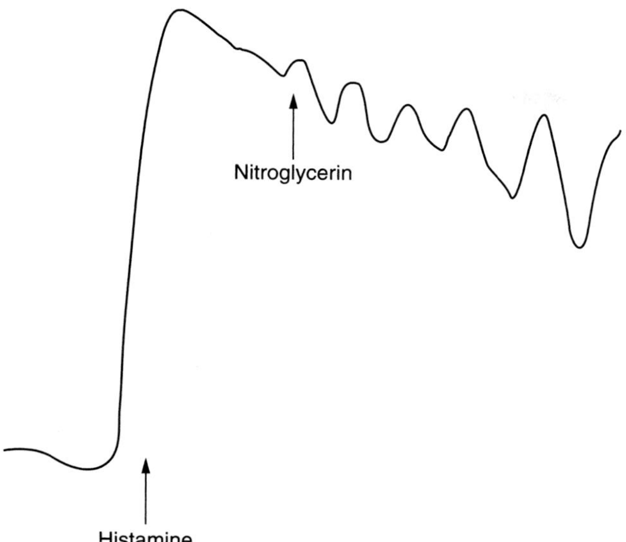


**FIG. 72-2** Histamine induced hypertonus followed by nitrite restoring rhythmical contractions.
SOURCE: Croft C. Contraction ring: treatment of amyl nitrite, with observations on the pharmacological action of nitrite. *Proc R Soc Med.* 1935;28:37–44.

muscular tone of the uterus or of the blood vessels (Fig. 72-2 and note that after nitroglycerin administration uterine tone remains and this is thought to decrease the risk of hemorrhage). Refer to the classic article by CR Groft published in 1935.

Thus, it is safer to use small doses of nitroglycerin (amyl nitrite) than the more prolonged effect of magnesium sulfate or terbutaline. Nitroglycerin has also been used for breech extraction of the second twin and to prevent head entrapment.

3. In rare cases, general anesthesia with halothane may be required to relax the cervix and uterus to correct the inversion.
4. Hydrostatic pressure is another method first used in the early 1900s and redescribed by O'Sullivan in 1945. Infusing warm saline into the vagina using the fist to trap the fluid in the vaginal cause distention of the upper vaginal, causing the cervix to relax. A more recent modification using a silicone cup (used for vacuum extraction) to trap the saline within the vagina was recently described.

## BIBLIOGRAPHY

Catanzarite VA, Moffitt KD, Baker ML, Awadalla SG, Arguibright KF, Perkins RP. New approaches to the management of acute puerperal uterine inversion. *Obstet Gynecol.* 1986;68 (Suppl. 3):7S–10S.

Creasy RK, Resnik R, Iams JD. *Maternal-Fetal Medicine Principals and Practice.* 5th ed. WB Saunders 2004:679–680.

Croft CR. Contraction ring: treatment by amyl nitrite, with observations on the pharmacological action of nitrite. *Proc R Soc Med.* 1935;28:37–44.

Dayan SS, Schwalbe SS. The use of small-dose intravenous nitroglycerin in a case of uterine inversion. *Anesth Analg.* 1996;82:1091–1093.

Hostetler DR, Bosworth MF. Uterine inversion: a life-threatening obstetric emergency. *J Am Board of Fam Pract.* 2000;13:120–123.

Ogueh O, Ayida G. Acute inversion: a new technique of hydrostatic replacement. *Br J Obstet Gynecol.* 1997;104:951–952.

Rosen DJD, Velez J, Greenspoon JS. Total breech extraction of the second twin with uterine relaxation induced by nitroglycerin sublingual spray. *Israel J Obstet Gynecol.* 1994;5:18–21.

Skinner GN, Louden KA. Non-puerperal uterine inversion associated with an atypical leiomyoma. *Aust NZJ Obstet Gynecol.* 2001;41:100–101.

Vaidyanathan G. Uterine inversion and corpus malignancies: a historical review. *Obstet Gynecol Surv.* 2000;55:703–707.

# 73 VAGINAL BIRTH AFTER CESAREAN AND UTERINE RUPTURE

*Kevin R. Justus*

## LEARNING POINT

The practice of planned vaginal birth after cesarean section (VBAC) or planned elective repeat cesarean section in women with a history of a previous cesarean birth are both associated with risk and benefits.

## VIGNETTE

A 36-year-old woman, G3P1, is at 38 weeks of gestation who presents today for a routine prenatal visit. Her pregnancy thus far has been uncomplicated. She has a history in 2003 of a cesarean delivery (low vertical uterine incision) of an 8-pound male fetus that was found to be breech at 39 weeks in early labor. That baby required admission to the neonatal intensive care unit for suspected respiratory distress syndrome (RDS) and was discharged on hospital day of life 6 and is now doing fine. She appears to be a bit anxious and asks you about an attempt at VBAC. She asks you to discuss the risk and benefits of VBAC as compared to repeat cesarean delivery.

## QUESTION 1

*What are the risk and benefits associated with VBAC?*

## ANSWER 1

Neither a trial of labor or a repeat cesarean section is risk free. When VBAC is successful, it is associated with less morbidity than with a repeat cesarean section. Advantages include fewer blood transfusions, fewer postpartum infections, and shorter postpartum stays, usually with no increased perinatal morbidity. However, women (and their infants) who have a failed trial of labor are at increased risk for infection and morbidity.

Rupture of the uterus is the most life-threatening complication faced by women undergoing a trial of labor. This can result in increased morbidity/mortality to both the patient and fetus. Occurrence of rupture is dependent on the type and location of the previous incision (see Table 73-1).

The most common sign of uterine rupture is a nonreassuring fetal heart rate pattern with variable decelerations that may develop into late decelerations, bradycardia, and a undetectable fetal heart rate. Other, more variable findings include: uterine/abdominal pain, loss of station of the presenting part, vaginal bleeding, and hypovolemia.

There are several factors that may increase the risk of uterine rupture including:

Prostaglandins, induction or augmentation of labor with pitocin, and protracted labor disorders. Although these factors have been associated with an increase in uterine rupture, none have been shown to directly cause uterine rupture.

**TABLE 73-1. Rates of Reported Uterine Rupture**

| | |
|---|---|
| Classical cesarean section | 4–9% |
| T-shaped incision | 4–9% |
| Low vertical incision | 1–7% |
| Low transverse incision | 0.2–1.5% |

## QUESTION 2

*What factors are associated with an increase risk of uterine rupture?*

## ANSWER 2

Multiple prior cesarean sections have a two to five times higher rate of uterine rupture than observed among patients who have only one prior cesarean section. An increased maternal age (defined as age greater than 30 years) has a 1.4% risk of uterine rupture compared to 0.5% in women less than 30 years of age. Short interdelivery interval, which is defined as less than 18 months, is associated with a three times higher rate of rupture.

In addition, the reported uterine rupture rate of 0.16% occurs among women who undergo repeat cesarean delivery without labor, 0.52% among women in spontaneous labor, 0.77% among women with labor induced without prostaglandins, and 2.45% for those women whose labor is induced with prostaglandins.

## QUESTION 3

*What selection criteria are used to identify candidates for VBAC?*

## ANSWER 3

The majority of the studies conducted to date support that most patients who have had a low transverse uterine incision from a previous cesarean delivery are candidates for a VBAC. ACOG recommends the following selection criteria when selecting a candidate for attempt at vaginal birth after cesarean delivery:

1. One or two prior low transverse cesarean deliveries
2. Clinically adequate pelvis
3. No other uterine scars or previous rupture
4. Physician immediately available throughout active labor capable of performing an emergency cesarean section
5. Availability of anesthesia and personnel for emergency cesarean delivery

## QUESTION 4

*What is the success rate for VBAC and what factors may influence the rate of VBAC?*

## ANSWER 4

Most published series report success rates of 56–82% for VBACs. The success rates for VBACs for women whose first cesarean section was for a nonrecurring cause are usually higher than those who had cesarean section for labor disorders. Additionally, the success rates are higher in women who have had a successful vaginal delivery at least once before or after their previous cesarean section. Furthermore, the rate of success for vaginal birth after cesarean delivery is reported to be higher (82%) in preterm infants compared to term (74%) infants.

Maternal age greater than 35 years may be associated with a lower VBAC rate. Additionally, higher maternal body mass index (BMI) (i.e., in the obesity range greater than 30 kg/m$^2$) is associated with a lower VBAC rate.

## BIBLIOGRAPHY

ACOG Committee Opinion No. 271. Induction of labor for vaginal birth after cesarean delivery. 2002.

ACOG Practice Bulletin No. 54. Vaginal birth after previous cesarean delivery. 2004.

Bujold E, Hammoud AO, Hendler I, Berman S, Blackwell SC, Duperron L, Gathier RJ. Trial of labor in patients with a previous cesarean section: does maternal age influence outcome? *Am J Obstet Gynecol.* 2004;190:1113–1118.

Caughey AB, Shipp TD, Repke JT, Zelop CM, Chen A. Rate of uterine rupture during a trial of labor in women with one or two prior cesarean deliveries. *Am J Obstet Gynecol.* 1999;181:872–876.

Dodd JM, Crowther CA, Huertas E, Guise JM, Horey D. Planned elective repeat cesarean section versus planned vaginal birth for women with a previous cesarean birth. Cochrane Database Syst Rev. 2005;1:1–23.

Durnwald CP, et al. The impact of maternal obesity and weight gain on vaginal birth after cesarean section success. *Am J Obstet Gynecol.* 2004;191:954–957.

Gregory K, Korst L, Cane PL, Platt L, Kahn K. Vaginal birth after cesarean and uterine upture rates in California. *Obstet Gynecol.* 1999;94:985–989.

Guise JM, Berlin M, McDonagh M, Osterweil B, Helfand M. Safety of vaginal birth after cesarean: a systematic review. *Obstet Gynecol.* 2004;103:420–429.

Lydon-Rochelle M, Holt VL, Easterling TR, Martin DP. Risk of uterine rupture during labor among women with a prior cesarean delivery. *N Engl J Med.* 2001;345:3–8.

Miller DA, Diaz FG, Paul RH. Vaginal birth after cesarean: a 10 year experience. *Obstet Gynecol.* 1994;84:255–258

Quinones J, Stamillo D, Pare E, Peipert J, Stevens E, Macones G. The effect of prematurity on vaginal birth after cesarean delivery: success and maternal morbidity. *Obstet Gynecol.* 2005;105: 519–524.

Shipp T. Trial of labor after cesarean: so, what are the risks? *Clin Obstet Gynecol.* 2004;47:365–377.

# 74 MIDTRIMESTER ABORTION

*Jane L. Davis*

## LEARNING POINT

Proper preabortion counseling and evaluation is important.

## VIGNETTE

A 28-year-old, G1, female with an intrauterine pregnancy at 18 weeks has an ultrasound that reveals a fetus with anencephaly. After extensive counseling, the patient elects to terminate the pregnancy. The patient denies any significant medical problems. She has never had any surgery.

The physical examination reveals a gravid Caucasian woman. Vital signs reveal blood pressure of 110/68 mm Hg, pulse of 82/min, respiratory rate of 18/min, and temperature of 98.6°F. Thyroid is nonpalpable, lungs are clear, heart has regular rate and rhythm without audible murmurs, and a gravid abdomen with a fundal height of 20 cm and fetal heart tones auscultated at 140/min. Pelvic examination reveals the cervix to be long and closed.

## QUESTION 1

*What are some reasons for delaying abortions until the second trimester?*

## ANSWER 1

About 1.5 million abortions are performed each year in the United States. Approximately 90% of these abortions are performed in the first trimester, and 10% are performed in the second trimester or later. Midtrimester abortions are performed most frequently for:

1. Fetal defects detected later on in pregnancy.
2. Abnormal fetal karyotype detected later on in pregnancy.
3. Fetal exposure to known teratogen.
4. Premature rupture of membranes prior to 24 weeks.
5. In utero fetal death.
6. Maternal medical/psychiatric illness detected later in pregnancy.
7. Change in maternal social situation.
8. Late diagnosis of pregnancy in women ≤15 years of age. Midtrimester abortions account for 22% of abortions in this young age group as opposed to 8% of abortions in women ages 30–34 years. This is most likely since adolescents often lack access to adequate contraception counseling, education regarding early signs of pregnancy, pregnancy testing, and abortion services, especially in states that require parental notification/consent prior to performing an abortion.

## QUESTION 2

*What is the risk of death from an abortion?*

## ANSWER 2

It is important to realize that the risk of death from an abortion increases with the gestational age of the pregnancy that is being terminated (0.4/100,000 procedures at 8 weeks gestation, 2.9/100,000 procedures at 13–15 weeks, and 9.3/100,000 at 16–20 weeks). Therefore, abortions should be performed as early as possible.

## QUESTION 3

*What sort of counseling and diagnostic procedures should be done prior to performing a midtrimester abortion?*

## ANSWER 3

Prior to performing a midtrimester abortion, the following should be obtained:

1. Careful medical/psychiatric history
2. Complete blood count
3. Blood type
4. Ultrasound to date pregnancy

## QUESTION 4

*What are types of procedures available for midtrimester termination?*

## ANSWER 4

1. Dilatation and evacuation (D&E)
2. Labor induction procedures:
   a. Hypertonic saline
   b. Hypertonic urea
   c. Intraamniotic prostaglandin combined with urea or saline
   d. Intraamniotic prostaglandin
   e. Systemic prostaglandin
   f. Misoprostol
   g. High dose oxytocin
3. Hysterotomy and/or hysterectomy
4. Intrauterine mechanical devices (catheters, plastic coils, laminaria, metreurynter-balloon)

## QUESTION 5

*What are potential problems associated with each type of midtrimester termination?*

## ANSWER 5

Potential problems of midtrimester termination include:

1. D&E
   a. Operator experience is required.
   b. May be restricted to early midtrimester.
   c. Preparation of cervix required with laminaria. This may increase risk of cervical lacerations and hemorrhage.
   d. General anesthesia often required.
   e. Disseminated intravascular coagulation (DIC) can be seen because tissue thromboplastins are released into maternal circulation. The use of oxytocin and intracervical vasopressin can reduce this risk.
   f. Uterine perforation with bowel and bladder injury.
   g. Amniotic fluid embolism.
2. Labor induction procedures
   a. Prolonged procedure increases the need for overnight hospital admission.
   b. Incomplete abortion/retained placenta.
   c. Hemorrhage.
   d. Infection.
   e. Embolic phenomena.
   f. Cardiovascular collapse (contraindicated in patients with cardiovascular disease), pulmonary and/or cerebral edema, renal failure, and DIC with hypertonic failure, particularly if injected intravenously.
   g. Muscle necrosis with intramyometrial injection of either hypertonic saline or urea.

h. Prostaglandin F2 alpha is contraindicated in patients with a history of asthma, epilepsy, glaucoma, pulmonary hypertension, and cardiovascular disease.
i. Prostaglandins may cause fever (temperature elevation of 1°C or more), nausea, vomiting, and diarrhea.

3. Hysterotomy and hysterectomy
   a. High morbidity/mortality
   b. Prolonged hospital stay

## BIBLIOGRAPHY

ACOG Technical Bulletin No. 109. Methods of Midtrimester Abortion. 1987.

Koonin, et al. Abortion surveillance in the United States. *Morb Mortal Wkly Rep.* 1993;42:29.

Lawson HW, et al. Abortion mortality in the United States. *Am J Obstet Gynecol.* 1994;171:1365.

## Section 5

# GYNECOLOGY/UROGYNECOLOGY

## 75 ADENOMYOSIS

*Ricardo Azziz*

### LEARNING POINT

To understand the diagnosis, prevalence, clinical features, and treatment options available for adenomyosis.

### VIGNETTE

A 38-year-old, G5P3023, presents to your office complaining of progressive heaviness with menstruation, increasing dysmenorrhea, and dyspareunia. Furthermore, she feels "heaviness" in her pelvis. Her cycles, despite being heavier than usual and with occasional clots, come at regular intervals and are accompanied by premenstrual breast tenderness and mood changes. She has had a tubal ligation following her last vaginal delivery.

On examination, the pelvis feels normal, as does the cervix, with the exception that the uterus is somewhat tender and appears to be enlarged without any discreet masses. There is no cervical motion tenderness. Transvaginal ultrasound is performed, which reveals what appears to be a relatively normal uterine cavity with an endometrial thickness of 6 mm. The myometrium appears to be somewhat heterogeneous, and the posterior wall of the uterus is significantly enlarged compared to the anterior wall, measuring 2.47 cm. There are no discreet fibroids encountered, but there appears to be irregularity in the posterior wall. The ovaries appear to be normal with occasional small cystic structures measuring 2–8 mm in diameter. There is no free fluid. You suspect, among other possible diagnoses, that the patient may suffer from adenomyosis.

### QUESTION 1

*What are the definition, etiology, and prevalence of adenomyosis?*

### ANSWER 1

Adenomyosis is the presence of endometrial glands and stroma deeper than the myometrium (Fig. 75-1). The exact pathologic definition has varied widely and has contributed to current confusion. The pathologic criteria for the diagnosis range from the presence of glands and stroma to greater than high power field from the endometrial surface to as deep as two low-power fields. Nonetheless, the majority of pathologists today will not make a diagnosis of adenomyosis unless the glands extend more than 2.5 mm below the endometrial-myometrial interface. Histopathologically, the posterior wall and fundus are more often affected by adenomyosis, with a general sparing of the cervix and anterior lower segment.

The prevalence of adenomyosis varies widely, although most series of patients undergoing hysterectomy for benign gynecologic disease suggest that between 10% and 35% of women demonstrate some degree of adenomyosis. The impact of the variation of diagnostic criteria is highlighted by recent study of 549 consecutive women undergoing hysterectomy between 1990 and 1991, where the prevalence of adenomyosis varied from 10% to 18.2%, depending on the diagnostic criteria used.

The exact etiology of adenomyosis is unknown, although it appears to be associated with increased estrogenization, and inflammation and/or damage to the endometrial myometrial interface. A recent study in mice using selective estrogen receptor modulators suggested that adenomyosis, at least in this animal model, might develop primarily secondary to inherited or intrauterine defects in the formation of the myometrium resulting from disordered stromal differentiation.

## QUESTION 2

*What are the signs and symptoms of adenomyosis?*

## ANSWER 2

The symptoms of adenomyosis vary widely. Up to one-third of patients with this disorder may be asymptomatic. Symptomatic patients whose pelvic pathology is limited to adenomyosis most often complain of menorrhagia (40–50%), dysmenorrhea (15–30%), metrorrhagia (10–12%), dyspareunia (7–15%), or a combination of these complaints. On physical examination, the uterus is enlarged in 60–80% of patients, but rarely exceeding 12 weeks gestation. On examination or palpation, the uterus may feel diffusely boggy or may be occasionally nodular, when there are significant adenomyomas present. Observed visually, the uterus may have a dusky appearance suggesting irregular hyperemia or congestion. While clinical suspicion remains the mainstay of preoperative diagnosis, it is also notoriously inexact. In fact, prior to the advent of magnetic resonance imaging (MRI) or ultrasonography, only 2–26% of cases were diagnosed preoperatively.

## QUESTION 3

*Other than clinical assessment, how can adenomyosis be diagnosed preoperatively?*

## ANSWER 3

While there are no currently available tests that have a high degree of accuracy in diagnosing adenomyosis preoperatively, the use of ultrasonography and MRI has provided additional tools for the practitioner who has clinical suspicion. In the study of 106 consecutive premenopausal women who underwent hysterectomy for benign reasons, and of which 21% had adenomyosis, the sensitivity and specificity of MRI was 0.70 and 0.86, and that of transvaginal ultrasonography was 0.68 and 0.65, respectively. In this study, the combination of MRI and transvaginal ultrasonography was the most sensitive method of diagnosis (0.89), although with the lowest degree of specificity (0.60). It should be noted that the diagnostic accuracy of MRI and transvaginal ultrasonography decreases as the uterine volume increases, particularly if greater than 400 $cm^3$.

Features of adenomyosis during MRI include high signal intensity myometrial spots, junctional zone (JZ) that is visible and greater than 12 mm in thickness, the presence of ill-defined low signal intensity myometrial areas, and a maximum JZ depth to entire myometrium ratio of greater than 40% (Fig. 75-2). Features during transvaginal ultrasonography include a fully defined focus of abnormal myometrial echo texture, distorted and heterogeneous myometrial echo texture, myometrial linear striations, and myometrial cysts.

Other tests have been proposed for the preoperative diagnosis of adenomyosis including hysteroscopic or laparoscopic directed needle biopsies, hysteroscopic resection, and even hysteroscopy. However, these diagnostic modalities are generally insensitive, and are invasive in nature.

## QUESTION 4

*What are the risk factors for the development of adenomyosis?*

## ANSWER 4

It appears that an increased estrogen effect, in combination with damage to the endometrium-myometrial interface may be associated with the development of adenomyosis. As such, patients who have had uterine trauma including those undergoing dilatation and curettage for

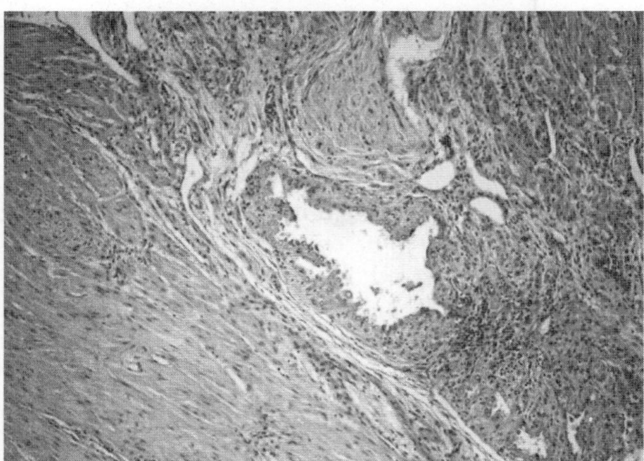

**FIG. 75-1** Adenomyosis is composed of stroma and glands embedded deep in the myometrium, resembling the basal layer of the endometrium (H&E stain, X40).
SOURCE: Courtesy of Dr. Hazel Gore.

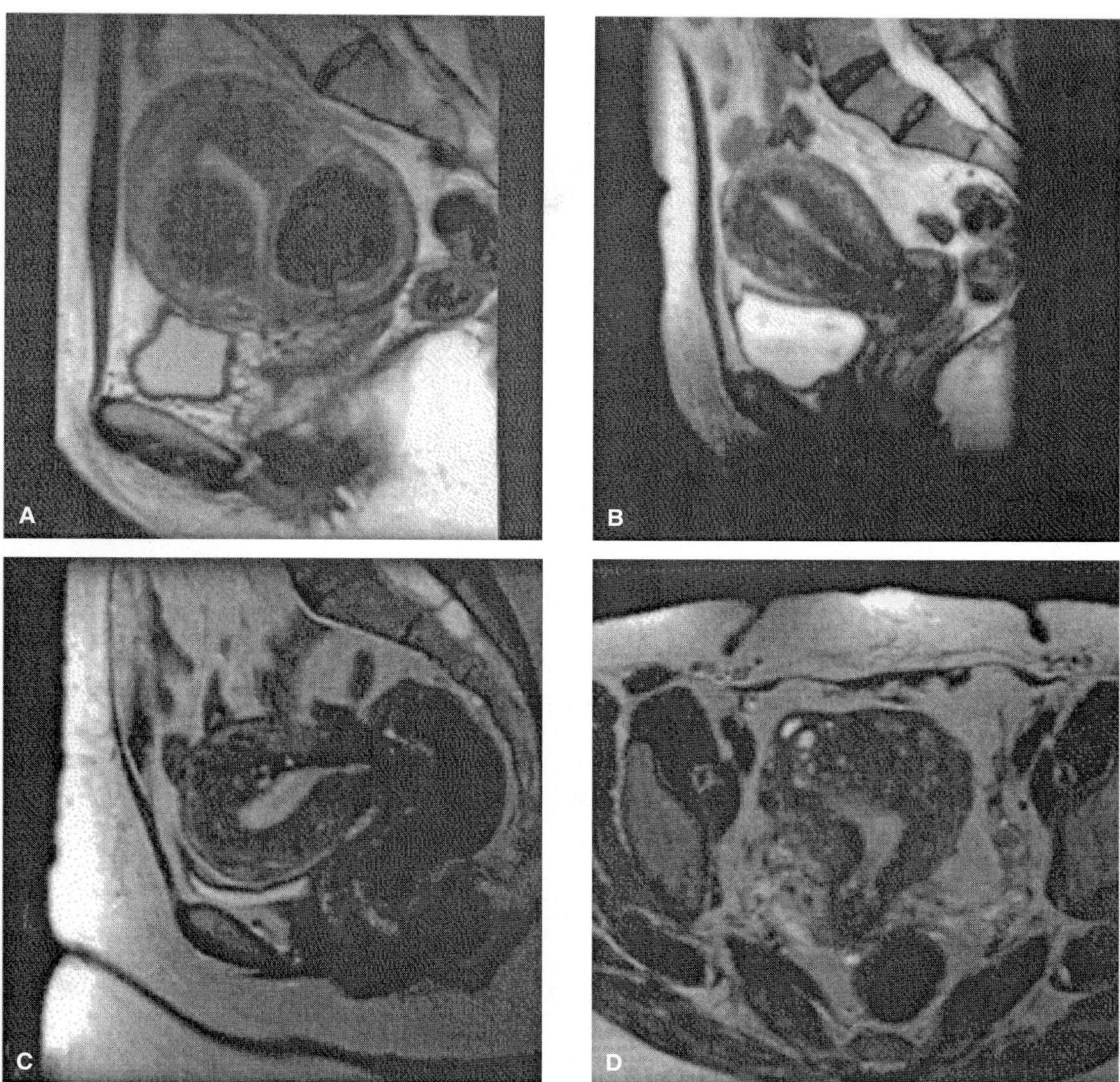


**FIG. 75-2** Magnetic resonance images of uteri with adenomyosis. The high intensity central signals represent the endometrium, whereas the low intensity inner myometrial layers are the junctional zones (JZ). (A) The difference between findings of myomas and adenomyosis are demonstrated. A myoma (posterior–inferior myometrial wall in right side of the picture) had well-defined borders and low-signal intensity, and findings of adenomyosis (posterior and anterior JZ) had not uniformly thickened, not well-demarcated JZ of low signal intensity in the myometrium. (B, C, D, E) Irregular thickened JZ. (C, D, E) Seen with small foci of high intensity. *(Continued)*

SOURCE: Reprinted with permission from Duelholm, et al. Magnetic resonance imaging and transvaginal ultrasonography for the diagnosis of adenomyosis. *Fertil Steril.* 2001;76:588–594.

spontaneous or elective abortions, cesarean section, and even vaginal deliveries have an increased risk of having adenomyosis. Multiparity is another risk factor. Chronic endomyometritis, which is increased in multiparous women and women with spontaneous abortions, is also a risk factor. Finally, hyperestrogenemia is also a risk factor, as evidenced by the frequency of endometrial hyperplasia found concomitantly in patients with adenomyosis. Furthermore, individuals who are smokers, and generally have lower circulating estrogen levels, have a decreased prevalence of adenomyosis.

## QUESTION 5

*What are the treatment options for patients suspected of having adenomyosis?*

## ANSWER 5

If the patients are significantly symptomatic, such that their pain and discomfort precludes them from having a

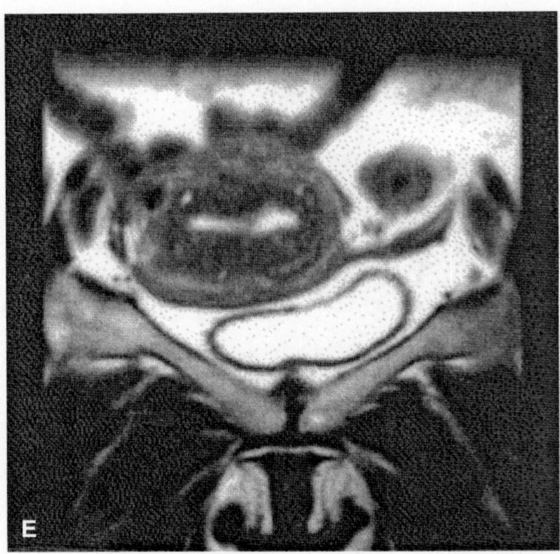


**FIG. 75-2** (*Continued*)

normal enjoyable life (e.g., chronic lower pelvic pain, dyspaerunia, and the like), and they have completed their childbearing, hysterectomy is the preferred treatment. Alternatively, hormonal suppression with either GnRH analogs or danazol has also been demonstrated to be partially effective. Anecdotally, continuous oral contraceptives, progestins or aromatase inhibitors have also been suggested as useful. Uterine artery embolization has also been proposed to ameliorate the symptoms of adenomyosis, although most results are preliminary. A small study of 18 women suspected of having symptomatic adenomyosis undergoing bilateral embolization of the uterine arteries indicated that the majority of the women treated had improved menorrhagia, although this fell sharply to 56% of women at 2 years follow-up, with almost 50% requiring additional treatment for their symptoms.

In patients who are significantly symptomatic and desire to preserve their fertility, a conservative resection using hysteroscopic endomyometrial resection, laparoscopic resection, or electric coagulation, or myometrial resection via laparotomy has been proposed. Nonetheless, these procedures are highly invasive, and outcomes are primarily anecdotal. Furthermore, it is clear that these procedures will weaken the uterine wall, something that patients who desire to carry a pregnancy need to be cautioned about.

## BIBLIOGRAPHY


Azziz R. Adenomyosis: current perspectives. *Obstet Gynecol Clin North Am.* 1989;16(1):221–235.

Bergholt T, Eriksen L, Berendt N, Jacobsen M, Hertz JB. Prevalence and risk factors of adenomyosis at hysterectomy. *Hum Reprod.* 2001;16(11):2418–2421.

Dueholm M, Lundorf E, Hansen E, Sorensen J, Ledertoug S, Olesen F. Magnetic resonance imaging and transvaginal ultrasonography for the diagnosis of adenomyosis. *Fertil Steril.* 2001;76(3):588–594.

Parrott E, Butterworth M, Green A, White IN, Greaves P. Adenomyosis—a result of disordered stromal differentiation. *Am J Pathol.* 2001;159(2):623–630.

Pelage JP, Jacob D, Fazel A, Namur J, Laurent A, Rymer R, Le Dref O. Midterm results of uterine artery embolization for symptomatic adenomyosis: initial experience. *Radiology.* 2005;234(3):948–953.

Wood C. Surgical and medical treatment of adenomyosis. *Hum Reprod Update.* 1998;4(4):323–336.


# 76 BARTHOLIN'S GLAND MASS

*Ilana Cass*

## LEARNING POINT

To understand the management of a Bartholin's gland mass.

## VIGNETTE

A 50-year-old, G2P1, presents with a painful left vulvar mass. She is postmenopausal and has never used hormone replacement therapy. She reports having had a similar left-sided mass, initially in her twenties and then again in her thirties that was managed with a Word catheter on each occasion. She has recently noticed this mass again over the past year, although it has been painless and was initially smaller until several weeks ago. She denies any other associated changes in her bowel or bladder habits, with no recent change in her weight. She has had some associated dyspareunia over the past several weeks, although she is rarely sexually active. She has had normal Pap smears in the past, although she has had irregular gynecologic care over the past 5 years. She denies any history of sexually transmitted disease.

She has well controlled hypertension and no prior surgeries. She denies any family history of cancer, but reports a maternal history of cardiovascular disease.

The physical examination reveals a thin woman in no apparent distress. Vitals signs: pulse 68 bpm, BP 100/60 mm Hg, and afebrile. Head, eyes, ears, nose, and throat (HEENT) examination reveals no adenopathy, chest is clear to auscultation, cardiac examination shows regular

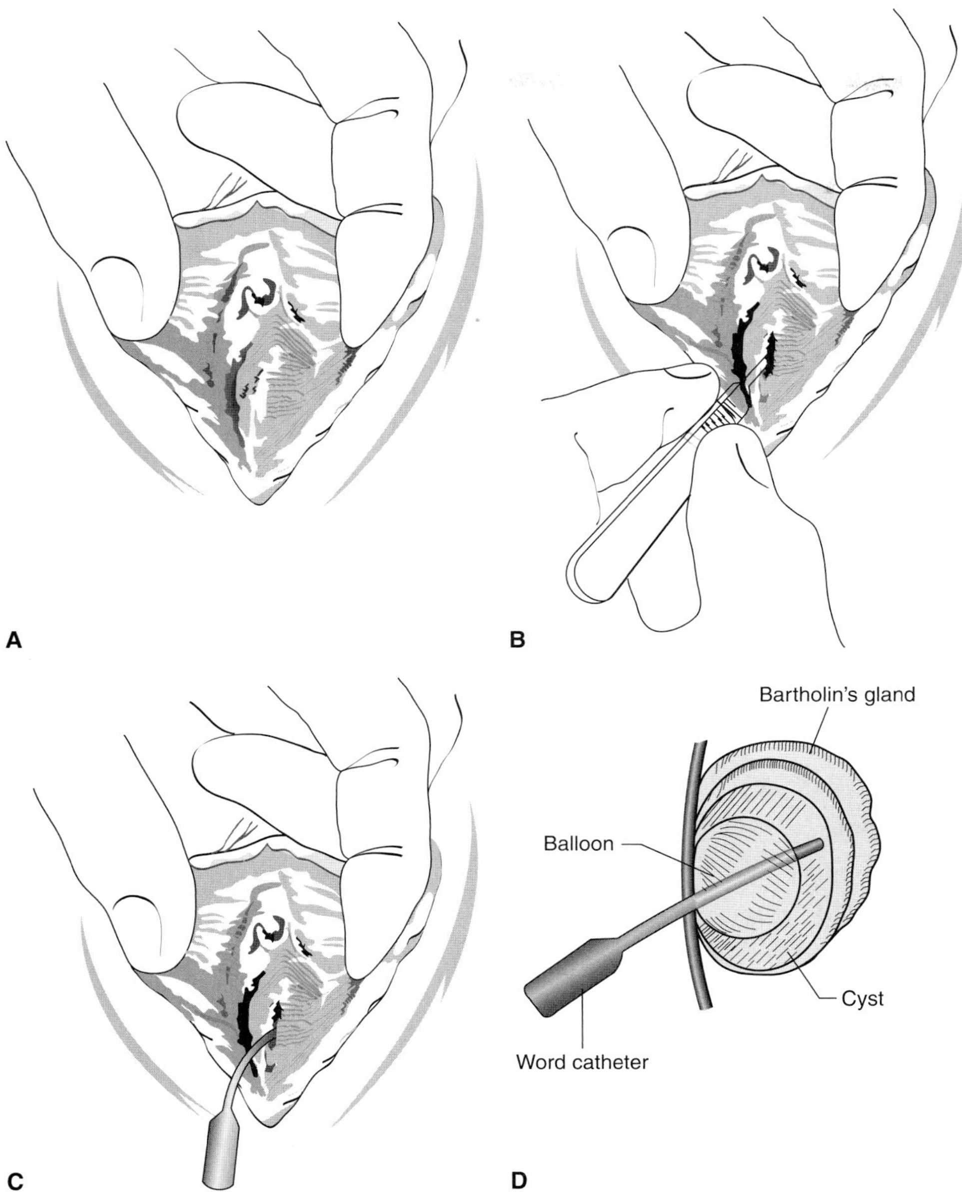


**FIG. 76-1** Incision and drainage of Bartholin's abscess. A. Inject local anesthetic into the mucosal surface of the abscess and the mucocutaneous junction of the labia minora. B. Make a 1-cm incision on the mucosal surface. C and D. Insert the word catheter and inflate the balloon with 5 mL normal saline solution.
Source: From Campbell CJ. Incision and drainage of Bartholin's cyst. In: Rosen P, et al. (eds.). *Atlas of Emergency Procedures.* St. Louis, MO: Mosby; 2001.

rate and rhythm, abdominal examination shows no inguinal adenopathy, pelvic examination reveals a tender, mobile left vulvar mass of the Bartholin's gland. The area is indurated, without any visible discharge. The remainder of the pelvic examination is normal.

## QUESTION 1

*What is the etiology of Bartholin's gland cysts and abscesses? What are the risk factors for Bartholin's duct cysts or abscesses?*

## ANSWER 1

The Bartholin's glands, major vestibular glands, are paired structures that empty into the posterolateral vestibule at the junction of the hymen and the labium minora. They contribute a minimal amount of secretions with sexual arousal. Ductal occlusion can occur secondary to inspissated mucous, inflammation, or rarely cancer. Ductal occlusion with infection results in an abscess. Risk factors for Bartholin's gland cysts or abscess are comparable to risks of sexually transmitted diseases—young, single women, low socioeconomic background. Two large series describe that >80% of patients with Bartholin's gland enlargements are <50 years old. The polymicrobial flora of Bartholin's gland cysts and abscesses include anaerobic and aerobic infection in the majority of patients which mirror vaginal flora, predominantly Bacteroides species, *Escherichia coli* and gonorrhea. Older series described gonorrhea and Chlamydial infection in 70–80% and 40% of patients, respectively. More recent series have described gonorrhea and/or Chlamydiae in <10% of patients.

## QUESTION 2

*What is the appropriate management of the Bartholin's gland cyst or abscess? Does this vary by age of the patient?*

## ANSWER 2

Historically, patients <40 years of age with asymptomatic small or stable Bartholin's gland cysts do not require any therapy. Therapy for symptomatic Bartholin's gland cysts and abscesses include surgical drainage with creation of a fistulous tract (possibly using a Word catheter), marsupialization, laser therapy, and silver nitrate insertion (see Fig. 76-1). Excision of the gland is recommended in patients with persistent deep infection, recurrence of abscesses, and debatably in patients >40 years of age because of the increased rate of Bartholin's gland carcinoma. Recent data; however, has questioned the need for excision in all patients >40 years of age, considering the rarity of this carcinoma, and statistically comparable rates of Bartholin's gland carcinoma in pre- and postmenopausal women, 0.023/100,000 woman/years *versus* 0.114/100,000 women/years. Authors agree that excision/biopsy is mandated in any patient with persistent Bartholin's gland mass unresponsive to conventional therapy. Routine antibiotics are not needed, but patients should have cervical cultures for gonorrhea and chlamydia and close follow-up for resolution of symptoms.

## QUESTION 3

*What are some of the clinical features of Bartholin's gland carcinoma?*

## ANSWER 3

Bartholin's gland carcinoma accounts for 3–5% of invasive vulvar cancer. The median age of women with Bartholin's gland carcinoma is 50–57 years, although up to 38% of patients are less than 50 at presentation. Patients present most commonly with a vulvar mass, and/or perineal pain. A minority of patients has a history of prior Bartholin's gland cyst or abscess, 8–27%, and 25–75% of patients were initially treated for an abscess before a biopsy was obtained, although patient numbers are small.

## BIBLIOGRAPHY


Aghajanian A, et al. Bartholin's duct abscess and cyst: a case-control study. *Southern Med J.* 1994;87(1):26–29.

Andersen PG, et al. Treatment of Bartholin's abscess. *Acta Obstet Gynecol Scand.* 1992;71:59–62.

Campbell CJ. Incision and drainage of Bartholin's cyst. In: Rosen P, et al. (eds.). *Atlas of Emergency Procedures.* St. Louis, Mosby, MO: 2001.

Cardosi RJ, et al. Bartholin's gland carcinoma: a 15 year experience. *Gynecol Oncol.* 2001;82:247–251.

Droegemueller W. Infections of the lower genital tract. *Comprehensive Gynecology.* St. Louis, MO: CV Mosby CO; 1987:567–613.

Leuchter RS, et al. Primary carcinoma of the Bartholin gland: a report of 14 cases and review of the literature. *Obstet Gynecol.* 1982;60:361–368.

Quentin R, et al. Frequent isolation of canophilic bacteria in aspirates of Bartholin's gland abscesses and cycts. *Eur J Clin Microbiol Infect Dis.* 1990;9(2):138–141.

Viscio AG, Del Priore G. Postmenopausal Bartholin gland enlargement: a hospital-based cancer risk assessment. *Obstet Gynecol.* 1996;87:286–290.


# 77 DES EXPOSURE

*Lee Kao*

## LEARNING POINTS

What is diethylstilbestrol (DES)? What are the health issues related to DES exposure and does DES exposure increase the risk for infertility?

# VIGNETTE

A 38-year-old Hispanic female, G2P0020, presents with her husband for secondary infertility consultation. The patient had previously seen some other provider about difficulty in achieving pregnancy and after some workup she was told that she might have been exposed to DES in utero. No detailed information was given to her and she's rather frustrated and would like to know more about, and eventually pursue, infertility treatment. She is now seeking further information from you and would like to know much more about this substance and her potential problems. What would you tell her?

## QUESTION 1

*What is DES?*

## ANSWER 1

DES is a synthetic estrogen originally developed to supplement natural estrogen production. First prescribed by physicians in 1938 for women who experienced miscarriages or premature deliveries, it was originally considered effective and safe for both the mother and the developing baby. In the United States, about 5–10 million persons were exposed to DES from 1938 to 1971, including the women who were prescribed DES while pregnant and the female and male children born of these pregnancies. In 1971, the U.S. Food and Drug Administration issued a drug bulletin advising physicians to stop prescribing DES to pregnant women. Despite efforts to identify DES-exposed women and men, many persons exposed to DES were not located. Unfortunately, no medical test can confirm DES exposure and these subjects may not realize that they had been exposed. After more than 30 years, research has confirmed significant health risks associated with DES exposure. However, not all exposed persons will experience the DES-related health problems.

## QUESTION 2

*What are the health issues related to DES exposure?*

## ANSWER 2

1. Women prescribed DES while pregnant are at a modestly increased risk (~30% greater risk) for breast cancer. That raises their lifetime breast cancer risk from one in eight unexposed women to one in six women prescribed DES during pregnancy.
2. Women exposed to DES before birth (DES daughters) are at increased risk for clear cell adenocarcinoma (CCA) of the vagina and cervix. Approximately 0.1% of DES daughters are expected to develop CCA. The highest risk for CCA has been reported to be in the teens and early twenties, but it has been detected later in the thirties and even forties.
3. DES daughters are at an increased risk for reproductive tract structural abnormalities. Up to one-third of DES daughters exhibit some form of reproductive tract abnormality of the cervix, uterus, or fallopian tubes. These include vaginal adenosis, cervical changes (hooded cervix, cervical collars, septae, cockscomb, or pseudopolyp), and T-shaped uterus (see Fig. 77-1).
4. DES daughters are at an increased risk for pregnancy complications such as ectopic pregnancies, miscarriages, and premature delivery. Their risk for an ectopic pregnancy ranges from three- to fivefolds higher than unexposed women. Almost 20% of DES

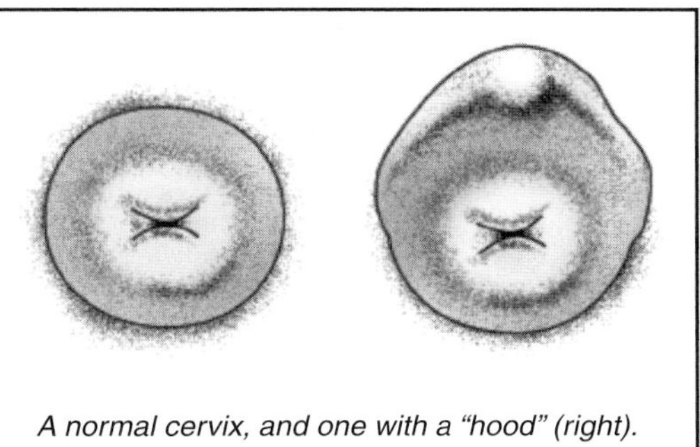

A normal cervix, and one with a "hood" (right).

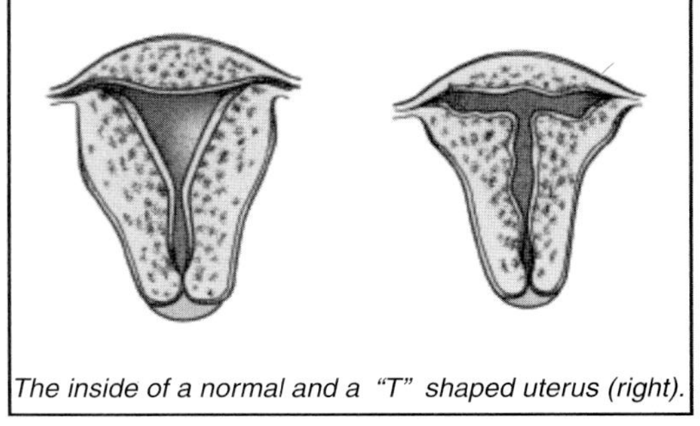

The inside of a normal and a "T" shaped uterus (right).

**FIG. 77-1** Reproductive tract differences in DES daughters.
SOURCE: Reproduced with permission from the Centers for Disease Control and Prevention. www.cdc.gov/DES

**FIG. 77-2** Infertility rates for DES daughters vs. unexposed population.
SOURCE: Adapted from Palmer JR. et al. Infertility among women exposed prenatally to diethylstilbestrol. *Am J Epidemiol.* 2001;154(4):316–321.

daughters miscarry during their first pregnancy, while about 10% of unexposed women have a miscarriage during their first pregnancy. Of DES daughters, 64% deliver full-term in their first pregnancy, compared with 85% of unexposed women, and approximately 20% of DES daughters experience preterm labor, compared with 8% of unexposed women.

5. DES daughters are at an increased risk for infertility (Fig. 77-2).
6. DES sons are at an increased risk for noncancerous epididymal cysts.

The National Cancer Institute (NCI) has published recommendations for what is an appropriate pelvic examination for DES daughters:

- Careful visual examination and palpation of the vagina and cervix with rotation of the speculum so that all vaginal walls can be inspected;
- Pap smears from the cervix and the surfaces of the upper vagina; and
- Iodine staining of the vagina and cervix or a colposcopy if abnormalities are detected during the examination.

## QUESTION 3

*Does DES exposure increase the risk for infertility?*

## ANSWER 3

Reasons for DES-related infertility vary. Recent research indicates that the primary reason for an increased risk of infertility among DES daughters results from abnormalities in the uterus or fallopian tubes that are associated with in utero DES exposure.

## BIBLIOGRAPHY

Barnes AB, Colton T, Gundersen J, et al. Fertility and outcome of pregnancy in women exposed in utero to diethylstilbestrol. *N Engl J Med.* 1980;302:609–613.

Jefferies JA, Robboy SJ, O'Brien PC, et al. Structural anomalies of the cervix and vagina in women enrolled in the Diethylstilbestrol Adenosis (DESAD) Project. *Am J Obstet Gynecol.* 1984;148:59–66.

Kaufman RH, Adam E, Binder GL, et al. Upper genital tract changes and pregnancy outcome in offspring exposed in utero to diethylstilbestro. *Am J obstet Gynecol.* 1980;137:299–308.

Palmer JR, Hatch EE, Rao RS, Kaufman RH, Herbst AL, Noller KL, Titus-Ernstoff L, Hoover RN. Infertility among women exposed prenatally to diethylstilbestrol. *Am J Epidemiol.* 2001;154(4):316–321.

# 78 ECTOPIC PREGNANCY: METHOTREXATE VERSUS SURGERY

*Margareta D. Pisarka*

## LEARNING POINT

There are different indications for surgical intervention versus medical management (methotrexate) for ectopic pregnancy.

## VIGNETTE

A 28-year-old, G1P0, comes in because she is having some vaginal spotting. She states that her last menstrual period was 7 weeks ago and a home pregnancy test was positive. She is concerned that she has been spotting for the last 3 days. A history reveals the following:

> Gynecologic history: Menarache at age 12 years, regular cycles every 28 days, with 5 days of bleeding. The patient states that she was treated for chlamydia at the age of 21. She has no history of fibroids or ovarian cysts.
> Obstetrics history: Present pregnancy only. Medical history is negative.
> Surgical history: Appendectomy for a ruptured appendix at the age of 16.
> Social history: She does not smoke, drink alcohol, or use illicit drugs. She is not taking any medications and has no allergies to medications. Her family history is noncontributory.

Physical examination reveals a healthy appearing female. Vital signs: blood pressure 110/70 mm Hg, pulse 80/min, respiratory rate 18/min, and temperature 98.6°F. Weight 105 lb and height 5 ft 6 in. Thyroid nonpalpable, lungs clear, heart regular rate and rhythm without audible murmurs. Abdomen normal bowel sounds, soft, nontender, no palpable masses. Pelvic examination: normal external genitalia, cervix nulliparous, no lesions, uterus anteverted normal size, right adnexa slightly tender, left adnexa nontender, no masses bilaterally. Rectovaginal confirms.

Blood work reveals the following: Beta human chorionic gandotropin ($\beta$-hCG) is 1500 mIU/ mL. An ultrasound reveals an empty uterus and a 2 cm left adnexal mass distinctly separate from the ovary.

### QUESTION 1

*What are the indications for surgical intervention for an ectopic pregnancy? What types of surgery are preferable?*

### ANSWER 1

Surgery is the preferred treatment for ectopic pregnancy when there is rupture, hypotension, anemia, diameter of the gestational sac greater than 4 cm on ultrasonography, or pain persisting beyond 24 hour. Surgery is also perhaps for patients who are likely to be noncompliant with follow-up visits after medical treatment. Laparoscopic surgery is generally preferred over laparotomy. It has benefits in terms of lower cost, blood loss, and analgesia requirements, and shorter postoperative recovery. Laparotomy is preferred; however, when the patient is hemodynamically unstable, the surgeon is not trained in operative laparoscopy, or when the laparoscopic approach is technically too difficult.

Laparoscopic linear salpingostomy is recommended for ampullary ectopic pregnancies. For isthmic pregnancies, the treatment is segmental excision followed by intraoperative or delayed microsurgical anastomosis. Salpingectomy is preferable in cases of uncontrollable bleeding, extensive tubal damage, or recurrent ectopic pregnancy in the same tube, and when the woman requests sterilization. A complication of laparoscopic salpingostomy is persistent ectopic pregnancy, which occurs at a frequency of 5–20%. It occurs as a result of incomplete removal of trophoblastic tissue. It is diagnosed during follow-up when $\beta$-hCG concentrations measured once a week plateau or rise. This can be treated successfully with a single-dose systemic methotrexate (50 mg/m$^2$).

### QUESTION 2

*What are the two types of methotrexate administration and how should you follow up?*

### ANSWER 2

Variable dose methotrexate is administered on alternate days with leukovorin. The dose of methotrexate is 1 mg/kg intramuscularly on alternate days (days 1, 3, 5, 7). The dose of leukovorin is 0.1 mg/kg, intramuscularly, on alternate days (days 2, 4, 6, 8). Therapy is continue until $\beta$-hCG falls $\geq$15% in 48 hours or four doses of methotrexate are given.

Single dose methotrexate is administered as 50 mg/m$^2$ intramuscularly. A repeat dose is given if $\beta$-hCG does not decline by at least 15% between day 4 and day 7 post injection.

For both treatment regimens, weekly $\beta$-hCG should be followed until <5 IU/L. No sexual intercourse, pelvic examinations, or ultrasound should be performed until resolved. If the ectopic pregnancy is not resolved, based on $\beta$-hCG levels a repeat course for persistant ectopic pregnancy is indicated. Single dose or a multidose course can be administered.

### QUESTION 3

*When is methotrexate contraindicated? What types of pretreatment blood work should be obtained?*

## ANSWER 3

Absolute contraindications include hepatic, renal, or hematologic dysfunction. This includes chronic liver disease or alcoholism, preexisting blood dyscrasias, such as bone marrow hypoplasia, leukopenia, thrombocytopenia, or significant anemia. Immunodeficiency is also a contraindication. High dose methotrexate can cause bone marrow suppression, acute and chronic hepatotoxic effects, stomatitis, gastritis, and enteritis. Thus, methotrexate is also contraindicated in peptic ulcer disease.

Methotrexate should not be used in patients with known pulmonary disease, since it has been associated with pneumonitis. Breast-feeding or known sensitivity to methotrexate is also contraindication. Relative contraindications include a gestational sac ≥3.5 cm and embryonic cardiac motion. These have been associated with a higher rate of failure or need for multiple courses of methotrexate.

Pretreatment blood work includes a complete blood count (CBC), renal and liver function tests. Pretreatment β-hCG should also be obtained. Blood type, Rh factor, and antibodies should be determined. Rh immune globulin should be administered to patients who are Rh negative. Folic acid supplements, including prenatal vitamins should be discontinued and the use of nonsteroidal inflammatory drugs avoided.

## QUESTION 4

*What are the success rates of the different treatment modalities?*

## ANSWER 4

The success rates of the different treatment modalities for an ectopic pregnancy is depicted in Table 78-1. A recent meta-analysis comparing single to multidose methotrexate revealed that there was a significant increase in success with multidose methotrexate compared to single dose methotrexate. The overall success rate for women managed with single-dose therapy was 88.1% (940 of 1067). The overall success rate for women managed with the multidose protocol was similar, 92.7% (241 of 260). However, the mean β-hCG value for those treated with a single-dose regimen was significantly lower than that of the multidose regimen women (2778 ± 2848 mIU vs. 5023 ± 5342 mIU, respectively; $P < .001$). A total of 14.5% of women who were scheduled to receive a single dose required more that one dose. The use of single dose was associated with a significantly greater chance of failed medical management than the use of the multidose, however the single dose was associated with fewer side effects.

In addition, women who experienced side effects were more likely to have successful treatment regardless of regimen.

## BIBLIOGRAPHY

ACOG Practice Bulletin No. 3, Medical Management of Tubal Pregnancy. 1998;1–7.

ASRM Practice Committee Report, A Technical Bulletin. Early Diagnosis and Management of Ectopic Pregnancy. 2001;1–4.

Barnhart KT, Gosman G, Ashby R, Sammel M. The medical management of ectopic pregnancy: a meta-analysis comparing "single dose" and "multidose" regimens. *Obstet Gynecol.* 2003;101:778–784.

Pisarska MD, Carson SA, Buster JE. Ectopic pregnancy. *Lancet.* 1998;351:1115–1120.

**TABLE 78-1. Evaluation of Various Publications Reveals the Following Success Rates**

| METHOD | STUDIES | PATIENTS | SUCCESSFUL RATE RESOLUTION | TUBAL PATENCY | SUBSEQUENT FERTILITY RATE INTRAUTERINE PREGNANCY | ECTOPIC PREGNANCY |
|---|---|---|---|---|---|---|
| Conservative laparoscopic surgery | 32 | 1626 | 1516 (93%) | 170/223 (76%) | 366/647 (57%) | 87/647 (13%) |
| Variable-dose methotrexate | 12 | 338 | 314 (93%) | 136/182 (75%) | 55/95 (58%) | 7/95 (7%) |
| Single dose methotrexate | 7 | 393 | 340* (87%) | 61/75 (81%) | 39/64 (61%) | 5/64 (8%) |

*For patients receiving single dose methotrexate, 8% required a second dose.

SOURCE: Pisarska MD, Carson SA, Buster JE. Ectopic pregnancy. *Lancet.* 1998;351:1115–1120.

# 79 ENDOMETRIAL ABLATION

*Lee Kao*

## LEARNING POINTS

Is there any benefit in treating anovulatory bleeding surgically rather than medically, in patients who have completed childbearing? In women who have completed childbearing, what is the efficacy among surgical techniques? Is there evidence supporting the use of medical management prior to surgical ablation?

## VIGNETTE

A 47-year-old African-American female, G2P0020, currently separated, presents for a second opinion regarding irregular vaginal bleeding. The patient had been enjoying relatively good health until about 6 months ago when she noticed her menstrual cycles had become irregular and bothersome. She subsequently visited her primary care physician and was told to have perimenopausal bleeding pattern and she was referred to gynecologic care. She visited two separate gynecologists by referral and has been offered different advice regarding surgery. The patient cannot decide based on the information she has been given and she also does not feel comfortable with either physician and is currently here seeking a third opinion and consultation regarding her situation.

### QUESTION 1

*In patients who have completed childbearing, what is the benefit of treating anovulatory bleeding surgically rather than medically?*

### ANSWER 1

The goals of medical therapy in women with excessive anovulatory bleeding are to avoid anemia, to reduce excessive heavy bleeding, and to increase predictability of bleeding. Success or failure of such therapy should be defined in partnership with the patient, in order to achieve the therapeutic goal. Surgical therapy is indicated for women with excessive anovulatory bleeding in whom medical management has failed and who have completed their childbearing. Currently, there are few randomized trials comparing medical versus surgical therapy for anovulatory uterine bleeding. One randomized trial comparing endometrial resection with medical management for women with menorrhagia found that medical management patients were less likely to be satisfied with their therapy. However, because of its reduced cost and risks, medical therapy still should be offered before surgical intervention unless it is otherwise contraindicated.

### QUESTION 2

*In women who have completed childbearing, what is the efficacy among surgical techniques?*

### ANSWER 2

The surgical options for the treatment of excessive anovulatory bleeding are hysterectomy or endometrial ablation. In general, morbidity rates for women undergoing hysterectomy for various indications have been reported at between 7% and 15% with an overall mortality rate of 12 deaths per 10,000 procedures, for all indications. Endometrial ablation, performed with or without the assistance of hysteroscopy, can be an alternative to hysterectomy. Hysteroscopically, this can be performed with the resectoscope and the endometrium removed/resected by electrocautery loop or ablated with the rollerball, or be accomplished with the Nd: yttrium aluminum garnet (YAG) laser. Alternatively, thermal balloon ablation can be done without hysteroscopy, in which the endometrium is ablated by heating saline inside an intrauterine balloon to approximately 85°C. The most frequently reported complications of hysteroscopy are uterine perforation, which occurs in approximately 14 per 1000 procedures, and fluid overload occurs in approximately 2 per 1000 cases.

About 45% of women after undergoing an endometrial resection using the resectoscope or laser ablation are amenorrheic, and the percentage of satisfaction at 12 months post-op approaches 90%. Thermal balloon endometrial ablation yields an amenorrhea rate of approximately 15% and a 12-month postoperative satisfaction rate of about 90%. Because women who undergo endometrial ablation can have residual active endometrium, they should receive progestin if they are to be given estrogen replacement. In a 5-year follow up study, 34% of patients who had undergone hysteroscopic ablation subsequently needed a hysterectomy.

## QUESTION 3

*Is there evidence supporting the use of medical management in preparation for surgical ablation?*

## ANSWER 3

Evidence from randomized trials supports the use of either a gonadotropin-releasing hormone agonist or danazol prior to endometrial ablation or resection with regard to improved intrauterine operating environment and short-term postoperative outcome. The choice of agents should be based on cost, efficacy, and side effects. There are insufficient data to assess the value of progestin therapy prior to endometrial ablation.

## BIBLIOGRAPHY

ACOG Committee on Practice Bulletins—Gynecology. ACOG Practice Bulletin No. 14. Management of anovulatory bleeding. *Int J Gynecol Obstet.* 2001;72(3):263–271.

Vilos GA. Hysteroscopic and nonhysteroscopic endometrial ablation. *Obstet Gynecol Clin North Am.* 2004;31(3):687–704.

# 80 FIBROIDS: CAUSE OF RECURRENT ABORTION

*Shahin Ghadir*

## LEARNING POINT

Fibroids can be a cause of recurrent abortion.

## VIGNETTE

A 33-year-old, G3P0030, female presents to her gynecologist's office with concerns about her three prior spontaneous abortions. She and her husband of 8 years had decided to have a baby 2 years ago and during this time she had become pregnant easily on three different occasions. All three pregnancies aborted spontaneously between 7 and 10 weeks of gestation and all three were noted to have normal fetal cardiac activity. The patient has already had a completely normal hormonal and thrombophilia evaluation and both the patient and her husband have had normal karyotyping. The patient denies any other significant medical problems and denies any previous surgeries. The patient takes prenatal vitamins and has no known drug allergies. The patient also denies the use of tobacco, alcohol, or drugs. Patient states that she has regular cycles every 28–29 days, with menses lasting 5–7 days.

The physical examination reveals a well-nutritioned, well-developed African American female. Vital signs: blood pressure 128/82 mm Hg, pulse 76/min, respiratory rate 18/min, temperature 98.6°F, weight 138 lb, height 5 ft 3 in. Thyroid: no enlargement, no masses, lungs: clear to auscultation bilaterally, heart: regular rate and rhythm, no murmurs, abdomen: soft, nontender, no masses. Pelvic examination: external genitalia within normal limits, vagina well estrogenized, no vaginal discharge, normal cervix, uterus anteverted, irregular and enlarged to 12 week size, adnexa nontender, without palpable masses. Rectovaginal confirms.

## QUESTION 1

*What additional diagnostic methods can be used for the workup of the patient with recurrent abortions and a possible fibroid uterus?*

## ANSWER 1

The principal methods used for anatomical evaluation of the uterus and the endometrial cavity include hysterosalpingography (HSG), transvaginal ultrasonography, and sonohysterography. There are some benefits to the HSG including the evaluation of tubal patency, although this is not necessarily indicated in this patient since she has had no trouble in achieving pregnancy. Transvaginal ultrasonography and sonohysterography may be more beneficial in the recurrent pregnancy patient because they also allow for visualization of the external uterine contour and are easier to perform and better tolerated than the HSG. Furthermore, sonohysterography is better for the evaluation of the endometrial cavity and allows for visualization of submucous myomas and endometrial polyps.

## QUESTION 2

*What type of fibroids does this patient most likely have?*

## ANSWER 2

Submucous fibroids are the most likely cause of this patient's recurrent pregnancy losses. There is no substantial data that support subserosal or intramural myomas under 5–7 cm in size from causing pregnancy loss. However, one study looking at women undergoing in vitro fertilization (IVF) showed a decreased implantation rate in women with distorted endometrial cavities.

## QUESTION 3

*What is the recommended method of treatment for a submucous myoma?*

## ANSWER 3

Hysteroscopic myomectomies are recommended when the fibroids are single and small. When there are many submucous fibroids or larger fibroids, the hysteroscopic resection may be technically more difficult and have greater risk for the patient. When the fibroids do not distort the endometrial cavity, surgery is not indicated unless the fibroid is causing other symptoms.

## QUESTION 4

*Is there any risk of the fibroids recurring after myomectomy?*

## ANSWER 4

Yes, the risk of recurrent myomas is fairly high and therefore, consideration of fertility desires, the size and location of the fibroids, severity of symptoms, and the patient's age should all be taken into account before attempting myomectomy.

## BIBLIOGRAPHY

ACOG Practice Bulletin No. 16. Surgical Alternatives to Hysterectomy in the Management of Leiomyomas. 2000.

Farhi J, Ashkenazi J, Feldberg D, Dicker D, Orvieto R, Ben Rafael Z. Effect of uterine leiomyomata on the results of in-vitro fertilization treatment. *Hum Reprod.* 1995;10:2576–2578.

Giatras K, Berkeley AS, Noyes N, Licciardi F, Lolis D, Grifo JA. Fertility after hysteroscopic resection of submucous myomas. *J Am Assoc Gynecol Laparosc.* 1999;6:155.

Speroff L, Fritz MA: Clinical gynecologic endocrinology and infertility. 7th ed. Philadelphia, PA: Lipincott Williams & Wilkins; 2005.

# 81 FIBROIDS: HYSTEROSCOPIC TREATMENT

*Amer K. Karam*

## LEARNING POINT

Indications, risks, and alternatives of hysteroscopic myomectomy.

## VIGNETTE

A 30-year-old female sought medical advice for menorrhagia for 2 years and two spontaneous abortions. Her obstetric history included a cesarean section 4 years prior, followed by two, first trimester spontaneous abortions, the second of which occurred 6 months previously. She had been diagnosed with a submucosal myoma of the uterus on diagnostic laparoscopy and hysteroscopy at another hospital. On bimanual pelvic examination, the uterus was enlarged irregularly to 10-week size. Pelvic ultrasonography revealed a submucosal myoma on the anterior wall of the uterus. The patient wished for transcervical resection of the myoma if possible.

## QUESTION 1

*What are contraindications to hysteroscopic myomectomy?*

## ANSWER 1

1. Patients with an enlarged uterus and three or more myomas
2. Intramural extension of the fibroid is greater than 50%
3. When malignancy is suspected
4. Patients with cardiac, pulmonary, or renal disorders

## QUESTION 2

*What are some of the complications associated with hysteroscopic myomectomy?*

## ANSWER 2

Hysteroscopic myomectomy (Fig. 81-1) is relatively safe, but, like any other surgical procedure, it is not free

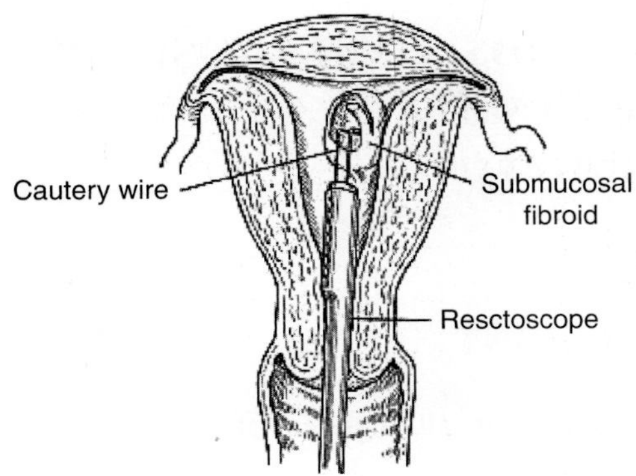


**FIG. 81-1** Hysteroscopic myomectomy using the resectoscope.
SOURCE: Glasser MH, Zimmerman JD. The HydroThermAblator system for management of menorrhagia in women with submucous myomas: 12- to 20-month follow-up. *J Am Assoc Gynecol Laparosc*. 2003;10(4):521–527.

of complications. Complication rates of 2% and 2.7% have been reported in the literature. These can be divided into perioperative and early or late postoperative complications.

1. Perioperative complications.
   a. Hemorrhage is generally caused by surgery and may be associated with uterine perforation. Heavy bleeding was reported in 0.65% in a review of 2116 cases of operative hysteroscopy.
   b. Uterine perforation can happen at any stage during the procedure and is estimated to occur in 0.4–1.6% of operative hysteroscopies. If suspected, perforation should be ruled out by laparoscopy. In a review of 547 cases, two bowel injuries were reported in association with seven uterine perforations.
   c. Fluid overload is the most common perioperative complication. An incidence rate between 0.38% and 3.3% has been reported. The commonly reported complications are pulmonary edema, cerebral edema, coagulopathy, and hyponatremia, especially when low-viscosity fluids such as glycine, glucose, sorbitol, and mannitol are used. Resection of myomas, greater than 3 cm in diameter is associated with increased risk distention media complications. High-viscosity distension fluids, popularly used in the past, caused anaphylactic reaction in 1 in 10,000 cases.
2. Early postoperative complications
   a. A postoperative infection rate of 1.42% was reported in a review of 1116 operative hysteroscopy cases, with two-thirds caused by endometritis and one-third caused by urinary tract infection. Intrauterine synechia develop in 13.4% of cases and can be divided at second-look hysteroscopy.
3. Late postoperative complications
   a. Uterine rupture has been reported antenatally and during labor in subsequent pregnancies following endometrial resections. In most of these cases, hysteroscopies were complicated by uterine perforation.

## QUESTION 3

*What are some recommendations used to optimize the outcome of hysteroscopic myomectomy?*

## ANSWER 3

1. A uterine size of 12 weeks or more can be detected clinically, and grossly enlarged uteri that are unsuitable for hysteroscopic surgery can be ruled out. Transvaginal ultrasonography is the most cost-effective method of localizing and measuring uterine myomas. Hysterosalpingography is considered the standard for diagnosing distortion of the uterine cavity caused by submucous myomas.
2. Administration of gonadotrophin releasing hormone (GnRH) analogues before hysteroscopic surgery significantly reduces the operating time and the volume of distension medium used. However, stated that small fibroids may shrink and be overlooked, increasing the risk of recurrence.
3. Aggressive attempts at resecting intramyometrial fibroids can lead to uterine perforation. Therefore monitoring with intraoperative transabdominal ultrasound has been suggested.
4. Several large studies on hysteroscopic myomectomy have recommended routine use of antibiotic coverage before, during, and after surgery.
5. It is generally agreed that when a nonelectrolyte fluid deficit reaches 1000 mL, the serum sodium level should be checked; if it is 120 mmol/L, or if the deficit is 1500–2000 mL, the procedure should be stopped immediately. Use of proper equipment for monitoring the intrauterine pressure and adjusting it just above the patient's diastolic blood pressure is vital. The intrauterine pressure should not exceed 80 mm Hg.
6. Patients with menorrhagia who are no longer desirous of fertility show better results if endometrial ablation is performed along with resection.

## QUESTION 4

*What are alternative therapies to hysteroscopic myomectomy?*

ANSWER 4

1. Hysterectomy is a reasonable alternative unless fertility is still desired.
2. Abdominal myomectomy either by laparoscopy or laparotomy is another option for those wanting to preserve the uterus but has the disadvantage of greater blood loss than a hysterectomy.
3. GnRH with add-back estrogen replacement therapy analogues can only provide relief for a limited duration.
4. Uterine artery embolization for the treatment of uterine fibroids was described by Ravina in 1994. Immediate cessation of menorrhagia with improvement in pain and pressure symptoms was noted in 70% of the patients.
5. Vaginal myomectomy is a relatively new approach developed for the removal of the larger fibroids considered unsuitable for hysteroscopic or laparoscopic removal and provides an alternative to open myomectomy. However, this technique has failed to gain popularity because of poor accessibility and difficulty in ensuring hemostasis.

## BIBLIOGRAPHY

Agostini A, et al. Hemorrhage risk during operative hysteroscopy. *Acta Obstet Gynecol Scand.* 2002;81(9):878–881.

Batra N, et al. Hysteroscopic myomectomy. *Obstet Gynecol Clin North Am.* 2004;31:669–685.

Corson SL, Brooks PG. Resectoscopic myomectomy. *Fertil Steril.* 1991;55:1041–1044.

Drews MR, Reyniak JV. Surgical approach to myomas: laparoscopy and hysteroscopy. *Semin Reprod Endocrinol.* 2001;10:367–377.

Emanuel MH, et al. Long term results of hysteroscopic myomectomy for abnormal uterine bleeding. *Obstet Gynecol.* 1999;93: 743–748.

Hart R, et al. Long term follow up of hysteroscopic myomectomy assessed by survival analysis. *Br J Obstet Gynecol.* 1999;106(7):700–705.

Indman PD. Hysteroscopic treatment of menorrhagia associated with uterine leiomyomas. *Obstet Gynecol.* 1993;81:716–720.

Magos A, et al. Vaginal myomectomy. *Br J Obstet Gynecol.* 1994;101:1092–1094.

Munro MG. Abnormal uterine bleeding: surgical management–part III. *J Am Assoc Gynecol Laparosc.* 2001;8(1):18–44.

Olive DL. Review of the evidence for treatment of leiomyomata. *Environ Health Perspect.* 2000;108(Suppl. 5):841–843.

Perino A, et al. Role of leuprolide acetate depot in hysteroscopic surgery: a controlled study. *Fertil Steril.* 1993;59:507–510.

Propst AM, Liberman RF, Harlow BL, Ginsburg ES. Complication of hysteroscopic surgery: predicting patients at risk. *Obstet Gynecol.* 2000;96(4):517–520.

Ravina JH, et al. Arterial embolisation to treat uterine myomata. *Lancet.* 1995;346:671–672.

Ubaldi F, et al. Fertility after hysteroscopic myomectomy. *Hum Reprod Update.* 1995;1(1):81–90.

# 82 FIBROIDS: MYOMECTOMY VERSUS UTERINE ARTERY EMBOLIZATION AND CRYOMYOLYSIS

*Susan Sarajari*

## LEARNING POINT

Understanding the surgical alternatives to hysterectomy in patients with uterine fibroids.

## VIGNETTE

A 37-year-old, G2P2002, presents to your office complaining of regular but very heavy periods that last up to 10 days and abdominal fullness. She states that she often is not able to go to work due to the heavy menstrual flow and she sometimes feels lightheaded during her period. She denies any urinary or gastrointestinal symptoms. She was told by another physician that she has uterine fibroids and wants to discuss treatment options with you. She has had one vaginal delivery and one prior cesarean section, but has not had any other surgeries. She is very interested in fertility. She has no other medical problems and takes no medications. On pelvic examination a 14-week size uterus is palpated that is irregular in shape. The adnexa could not be palpated. An ultrasound examination reveals a $14 \times 9 \times 6$ cm uterus with multiple leiomyomata and the ovaries appear normal. No ureteral dilation is noted.

QUESTION 1

*What factors should be considered in the selection of treatment for uterine fibroids?*

ANSWER 1

The type and timing of any intervention for uterine fibroids should be based on:

- Symptoms
- Size of myomas
- Location of myomas (see Fig. 82-1)

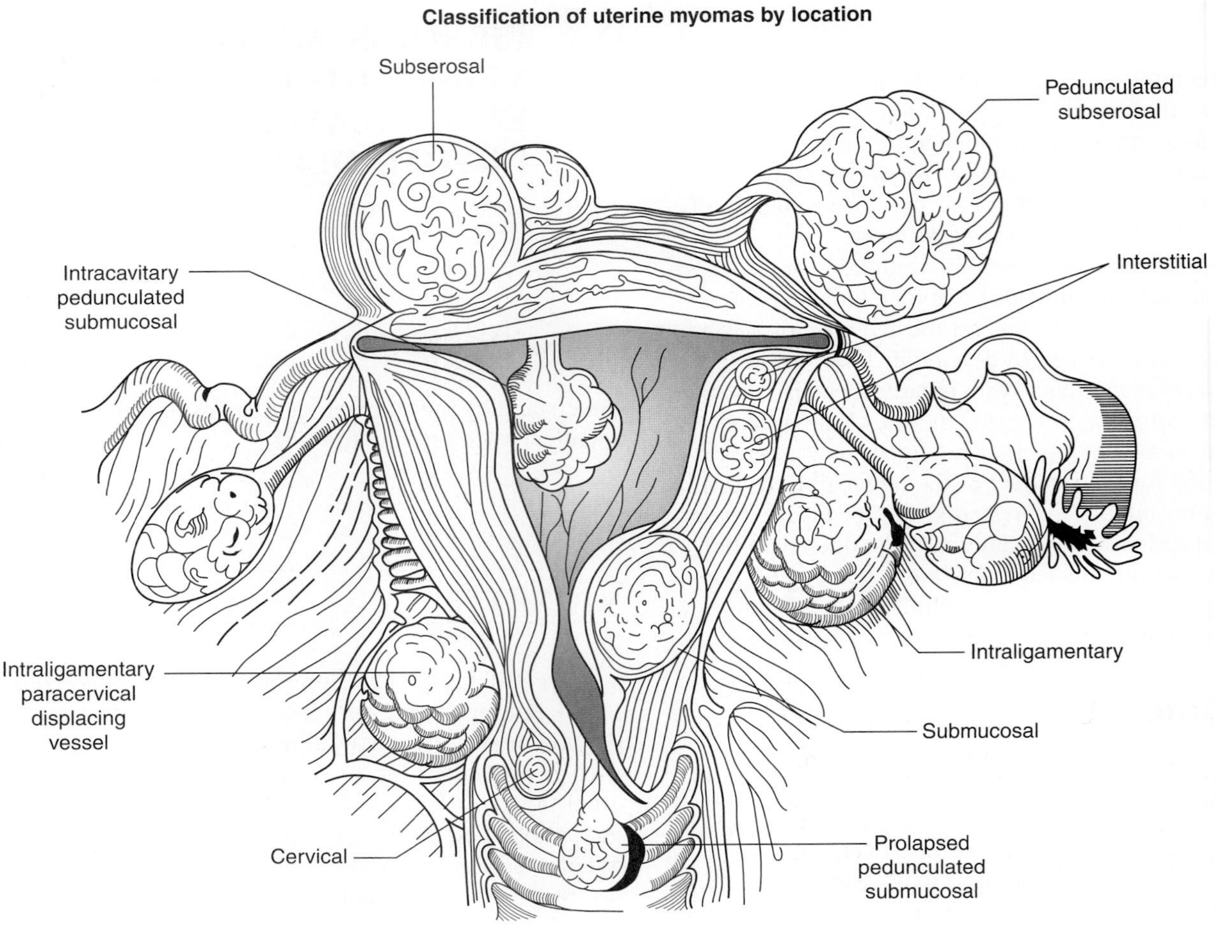

**FIG. 82-1** Classification of uterine myomas by location.
SOURCE: Stoval TG, Mann WJ. Myomectomy. In: Rose BD (ed.). *UpToDate*. Waltham, MA: UpToDate;2006. www.Uptodate.com

- Reproductive plans and obstetrical history (does patient still desire fertility?)
- Woman's age (is patient near menopause?)

## QUESTION 2

*What are the advantages and disadvantages of a myomectomy?*

## ANSWER 2

Advantages:

- One option for the removal of fibroids in patients who desire future fertility since only the myomas are removed.
- Effective therapy for menorrhagia and pelvic pressure.
- Can be performed by laparotomy, laparoscopy, and hysteroscopy.

Disadvantages:

- Significant risk that leiomyomas will recur. About 50% of patients will have recurrence after 5 years and 11–26% of patients require a second surgery.
- Myomectomy near the oviduct can cause adhesions that may affect fertility.
- Risk of uterine rupture in a subsequent pregnancy.

## QUESTION 3

*What approaches to myomectomy are available?*

## ANSWER 3

- Laparotomy: Treatment of choice when there are multiple myomas, the uterus is greater than 16-week size, or the myomas are deep and intramural. Operative time, blood loss, and hospital stay are similar to abdominal hysterectomy.

- Laparoscopy: Indicated for patients with a uterus less than 17-week size or with a small number of subserosal or intramural fibroids. The uterus must be small enough to allow visualization through the endoscope.
- Hysteroscope: Indicated for resection of submucous myomas. Can be performed as outpatient surgery and the recovery period is short. Excellent fertility rates.

### QUESTION 4

*What is uterine artery embolization (UAE) and what factors need to be considered before performing the procedure?*

### ANSWER 4

- UAE is performed by inserting a catheter through the femoral artery to access the uterine arteries. Polyvinyl alcohol particles or tris-acryl gelatin microspheres are then used to embolize the uterine arteries. Metal coils may also be used to assist with vascular occlusion.
- May be performed in premenopausal women but is not indicated in postmenopausal women.
- Reports have shown a short-term reduction in myomas, a short-term clinical improvement in bulk-related symptoms, and decrease in menstrual bleeding.
- Several pregnancies have been reported after UAE, however further data regarding fertility outcome are needed. Loss of ovarian function has been reported to occur in 14% of the patients. UAE is relatively contraindicated in patients who want to preserve fertility.
- Risk of performing procedure on a malignancy since preoperative evaluation cannot distinguish with certainty between benign and malignant lesions.
- Complications from UAE include infection, abscess, sepsis, labial necrosis, permanent amenorrhea, hysterectomy, groin hematoma, focal bladder necrosis, vesicouterine fistula, uterine wall defects, and pulmonary emboli.

### QUESTION 5

*What is myolysis and which patients are candidates for the procedure?*

### ANSWER 5

Myolysis is the laparoscopic thermal coagulation or cryoablation (cryomyolysis) of uterine myomas. Women with fewer than four fibroids with the largest fibroid less than 10 cm in diameter are candidates for this procedure. Fertility and pregnancy outcome after this procedure are not known and it should therefore be reserved for patients who no longer desire fertility. Three to six months following the procedure, myomas regress by 50–90% and recurrences are rare.

## BIBLIOGRAPHY

ACOG Committee Opinion. Committee on Gynecologic Practice. Uterine artery embolization. 293. 2004.

ACOG Committee on Practice Bulletins-Gynecology. ACOG Practice Bulletin. No. 16, May 2000. Surgical alternatives to hysterectomy in the management of leiomyomas. *Int J Gynecol Obstet*. 2001;73(3):285–293.

TJ Stovall, WJ Mann. Myomectomy. In: Rose, BD (ed.). *UpToDate*. Waltham, MA;200. www.Uptodate.com.

Stewart EA. Treatment of uterine leiomyomas, In: Rose, BD (ed.). *UpToDate*. Waltham, MA; 2006. www.Uptodate.com.

# 83 SUPRACERVICAL HYSTERECTOMY

*Ilana Cass*

## LEARNING POINT

To understand the rationale and data regarding supracervical hysterectomy.

## VIGNETTE

A 40-year-old, G3P2, presents with pelvic pressure and progressive menorrhagia. She is sexually active and has had a prior tubal ligation. Her last menstrual period was 2 weeks ago and lasted 14 days. She reports feeling lightheaded during her menses, and had to take 3 days off from work during her last menses. She was found to have hemoglobin of 9.1 g/dL at her internist's office, and she started the patient on iron. She denies any change in her bowel habits, but she does report urinary frequency and a sense of incomplete voiding.

She has a significant gynecologic history of uterine fibroids and has had two prior myomectomies and cesarean sections at term. She has no significant past medical history. She denies any family history of cancer.

The physical examination reveals a thin woman in no apparent distress. Vitals signs: pulse 68/min, BP 100/60 mm Hg, and afebrile. Head, eyes, ears, nose, and throat examination reveals no adenopathy, chest is clear to auscultation; cardiac examination shows regular rate and rhythm; abdominal examination shows no ascites of distention there is slight tenderness to deep palpation in the left lower quadrant without any masses or inguinal adenopathy, and pelvic examination reveals normal anatomy with a palpable, slightly tender, mobile mass approximately 6 cm on bimanual examination on the left, with no masses in the rectovaginal septum.

A pelvic ultrasound is performed 3 days after her next menses begins, which shows an enlarged uterus consistent with multiple fibroids, the largest of which measures 9 × 8 × 8 cm and 7 × 5 × 6 cm. The adnexa are visualized and are normal, and the endometrial echo is 6 mm. There is no pelvic fluid noted in the cul-de-sac. A repeat hemoglobin is 11 g/dL.

## QUESTION 1

*What are the historic reasons cited for performing a supracervical hysterectomy, and why did they fall out of favor?*

## ANSWER 1

Supracervical hysterectomy was the procedure of choice in the nineteenth and early twentieth century when surgical technique was limited by rudimentary anesthesia, and blood banks and antibiotics did not exist. Most of the visceral and hemorrhagic complications associated with hysterectomies resulted from the cervicectomy portion of the surgery. Studies at the time described that the mortality of supracervical hysterectomy was half that of total hysterectomy. Ninety five percent of all hysterectomies performed before 1950 were supracervical. In the 1940s, the role of total hysterectomy in preventing cervical cancer, which was very common and undetectable in the preinvasive state, was understood, and total hysterectomy became the procedure of choice.

## QUESTION 2

*What are the observed differences in outcome for women who have supracervical abdominal hysterectomy versus total abdominal hysterectomy?*

## ANSWER 2

Large prospective randomized trials of women with benign disease have shown similar rates of bladder, bowel, and sexual function between patients who have had subtotal and total abdominal hysterectomies. A recent study that focused on sexual function 2 years after surgery found no differences in sexual function or quality-of-life outcomes between the two groups of patients. Although follow-up was only 6–24 months after surgery, sexual function tended to improve after hysterectomy as did urinary frequency, irrespective of the type of hysterectomy. Supracervical hysterectomy has been associated with less operative time, less blood loss, and shorter hospital stay. Total abdominal hysterectomy has been associated with higher rates of postoperative complications including urinary complications and wound infections. Cyclical bleeding has been reported to occur in 7–8% of patients after supracervical hysterectomy.

## QUESTION 3

*What are the relative contraindications to performing a supracervical hysterectomy? What is the cited incidence of cervical stump carcinoma and do patients have the same outcome?*

## ANSWER 3

Contraindications: endometrial cancer, patients with a history of abnormal cervical cytology or those with no access to cytologic screening, patients with unexplained abnormal uterine bleeding. The cited incidence of cervical stump carcinoma is 1/1000. As a group, stage for survival is the same, but surgical and radiation induced complications are higher due to previous adhesive disease and absence of the uterus to protect pelvic organs.

## BIBLIOGRAPHY

Johns A. Supracervical versus total hysterectomy. *Clin Obstet Gynecol.* 1997;49(4);903–913.

Kuppermann M, Summitt RL, Varner RE, McNeeley SG, Goodman-Gruen D, Learman LA, et al. *Obstet Gynecol.* 2005; 105:1309–1318.

Metler L. Endometrial cancer represents a contraindication for classic intrafascial supracervical hysterectomy by laparoscopy. *Am J Obstet Gynecol* 1998;178(3):628.

Munro M. Supracervical hysterectomy: a time for reappraisal. *Obstet Gynecol.* 1997;89(1).

Roovers J, van der Bom JG, can der Vaart CH, Heintz PM, et al. Hysterectomy and sexual wellbeing: prospective observational study of vaginal hysterectomy, subtotal abdominal hysterectomy and abdominal hysterectomy. *BMJ.* 2003;327:774–778.

Thakar R, Ayers S, Clarkson P, Stanton S, Manyonda I. Outcomes after total versus subtotal abdominal hysterectomy. *New Engl J Med.* 2002;347(17):1318–1325.

# 84 COMPLICATIONS OF HYSTEROSCOPY

*Lee Kao*

## LEARNING POINTS

What are the potential complications during hysteroscopy? What are the media you would use in hysteroscopy, and is there any specific reason for you to prefer a particular one? How can you minimize the patient's risk for air emboli during hysteroscopy? What would you do if you think you have perforated the uterus during a hysteroscopy?

## VIGNETTE

A 37-year-old Hispanic female, G1P0010, presents desiring fertility. In 1998 she had sought infertility treatment without success. Subsequently in 2002, the patient had a laparoscopy performed and was told postoperatively that her right side tube was blocked and also there were ovarian cysts.

She achieved a spontaneous pregnancy in late 2002, which ended as a spontaneous miscarriage, for which she did not undergo a dilation and curettage (D&C). In 2004, a hysterosalpingogram revealed: (1) left-sided proximal tubal occlusion, (2) right-sided normal caliber fallopian tube with no free spill documented, and (3) questionable uterine lower segment filling defect. Upon follow-up, a transvaginal ultrasound (TV-US) reported a normal sized uterus, normal sized bilateral ovaries, and a single left lateral submucous uterine fibroid, measuring about 1.3 cm in diameter. The patient is now requesting a hysteroscopic surgery.

### QUESTION 1

*What are the media you would use in hysteroscopy, and is there any specific reason for you to prefer a particular one?*

### ANSWER 1

Currently available distention media include $CO_2$, high-viscosity fluids, and low-viscosity fluids. $CO_2$ gas is mainly limited to diagnostic hysteroscopy because it does not allow for clearing of debris during operative procedures. Though the most significant potential complication of $CO_2$ is gas embolism, it is much more soluble in plasma than room air and provides a wide margin of safety from embolic complications.

*High-viscosity fluid:* Dextran 70 (Hyskon) is a clear, viscous solution with 32% dextran 70 in 10% dextrose/water. It is immiscible with blood and allows clear visualization in the presence of bleeding and becomes the favorite distention medium for some. However, dextran 70 is not the ideal distention medium for operative hysteroscopy. It has an average molecular weight (MW) of 70, and dextrans less than MW 50 are excreted by the kidney without difficulty. In patients with normal renal function, 50% of dextrans is excreted within 24 hours. However, larger dextran molecules need to be metabolized to $CO_2$ and water by the liver and reticuloendothelial systems and have a half-life of several days. When using dextran 70 for operative hysteroscopy, the operator must be vigilant to prevent complications, be cognizant of operative time, absorbed volume, and intrauterine pressures. Patients requiring an extensive procedure should be counseled about the possibility of a two-stage process if the surgeon cannot complete all operative goals without risking excessive dextran absorption.

Low-viscosity fluids are the most commonly used distention media because of their relative safety and ability to be used with the continuous-flow resectoscope. The major complications of low-viscosity media result from excessive absorption and consequent fluid overload. Low-viscosity media are best divided into two groups based on their tonicity and electrolyte content (Table 84-1): (1) hypotonic/electrolyte-free media that can lead to hypotonic fluid overload, and (2) isotonic-/electrolyte-containing media that cause isotonic fluid overload, which can be easily treated.

The hypotonic group includes glycine and sorbitol solutions. They are electrolyte-free and relatively nonconductive. They are the preferred distention media for

**TABLE 84-1. Osmolality and Electrolyte Content of Hysteroscopic Distention Media**

| MEDIUM | OSMOLALITY (mOsm/kg $H_2O$) | SODIUM CONCENTRATION (mEq/L) |
|---|---|---|
| Normal saline | 308 | 154 |
| Serum | 290 | 135–145 |
| Mannitol 5% | 280 | — |
| Ringer's lactate | 273 | 130 |
| Glycine 1.5% | 200 | — |
| Sorbitol 3% + mannitol 0.5% | 178 | — |

conventional electrosurgical operative hysteroscopy because electrolytes disperse electrical energy and prohibit conventional electrosurgical instruments from achieving current densities needed for effective surgery. When absorbed in large volumes, glycine and sorbitol are easily metabolized leaving free water in the intravascular space, which may lead to fatal hyponatremic hypervolemia. Recently, 5% mannitol has been gaining popularity as a distention medium that is isotonic and electrolyte poor, compatible with conventional electrosurgical tools yet carries less risk for encephalopathy.

The isotonic media commonly used are normal saline and Ringer's lactate. As with the hypotonic media, excessive absorption is their main complication. Since these contain electrolytes, their use is limited to operative hysteroscopy with use of mechanical, rather than electrosurgical, instrumentation. In general, fluid overload from normal saline or Ringer's lactate is less dangerous and treated more easily than fluid overload from glycine or sorbitol solutions.

Three new electrosurgical instruments compatible with normal saline and Ringer's lactate, have been created to avoid the inherent complications of hypotonic media by making use of physiologic distention media. The Versapoint uses a 1.7-mm diameter bipolar electrode operating system that conducts electric current between two electrodes that are in close proximity in isotonic media. The ERA sleeve is a monopolar system using a disposable outer sheath that fits over standard resectoscope to function as a return electrode in isotonic media. The OPERA Star system is another modification of monopolar technology that facilitates tissue cutting and coagulation in isotonic media.

## QUESTION 2

*What are the potential complications during hysteroscopy?*

## ANSWER 2

Complications from distention media, depending on the media that is used, include gas embolism, anaphylactic reactions, fluid overload, and coagulopathy, pulmonary edema, and potential complications of increasing free ammonia. The use of high-viscosity distension media is associated with the development of anaphylactic reactions, fluid overload, and pulmonary edema.

Pulmonary edema can occur with dextran 70 (Hyskon) as a result of simple fluid overload from excess absorption or from direct pulmonary capillary toxic effect. Anaphylactic reactions, fluid overload, and coagulopathy occur in about 1:1500– 1:300,000 patients receiving dextran-70. Treatment consists of diphenhydramine, epinephrine, steroids, and fluid and ventilatory support as necessary, as well as removing or irrigating all dextran from the patient's body. Diuretics are likely to be ineffective because the persistent intravascular high-molecular-weight dextrans, and plasmapheresis may be needed. The manufacturer recommends vigilance for pulmonary edema, especially when procedures last more than 45 minutes, deficit is greater than 250 mL of dextran 70, resection of large areas of endometrium, or administration of intravenous fluids at more than a maintenance rate. Special mention is made in the package insert for measuring the running volumes of infused and recovered dextran 70 every 15 minutes to recognize dextran absorption.

When using low-viscosity distention media, risk factors for excessive absorption include excessive intrauterine pressure, prolonged operating time, procedures that open vascular channels on the endometrial surface, and uterine perforation or cervical laceration. In the majority of the cases, 60–75 mm Hg of infusion pressure creates approximately an intrauterine pressure of 10–15 mm Hg and is sufficient to achieve a clear view. Greater than 100 mm Hg infusion pressure should never be necessary because the risk for fluid overload is markedly increased when the mean infusion pressure exceeds mean arterial pressure. When using gravity feed, 75 and 100 mm Hg infusion pressures are achieved by suspending the bag of media 39 and 52 in. over the uterus, respectively. Operative procedures lasting longer than 1 hour are more likely to have fluid overload. When 1000 mL of fluid has been absorbed, the operator should move toward a rapid conclusion of the procedure and consider monitoring serum electrolytes. If the fluid deficit reaches 1500 mL or the serum sodium is less than 125 mmol/L, the procedure should be terminated. When using glycine, deamination by the liver and kidney creates glycolic acid and ammonia, which carries additional potential complication of elevating blood-free ammonia concentrations that may cause muscle aches, visual disturbances, and encephalopathy.

*Mechanical complications:* Mechanical complications include cervical laceration, uterine perforation, and the potential dissemination of malignant endometrial cells. Nulliparity, postmenopausal status, cervical stenosis, diethylstilbestrol (DES) exposure, or past history of difficult cervical dilation, are risk factors for cervical laceration. Preparatory use of osmotic dilators and the use of a double-toothed tenaculum or ring forceps, instead of single-toothed tenaculum, can lessen the risk for cervical trauma. The use of small-diameter (5 mm) rigid hysteroscope or a flexible hysteroscope, commonly less than 5 mm, also reduces this risk. Uterine perforation is the most common complication of hysteroscopy and occurs about 14 per 1000 cases. Stenotic os, severe uterine anteflexion or retroflexion, lower uterine segment myomas, Asherman's syndrome, and operator inexperience are known risk factors. It can also occur during intramural myoma resection, septa division, endometrial resection, or adhesiolysis. Prompt recognition and appropriate exploration are keys to limiting further complication. If electrocautery or laser were used, monitoring serial WBC, temperatures, observation for any signs or symptoms of developing visceral injury, and laparoscopy/laparotomy exploration, may be necessary.

*Bleeding:* Hemorrhage is the second most common complication of hysteroscopy and occurs in 2.5 of every 1000 cases. Resection of myomas with a transmural component carries the highest risk of 2–3%, and 0.2–2.2% for endometrial ablation. Bleeding during operative hysteroscopy is rare because the pressure suppresses venous blood loss, visualization of the entire cavity with reduced pressure at the end of a procedure is important. If bleeding continues, an intrauterine Foley catheter with 20–30 mL of saline filling its balloon may be used, this can be removed in 2–24 hours. Vasopressin (20 U in 20 mL normal saline) injected into the cervix, rectal misoprostol, or vasopressin-soaked gauze packing can be given if bleeding continues. Other alternatives for continuing bleeding would be uterine artery embolization or hysterectomy.

*Anesthetic complications:* Lidocaine is the most frequently used agent for paracervical or intracervical anesthesia. Maximum dosage is 4.5 mg/kg (not to exceed 300 mg) for lidocaine without epinephrine, or 7 mg/kg (not to exceed 500 mg) for lidocaine with epinephrine. Usually no more than 20 mL of 1% lidocaine, or 200 mg, is required. Central nervous system (CNS) toxicity can present as anxiety, restlessness, dizziness, nausea, tremors, or seizures. Alternatively, hypotension, sinus bradycardia or other arrhythmia, cardiovascular collapse, and death, may occur.

*Laser and electrosurgical complications:* When using laser or electrosurgical devices, thermal injuries can happen subsequent to uterine perforation, and present with delayed manifestations such as peritonitis, sepsis, and death. The Nd:yttrium aluminum garnet (YAG) laser penetrates only 4–5 mm depth of endometrium, yet thermal bowel injury without perforation has been reported. Potential problems of monopolar electrical energy are caused by stray current, secondary to faulty insulation of electrodes, capacitative coupling, or direct coupling, and can damage tissue outside the view of the scope. When the active electrode of a monopolar device is electrically separated from the tissue by a nonconductive plastic sleeve, a capacitor is formed and capacitative coupling current can occur unpredictably out of the view of the scope. Direct coupling is not an issue in single instrument operation such as hysteroscopy.

*Infection:* Infection is uncommon at about 1.6%, most are uncomplicated cystitis, endometritis, or parametritis, and about 0.3–0.4% for hysteroscopic endometrial ablation. Prophylactic antibiotics have not been demonstrated to be effective. Toxic shock syndrome, pyometria, tubo-ovarian abscesses, broad ligament abscess, had all been reported. Patients with history of pelvic inflammatory disease or with valvular heart diseases likely will benefit from prophylactic antibiotics.

*Air embolism:* During surgery, venous channels in the cervix or endometrium can allow ambient air or pressurized gas to enter the circulation. The intravasated gas can travel to the right side of the heart, and cause ineffective pumping cue to the compressibility of gas. The right outflow tract is thus functionally occluded, and pulmonary blood flow drops acutely. Subsequently, cardiac output and blood pressure drop, tachycardia and tachypnea develop, and electrocardiogram (ECG) changes immediately before cardiovascular collapse. As pressure in the right side of the heart increases, the foramen ovale can be reopened in 15% of adults, which results in passage of air to the left side of the heart and paradoxic emboli through the arterial tree to the brain and other organs.

## QUESTION 3

*How can you minimize the patient's risk for air emboli during hysteroscopy?*

## ANSWER 3

Prevention of air embolism relies on understanding the pathophysiology and the risk factors. Trendelenburg position places the uterus above the heart and creates a venous vacuum, potentially sucking air through the open venous sinuses. Difficult cervical dilation and operative procedures create more trauma and more portals for air entry. Operators should exercise preventive measures: (1) avoiding Trendelenburg positioning or at least use the minimum possible; (2) minimizing cervical trauma; (3) keeping the os occluded; (4) flushing the hysteroscope and tubings of all air bubbles; and (5) communicating with the anesthesiologist and monitor end-tidal $CO_2$ and pulse oximetry as standard protocol.

## QUESTION 4

*What would you do if you think you have perforated the uterus during a hysteroscopy?*

## ANSWER 4

Preoperative examination for uterine position and application of ultrasound during cervical dilatation can prevent creation of false passage and subsequent perforations of the anterior or posterior uterine wall. A fundal perforation with a uterine sound or a narrow dilator and absence of bleeding can be managed expectantly with observation. A short course of antibiotics may be considered. Fundal perforations with detectable bleeding or those caused by larger dilators or hysteroscopes should be considered candidates for diagnostic hysteroscopy to rule out significant bleeding or visceral injury. Anterior wall perforations may lead to bladder injury. When the defect is small, repair is not necessary. If the defect is large or was created with electrical/laser energy, it must be meticulously repaired. Cystoscopy should be performed whenever the surgeon is not certain about the presence of bladder injury. Posterior wall perforations can involve the rectum or large bowel; thus, whenever the uterine serosa is perforated, diagnostic laparoscopy is warranted. When there is posterior or lateral perforation concomitant ureteral injury may exist, mandating vigilant laparoscopic inspection of the ureters and possible urologic consultation. Perforations in the lateral uterine wall are most likely to cause vascular injury of the iliac vessels, mesenteric artery, aorta, or presacral vessels. Diagnostic laparoscopy or even laparotomy should be performed promptly.

## BIBLIOGRAPHY

Cooper JM, Brady RM. Intraoperative and early postoperative complications of operative hysteroscopy. *Obstet Gynecol Clin North Am.* 2000;27(2):347–366.

# 85 LAPAROSCOPIC COMPLICATIONS: PREDICTION AND AVOIDANCE

*Ricardo Azziz*

## LEARNING POINT

To understand the risks of laparoscopic complications during operative laparoscopy and to undertake maneuvers to minimize these risks.

## VIGNETTE

A 34-year-old woman, with a long history of endometriosis, is found to have a persistent left ovarian cyst measuring approximately 4 × 4 × 3 cm. Sonographic evidence suggests that it is an endometrioma. The patient is 5 ft 5 in. tall and weighs 186 lb. Her only prior surgery for endometriosis, performed some 10 years, was carried out through a laparotomy using a transverse skin incision. In her preoperative counseling, you discuss the possibility and risk of complications, and the patient has multiple questions in this regard.

### QUESTION 1

*What is the prevalence and type of complications occurring during operative laparoscopy?*

### ANSWER 1

The overall complication rate of patients undergoing operative laparoscopy for gynecologic procedures ranges from 1.5 to 3.0%. Only a minority of these requires conversion to laparotomy for management of the complication. Roughly, complications can be divided into those that are hemorrhagic following vascular injury, those that are related to intestinal injury, and those related to urologic injuries. Approximately one-third of complications fall into each of these categories. Approximately 50% of all complications are associated with trocar or Veress needle insertion, and the remaining occur during the operative procedure. While approximately 60% of all complications are recognized at the time of the surgery, up to 40% may go unrecognized and present postoperatively.

### QUESTION 2

*What are predictors of complications during operative gynecologic laparoscopy and conversion of laparoscopy to laparotomy?*

### ANSWER 2

A number of factors are associated with an increased risk for laparoscopic complications. In some studies, age greater than 35 years or parity greater than two live births was associated with an increased risk of operative injuries or abdominal bleeding. Prior laparotomy does increase the overall risk of complications by 20–40%. It is less clear how body mass impacts on the complication rate, with some investigators noting that increasing body mass actually was protective against complications, while others reporting that complications actually increased with body mass. It is clear that extremes in body weight will predispose the patient to laparoscopic complications, as the thin patient will have little protection against trocar and other related injuries, and the very overweight patient may require heroic and often uncontrolled efforts to enter her abdomen.

An important predictor of laparoscopic complications is surgeon inexperience, with the complication rate decreasing proportionate to the amount of surgical experience. An analysis of most procedures indicates that complication rates begin to level off after the surgeon has performed between 20 and 50 of a specific type of procedure (e.g., laparoscopic-assisted vaginal hysterectomy).

The level of complexity of the procedure is also a determinant of the prevalence of laparoscopic complications, a factor whose impact is not fully offset by increasing surgeon experience. Finally, some procedures are more prone to complications than others. In general, treatment of endometriosis or ovarian cystectomy generally have lower rates of operative complications, while laparoscopic-assisted vaginal hysterectomies have higher rates of complications, notably ureteral injuries.

## QUESTION 3

*What techniques can be used to minimize the rate of complications associated with trocar insertion?*

## ANSWER 3

Trocar insertion during the performance of laparoscopy accounts for between 20% and 50% of all laparoscopic surgery-associated complications. Steps that can be taken to minimize these include; (a) maintaining the patient horizontal when the umbilical trocar is inserted, (b) lowering the operating table to the level of the surgeon's elbows so that excessive pressure is not applied and full control is maintained, (c) extending the index finger to within 3 cm of the trocar tip when inserting it through the umbilicus, (d) using a controlled twisting motion, directing the trocar toward the sacral hollow, and (e) when abdominal entry is achieved, advancing the trocar no more than 2 cm beyond peritoneum. While the use of shielded trocars has provided some degree of protection, these trocars are not fail-safe and, in fact, can often lead to a false sense of security, which can actually result in more complications.

The insertion of the auxiliary trocars can also be associated with complications. Minimization of complications with the insertion of these ports can be achieved by: (a) placing the patient in Trendelenburg position at the time of insertion, (b) transilluminating the abdomen to visualize the superficial epigastric vessels, (c) identifying at laparoscopy the course of the inferior epigastric vessels in order to avoid them, (d) placing the trocars as high above the symphysis as cosmetically possible but certainly not less than 3 cm from the symphysis pubis, and (d) inserting the ports under direct laparoscopic visualization. The placement of larger ports through these auxiliary incisions can be safely achieved with the use of radially expanding sleeves.

## QUESTION 4

*How can gastrointestinal injuries be minimized and, if they occur, detected promptly?*

## ANSWER 4

Gastrointestinal injuries can be caused by burns, Veress needle or trocar insertion, and endoscopic dissection. Approximately 50% of bowel injuries occur in patients without prior risk factors. In some cases, bowel entrapment may occur at the umbilical or other 8–12 mm ancillary port sites, as instruments are withdrawn (Fig. 85-1).

Strategies to minimize gastrointestinal injuries include the use of alternative trocar insertion sites, particularly in patients who have had prior laparotomies. The risk of bowel entrapment may be minimized by:

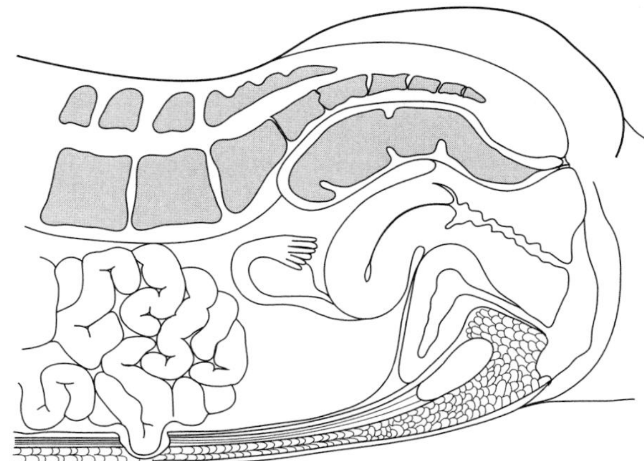

**FIG. 85-1** Herniation of the small intestine at the site of the umbilical trocar may be prevented by withdrawing the laparoscope while observing closure of the peritoneum and suturing the fascia closed.

SOURCE: Reprinted with permission from Smith S. Minimizing, recognizing, and managing laparoscopic complications. In: Azziz R, Murphy AA (eds.). *Practical Manual of Operative Laparoscopy and Hysteroscopy,* 2nd ed. New York, NY: Springer–Verlag; 1992:248–269.

(a) using smaller diameter trocars, (b) using expanding sleeves to switch from a small diameter to a large diameter port, (c) closing the fascia for trocar incisions that are greater than 10 mm in size, (d) reducing excessive postoperative vomiting or retching, which can force bowel up into a port site, and (e) replacing the laparoscope into the sleeve when withdrawing the trocar sleeve.

If a Veress needle is observed to have entered bowel (e.g., because of the aspiration of intestinal fluids), the needle may be withdrawn and an alternative site for placement chosen. Veress needle injuries may be watched for 48 hours and generally do not lead to further infection or problems. Alternatively, if a trocar transverses bowel wall, the injury requires immediate repair and a delay in performing a laparotomy increases the risk of nonviable bowel, and infection and/or septic shock. Some patients may present with evidence of sepsis as late as 24–72 hours postoperatively following bowel injury. A high mortality can be expected if the bowel injury goes unrecognized and the patient develops septic shock, hence a high degree of clinical suspicion should be maintained. In general, patients should progressively improve postoperatively following laparoscopic surgery, and if this is not the case then a careful evaluation of the patient for the possibility of complications, particularly gastrointestinal, should be performed.

## BIBLIOGRAPHY

Chapron C, Querleu D, Bruhat MA, Madelenat P, Fernandez H, Pierre F, Dubuisson JB. Surgical complications of diagnostic and operative gynaecological laparoscopy: a series of 29, 966 cases. *Hum Reprod.* 1998;13:867–872.

Harkki-Siren P, Kurki T. A nationwide analysis of laparoscopic complications. *Obstet Gynecol.* 1997;89:108–112

Hulka J, Peterson HB, Phillips JM, Surrey MW. Operative laparoscopy: American Association of Gynecologic Laparoscopists' 1993 membership survey. *J Am Assoc Gynecol Laparosc.* 1995;2:133–136.

Jansen FW, Kapiteyn K, Trimbos-Kemper T, Hermans J, Trimbos JB. Complications of laparoscopy: a prospective multicentre observational study. *Br J Obstet Gynecol.* 1997;104:595–600.

Mirhashemi R, Harlow BL, Ginsburg ES, Signorello LB, Berkowitz R, Feldman S. Predicting risk of complications with gynecologic laparoscopic surgery. *Obstet Gynecol.* 1998;92: 327–331.

Ostrzenski A, Radolinski B, Ostrzenska KM. A review of laparoscopic ureteral injury in pelvic surgery. *Obstet Gynecol Surv.* 2003;58:794–799.

Smith S. Minimizing, recognizing, and managing laparoscopic complications. In: Azziz R, Murphy AA (eds.). *Practical Manual of Operative Laparoscopy and Hysteroscopy.* 2nd ed. New York, NY: Springer–Verlag; 1992:248–269.

Sokol AI, Chuang K, Milad MP. Risk factors for conversion to laparotomy during gynecologic laparoscopy. *J Am Assoc Gynecol Laparosc.* 2003;10:469–473.

# 86 ADNEXAL TORSION

*Shahin Ghadir*

## LEARNING POINT

To understand the differential diagnosis, work up, and treatment of adnexal torsion.

## VIGNETTE

A 22-year-old, G0, female presents to the emergency room with 2 hour history of severe left adnexal pain and nausea that had a sudden onset during her aerobics class. The patient has not been sexually active for the past 8 months. She has regular menstrual cycles every 28–30 days and had a recent Pap smear with normal results 1 month ago. The patient denies any significant medical problems and denies any previous surgeries. The patient takes a multivitamin daily and has no known drug allergies. The patient also denies the use of tobacco, alcohol, or drugs.

The physical examination reveals a well-nutritioned, well-developed Caucasian female. Vital signs: blood pressure 138/88 mm Hg, pulse 97/min, respiratory rate 22/min, temperature 100.1°F, weight 122 lb and height 5 ft 3 in. Thyroid: no enlargement, no masses; lungs: clear to auscultation bilaterally, heart: regular rate and rhythm, no murmurs; abdomen: tender to deep palpation with left much more tender than the right, no gross masses palpated; and pelvic examination: external genitalia within normal limits, vagina well estrogenized, no vaginal discharge, normal cervix, uterus anteverted with normal shape and size, right adnexa mildly tender without palpable masses, left adnexa very tender to palpation, and adnexal fullness is noted. Rectovaginal confirmed.

### QUESTION 1

*What is the differential diagnosis of acute adnexal pain?*

### ANSWER 1

The differential diagnosis of acute adnexal pain includes:

1. Complications of pregnancy, including a ruptured ectopic pregnancy, a spontaneous abortion, or a degenerating fibroid.

2. Acute infections including endometritis, pelvic inflammatory disease (PID), or tubo-ovarian abscesses.
3. Hemorrhagic functional ovarian cysts.
4. Torsion of adnexa.
5. Twisted paraovarian cyst.
6. Ruptured ovarian cyst.

## QUESTION 2

*What are the most important signs to diagnose adnexal torsion?*

## ANSWER 2

Important clinical and laboratory signs suggesting adnexal torsion include:

1. Very tender abdomen.
2. Localized rebound tenderness.
3. Palpable pelvic mass on physical examination.
4. Mild temperature elevation.
5. Leukocytosis (may accompany infarction).
6. Acute pain that is unilateral.

## QUESTION 3

*How can Doppler flow studies help in the diagnosis of adnexal torsion?*

## ANSWER 3

First, Doppler flow studies that indicate a reduced flow are highly predictive of ovarian torsion. Second, the lack of findings of internal flow to the ovary is not specific to torsion and may represent other etiologies, such as cyst rupture. Visualization of a twisted vascular pedicle is very predictive of torsion. Finally, it is important to understand that a lack of normal flow to the ovary does not exclude torsion and up to 60% of surgically confirmed adnexal torsion have normal Doppler flow.

## QUESTION 4

*What is the recommended method of treatment for adnexal torsion?*

## ANSWER 4

The recommended treatment for adnexal torsion is prompt surgical intervention. Either laparotomy or laparoscopy may be performed. The decision to perform laparotomy versus laparoscopy depends on the size of the adnexa and expertise of the surgeon. In one study up to 75% of the adnexal torsions were treal by laparoscopy. If necrosis has occurred, an oophorectomy must be performed. In the past removal of the ovary was the standard treatment. However, many reports have shown that it is safe to detorse the ovary and evaluate for blood flow prior to deciding to perform an oophorectomy. An additional tool which has been used to assist in determination of the perfusion of the ovary is the use of fluorescein dye. The dye is injected intravenously and ultra violet (UV) light is used to assess if yellow green florescence is present in the ovary indicating viable tissue and adequate perfusion.

## BIBLIOGRAPHY

Berek JS. *Novak's Gynecology*. 13th ed, Philadelphia, PA: Lipincott Williams & Wilkins; 2002.

Bouguizane S, et al. Adnexal torsion: a report of 135 cases. *J Gynecol Obstet Biol Reprod.* 2003;32(6):535–540.

Chapron C, Capella-Allouc S, Dubuisson JB. Treatment of adnexal torsion using operative laparoscopy. *Hum Reprod.* 1996; 11(5):998–1003.

McHutchinson LL, Koonings PP. Ballard CA, et al. Preservation of ovarian tissue in adrezal torsion with fluorescein. *Am J Obstet Gynecol.* 1993;168(5):1386–1388.

Penna JE, Ufberg D, Cooney N, et al. Usefulness of Doppler sonography in the diagnosis of ovarian torsion. *Fertil Steril.* 2000;73:1047–1050.

Speroff L, Fritz MA. *Clinical Gynecologic Endocrinology and Infertility*. 7th ed. Philadelphia, PA: Lipincott Williams & Wilkins; 2005.

# 87 URETHRAL DIVERTICULUM

*Cynthia D. Hall*

## LEARNING POINT

A urethral diverticulum can present as a vaginal mass, with recurrent urinary tract infections (UTIs) and/or dyspareunia.

## VIGNETTE

A 33-year-old, G7P2052, female who presents with complaints of dysuria and purulent discharge from the urethra for 3 days duration. She reports significant entry dyspareunia and a history of four courses of antibiotic therapy for UTI in the past year. She noticed a protruding mass at the introitus, which she believes has increased in size.

Her past gynecologic history is significant for gonorrhea infection and cervical dysplasia, treated by a loop electrosurgical excision procedure (LEEP). Obstetric history is significant for one normal spontaneous vaginal delivery, one forceps-assisted vaginal delivery, and five first trimester elective terminations.

Physical examination reveals a midline suburethral mass that is tender. She has an otherwise benign pelvic examination. Urinalysis is significant for multiple white blood cells (WBCs) and leukocyte esterase.

Urodynamic evaluation demonstrates a drop in urethral pressure in the midurethral region. A pelvic ultrasound is performed and a urethral diverticulum is strongly suspected. A magnetic resonance imaging (MRI) confirms a posterior diverticulum. Antibiotics are prescribed, and the patient is scheduled for diverticulum excision with Martius graft.

## QUESTION 1

*What is the incidence and etiology of urethral diverticuli?*

## ANSWER 1

A diverticulum is a sacular out-pouching from a hollow organ. A urethral diverticulum is found in 0.6–6% of women and occurs mostly in the third to fifth decades of life. A higher prevalence in African-American females was found in earlier studies, although this is not supported by more recent reports. The most common location for a urethral diverticulum is posteriorly (anterior vagina) anywhere along the urethra, most often in the midline.

A urethral diverticulum is most likely caused by repeat infections within the periurethral and urethral glands, which lead to abscess formation and eventual rupture into the urethra. The most common infectious agent is gonorrhea, although many patients give no antecedent history of sexually transmitted disease. Other factors that can lead to urethral diverticula formation are obstetric trauma, urethral instrumentation, periurethral collagen injection, and other anti-incontinence procedures that result in urethral handling.

## QUESTION 2

*How do urethral diverticuli commonly present, and how is the patient evaluated?*

## ANSWER 2

Urethral diverticuli commonly present as recurrent UTI and voiding dysfunction, most notably postvoid dribbling. Women with this condition may also experience dysuria, frequency and urgency, and hematuria. A suburethral cyst or a vaginal mass may be found on physical examination and cause pain to the patient. Occasionally pus can be expressed by compression of the mass, however the examination is often benign. Dyspareunia is a frequent complaint. Occasionally, a diverticulum can present as chronic pelvic pain.

The presentation and symptoms of a urethral diverticulum can vary according to its size. For instance, small diverticuli can present with pain and recurrent UTI, whereas larger ones may be a cause of urinary incontinence and dribbling.

A strong index of suspicion is required when approaching the patient with recurrent UTIs, dyspareunia, or urinary dribbling. The diagnosis is commonly confused with and treated as any of the following conditions: UTI, stress urinary incontinence, interstitial cystitis, urethral syndrome, vulvovestibulitis, cystocele, and sensory urgency. In a retrospective cohort of 46 patients, Romanzi and colleagues found the mean interval from onset of symptoms to diagnosis to be 5.2 years.

## QUESTION 3

*What is the differential diagnosis of benign anterior vaginal cystic lesions?*

## ANSWER 3

Benign cystic lesions of the anterior wall of the vagina can be the result of residual tissue from embryological development such as: (1) mullerian cysts (a persistent epithelial tissue within the vaginal wall); (2) Gartner's duct cysts (vestigial remnants of mesonephric ducts); or (3) vaginal adenosis (presence of glandular epithelium within the vagina).

They can likewise have an infectious etiology such as an abscess in Skene's glands, which are prostatic homologues located beneath the urethra. Rarely, a vaginal cyst may be due to vaginitis emphysematosa, which results in gas-filled cysts in the vaginal wall associated with Trichomonas infection. Endometriosis-filled cysts in the anterior vaginal wall have also been described.

Furthermore, what appears to be an anterior vaginal cyst can be the result of anatomic defects such as urethral caruncle, which is an ectropion of urethral wall or an anterior wall prolapse leading to ureterocele or cystocele.

## QUESTION 4

*What are the available modalities for diagnosing a urethral diverticulum and some advantages and disadvantages of these studies?*

## ANSWER 4

A voiding cystourethrogram has been utilized as an initial tool in the evaluation of suspected urethral diverticula. The accuracy in diagnosis was found to be between 65–77%, depending both on operator technique and the size of the neck of the diverticulum, which has to be sufficiently large for contrast media to pass through into the sac under low pressure. Positive pressure urethrography (with a double balloon to seal off the urethra) provides one of the highest accuracies and sensitivities (Fig. 87-1). However, it is an invasive test causing significant patient discomfort, and many radiology departments do not perform the test.

MRI has the highest sensitivity, with little radiation exposure, and is a superior examination for surgery planning. The best-documented technique requires external coil, T-2-weighted images, as well as sagittal and axial views. The drawback of this test is its cost. Transvaginal ultrasound is the least expensive and least invasive method and has been reported to have a diagnostic accuracy of up to 90%.

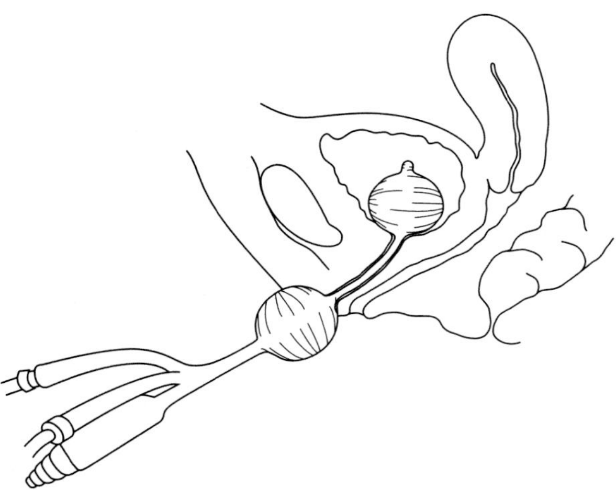

**FIG. 87-1** Trattner double-balloon catheter. Proximal balloon inflates within bladder neck, anchoring catheter, and distal balloon occludes external meatus. Contrast fills urethra slit between balloons.
SOURCE: Reprinted with permission from Greenberg M, Stone D, Cochran ST, et al. *AJR* 1981;136:259.

Urethroscopy is another appropriate method of evaluation and can be done in the office setting. Some investigators found it to provide up to 90% diagnostic accuracy, allowing for direct visualization of the lesion.

Urodynamics can identify a urethral diverticulum if located within the functional sphincter zone a drop in urethral pressure. However, the diagnostic accuracy is only 72%. Nevertheless, this test is often recommended prior to surgical correction to rule exclude concurrent stress urinary incontinence.

## QUESTION 5

*What are the options for treatment?*

## ANSWER 5

Conservative management is reserved for small diverticula with only minor symptoms or if the patient considers the risks associated with surgery too great. In these cases, symptomatic relief with antibiotics and anticholinergics can accompany close observation. Postvoid digital decompression can also be employed.

Midurethral, larger, or symptomatic diverticula require surgical excision with careful dissection to create several layers. A Martius (bulbocavernosus) graft is an option to bring in blood supply to the area to reduce the risk of wound breakdown and fistula formation.

The patient with a diverticulum will often have coexistent stress urinary incontinence, and a sling placement can be appropriate, which would be placed after the closure of the periurethral fascia. Many practitioners recommend this as a two-step procedure, with the repair of the diverticulum and treatment of the urinary incontinence performed separately.

For distally located diverticulum (not in the functional urethral sphincter zone), a Spence procedure may be used, where the diverticulum is marsupialized and the defect is closed with 3-0 or 4-0 absorbable suture.

To facilitate recovery, a Foley catheter is left in place for 2 weeks along with antibiotic prophylaxis. Some surgeons perform a voiding cystourethrogram before the Foley is removed to evaluate for extravasation.

The main intraoperative complication is bleeding, especially if extensive dissection is necessary and if the surrounding tissue is of poor quality after long-standing infection. Postoperative complications include fistula formation, recurrence, urethral stricture, and new onset urinary incontinence.

## BIBLIOGRAPHY

Aspera AM, Rackley RR, Vasavada SP. Contemporary evaluations and management of the female urethral diverticulum. *Urol Clin N Am.* 2002;29:617–624.

Eilber KS, Raz S. Benign cystic lesions of the vagina: a literature review. *J Urol.* 2003;170:717.

Gerrard ER Jr, Lloyd LK, Kubricht WS, Kolettis PN. Transvaginal ultrasound for the diagnosis of urethral diverticulum. *J Urol.* 2003;169:1395.

Leach GE, Bavendam TG. Female urethral diverticula. *Urology.* 1987;30:407.

Leach GE, Trockman BA. Surgery for vesicovaginal and urethrovaginal fistula and urethral diverticulum. In: *Campbell's Urology.* 7th ed. WB Saunders: 1998;1135–1153.

Neitlich JD, Foster HE Jr, Glickman MG, Smith RC. Detection of urethral diverticula in women: comparison of a high-resolution fast spin echo technique with double balloon urethrography. *J Urol.* 159;408:1998.

Romanzi LJ, Groutz A, Blaivas JG. Urethral diverticulum in women: diverse presentations resulting in diagnostic delay and mismanagement. *J Urol.* 2000;164:428–433.

Scotti RJ, Ostergard DR. Disorders of the urethra. In: Bent AE, Ostergard DR, et al. (eds.). *Ostergard's Urogynecology and Pelvic Floor Dysfunction.* 5th ed. Lippincott, Williams & Wilkins; 2003.

Vakili B, Wai C, Nihira M. Anterior urethral diverticulum in the female: diagnostic and surgical approach. *Obstet Gynecol.* 2003;102:1179.

# 88 STRESS URINARY INCONTINENCE

*Cynthia D. Hall*

## LEARNING POINT

Stress urinary incontinence (SUI) is a common condition in women. Although conservative management can improve symptoms, surgery is one of the mainstays of treatment.

## VIGNETTE

A 53-year-old, G3P3, female complaining of urinary leakage with exercise presents to the office. Urinary incontinence began after the birth of her second child but has worsened significantly over the past 2 years. As a result, she has begun to limit her activity. She also leaks with coughing and sneezing. She urinates every 3–4 hours and gets up once at night to urinate. She has no urgency or urge incontinence. She has no symptoms of prolapse or defecatory problems and is sexually active without problems. Her past medical and surgical histories are negative. She had three vaginal deliveries, the first of which was delivered by forceps. She is a nonsmoker.

### QUESTION 1

*What are the causes of stress incontinence?*

### ANSWER 1

SUI is urinary leakage (usually small amounts) concurrent to an increase in intra-abdominal pressure (such as coughing, sneezing, and exercise). SUI is caused by a combination of a lack of support to the bladder neck and inadequate urethral closure. One or the other mechanism may be predominant in a particular patient. In a normal woman, the bladder neck is suspended above the level of the levator ani musculature. Additionally, the pelvic floor and the urethral sphincter should contract reflexively with increases in intra-abdominal pressure. In a woman with SUI, these mechanisms fail and the result is urine leakage.

Risk factors for SUI include childbearing, especially vaginal birth with a prolonged second stage, increased fetal weight, and an instrumental delivery. Cesarean section appears protective, but any pregnancy increases a woman's risk. Other factors include obesity, chronic straining such as in constipation and pulmonary disease, and previous surgery. There probably is a genetic component, but it is poorly defined.

### QUESTION 2

*What nonsurgical options are available for SUI treatment?*

### ANSWER 2

Pelvic floor (Kegel's) exercises can be effective to lessen leakage in patients with SUI. Studies have shown that voluntarily contracting the pelvic musculature at the same time as an increase in intra-abdominal pressure can raise the threshold for urine leakage.

Bump demonstrated that only 50% of college-educated women with verbal and written instruction correctly isolated and contracted the pelvic floor. Biofeedback (showing patients visually what is going on with the pelvic floor) and electrical stimulation to passively contract the muscles are often helpful in these women.

There are intravaginal and intraurethral devices that have been designed to improve SUI in women. These include specialized pessaries, which give extra support to the urethra such as the Introl or Mylex incontinence ring or dish. Occlusive devices placed in or over the urethra are not well tolerated because of urethral irritation and/or recurrent UTIs. Imipramine works through its alpha-agonist effects on urethral tone. Duloxetine increases rhabdosphincter contractility via alpha-agonist and serotonin stimulation of the pudendal nerve.

## QUESTION 3

*What surgeries are available to treat SUI?*

## ANSWER 3

Retropubic colposuspensions are performed abdominally through either a pfannensteil or a low vertical incision. The space of Retzius is exposed, and the bladder is swept medially off the pubocervical fascia, with a hand in the vagina to fascilitate dissection. For the Burch procedure, sutures are placed through the paravaginal fascia and suspended to Cooper's ligament. These are then suspended loosely in a "banjo string" manner to support but not overelevate the bladder neck. In the Marshall-Marchetti-Krantz procedure (MMK), sutures are placed adjacent to the urethra and then suspended to the periosteum of the pubic bone (see Fig. 88-1). There is a risk of osteitis pubis with this procedure, and it tends to cause more overelevation, voiding dysfunction, and irritative symptoms.

Classic retropubic slings were commonly performed with a combined vaginal and abdominal dissection. The sling (either synthetic or biologic) was at least 2 cm in width and placed under most of the urethra, including the bladder neck. These procedures had excellent success rates, but the patients had moderate recovery times and often had delayed voiding and irritative symptoms. The newer *midurethral, minimally invasive slings* (such as the

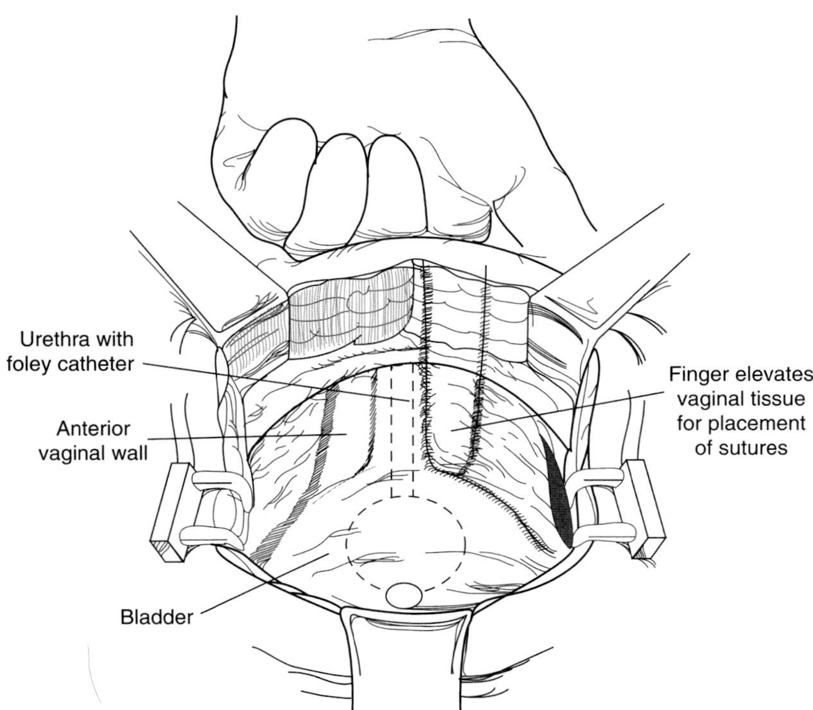


**FIG. 88-1** Dissection for Marshall-Marchetti-Krantz (MMK) or Burch procedure.
SOURCE: In: Mann WM, Stovall TG (eds.). *Gynecologic Surgery.* Churchill Livingstone; New York: 1996:716.

TVT, Sparc, Monarch, and the like) have become the procedure of choice in women with straightforward SUI as an initial procedure. There is no abdominal dissection, limited vaginal dissection, and they can be performed in an outpatient setting. Voiding difficulties are few. Transobturator slips are the newest modification, avoid the retropubic area altogether, but may not be as effective in patients with a significant urethral component or intrinsic sphincter deficiency (see Question 4).

Anterior repairs are no longer considered continence procedures because of abysmal success rates of 30–40% at 5 years. Needle suspensions have only 60–70% success rates at 3–5 years. Paravaginal repairs to reattach the pubocervical fascia to the arcus tendineus fascia pelvis (ATFP) results in an anatomic repair. However, the success rates for paravaginal repair are inferior to the Burch or MMK, likely because the ATFP is not as consistent a suspension point.

## QUESTION 4

*How does the physician decide which surgical procedure is most appropriate?*

## ANSWER 4

Choice of procedure depends on physician preference, the patient's anatomy, the need to perform concurrent procedures, and often urodynamic indices (see Table 88-1). If the problem is predominantly lack of support, surgeries to restore support (retropubic procedure or sling) are usually successful (85%). If urethral coaptation is the problem, periurethral injectable therapies usually improve the leakage. In a patient with a combined problem, a suburethral sling is indicated, as it provides support and improves coaptation.

Both the leak point pressure (LPP) and the maximum urethral closure pressure (MUCP) have been used to diagnose "intrinsic sphincter deficiency" (ISD). LPPs are measured by having the patient perform incremental coughs and valsalva and noting the smallest pressure necessary to cause leakage. McGuire noted that there was a high correlation of open bladder necks on fluoroscopy in patients with LPP <60 cm $H_2O$.

**TABLE 88-1. Choice of Procedure Based on Q-Tip Test and Urethral Function (ISD)**

| | NO ISD (NORMAL LPP OR MUCP) | ISD (LOW LPP OR MUCP) |
|---|---|---|
| Hypermobility (Q-Tip >30°) | Retropubic colposuspension or sling | Sling |
| No hypermobility (Q-Tip <30°) | | Sling or periurethral injection |

The MUCP is measured by slowly pulling the transducer past the high-pressure zone of the urethra and substracting the bladder pressure from the urethral pressure. Sand noted that Burch procedures were much less successful in patients who had an MUCP <20 cm $H_2O$ (54%) as compared to patients who had an MUCP >20 cm $H_2O$ (18%).

Currently, ISD is felt to be a continuum, and therefore these numbers should not be used as absolute indications for selecting a particular procedure.

## BIBLIOGRAPHY


Bergman A, Elia G. Three surgical procedures for genuine stress incontinence: five-year follow up of a prospective randomized study. *Am J Obstet Gynecol.* 1995;173:66.

Bump RC, Hurt WG, Fantl JA, et al. Assessment of Kegel pelvic muscle exercise performance after brief verbal instruction. *Am J Obstet Gynecol.* 1991;165(2):322.

Ertunc D, Tok EC, Pata O, Dilek U, Ozdemir G, Dilek S. Is stress urinary incontinence a familial condition? *Acta Obset Gynecol Scand.* 2004;83(10):912.

Handa VL, Harvey L, Fox HE, et al. Parity and route of delivery: does cesarean delivery reduce bladder symptoms later in life? *Am J Obstet Gynecol.* 2004;191(2):463.

Mcguire EJ, Cespedes RD, Cross CA, et al. Videourodynamic studies. *Urol Clin North Am.* 1996;23(2):309.

Miller JM, Ashton-Miller J, DeLancey JO. A pelvic muscle precontraction can reduce cough-related urine loss in selected women with mild SUI. *J Am Geriatr Soc.* 1998;46(7):870.

Rezapour M, Ulmsten U. TVT in women with mixed urinary incontinence. *Int Urogyn J.* 2001;(Suppl.) 2:S15.

Sand PK, Bowen LW, Panganiban R, et al. The low-pressure urethra as a factor in failed retropubic urethropexy. *Obstet Gynecol.* 1987;69(3 Pt. 1):399.

Van Kerrelbroek P, Abrams P, Lange R, et al. Duloxetine versus placebo in the treatment of European and Canadian women with stress urinary incontinence. *BJOG.* 2004;111:249.


# 89 URGE AND OVERFLOW URINAL INCONTINENCE

*Cynthia D. Hall*

## LEARNING POINT

Different types of urinary incontinence (UI) may present similarly, so it is important to perform a detailed history and physical in order to implement appropriate treatment.

## VIGNETTE

A 77-year-old woman presents with frequency, urgency, and urge incontinence, which have become progressively worse over the last 5 years to the point that she needs to wear an adult diaper at all times. She urinates every 1–2 hours despite drinking very little fluid. She has to get up three to four times at night and has had a few episodes of nocturnal enuresis. She denies urine leakage during coughing and sneezing, but will often have dribbling after voiding without an urge to urinate. She has mild symptoms of fullness in the vagina and *feels something* at the vaginal entrance sometimes after urinating. She denies fecal incontinence.

Her past medical history is significant for hypertension hypercholesterolemia. She takes furosemide and and a statin every morning. She had an abdominal hysterectomy at the age of 45 for bleeding and fibroids.

On examination, she is a healthy-appearing woman who is thin and has a normal gait. She has no palpable abdominal masses. The anterior vaginal wall descends to the introitus, and the vaginal vault descends about halfway to the hymen. Her targeted neurologic examination is normal.

### QUESTION 1

*What is meant by "urge incontinence," and what is its etiology?*

### ANSWER 1

Urge incontinence is the symptom of urinary leakage occurring while having urgency to urinate. Urge incontinence can be a small amount of urine just as someone removes his or her clothing. Alternatively, urge incontinence can be a large amount of urine with little warning. Urge incontinence, the *symptom*, is usually caused by the condition of detrusor overactivity (DO). The International Continence Society (ICS) defines DO as spontaneous or provoked bladder contractions during the filling phase of cystometry. It is considered idiopathic if there is no definable cause (90% of cases) and neurogenic if associated with a relevant neurologic disorder, such as multiple sclerosis, Parkinson's disease, cerebrovascular disease, or spinal cord injury.

Other terms used to describe involuntary detrusor contractions include unstable, spastic, hypertonic, systolic, uninhibited, irritable, or dyssynergic bladder. The ICS terms are preferable because they classify patients into two clinically useful categories.

Patients with DO often have other symptoms such as urinary frequency, urgency, and nocturia. Overactive bladder (OAB) is a term used to describe the *symptoms* of urinary frequency, urgency, and nocturia, with or without the symptoms of urge incontinence.

### QUESTION 2

*What are other types of UI, and how common are they?*

### ANSWER 2

Stress incontinence is the involuntary leakage of urine during increases of intra-abdominal pressure such as coughing, sneezing, and exercise. Mixed incontinence is a combination of stress and urge incontinence.

Overflow incontinence is when the bladder has been filled beyond capacity. This may result from lack of a bladder contraction (atonic bladder), outlet obstruction, or a combination of the two. Overflow incontinence is common in men because of the high incidence of benign prostatic hypertrophy and subsequent outlet obstruction. Reasons for outlet obstruction in women are previous continence surgery, severe prolapse with kinking of the urethra, urethral strictures, or partial obstruction due to inability to relax the pelvic floor.

Functional incontinence is a term to describe leakage due to factors outside the urinary tract such as delirium or decreased mobility. UI can also result from a vesicovaginal, urethrovaginal, or ureterovaginal fistula, which effectively bypass the usual continence mechanism.

UI is estimated to affect at least 13 million Americans. In one series of almost 300 consecutive women, the proportion of stress incontinence, DO, and mixed incontinence were 35%, 32%, and 29%, respectively (4% had normal results). These relative percentages are different for different age groups, with urge and mixed incontinence increasing in the older age groups (Fig. 89-1).

### QUESTION 3

*What should be the initial evaluation for this patient?*

### ANSWER 3

The history should include assessment for any prolapse symptoms or fecal complaints. The pelvic examination begins with an assessment of the urogenital estrogenization. Then each compartment must be evaluated

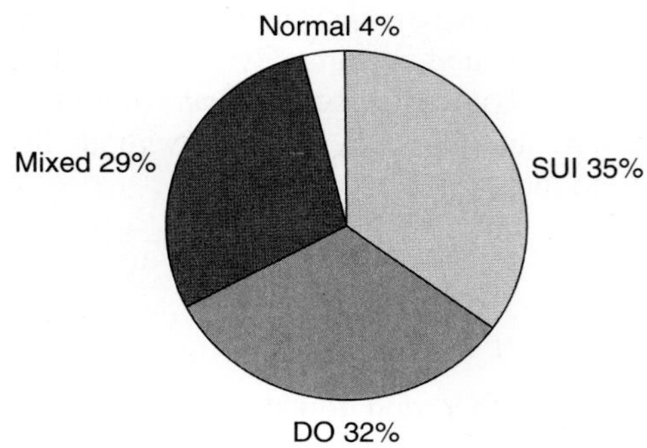


**FIG. 89-1** Percentages of various types of incontinence in a group of 300 women. SUI = stress urinary incontinence, DO = detrusor activity, mixed = combined SUI and DO.

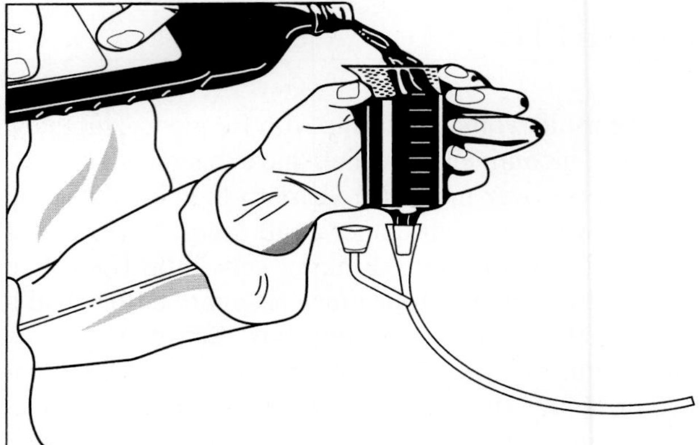

**FIG. 89-2** Simple cystometrogram. Multichannel urodynamic testing can be done to further elucidate the diagnosis.

individually by dissembling a bivalve speculum. A urine culture should always be sent as a UTI can be longstanding and present either as UI (more commonly) or SUI. A screening neurologic examination should be performed to assess orientation, the lower back, perineal sensation, anal sphincter tone, and motor reflexes of the anal and bulbocavernosus muscles. These reflexes can be elicited by stroking the areas near the clitoris and perianal skin with a cotton-tipped swab. Any neurologic abnormality requires consultation with a neurologist.

A simple cystometrogram can reveal much information (see Fig. 89-2) and is performed as follows:

- Insert a 16F red rubber catheter.
- Record the postvoid residual (PVR) to rule out urinary retention.
- Attach a Toomey syringe and fill the bladder by pouring sterile water into the syringe while watching the meniscus.
- Note bladder sensation (first sensation of filling, first urge, strong urge, and maximum capacity).
- Cessation of filling or a rise in the meniscus without bearing down indicates a bladder contraction.
- Remove catheter and with the bladder full, perform a stress test.
- Have the patient void and calculate a repeat PVR (fill minus voided volume).

## QUESTION 4

*What nonsurgical, nonpharmacologic options are available for treatment of DO?*

## ANSWER 4

Bladder training to reestablish cortical control over the OAB can be accomplished in an outpatient program with weekly office visits to provide positive reinforcement, monitor progress, and adjust voiding intervals. Usually this involves gradually increasing the interval between voids.

Biofeedback training uses a visual or auditory signal to give the patient information about physiologic processes that are normally unconscious. Perineal skin and vaginal or anal electrodes can provide feedback to encourage the patient with DO to voluntarily contract the levator ani muscle and the external anal and urethral sphincters in response to a sensation of urinary urgency or a rise in bladder pressure.

Intravaginal or perianal electrical stimulation of sacral somatic afferents can inhibit detrusor contractions by activation of sympathetic inhibitory fibers to the detrusor, central inhibition of the motor outflow to the bladder, and stimulation of pudendal afferents leading to reflex contraction of pelvic floor striated muscle.

## QUESTION 5

*What pharmacologic or surgical therapies are available for the treatment of DO?*

## ANSWER 5

There are now multiple drugs available for the treatment of DO. They all have antimuscarinic properties and work by blocking acetylcholine-mediated detrusor contractions. They have all been shown to be more effective than placebo but anticholinergic side effects (dry mouth, dry eyes, blurred vision, constipation) sometimes limit their tolerability (see Table 89-1).

**TABLE 89-1. Drugs Available to Treat Detrusor Overactivity (DO)**

| MEDICATION | DOSE | INTERVAL |
|---|---|---|
| Oxybutynin (short-acting) | 2.5–5 mg | Bid to tid |
| Tolterodine (Detrol) | 4 mg | Daily |
| Extended release Oxybutynin (Ditropan XL) | 5–15 mg | Daily |
| Oxybutynin patch (Oxytrol) | | Biw |
| Trospium chloride (Sanctura) | 5–10 mg | Bid |
| Solifenacin (Enablex) | 7.5–15 mg | Daily |
| Darifenacin (Vesicare) | 5–10 mg | Daily |
| Imipramine (Tofranil) | 25–75 mg | q hs |

If medications fail, nerve stimulation by implantable electrodes near the S2 and S3 nerve roots is effective in patients with neurogenic DO due to spinal cord injury as well as severe idiopathic DO. More invasive surgery is limited to rare cases where all conservative measures have failed. One of the most effective procedures is augmentation enterocystoplasty, the addition of a patch of ileum to a bisected bladder

## BIBLIOGRAPHY


Abrams P, Cardozo L, Fall M, et al. The standardization of terminology of lower urinary tract function: report from the Standardization Sub-committee of the International Continence Society. *Am J Obstet Gynecol.* 2002;187:116.

Bhatia NN, Rosensweig B. The urologically oriented neurologic examination. In: Ostergard D, Bent A (eds.). *Urogynecology Urodynamics*. Williams & Wilkins; 1991.

Cardozo LD. Biofeedback in overactive bladder. *Urology.* 55;24: 2000.

Haeusler G, Leitich H, van Trotsenburg M, et al. Drug therapy of urinary urge incontinence: a systematic review. *Obstet Gynecol.* 2002;100:1003.

Klingele CJ, Carley ME, Hill RF. Patient characteristics that are associated with urodynamically diagnosed detrusor instability and geniune stress incontinence. *Am J Obstet Gynecol.* 2002;186(5):866.

Marinkovic SP, Stanton SL. Incontinence and voiding difficulties associated with prolapse. *J Urol.* 2004;171:1021.

Schmidt RA, Jonas U, Oleson KA, et al. Sacral nerve stimulation for treatment of refractory urinary urge incontinence. Sacral Nerve Stimulation Study Group. *J Urol.* 1999;162:352.

Wall LL, Wiskind AK, Taylor PA. Simple bladder filling with a cough stress test compared with subtracted cystometry for the diagnosis of urinary incontinence. *Am J Obstet Gynecol.* 1994;171:1472.

Wyman JF, Fantl JA, McClish DK, et al. Comparative efficacy of behavioral interventions in the management of female urinary incontinence. Continence Program for Women Research Group. *Am J Obstet Gynecol.* 1998;179:999.


# 90 URINARY TRACT INFECTIONS

*Cynthia D. Hall*

## LEARNING POINT

Urinary tract infections (UTIs) are common in women and are usually easily diagnosed and treated.

## VIGNETTE

A 22-year-old nulliparous woman presents to the office complaining of urinary frequency, dysuria, and suprapubic discomfort for the past 2 days. She is not experiencing urinary incontinence. She has no fever or chills and denies back pain. She has no vaginal discharge or odor. Her last menstrual period was 2 weeks ago. She is sexually active and uses a diaphragm for contraception. She has been with her current partner for 9 months and is mutually monogamous. Her last sexual activity was 2 days ago. Her past medical and surgical histories are negative. She is a nonsmoker and drinks alcohol socially.

### QUESTION 1

*How common are UTIs in young healthy women? How common are recurrences?*

### ANSWER 1

Approximately 50–60% of adult women report that they have had a UTI at some time during their life. Young sexually active women have approximately 0.5 episodes of acute cystitis per person per year, and it is estimated that many millions of episodes of acute cystitis probably occur annually among women in the United States. In young college women, 27% experienced one recurrence within 1 month, and 2.7% had two or more recurrences in 6 months.

Recurrences were more common if the first infection was due to *Escherichia coli*. In a Finnish study of women 17–82 years of age who had *E. coli* cystitis, 44% had a recurrence within 1 year.

## QUESTION 2

*What are the usual signs and symptoms of a UTI?*

## ANSWER 2

Acute uncomplicated cystitis is manifested primarily by dysuria, usually in combination with frequency, urgency, suprapubic pain, and/or hematuria. Patients with urethritis and vaginitis also may complain of dysuria, thereby presenting a diagnostic challenge. Urethritis caused by *Neisseria gonorrheae* or *Chlamydia trachomatis* is relatively more likely to be present if the setting is a sexually transmitted disease (STD) clinic, there is a past history of an STD, the woman has had a new sex partner in the past few weeks, her sex partner has urethral symptoms, or symptoms were of gradual onset over several weeks. Vaginitis should be considered in the presence of vaginal discharge or odor, pruritus, dyspareunia, external dysuria, and the absence of frequency or urgency. Fever (>38°C), flank pain, costovertebral angle tenderness, and nausea or vomiting suggest upper tract infection and warrant more aggressive diagnostic and therapeutic measures.

## QUESTION 3

*How are UTI's diagnosed?*

## ANSWER 3

A directed history and physical examination provide sufficient data to make an accurate diagnosis in most cases of acute dysuria. The examination should include temperature, abdominal examination, and assessment of the costovertebral angle examination for tenderness.

The pelvic examination should include a careful evaluation for vaginitis, urethral discharge, or herpetic ulcerations. A cervical examination for evidence of cervicitis and cervical and urethral cultures for *N. gonorrheae* and *C. trachomatis* are indicated if there are any of the factors suggesting urethritis or vaginitis present.

Dysuria and frequency without vaginal discharge or irritation raise the probability of UTI in a woman to more than 90%, effectively ruling in the diagnosis based upon history alone. This suggests that it may be reasonable to offer empiric treatment for UTI when the probability of infection is high.

Evaluation of midstream urine for pyuria is the most valuable laboratory diagnostic test for UTI. Pyuria is present in almost all women with acute cystitis. The presence of hematuria is helpful since it is common in women with UTI, but not in women with urethritis or vaginitis.

Urine cultures were generally not thought to be necessary in women with uncomplicated cystitis, since the causative organisms and their antimicrobial susceptibility profiles were so predictable. However, recommendations for obtaining pretherapy urine cultures should be reassessed given the increasing prevalence of antimicrobial resistance among uropathogens. The standard definition of a positive urine culture is ≥10(5) CFU/mL. However, this definition does not apply to all patients. If fecal contamination has been ruled out, a lower colony count (>$10^2$/mL) may be indicative of UTI.

## QUESTION 4

*What are the usual pathogens in UTIs in young women?*

## ANSWER 4

*E. coli* is the causative pathogen in approximately 80–85% of episodes of acute uncomplicated cystitis. While *E. coli* is by far the most common etiology, increasing drug resistance has complicated therapy. Other pathogens include Enterococcus, *Staphylococcus saprophyticus, Proteus mirabilis,* Klebsiella species, and others. In addition, among women with dysuria and pyuria but a negative standard culture (a condition that had been called the acute urethral syndrome), chlamydia may be causative in some cases.

Knowledge of the antimicrobial susceptibility profile of uropathogens causing uncomplicated UTIs in the community, if known, should guide therapeutic decisions for the treatment of acute uncomplicated cystitis.

*E. coli* are resistant to ampicllin in 33%, trimethoprim-sulfamethoxazole (TMP-SMX) in 10–22%, and nitrofurantoin or the flouroquinolones only 5% or less. Enterococcus is not responsive to TMP-SMX and is best treated with ampicillin or nitrofurantoin. Nitrofurantoin is not effective against many uropathogens such as Proteus and Klebsiella.

## QUESTION 5

*What treatments are most appropriate as first line therapy?*

## ANSWER 5

Three-day short course regimens are generally recommended for the treatment of acute uncomplicated cystitis

**TABLE 90-1. Suggested Therapy for Acute Uncomplicated UTIs**

| DRUG | DOSE/INTERVAL | DURATION |
|---|---|---|
| TMP-SMX | 160/800 mg (DS) bid | 3 days |
| TMP | 100 mg bid | 3 days |
| Levofloxacin | 250 mg qd | 3 days |
| Ciprofloxacin | 250 mg bid or 500 mg qd | 3 days |
| Nitrofurantoin | 50 mg qid | 7 days |
| Nitrofurantoin macrocrystals (Macrobid) | 100 mg bid | 7 days |
| Amoxicillin/clavulanate (Augmentin) | 500 mg bid | 7 days |

because of better compliance, lower cost, and lower frequency of adverse reactions than with 7- to 10-day regimens. Several studies and clinical experience have confirmed the effectiveness of 3-day regimens of trimethoprim, TMP-SMX, or a fluoroquinolone for the treatment of acute uncomplicated cystitis (Table 90-1). Nitrofurantoin should be administered for 7 days. Patients undergoing effective treatment with an antimicrobial to which the infecting pathogen is susceptible should show definite signs of improvement within 24–48 hours; if not, a repeat urine culture and imaging studies such as ultrasound or computerized tomography should be considered to rule out urinary tract pathology.

## QUESTION 6

*What factors play a part in acute cystitis and recurrences in young women?*

## ANSWER 6

For acute infections, most uropathogens originate in the rectal flora, colonize the introitus, and ascend into the bladder. Bacterial virulence factors are directly related to the ability to adhere and colonize the urethra, bladder, and upper urinary tract. Specific virulence factors include fimbria (i.e., pili), flagella, production of hemolysin or urease, and resistance to plasma bacteriocidal properties.

Acute and recurrent cystitis is linked to sexual activity and diaphragm and spermicide use in young sexually active women. In one study, the risk of UTI in young women who had intercourse three times in 1 week is 2.6 times that of women not sexually active that week. Frequent sexual activity is a predisposing factor, likely due mostly to mechanical factors but possibly due to alterations in vaginal pH. Spermicides (Nonoxynol-9) alter the vaginal flora in favor of colonization of uropathogens. Other risk factors for recurrence include an alteration of the normal vaginal flora (with decrease in lactobacillus), genetic factors such as secreter versus nonsecreter status and interleukin receptor types. Recent antibiotic use is an independent risk factor likely due to its alteration of vaginal flora.

## QUESTION 7

*What are strategies for prevention in patients with recurrent UTIs?*

## ANSWER 7

Changing one's contraceptive method, voiding after coitus (theoretically to flush bacteria out of the bladder) and good hygiene are good first steps. However, the only two strategies that have been proven to limit recurrences in large cohorts of women are use of prophylactic antibiotics and hormone replacement in estrogen-deficient women.

Prophylactic antibiotics can be given daily or postcoitally. Daily prophylaxis was shown to decrease recurrences by 95% compared to placebo in one study. Both TMP-SMX and nitrofurantoin have been shown to be effective. Depending on the relation of infection to sexual intercourse or the frequency of intercourse, postcoital antibiotics may make more sense for some women.

Self-treatment is also an acceptable management technique for some women. UTIs can be accurately self-diagnosed in 85–95% of women. Recurrences must be clearly documented, and this approach requires a compliant and motivated patient who agrees to call her provider if symptoms do not resolve in 48 hours.

In postmenopausal women, the use of topical estrogen significantly reduced the incidence of UTI. These patients had an increase in lactobacillus and a decrease in uropathogen colonization of the vagina.

The results of studies of exogenous lactobacillus and cranberry juice or tablets to prevent UTIs are small or of poor quality. Other strategies under investigation are colonization with an avirulent *E. coli* instilled into the bladder and either whole cell vaccines or a vaccine based on a fimbrial protein.

## BIBLIOGRAPHY

Albert X, Huertas I, Pereiro I, et al. Antibiotics for preventing recurrent urinary tract infection in non-pregnant women. *Cochrane Database Syst Rev.* 2004;3:CD001209.

Bent S, Nallamamothu BK, Simel DL, et al. Does this woman have an acute uncomplicated urinary tract infection? *JAMA.* 2002;287:2701.

Fairley KF, Cavon NE, Gutch RC, et al. Site of infection in acute urinary tract infection in general practice. *Lancet.* 1971;2:615.

Foxman B, Barlow R, D'Arcy, H, et al. Urinary tract infection: self-reported incidence and associated costs. *Ann Epidemiol.* 2000;10:509.

Foxman B. Recurring urinary tract infection: incidence and risk factors. *Am J Public Health.* 1990;80:331.

Gupta K, Hooton TM, Roberts PL, Stamm WE. Patient-initiated treatment of uncomplicated recurrent urinary tract infections in young women. *Ann Intern Med.* 2001;135:9.

Gupta K, Sahm DF, Mayfield D, et al. Antimicrobial resistance among uropathogens that cause community-acquired urinary tract infections in women: a nationwide analysis. *Clin Infect Dis.* 2001;33:89.

Hooton TM, Besser R, Foxman B, et al. Acute uncomplicated cystitis in an era of increasing antibiotic resistance: a proposed approach to empirical therapy. *Clin Infect Dis.* 2004;39:75.

Johnson JR. Virulence factors in Escherichia coli urinary tract infection. *Clin Microbiol Rev.* 1991;4:80.

Komaroff AL. Acute dysuria in women. *N Engl J Med.* 1984;310: 368.

Kontiokari T, Sundqvist K, Nuutinen M, et al. Randomized trial of cranberry-ligonberry juice and lactobacillis GG drink for the prevention of urinary tract infection in women. *BMJ.* 2001; 322:1571.

Nicolle LE, Ronald AR. Recurrent urinary tract infection in adult women: diagnosis and treatment. *Infect Dis Clin North Am.* 1987;1:793.

Norrby SR. Short-term treatment of uncomplicated lower urinary tract infections in women. *Rev Infect Dis.* 1990;12:458.

Warren JW, Abrutyn E, Hebel JR, et al. Guidelines for antimicrobial treatment of uncomplicated acute bacterial cystitis and acute pyelonephritis in women. *Clin Infect Dis.* 1999;29:745.

Wilson ML, Gaido L. Laboratory diagnosis of urinary tract infections in adult patients. *Clin Infect Dis.* 2004;38:1150.

# 91 URODYNAMIC STUDIES

*Cynthia D. Hall*

## LEARNING POINT

Urodynamics can help with diagnosis of and treatment for urinary incontinence and voiding dysfunction.

## VIGNETTE

A 45-year-old, G3P2, female complaining of urine leakage with coughing, sneezing, and exercise such as jogging, presents to the office. These symptoms began after the birth of her second child and have worsened significantly in the past year to the point that she needs to wear a mini pad. She also has urinary urgency and occasional leakage of a few drops when arriving to the toilet. She does not have symptoms of prolapse or fecal evacuation difficulties.

Her past medical history includes asthma, which is well controlled with an inhaler. Surgical history is negative. Obstetric history includes two spontaneous vaginal deliveries with minor lacerations at both.

## QUESTION 1

*What is "urodynamic testing"?*

## ANSWER 1

Technically, urodynamic testing is any test that provides objective information about lower urinary tract function. They do not necessarily require the use of sophisticated electronic equipment.

Simple and useful urodynamic tests include:

- Stress test (the observation of urine leakage at the same time as a cough or valsalva)
- Measurement of postvoid residual (PVR) urine volume
- Voiding diary kept by the patient
- Simple or "eyeball" cystometrogram

When most practitioners refer to urodynamic testing, they are talking about the following tests that require electronic equipment and multiple simultaneous measurements such as:

- Complex cystometrogram
- Measurement of leak point pressures (LPP)
- Urethral pressure profiles (UPP)
- Complex uroflowmetry
- Pressure voiding studies
- Electromyogram (EMG) of the pelvic floor
- Fluoroscopic visualization of the bladder and urethra

## QUESTION 2

*What information are you hoping to obtain with urodynamic testing for this particular patient?*

## ANSWER 2

The objective of all urodynamic testing is to reproduce the patient's symptoms under controlled conditions.

Urodynamic studies that fail to do this are of little clinical value. Numerous pitfalls in urodynamic testing limit its value. Some fundamental problems include:

- Lack of standardization of technical details, such as patient position, type of pressure sensor, and filling rate. These variables significantly affect results.
- The artificial situation of the urodynamic laboratory, which produces nonphysiologic results in some patients.
- Inconsistent reproducibility of test results in the same patient.
- The wide range of physiologic values in normal, asymptomatic patients.
- The absence of a specific abnormality during urodynamic testing does not exclude its existence, and not all abnormalities found during urodynamics are clinically significant.

Thus, urodynamic testing cannot be considered definitive without placing the results in the context of other findings.

In this patient, we hope that urodynamic studies will:

- Confirm the urodynamic diagnosis of "genuine stress urinary incontinence" (involuntary loss of urine occurring during a rise in intra-abdominal pressure without evidence of a detrusor contraction).
- Provide some information regarding urethral sphincteric function (LPP and/or UPP—see next question).
- Evaluate for detrusor overactivity (rise in intravesical pressure without a rise in abdominal pressure when the patient is not attempting to void) in this patient with occasional urge incontinence.
- Evaluate voiding function (complex uroflow and/or pressure voiding study) to try to anticipate postoperative bladder emptying problems.

## QUESTION 3

*Describe the performance of a multichannel cystometrogram, LPP, UPP, and pressure voiding study.*

## ANSWER 3

Appropriate technique leads to correct diagnosis and appropriate treatment.

1. The patient should arrive with a full bladder to void on a calibrated uroflowmeter to evaluate voiding function in the noninstrumented state.
2. Catheterize to measure PVR volume.
3. Place intravesical pressure catheter and filling port.
4. Place intrarectal catheter to measure concurrent abdominal pressure.
5. Zero transducers are placed at the level of the symphysis pubis.
6. Check calibration by having the patient cough.
7. Have patient in semirecumbent or sitting position and begin filling at constant rate (60–80 cc/min) using sterile water at room temperature (see Fig. 91-1).
8. Make note of the first sensation of bladder filling, first desire to void, urgency, and cystometric capacity. Look for detrusor overactivity.

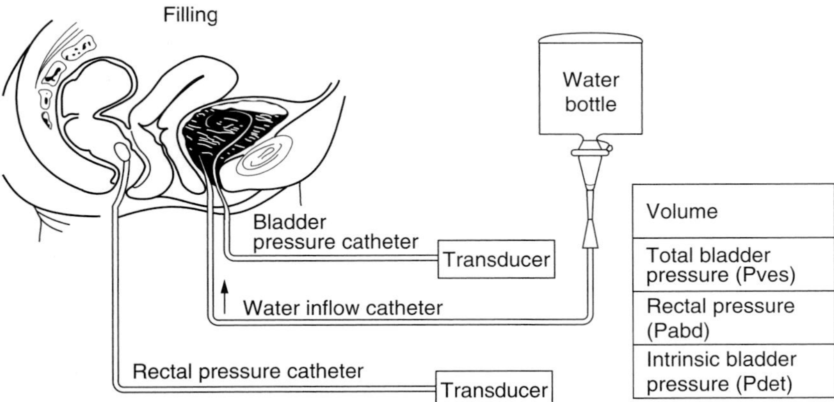


**FIG. 91-1** Complex cystometry: filling phase. Three catheters are generally used: a filling catheter through which sterile water will flow, a bladder pressure catheter, and a rectal pressure catheter. Intronsic detrusor pressure (Pdt) is calculated electronically by substracting rectal pressure (Pabd) from total bladder pressure (Pves).

SOURCE: From Wall and Addison. Post hysterectomy vaginal vault prolapse with emphasis on management by transabdominal sacral colpoexy. *Postgrad Obstet Gynecol.* 1988;8(26):1–7, with permission.

9. Stop filling at 250 cc to perform incremental coughs and valsalva and check for urine loss. The LPP is the lowest pressure that results in leakage.
10. Perform a urethral pressure profile, as indicated. This is done by slowly withdrawing the urethral and/or bladder catheter so that it traverses the high-pressure zone of the urethra.
11. Continue filling to capacity, periodically reevaluating LPP.
12. Seat patient on commode, zero transducers again to symphysis pubis, and have patient void.
13. Note presence or absence of bladder contraction during voiding and calculate PVR (filling volume minus voided volume).

## QUESTION 4

*Which patients need multichannel urodynamic testing?*

## ANSWER 4

The indications for urodynamic testing remain controversial. Current consensus statements and practice recommendations do not recommend urodynamic testing prior to conservative treatment of stress incontinence. However, some situations in which such testing may be useful include:

- Unclear diagnosis, after the initial history and physical examination, especially with respect to type of urinary incontinence.
- The patient's symptoms do not correlate with objective physical findings.
- The patient fails to improve with treatment.
- Clinical trials where objective confirmation of diagnosis is important.
- Surgical intervention is planned.

The last indication is the most controversial. An uncertain diagnosis may be acceptable if the recommended therapy has little or no risk (e.g., pelvic floor exercise, biofeedback, bladder training, pessary, or anticholinergic drugs), but most practitioners feel urodynamic confirmation of the diagnosis is desirable before a surgical treatment.

## BIBLIOGRAPHY


Anonymous. Assessment and treatment of urinary incontinence. Scientific Committee of the First International Consultation on Incontinence. *Lancet.* 2000;355(9221):2153.

Gupta A, Defreitas G, Lemack GE. The reproducibility of urodynamic findings in healthy female volunteers: results of repeated studies in the same setting and after short-term follow-up. *Neurourol Urodyn.* 2004;23(4):311.

Homma Y, Batista JE, Bauer SB, et al., (eds.). Incontinence. First International Consultation on Incontinence. Recommendations of the International Scientific Committee: the evaluation and treatment of urinary incontinence. Plymouth, UK, Health Publication Ltd, 1999.

Lemack GE. Urodynamic assessment of patients with stress incontinence: how effective are urethral pressure profilometry and abdominal leak point pressures at case selection and predicting outcome? *Curr Opin Urol.* 2004;14(6):307.

McLellan A, Cardozo L. Urodynamic techniques. *Int Urogynecol J Pelvic Floor Dysfunct.* 2001;12(4):266.

Schafer W, Abrams P, Liao L, et al. Good urodynamic practices: uroflowmetry, filling cystometry, and pressure-flow studies. *Neurourol Urodyn.* 2002;21(3):261.

Vereecken RL. A critical view on the value of urodynamics in non-neurogenic incontinence in women. *Int Urogynecol J Pelvic Floor Dysfunct.* 2000;11:188.

Wall LL, Wiskind AK, Taylor PA. Simple bladder filling with a cough stress test compared with subtracted cystometry for the diagnosis of urinary incontinence. *Am J Obstet Gynecol.* 1994; 171:1472.


# 92 UTERINE PROLAPSE

*Alison C. Madden*

## LEARNING POINT

Evaluation and treatment of uterine prolapse.

## VIGNETTE

An 85-year-old woman with medical history significant for chronic obstructive pulmonary disease and coronary artery disease presents to the emergency room complaining of a mass protruding through her vagina. She states she has felt pressure on and off for several years but over the last few months this sensation of pressure has increased. The patient states she noticed a mass this evening in the bath and is very anxious she may have cancer.

On pelvic examination her cervix is visible at the hymenal ring and the surface of her cervix is somewhat ulcerated. A small uterus is palpable on bimanual examination with no palpable adnexal masses. Upon valsalva, the cervix protrudes 1 cm beyond the hymenal ring. Upon standing and valsalva the cervix protrudes 3 cm past the hymenal ring.

## QUESTION 1

*What is the definition of uterine prolapse and how does it present?*

## ANSWER 1

Uterine prolapse occurs when the uterus and cervix descend into the vaginal canal. The descensus can occur due to defects in the uterosacral/cardinal ligaments or endopelvic fascia as well as relaxation of the musculature of the pelvic floor. Often patients are multigravid and postmenopausal. Other risk factors include obesity, collagen vascular disease, and chronic pulmonary disease causing increased intraabdominal pressure.

Patients with uterine prolapse often complain of a sense of pressure; a mass at the introitus or bowel/bladder changes. If the cervix and/or uterus is exteriorized the epithelium can become denuded and ulcerated and the patient may present with discharge or bleeding.

## QUESTION 2

*How can uterine prolapse be classified?*

## ANSWER 2

The older classification of uterine prolapse was based on a scale of 0–4 with 0 being no prolapse and 4 being procidentia (complete exteriorization of the uterus and cervix). The pelvic organ prolapse quantification (POPQ) system was designed to more accurately describe and quantitate the anatomic disturbances that occur with pelvic organ prolapse. It is useful for research and to better quantify defects for evaluation of treatment outcomes. Using the POPQ system, a clinician notes the position of six points in the vagina in relation to the hymenal ring. The locations of these points can be recorded in supine and standing positions with and without valsalva and recorded for future comparison (Figs. 92-1 and 92-2).

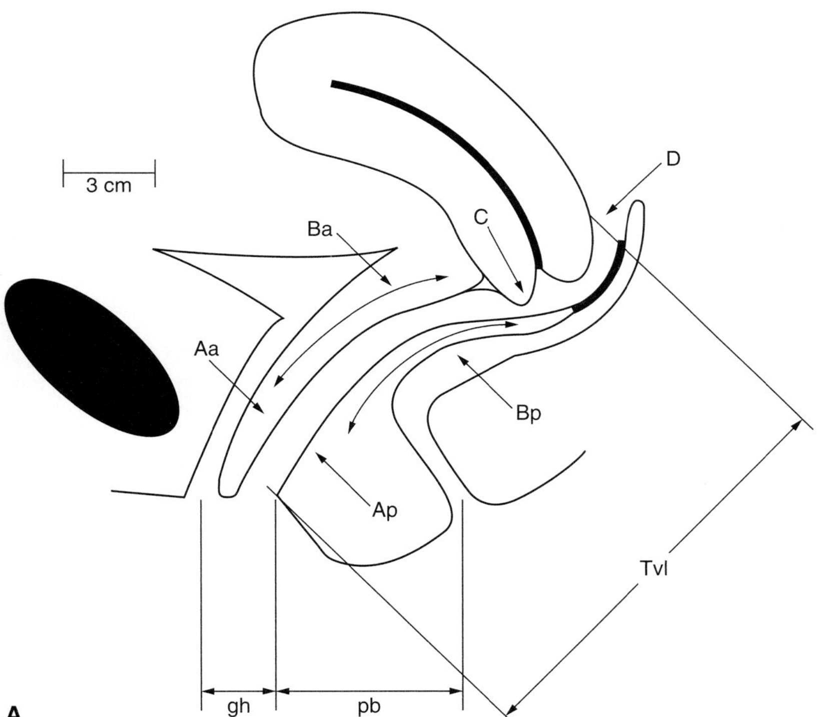


B

| Aa | Ba | C |
|---|---|---|
| gh | Pb | tvl |
| Ap | Bp | D |

**FIG. 92-1** (a) Pelvic organ prolapse quantitation (POPQ). Six sites (points Aa, Ba, C, D, Bp, Ap), genital hiatus (gh), perineal body (pb), and total vaginal length (tvl), are used for pelvic organ support quantitation.

SOURCE: Reproduced with permission from Bump, RC, Mattiasson, A, Bo, K, et al. The standardization of terminology of female pelvic organ prolapse and pelvic floor dysfunction. *Am J Obstet Gynecol;* 1996:175:10. Copyright © 1996 Mosby, Inc.

(b) Three-by-three grid used to express the quantified pelvic organ prolapse (POP-Q) system. Aa = point A of the anterior wall; Ba = point B of the anterior wall; C = cervix or cuff; D = posterior fornix; h = genital hiatus; pb = perineal body; tvl = total vaginal length; Ap = point A of the posterior wall; Bp = point B of the posterior wall.

SOURCE: Reproduced with permission from Harvey, M-A, Versi, E. Urogynecology and pelvic floor dysfunction. In: Ryan, KJ, Berkowitz, RS, Barbieri, RL, Dunaif, A (eds.). *Kistner's Gynecology and Women's Health*, 7th ed. St. Louis, Mosby, MO: Elsevier; 1999. Copyright © 1999 Elsevier.

**Pelvic organ prolapse staging**

| | |
|---|---|
| Stage 0 | No prolapse<br>Aa, Ba, Ap, Bp are −3 cm and C or D ≤ −(tvl − 2) cm |
| Stage 1 | Most distal portion of the prolapse −1 cm (above the level of hymen) |
| Stage 2 | Most distal portion of the prolapse ≥ − 1 cm but ≤ + 1 cm (≤ 1 cm above or below the hymen) |
| Stage 3 | Most distal portion of the prolapse > + 1 cm but < + (tvl − 2) cm (beyond the hymen; protrudes no farther than 2 cm less than the total vaginal length) |
| Stage 4 | Complete eversion; most distal portion of the prolapse ≥ + (tvl − 2) cm |

Note: Aa = Point A of anterior wall; Ba = Point B of anterior wall; Ap = Point A of posterior wall; Bp = Point B of posterior wall; −, above the hymen; +, beyond the hymen; tvl = total vaginal length.

**FIG. 92-2** Pelvic organ prolapse staging.
SOURCE: Reproduced with permission from Harvey, M-A, Versi, E. Urogynecology and pelvic floor dysfunction. In: Ryan, KJ, Berkowitz, RS, Barbieri, RL, Dunaif, A (eds.). *Kishner's Gynecology and Women's Health*. 7th ed. St. Louis, Mosby, MO: Elsevier; 1999. Copyright © 1999 Elsevier.

## QUESTION3

*What are the treatment options for uterine prolapse?*

## ANSWER 3

Treatment options include observation, pelvic floor exercises, pessaries, or surgical treatment including vaginal or abdominal hysterectomy; uterine fixation; or colpoclesis. Observation can be performed annually or as needed based on symptoms. Pelvic floor physical therapy can be useful with directed Kegel exercises. Pessaries can be very successful for treatment of uterine prolapse but requires careful patient selection and fitting. Surgery is frequently performed for treatment of uterine prolapse and can be combined with treatment of other symptoms such as urinary incontinence.

## QUESTION 4

*What factors should be taken into consideration when considering options for treatment?*

## ANSWER 4

For mild prolapse with no symptoms, observation and pelvic floor physical therapy combined with Kegels exercises may be all that is needed. If prolapse is more symptomatic, treatment options must be balanced with risks and benefits on an individual basis. Patients with hydronephrosis from uterine prolapse must be treated to prevent recurrent infections and renal injury. Pessary use is noninvasive and can be very successful for appropriate candidates. Such candidates may be young women who desire fertility and are comfortable removing and replacing a pessary or an older woman who is a poor surgical candidate. Pessary type depends on the degree of prolapse and the support structure of the perineum. Use of estrogen cream should be considered if appropriate. Surgical therapy can be performed either vaginally or abdominally. A hysterectomy can be performed with a suspension procedure as well as incontinence procedure if indicated. Uteropexy is also an option primarily for treatment of proplapse in a woman who wishes to preserve fertility. In these procedures the ligamentous attachments of the uterus are fixed to suspend the uterus to adjacent structures such as the anterior abdominal wall or sacrospinous ligament. Another surgical option for an elderly female who is not sexually active is the LeFort colpocleisis procedure which involves suturing the vaginal musculature and fascia together to prevent prolapse of the pelvic organs.

## BIBLIOGRAPHY


Benson JT, Lucente V, McClellan E. Vaginal versus abdominal reconstructive surgery for the treatment of pelvic support defects: a prospective randomized study with long-term outcome evaluation. *Am J Obstet Gynecol.* 1996;175(6):1418–1421.

Brubaker L, Norton P. Current clinical nomenclature for description of pelvic organ prolapse. *J Pelvic Surg.* 1996;2:257.

Bump RC, Mattiasson A, Bo K, et al. The standardization of terminology of female pelvic organ prolapse and pelvic floor dysfunction. *Am J Obstet Gynecol.* 1996;175:10.

Clemons JL, Aguilar VC, Tillinghast TA, et al. Patient satisfaction and changes in prolapse and urinary symptoms in women who were fitted successfully with a pessary for pelvic organ prolapse. *Am J Obstet Gynecol.* 2004;190(4):1025–1029.

Hall AF, Theofrastous JP, Cundiff GW, et al. Interobserver and intraobserver reliability of the proposed International Continence Society, Society of Gynecologic Surgeons, and American Urogynecologic Society pelvic organ prolapse classification system. *Am J Obstet Gynecol.* 1996;175:1467.

Kobashi KC, Leach GE. Pelvic prolapse. *J Urol.* 2000;164(6): 1879–1890.

Maher C, Baessler K, Glazener CM, et al. Surgical management of pelvic organ prolapse in women. *Cochrane Database Syst Rev.* 2004;4:CD004014.

Nygaard IE, McCreery R, Brubaker L, et al. Pelvic Floor Disorders Network. Abdominal sacrocolpopexy: a comprehensive review. *Obstet Gynecol.* 2004;104(4):805–823.

Swift S, Woodman P, O'Boyle A. Pelvic Organ Support Study (POSST): the distribution, clinical definition, and epidemiologic condition of pelvic organ support defects. *Am J Obstet Gynecol.* 2005;192(2):426–432.

Thakar R, Stanton S. Management of genital prolapse. *BMJ.* 2002;324(7348):1258–1262.

# 93 VAGINAL VAULT PROLAPSE

*Cynthia D. Hall*

## LEARNING POINT

Vaginal vault prolapse commonly accompanies other pelvic support defects and can be corrected surgically by different approaches.

## VIGNETTE

A 79-year-old, G4P4, female is seen complaining of a bulge in the vagina, especially late in the day. It is uncomfortable to sit and walk. She has also noticed progressive difficulty in urination and has to push the bulge in to empty the bladder. She does not currently complain of stress incontinence but recalls that it used to be an issue for her. She urinates infrequently, denies nocturia, and has no urgency or urge incontinence. She reports three urinary tract infections in the past year. She denies fecal incontinence; however, she will often strain to defecate and still feels as though she is unable to evacuate the rectum fully, even when the stools are soft. She is not sexually active.

Past medical history is significant for hypertension, hypercholesterolemia, and a history of previous myocardial infarction. Her previous surgeries include a vaginal hysterectomy at age 52 years for prolapse, an umbilical hernia repair at age 45 years, and an appendectomy. Her medications include furosemide, atenolol, lovostatin, and aspirin.

On examination, she is a frail, thin woman who appears her stated age. The vagina is completely everted (protruding about 7 cm from the introitus) with no support anteriorly, posteriorly, or apically. Her perineal body is extremely poor (1 cm), and the urogenital hiatus is widened (4 cm). There is significant urogenital atrophy and superficial erosion at the leading edge of the prolapse. The anal sphincter feels intact and of normal tone. Her postvoid residual is 250 cc, and she has cough-induced leakage of urine when the prolapse is reduced.

## QUESTION 1

*What is vaginal vault prolapse, and why does it occur?*

## ANSWER 1

Vaginal vault prolapse refers to the downward displacement of the vaginal fornix due to loss of apical support. This support is primarily derived from the integrity of the uterosacral and cardinal ligaments, thus vault prolapse often follows a hysterectomy for uterine descensus in which apical support was not reconstructed. The incidence of posthysterectomy vaginal prolapse has been shown to be several-fold higher after hysterectomies performed for pelvic relaxation than for those performed for other types of benign disease. Attempts directed solely at repairing the anterior and posterior vaginal walls will not solve the problem of apical support loss.

In most patients, vaginal vault prolapse is not an isolated finding and other defects must be assessed for and addressed concurrently. The terms anterior vaginal wall prolapse and posterior vaginal wall prolapse are preferred to cystocele and rectocele because vaginal topography does not reliably predict the location of the associated viscera in pelvic organ prolapse.

## QUESTION 2

*Using the pelvic organ prolapse quantification (POPQ) grading system, what is the stage of prolapse for this patient?*

## ANSWER 2

The POPQ system was devised in 1997 by members of the International Continence Society as a way to communicate objectively about pelvic floor defect anatomy. It consists of 9 measurements as follows (see Fig. 92-1):

Aa: anterior wall, 3 cm from hymen (can be −3 to +3)
Ba: anterior wall, most distal point
C: cervix or vaginal cuff
gh: genital hiatus on straining
pb: perineal body

| +3 Aa | +7 Ba | +7 C |
| --- | --- | --- |
| 4 gh | 1 Pb | 7 tvl |
| +3 Ap | +7 Bp | – D |

**FIG. 93-1** The overall stage of this woman's prolapse is a Stage IV.

tvl: total vaginal length
Ap: posterior wall, 3 cm form hymen (can be –3 to +3)
Bp: posterior wall, most distal point
D: posterior fornix

For this patient, these measurements can be depicted in a grid (Fig. 93-1) or with a line diagram (Fig. 93-2). Using the POPQ system, the severity of pelvic organ prolapse can be staged (see Fig. 92-2).

## QUESTION 3

*What are the usual symptoms of vault prolapse?*

## ANSWER 3

Pelvic organ prolapse of any organ can be asymptomatic or extremely uncomfortable for the patient. Other related symptoms may also occur.

Most commonly, pelvic organ prolapse is sensed by the patient as a bulge, fullness, or protuberance from the vagina. It is important to obtain an idea of what the maximum prolapse is from the patient (to the vaginal entrance, beyond the vaginal entrance) as the degree of prolapse can vary from day to day, and therefore the maximum descent may not be seen on examination. To observe maximal descent, the patient may be examined standing or reexamined late in the day.

The patient should be questioned regarding urinary and rectal function. Often there is a lack of support to the urethra that can result in stress urinary incontinence (SUI). However, if the prolapse is beyond the introitus, this can result in kinking of the urethra and difficulty voiding. With kinking of the urethra, "potential" or "occult" SUI can be a problem and therefore the patient should be examined after reducing the prolapse with a full bladder and having the patient strain or cough. Similarly, rectoceles can result in fecal trapping and give the patient the sensation of incomplete evacuation. Often such patients will push in (splint) the rectum or bladder in order to defecate and urinate.

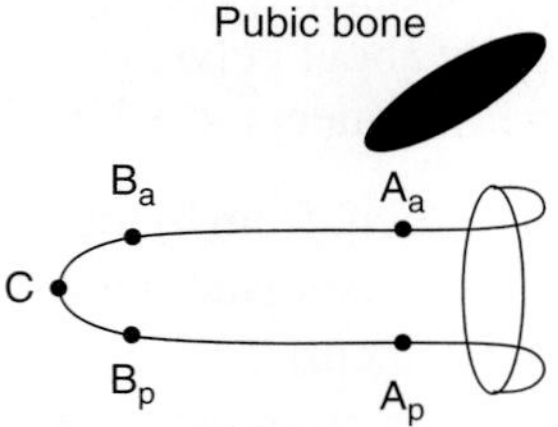


**FIG. 93-2** Grid and line diagram of complete vaginal eversion.

## QUESTION 4

*What are your treatment options?*

## ANSWER 4

Treatment options depend upon the type and degree of the defect and the patient's symptoms, but generally can range from reassurance to pelvic floor exercises, which can be effective in mild to moderate cases (Stage I–II), to the use of a pessary, or to reconstructive surgery.

For anterior compartment (cystocele) defects, surgery would include anterior repair (vaginal plication of the pubocervical fascia) and paravaginal repair (attachment of the fascia laterally to the araus tendineus fascia pelvis (ATFP) performed vaginally or abdominally). A Burch procedure performed for the treatment of SUI will often also correct the cystocele.

For posterior defects, plication of the rectovaginal fascia and/or levator ani musculature represents the traditional *posterior repair*. Many pelvic floor surgeons are now moving to a *site-specific* repair, identifying the specific fascial defects and repairing them individually without plication. Most studies report decreased rates of dyspareunia with this technique, although success rates may be decreased as well. The use of grafts in either compartment is becoming more widely embraced, although there are concerns regarding which is the optimum material to use and the risk of mesh erosion.

Apically, an enterocele must be reduced and the apex supported. Abdominally this can be accomplished by an abdominal sacral colpopexy (using mesh), an uterosacral suspension, or, rarely, a round ligament suspension in women who decline hysterectomy. Vaginally, a sacrospinous ligament suspension or high uterosacral plication suspends the vault. Finally, for a global prolapse in a woman who does not desire coital ability, a LeFort or total vaginal colpocleisis is a compensatory operation with excellent success rates and low morbidity. It is performed by sewing the pubocervical to the rectovaginal fascia in a layered fashion.

Of note, a patient with *potential* SUI must have a concomitant continence procedure.

## BIBLIOGRAPHY

Benson JT, Lucente V, McClellan E. Vaginal versus abdominal reconstructive surgery for the treatment of pelvic support defects: a prospective randomized study with long-term outcome evaluation. *Am J Obstet Gynecol.* 1996;175(6):1418.

Benson JT. Rectocele, descending perineal syndrome, enterocele. In: *Female Pelvic Floor Disorders: Investigation and Management.* Benson JT. (ed.). New York: Norton; 1992;384.

Bump RC, Fantl JA, Hurt WG, et al. The mechanism of urinary continence in women with severe uterovaginal prolapse: results of barrier studies. *Obstet Gynecol.* 1988;72:291.

Bump RC, Mattiasson A, Bo K, et al. The standardization of terminology of female pelvic organ prolapse and pelvic floor dysfunction. *Am J Obstet Gynecol.* 1996;175(1):10.

DeLancey JO, Morley GW. Total colpocleisis for vaginal eversion. *Am J Obstet Gynecol.* 1997;176:1228.

Kenton K, Shott S, Brubaker L. Vaginal topography does not correlate well with visceral position in women with pelvic organ prolapse. *Int Urogynecol J Pelvic Floor Dysfunct.* 1997;8:336.

Mant J, Painter R, Vessey M. Epidemiology of genital prolapse: observations from the Oxford Family Planning Association Study. *Br J Obstet Gynecol.* 1997;104:579–585.

Meschina M, Pifarotti P, Spennacchio M, et al. A randomized comparison of the tension-free vaginal tape and endopelvic fascia plication in women with genital prolapse and occult stress urinary incontinence. *Am J Obstet Gynecol.* 2004;190(3):609.

# 94 VULVAR LACERATION IN PEDIATRIC PATIENTS

*Alison C. Madden*

## LEARNING POINT

Evaluation and treatment of vulvar lacerations in a pediatric patient.

## VIGNETTE

A 5-year-old girl is brought to the emergency room by her mother after a fall in the playground. The mother states that she fell while climbing on monkey bars and landed in a position where she was straddling the bars. Immediately after she began to cry but then seemed fine until a few hours later when she complained it hurt to go to the bathroom. The mother found her daughter to have markedly swollen labia and brought her to the emergency room.

The girl began to kick and scream when an examination was attempted. Lidocaine jelly was applied using a gauze pad by the girl's mother and a second attempt at the examination was performed. An erythematous area was noted involving the left labia majora and mons with swelling and a 4 cm hematoma was noted involving the left labia majora and minora and spreading to the clitoral hood. A small laceration was present over this area but was not actively bleeding and only minimal blood was noted on the girls clothing. The hymen was found to be intact. After application of the lidocaine the girl was able to void with some discomfort.

### QUESTION 1

*What is the most common cause of vulvar lacerations in a pediatric population?*

### ANSWER 1

Straddle injuries are the most common cause of vulvar injury. Straddle injuries occur when a child falls onto an object he or she is straddling such as a bicycle, monkey bar, or other playground structure. Nonpenetrating straddle injuries result from blunt trauma to the soft tissues in the pelvis and can involve any of the structures in the pelvis but most commonly involve the anterior portion of the genitalia in girls, including the mons; clitoral hood, and labia minora. Vulvar hematomas can result, which may affect the ability to void. Penetrating straddle injuries can be more severe and cause vaginal or rectal perforation among other injuries. Lacerations can be present with either penetrating or nonpenetrating straddle injuries (see Fig. 94-1).

### QUESTION 2

*How should pediatric vulvar injuries be evaluated?*

### ANSWER 2

A careful history of the event should be obtained. The child should be examined with care in a calm and

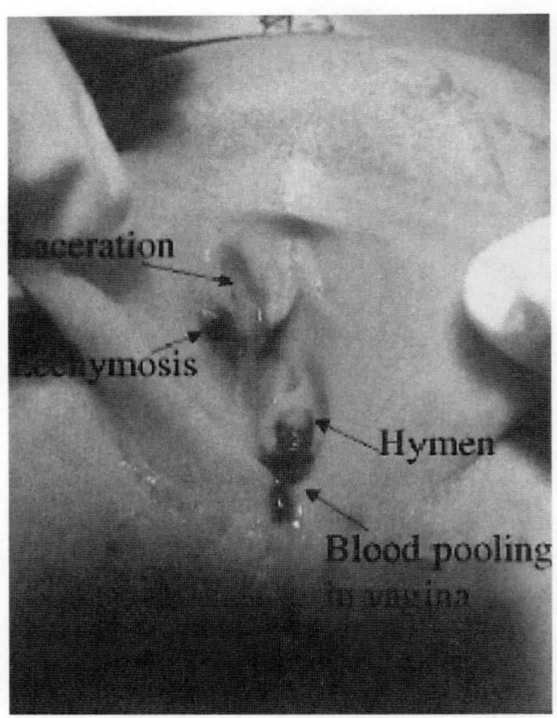


**FIG. 94-1** Straddle injury with laceration of right labia minora and superficial ecchymosis and blood pooling in vagina.

SOURCE: Merrit DF. Management quandary. Vulvar trauma in a young girl. *J Pediatr Adolescent Gynecol.* 2003;16(5):325–326.

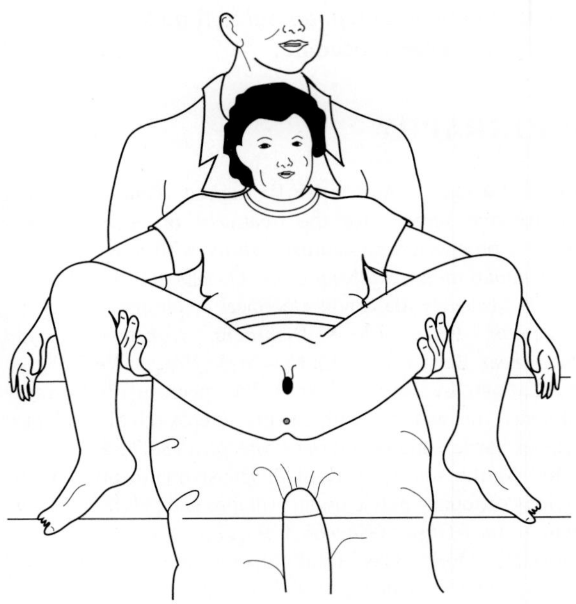

**FIG. 94-2** Recommended "frog leg" position to examine children.

SOURCE: Sachs C, Waddell M. Examination of the sexual assault victim. Chapter 59. In: Roberts JR and Hedges J (eds.). Clinical Procedure in Emergency Medicine. 4th ed. Philadelphia, PA: Saunders;2004.

relaxed setting. A *frog leg* position is often the best position for examination (see Fig. 94-2). Lidocaine jelly can be applied by the child or parent to the area prior to performing an examination to help numb the area. Sometimes sedation is needed to perform and adequate evaluation. The size and nature of the injury should be recorded and any hematomas should be measured to monitor their progression. Lacerations should be evaluated for location, depth, and active bleeding.

## QUESTION 3

*How should they be treated?*

## ANSWER 3

The child should be kept inactive for 24 hours. Vulvar hematomas should be monitored for growth and treated with ice packs for 24 hours. After this, sitz baths can be used to keep the area clean and help with voiding. If a girl is unable to void due to a large hematoma a urinary catheter should be placed. Surgical drainage of hematomas is generally avoided. Vulvar lacerations should be allowed to heal by secondary intention unless significant bleeding is present. If repair is needed due to heavy bleeding, the patient should be taken to the OR for adequate anesthesia and visualization.

Vaginal hematomas must be closely monitored. If bleeding continues, they should be opened and sutured under anesthesia. If a laceration or penetrating vaginal injury is sustained, it may be necessary to perform an exploratory laparotomy to rule out retroperitoneal or intraperitoneal hemorrhage.

## QUESTION 4

*What should be included in the differential diagnosis?*

## ANSWER 4

Sexual abuse should always be included in the differential diagnosis of a straddle injury. Certain physical findings are more concerning for possible sexual abuse and include posterior perineal injury including injury to the hymen; penetrating injury to vagina or rectum; incongruency between history and findings, and severe trauma.

## BIBLIOGRAPHY

Dowd MD, Fitzmaurice L, Knapp JF, Mooney D. The interpretation of urogenital findings in children with straddle injuries. *J Pediatr Surgery.* 1994;29(1):7–10.

Johnson CF. Child sexual abuse. *Lancet.* 2004;364(9432): 462–470.

Virgili A, Bianchi A, Mollica G, Corazza M. Serious hematoma of the vulva from a bicycle accident. A case report. *J Reprod Med.* 2000;45(8):662–664.

Waltzman ML, Shannon M, Bowen AP, et al. Monkeybar injuries: complications of play. *Pediatrics.* 2000;105(5):1174–1175.

# Section 6

# REPRODUCTIVE DISORDERS

## 95 RECURRENT ABORTION

*Magareta D. Pisarska*

### LEARNING POINT

Although many causes of recurrent pregnancy loss are unexplained, an evaluation should be conducted to determine any known causes that can be treated.

## VIGNETTE

A 35-year-old, G3P0030, comes in because she cannot keep a pregnancy. She had three previous losses with her current partner. Her obstetric history is as follows: first pregnancy resulted in a loss at 6 weeks gestation and a second pregnancy resulted in a loss at 8 weeks after a heartbeat was seen on ultrasound at 6 weeks. A D&C was performed. A third pregnancy resulted in a loss at 6 weeks. A heartbeat was not seen at the time. A D&C was not performed.

Gynecologic history: Menarche at 12 years, regular cycles every 28 days with 5 days of flow. No history of fibroids, ovarian cysts, or sexually transmitted diseases.

Medical history and surgical history are negative. Social history: She does not smoke, drink alcohol, or use illicit drugs. She is not taking any medications and has no allergies to medications. Her family history is noncontributory.

Physical examination reveals a healthy appearing female. Vital signs: blood pressure 110/70 mm Hg, pulse 80/min, respiratory rate 18/min, and temperature 98.6°F. Thyroid: nonpalpable, lungs clear, heart: regular rate and rhythm without audible murmurs. Abdomen: normal bowel sounds, soft, nontender, no palpable masses. Pelvic examination: normal external genitalia, cervix multiparous, no lesions, uterus anteverted normal size, adnexa nontender, no masses bilaterally. Rectovaginal confirms.

Workup reveals: normal female and male karyotypes, lupus anticoagulant is negative, anticardiolipin antibody testing is negative. Hysterosalpingogram reveals a uterine septum with patent fallopian tubes bilaterally.

### QUESTION 1

*What is the definition of recurrent pregnancy loss?*

### ANSWER 1

Traditionally recurrent pregnancy loss has been defined as three consecutive spontaneous abortions; however, the risk of a subsequent loss after two recurrent pregnancy losses is similar to the risk of three consecutive losses. Thus evaluation is appropriate after two consecutive losses. Most women will have recurrent preembryonic or embryonic losses.

### QUESTION 2

*What are the different causes of recurrent pregnancy loss?*

## ANSWER 2

There are a number of different genetic causes that may account for recurrent pregnancy loss (see Table 95-1). In approximately 2–4% of couples with recurrent pregnancy loss, one partner will have a chromosomal abnormality. Most are balanced translocations but chromosomal inversions may also be a factor. There is some evidence suggesting that recurrent aneuploidy in the conceptus may be a cause of recurrent pregnancy loss. In women with a history of recurrent pregnancy loss, up to 48% of cases had an abnormal karyotype in the subsequent pregnancy loss.

In addition a number of genetic mutations may also be associated with recurrent pregnancy losses, via vascular mechanisms, including those of factor V (Leiden factor) and factor II (G20210A). Endocrinologic abnormalities have been implicated. Women with poorly controlled type 1 (insulin-dependent) diabetes have an increased rate of abortion. However, glucose intolerance or mild thyroid disease has not been found as a cause of recurrent pregnancy loss.

Up to 10–15% of women with recurrent early pregnancy loss have uterine anomalies. Many congenital uterine anomalies are associated with second trimester losses. The most common malformations associated with pregnancy loss are bicornuate, septate, or didelphic uteri. Intra uterine synechiae and in utero diethylstilbestrol (DES) exposure with resultant uterine abnormalities may also be associated with recurrent pregnancy loss.

Antiphospholipid syndrome (APS) is associated with pregnancy loss in 3–15% of women with recurrent pregnancy loss. These women are at risk of early as well as late pregnancy loss. APS is an autoimmune disorder defined by the presence of significant antiphospholipid antibodies (anticardiolipin antibodies [ACL] or lupus anticoagulant [LAC]) and one or more of the following clinical features such as thrombosis, recurrent pregnancy loss, or fetal death.

Approximately half of couples with recurrent pregnancy loss will have no specific diagnosis following an evaluation for recurrent pregnancy loss.

**TABLE 95-1. Causes of Recurrent Pregnancy Losses**

| | |
|---|---|
| Genetic (40–50% fetal; 2–4% parental) | Usually aneuploidies, X0 and trisomies<br>Random errors<br>Parent with balanced translocation |
| Endocrine (2–5%) | Severe thyroid disease or diabetes<br>Luteal defect controversial |
| Anatomic (10–15%) | Usually lead to second trimester losses, i.e., cervical incompetence<br>Septate uterus most common<br>DES exposure<br>Uterine synechiae |
| Immunologic (3–15%) | Autoimmune diseases with antiphospholipid antibodies<br>Lupus anticoagulant (LAC), anticardiolipin antibody (ACL) |
| Microbiologic (1–5%) | Inconclusive (mycoplasmas?) |
| Unexplained (~50%) | Female age (often genetic), caffeine, smoking, other |

## QUESTION 3

*What type of evaluation should be considered for a couple with recurrent pregnancy loss?*

## ANSWER 3

Cytogenetic analysis (karyotype) of both the male and female partner should be offered. A search for uterine cavity abnormalities should be conducted by hysterosalpingography, hysteroscopy, or sonohysterogram. Women with recurrent pregnancy loss should be evaluated for APS, assessing for LAC or $\beta$2-glycoprotein I-dependent ALC. They should be positive on two occasions at least 6 weeks apart. In addition, measurement of homocystein levels (to exclude Leiden factor mutations) and exclusion of the prothrombin 20210G. A mutation by polymerase chain reaction (PCR) may be considered.

## QUESTION 4

*What types of treatment alternatives are available for couples with a history of recurrent pregnancy loss?*

## ANSWER 4

In women with unexplained recurrent pregnancy loss, up to 35–85% will have a live birth without any intervention. In couples with cytogenetic abnormalities, preimplantation genetic diagnosis can be used to screen embryos for cytogenetic abnormalities. Donor gametes can also be used. In women with uterine anatomic abnormalities, retrospective series suggest that a successful pregnancy can occur in up to 70–85% of women surgically treated for a bicornuate or septate uterus. However, these studies lack controls. Hysteroscopic resection, an outpatient procedure with low morbidity, can be used to treat a uterine septum. Success rates are comparable to metroplasty with less morbidity including a trial of labor with vaginal delivery. Women with APS benefit from treatment with heparin and low-dose aspirin. Successful pregnancy rates for women with APS treated with heparin and low-dose aspirin are 70–75% compared to less than 50% in untreated women.

## BIBLIOGRAPHY

ACOG Practice Bulletin No. 24. Management of Recurrent Early Pregnancy Loss. 2001;1–12.

Carr BR, Blackwell RE, Azziz R, Kutteh WH. Essential reproductive medicine. Recurrent pregnancy loss. 2005; 24:585–592.

Fausett MB, Branch DW. Autoimmunity and Pregnancy Loss. *Seminars in Reproductive Medicine*. 2000;18:379–392.

Verlinsky Y, Cohen J, Munne S, Gianaroli L, Simpson JL, Ferraretti AP, Kuliev A. Over a decade of experience with preimplantation genetic diagnosis: a multicenter report. *Fertil Steril*. 2004; 82(2):292–294.

# 96 AMENORRHEA EVALUATION

*Magareta D. Pisarska*

## LEARNING POINT

Primary and secondary amenorrhea requires a careful evaluation including history and physical and laboratory testing.

## VIGNETTE

A 16-year-old, G0P0, comes in because she has not had a period. She states that she had some pubic hair development that began at the age of 11 years. She also states that she had some breast development at the age of 12 years but her breasts are much smaller than her friends.

Gynecologic history: never menstruated. Pubic hair development began at age 11 years. Breast development began at age of 12 years. No history of fibroids, ovarian cysts, or sexually transmitted diseases.

Obstetrics history: none.

Medical history and surgical history is negative. Social history: she does not smoke, drink alcohol, or use illicit drugs. She is not taking any medications and has no allergies to medications. Her family history is noncontributory.

Physical examination reveals a healthy appearing female. Vital signs: blood pressure 110/70 mm Hg, pulse 80/min, and respiratory rate 18/min, and temperature 98.6°F. Weight 105 lb and height 4 ft 10 in. Thyroid: nonpalpable, lungs clear, heart: regular rate and rhythm without audible murmurs. Breasts: Tanner stage 3. Abdomen: normal bowel sounds, soft, nontender, no palpable masses. Pelvic examination: normal external genitalia, Tanner stage 3, internal examination deferred.

Blood work reveals the following: beta-human chorionic gonadotropin ($\beta$-hCG) is negative, follicle-stimulating hormone (FSH) is 40 mIU/mL, LH is 30 mIU/mL, thyroid-stimulating hormone (TSH) is 2 mIU/mL, and prolactin is 10 ng/mL.

Transabdominal ultrasound: infantile uterus, small ovaries bilaterally.

Karyotype reveals 46 XX/45 XO.

### QUESTION 1

*When should the evaluation of amenorrhea be initiated?*

### ANSWER 1

The evaluation of primary amenorrhea is indicated in an individual without menses by the age of 15 years but with the presence of secondary sexual characteristics. This is two standard deviations above the mean age of menses of 13 years. In addition, if menses has not occurred within 5 years after breast development if breast development began before age 10 years. In adolescents who do not develop breasts by age 13 years, on evaluation should also be initiated. Age 13 is two standard deviations above the mean of 10 years for the initiation of breast development. In women with regular menstrual cycles, delayed menses after 1 week should be evaluated for pregnancy. However, a complete workup should be initiated if amenorrhea is present for 3 months in normally cycling women or if there are less than nine cycles in a year.

### QUESTION 2

*What is the primary evaluation for amenorrhea?*

### ANSWER 2

Initially, a history and physical examination should be conducted. Breast development demonstrates that estrogen has been present at some point in time. Hirsutism and virilization indicates excessive testosterone or other androgen secretion. The external and internal genitalia should be properly examined. An abdominal ultrasound

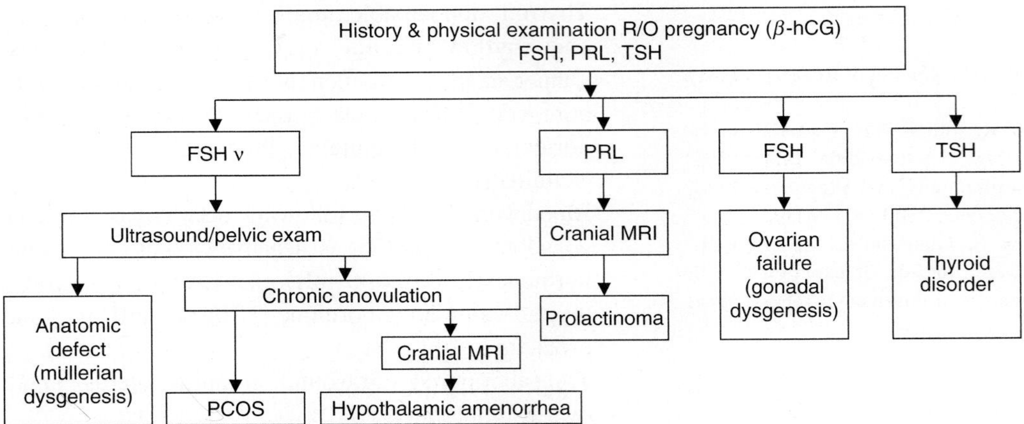


**FIG. 96-1** Flow diagram aiding in the evaluation of women with amenorrhea.

can be used in place of an internal examination as deemed appropriate. Up to 15% of women with primary amenorrhea will have an abnormal genital examination. Müllerian agenesis, transverse vaginal septum, or androgen insensitivity syndrome should be considered in women with a blind or absent vagina with breast development. It is also important to evaluate the genitalia for an imperforate hymen.

Laboratory testing for pregnancy ($\beta$-hCG FSH, TSH, and prolactin) should be the initial tests for evaluation. Along with the physical examination, these tests will determine the most common causes of amenorrhea (see Fig. 96-1).

## QUESTION 3

*What additional testing should be performed in women diagnosed with particular causes of amenorrhea?*

## ANSWER 3

If müllerian agenesis is diagnosed, evaluation of the renal system should be performed. Müllerian agenesis is associated with urogenital malformations such as unilateral renal agenesis, pelvic kidney, horseshoe kidney, hydronephrosis, and ureteral duplication. A serum testosterone will distinguish androgen insensitivity syndrome (AIS) from müllerian agenesis. A karyotype analysis will be confirmatory.

A karyotype should be performed for all women with premature ovarian failure. Although more prevalent in women with primary amenorrhea, the presence of Y chromosomal material requires extirpation of the gonadal tissue secondary to an increased risk of gonadal tumors. A karyotype will also determine if there is an X chromosome abnormality. Of particular importance, are chromosomal abnormalities resulting in Turners syndrome. These women should be screened for associated abnormalities. Additional evaluation including specific genetic defects as well as associated autoimmune disorders should be considered (see Chap. 117, Premature Ovarian Failure).

In the presence of hyperprolactinemia on more than one occasion and the absence of hypothyroidism, an MRI of the pituitary is indicated. Even mildly elevated prolactin levels can be present in women with pituitary adenomas, some may be nonfunctioning. Additionallly, other central nervous system lesions that can cause pituitary stalk compression should be ruled out. Congenital aqueductal stenosis should also be ruled out.

In women with normal or low FSH values, amenorrhea is frequently unexplained. The most common are hypothalamic amenorrhea and polycystic ovary syndrome (PCOS). Clinical characteristics may help distinguish between these two categories. The presence of hyperandrogenism is characteristic of PCOS.

The progesterone challenge test used to determine estrogen production correlates poorly with estrogen status. Up to 20% of women with oligomenorrhea or amenorrhea in whom estrogen is present have no withdrawal bleeding and withdrawal bleeding occurs in up to 40% of women with hypoestrogenic amenorrhea due to stress, weight loss, exercise, or hyperprolactinemia and in up to 50% of women with ovarian failure.

## BIBLIOGRAPHY

American College of Gynecology Practice Bulletin No. 34. Management of infertility caused by ovulatory dysfunction. 2002.

Hecht H, Jaff MR, Harman SM, Current evaluation of amenorrhea. *Fertil Steril.* 2004;82:266–272.

Nelson, LM, Covington SN, Rebar RW. An update: spontaneous premature ovarian failure is not an early menopause. *Fertil Steril.* 2005;83(5):1327–1332.

Rarick LD, Shangold MM, Ahmed SW. Cervical mucus and serum estradiol as predictors of response to progestin challenge. *Fertil Steril.* 1990;54:353–355.

# 97 HYPOTHALAMIC AMENORRHEA

*Magareta D. Pisarska*

## LEARNING POINT

Hypothalamic amenorrhea is frequently associated with stress, weight changes, poor nutrition, and excessive exercise, it is essentially a diagnosis of exclusion and other causes of amenorrhea need to be ruled out.

## VIGNETTE

A 28-year-old, G0P0, comes in because she has not had a period since she discontinued oral contraceptive pills 7 months ago. She started taking the oral contraceptive pill (OCP) when she was 16 years old because she had very irregular cycles, every 4–6 months. She states that she has not been sexually active in the last 8 months. She did a home pregnancy test, which was negative. She also complains that she has been feeling irritable and occasionally wakes up in a cold sweat. She states that her job has become more stressful in the past 12 months and she is working 10-hour days. She also states that the stress has caused her to lose approximately 15 lb over the last year.

Gynecologic history:
In addition to the above history, menarche occured at age 14 years. She states that she had normal breast and pubic hair development around the age of 11 years.
No history of fibroids, ovarian cysts, or sexually transmitted diseases.
Obstetrics history: none.
Medical history and surgical history are negative.
Social history: She does not smoke, drink alcohol, or use illicit drugs. She is not taking any medications and has no allergies to medications. Her family history is noncontributory.
Physical examination reveals a thin appearing female. Vital signs: blood pressure 110/70 mm Hg, pulse 80/min, respiratory rate 18/min, and temperature 98.6°F. Weight 105 lb. Height 5 ft 6 in. Thyroid: nonpalpable, lungs clear, heart: regular rate and rhythm without audible murmurs. Abdomen: normal bowel sounds, soft, nontender, no palpable masses. Pelvic examination: normal external genitalia, cervix nulliparous, no lesions, uterus anteverted normal size, adnexa nontender, no masses bilaterally. Rectovaginal confirms.
Blood work reveals the following: beta-human chorionic gonadotropin ($\beta$-hCG) is negative, follicle-stimulating hormone (FSH) is 3 mIU/mL, LH is 3 mIU/mL, thyroid-stimulating hormone (TSH) is 2 mIU/mL, and prolactin is 10 ng/mL.

### QUESTION 1

*What are the causes of hypothalamic amenorrhea?*

### ANSWER 1

The most common causes of amenorrhea is hypothalamic amenorrhea. Although the specific pathophysiologic mechanisms are unclear, stress, weight changes, poor nutrition, and excessive exercise are frequently associated with hypothalamic amenorrhea. However, it is essentially a diagnosis of exclusion and therefore other causes of amenorrhea need to be ruled out. Although weight loss is more common than anorexia nervosa in women with amenorrhea, anorexia nervosa has additional significant health implications that need to be addressed. Competitive athletes, particularly competitive runners are at higher risk of developing amenorrhea. Individuals with chronic diseases such as uncontrolled juvenile diabetes, end-stage kidney disease, malignancy, acquired immune deficiency syndrome, or malabsorption may also develop amenorrhea.

Rare causes of hypothalamic amenorrhea include genetic abnormalities leading either to isolated gonadotropin deficiencies or gonadotropin-releasing hormone receptor mutations. Kallmann syndrome, the most common gonadotropin deficiency, is associated with anosmia, secondary to defects in olfactory bulb development.

QUESTION 2

*How do you make the diagnosis of hypothalamic amenorrhea?*

ANSWER 2

A history and physical examination should be initially conducted. Breast development demonstrates that estrogen has been present at some point in time. Hirsutism and possibly virilization indicates excessive testosterone secretion. The external and internal genitalia should be properly examined for any abnormalities that can be the cause of amenorrhea. An abdominal ultrasound can be used in place of an internal examination as deemed appropriate.

Laboratory testing for pregnancy ($\beta$-hCG, FSH, TSH, and prolactin) should be the initial tests for evaluation. Low or normal gonadotropins in the presence of a normal examination and other laboratory tests are suggestive of hypothalamic amenorrhea. A cranial magnetic resonance imaging (MRI) should be considered to rule out any cranial abnormalities, particularly pituitary, that may mimic hypothalamic amenorrhea. Some pituitary disorders that can cause amenorrhea include Sheehan's syndrome, necrosis of the pituitary gland, empty sella syndrome, and nonfunctioning adenomas.

QUESTION 3

*What type of therapy is appropriate for a woman with hypothalamic amenorrhea?*

ANSWER 3

Women not desiring pregnancy should be treated with cyclic estrogen-progestin therapy either in the form of oral contraceptives or hormone therapy, since they are prone to develop osteoporosis. If pregnancy is desired, it is important to address proper nutrition and weight gain. In addition, ovulation induction should also be offered. Most women will need exogenous gonadotropins to induce ovulation (see Fig. 96-1).

## BIBLIOGRAPHY

American Society for Reproductive Medicine. Practice Committee. Current evaluation of amenorrhea. *Fertil Steril.* 2004;82:1.

Bradshaw KD, Carr BR. Disorders of puberty and amenorrhea. In: Carr BR, Blackwell RE, Azziz R (eds.). *Essential Reproductive Medicine*. New York, NY:McGraw-Hill; 2004:203–238.

# 98 HIRSUTISM

*Ricardo Azziz*

## LEARNING POINT

To understand the evaluation of the patient who complains of hirsutism and formulate a treatment plan.

## VIGNETTE

A 21-year-old female, G0, presents to your office complaining of acne and unwanted hair growth. She feels that she is turning into a "man." The hair growth is sufficient to inhibit her from participating in social events, most notably dating, and she feels that the excess hair growth and acne are "ruining her life." On questioning, you find that her menstrual cycles appear to be regular, approximately once per month, and that she is currently not sexually active and is not using contraceptive or hormonal therapy. She has seen a dermatologist who prescribed tetracycline 500 mg once daily and topical facial washes for her acne. Past medical history is otherwise not significant. Family history indicates that the patient has two maternal aunts who also had excess hair growth, and her father has diabetes. On physical examination the patient demonstrates moderate inflammatory acne of the face, back, and chest. She also demonstrates dark, coarse hairs on her chin, upper lip, sideburn area, and lower abdomen. She has shaved her thighs, and it is difficult to ascertain hair growth in this area.

QUESTION 1

*What is hirsutism and what is its prevalence?*

ANSWER 1

By some estimates unwanted hair growth affects approximately 14–15 million women in the United States. However, not all patients who complain of unwanted hair growth will have hirsutism. By definition, hirsutism is the excessive growth of terminal hairs in a male-like pattern in women. Terminal hairs can be recognized on clinical examination by generally being pigmented and greater than 5 mm in length (if allowed to freely grow); they generally feel coarser (because they are structurally medullated) than the surrounding vellus hairs. Hirsutism is usually defined by a clinical evaluation assessing the presence of terminal hairs in areas that are primarily masculine. These may include the chin, upper lip, side burn area, chest, upper abdomen, lower abdomen (also called male escutcheon), buttocks, thighs, upper and lower back, and upper arms. Excessive terminal hair growth in the forearms or the lower legs alone is not indicative of hirsutism and is not included in the general classifications. The most commonly used clinical assessment method is the modified Ferriman-Gallwey scoring system, where nine body areas are scored from 0 to 4, depending on their content of terminal hair growth (Fig. 98-1). In this visual system, a score of 0 indicates the absence of terminal hairs in the areas examined, 1 is barely visible excess terminal hair, 2 is moderate excess terminal hair growth (but significantly less than that of a male), 3 is moderate to severe terminal hair growth (reminiscent of a male), and a score of 4 is assigned to those body areas with severe terminal hair growth (consistent with that of a male).

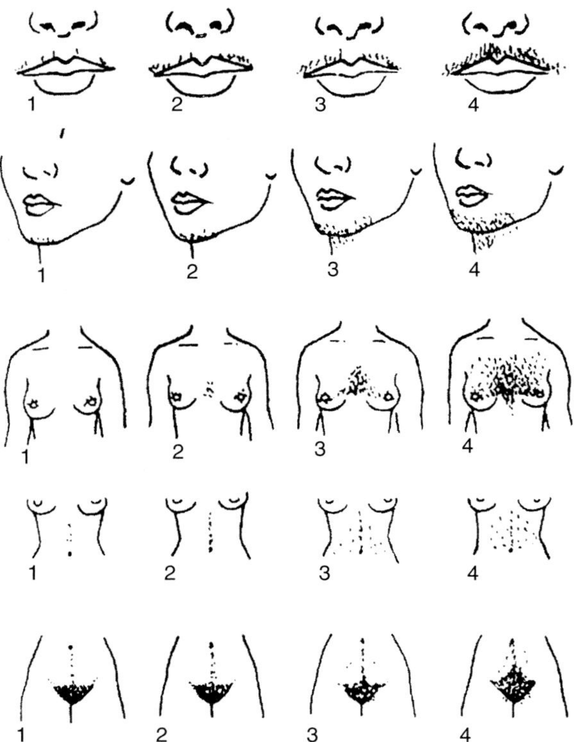


**FIG. 98-1** Visual method of scoring hair growth in women, modified from the system originally reported by Ferriman and Gallwey in 1961. Each of the nine body areas depicted is scored from 0 (absence of terminal hairs) to 4 (extensive terminal hair growth), and the scores in each area are summed for a total hair growth score. Hair growth scores of 6–8 or greater are generally considered to represent hirsutism.
SOURCE: Reprinted with permission from Azziz R. The evaluation and management of hirsutism. *Obstet Gynecol.* 2003;101:995–1007.

Between 7% and 10% of the U.S. population of reproductive-aged women, at least those of White and Black race, suffer from hirsutism, although the exact prevalence will certainly vary according to definition. Individuals of Asian descent generally have less hair growth and consequently a lower prevalence of hirsutism than other races.

## QUESTION 2

*What is the differential diagnosis of hirsutism?*

## ANSWER 2

The majority of patients with hirsutism demonstrate an underlying androgen excess disorder, which may include polycystic ovary syndrome (PCOS; 75–85%), 21-hydroxylase deficient nonclassic adrenal hyperplasia (NCAH; 1–8% depending on ethnicity), idiopathic hirsutism (IH; 5–15%, depending on definition), the hyperandrogenic insulin resistant-acanthosis nigricans (HAIRAN) syndrome (2–4%), androgen-secreting tumors (ASNs; 1 in 300 to 1 in 1000), and the use or abuse of androgenic drugs.

## QUESTION 3

*How is the hirsute patient evaluated?*

## ANSWER 3

Firstly, the examiner must confirm that the patient actually does have hirsutism, i.e., the presence of excessive terminal hairs in a male-like pattern. Many patients complaining of unwanted hair growth either complain of excessive hair growth that affects the pubic and inner thighs area or the lower legs or lower arms, which in and of itself may not suggest an androgen excess disorder. Likewise, many patients may complain of excessive growth of vellus hairs, which is often the result of ethnic predisposition (e.g., women of Mediterranean or Scandinavian extraction), although some drugs may result in excessive growth of vellus hairs (e.g., certain antiseizure drugs, such as phenytoin).

Second, once the presence of hirsutism is confirmed, the practitioner needs to proceed in a systematic fashion to exclude specific disorders and other associated dysfunctions. In patients who are hirsute and have frank menstrual irregularity and/or oligomenorrhea (e.g., episodes of vaginal bleeding at greater than 35-day intervals or occurring less than eight times per year) no further testing of ovulatory function is required, since by definition the patients would be considered oligo-ovulatory.

Alternatively, between 20–50% of hirsute patients may relate a history of what appears to be *regular* vaginal bleeding episodes or *menses*. In these latter patients, ovulatory function must be confirmed by objective testing, as 40% of hirsute eumenorrheic women actually have ovulatory dysfunction. Confirmation of ovulatory function can be easily accomplished by measuring a serum progesterone (P4) level on days 22–24 (luteal phase) of the menstrual cycle in one, or preferably two, consecutive cycles may be sufficient to confirm ovulatory function. While the use of a basal body temperature chart may be helpful to the practitioner to identify approximately when the patient ovulated, it is not absolutely necessary for the confirmation of ovulation.

In patients who demonstrate ovulatory dysfunction, the measurement of a basal third generation thyroid stimulating hormone (TSH) and a prolactin level (to exclude thyroid dysfunction and hyperprolactinemia, respectively) should be considered, although the prevalence of these disorders in patients with frank evidence of hyperandrogenism is generally less than 2%.

In addition to ascertaining whether the patient is ovulatory, either by history or by luteal phase P4 measurements, specific disorders that may result in hirsutism should be excluded. A careful history may reveal the use of drugs that have androgenic potential. Screening for 21-hydroxylase NCAH can be performed by measuring the basal serum 17-hydroxyprogesterone level in the follicular phase (see also Chap. 99, 21-Hydroxylase Deficient Nonclassic Adrenal Hyperplasia). Androgen-secreting neoplasms are generally suspected by physical examination (severe virilization or masculinization, potentially in association with cushingoid features if an adrenocortical process, most notably adrenocortical carcinoma). Confirmation of the diagnosis is generally obtained radiologically, using transvaginal ultrasonography and adrenal imaging.

There is currently controversy regarding whether the HAIRAN syndrome is actually a disorder distinct from PCOS or whether patients with the HAIRAN syndrome are actually individuals with PCOS who have extreme levels of insulin resistance. Nonetheless, because HAIRAN syndrome patients often demonstrate other associated abnormalities not seen in PCOS patients, e.g. lipodystrophy, we tend to consider it as a separate abnormality. Patients with HAIRAN syndrome can be clinically identified by the presence of significant degrees of acanthosis nigricans. The diagnosis can be confirmed by either the basal measurement of a circulating fasting insulin level, which is generally greater than 80 mIU/mL, or by the response of insulin to a glucose challenge, which generally exceeds 300–500 mIU/mL. Individuals with HAIRAN syndrome are at significantly greater risk for developing vascular and metabolic abnormalities, including cardiovascular disease and diabetes.

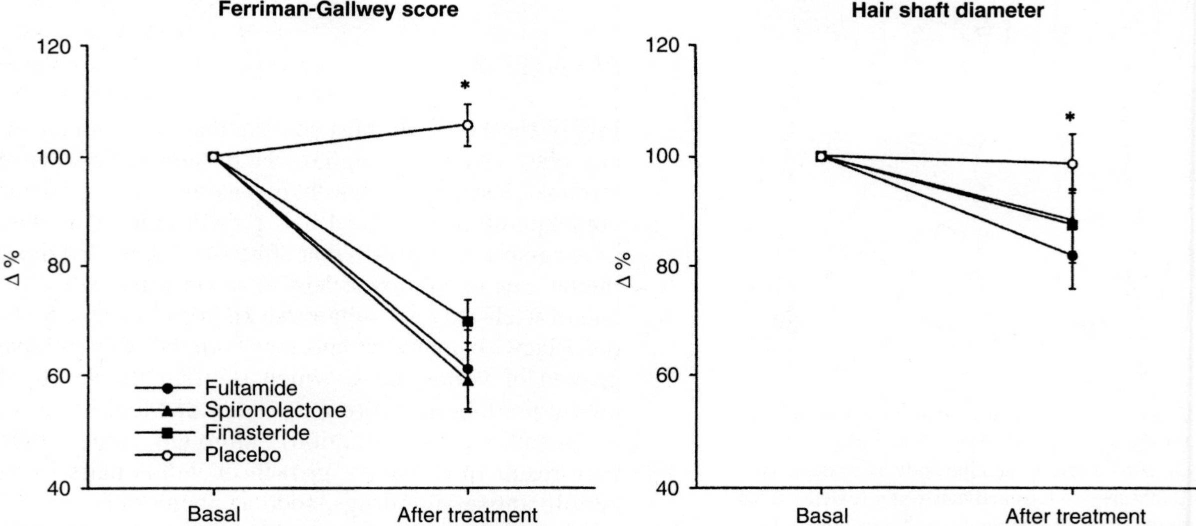


**FIG. 98-2** Changes after therapy (Δ%) in modified Ferriman-Gallwey (F-G) hirsutism score and mean hair shaft diameter in 40 hirsute women randomly assigned to double blind treatments with spironolactone (100 mg/day), flutamide (250 mg/day), finasteride (5 mg/day), or placebo for 6 months.

SOURCE: Reprinted with permission from Moghetti P, et al. Comparison of spironolactone, flutamide, and finasteride efficacy in the treatment of hirsutism: a randomized, double blind, placebo-controlled trial. *J Clin Endocrinol Metab.* 2000;85:89–94.

Third, after specific disorders that may lead to androgen excess or the associated ovulatory dysfunction (e.g., NCAH, HAIRAN syndrome, ASNs, hyperprolactinemia, thyroid dysfunction, and androgenic drug use or abuse) are excluded, the remaining patients (which are the majority) will need to be classified further into either patients with PCOS or patients with IH. Patients with PCOS are those individuals who demonstrate clinical (e.g., hirsutism) and/or biochemical (e.g., excess total or free testosterone levels) hyperandrogenism in conjunction with ovulatory dysfunction. Patients with IH generally are those individuals who demonstrate obvious hirsutism, but without evidence of ovulatory dysfunction or elevated androgen levels. Recently, the use of transvaginal ultrasonography has been incorporated into the evaluation of the androgen excess patients, such that some patients with PCOS may not demonstrate ovulatory dysfunction at the time of their evaluation, but may demonstrate polycystic-appearing ovaries. Likewise, the definition of IH is becoming increasingly stricter, as many investigators and clinicians consider that IH patients should also have normal ovarian morphology on ultrasonography.

A few caveats should be considered when establishing the diagnoses of PCOS or IH. First, the definition of polycystic ovaries on ultrasonography is relatively strict, generally including the presence of greater than 12 follicles measuring 2–9 mm in diameter or an ovarian volume (obtained from three dimensional measurement) greater than 11 $cm^3$, in at least one ovary. Second, between 5–15% of hirsute patients evaluated may fall outside of the specific diagnoses and may present with hirsutism, and elevated androgen levels, but normal ovulatory function and ovarian morphology. Hence, our current classification of functional disorders of androgen excess (i.e., those in which specific disorders have been excluded) is still far from complete.

## QUESTION 4

*What are the therapeutic options for hirsutism available to this patient?*

## ANSWER 4

Certainly, if specific underlying disorders are identified (e.g., ASNs, hypothyroidism, hyperprolactinemia, and the like), the therapy should be targeted toward these disorders. Patients with PCOS and the HAIRAN syndrome will generally benefit from the use of oral contraceptive medications and/or insulin sensitizers for suppression of circulating androgen levels and the protection of the endometrium, while women with NCAH may benefit from low-dose corticosteroid therapy with or without an oral contraceptive.

The vast majority of hirsute patients, regardless of underlying etiology, will benefit from the use of systemic antiandrogen therapy, including the use of spironolactone, flutamide, cyproterone acetate (CPA) (not available in the United States), or less often, finasteride (Fig. 98-2). Spironolactone, CPA, and flutamide are medications that block the androgen receptor and reduce the overall effect of circulating androgens.

Spironolactone is an aldosterone antagonist and is FDA-approved as an antihypertensive agent. Consequently, side effects of spironolactone will include mild hypotension, polyuria and nocturia, fatigue, and rarely syncope. In addition, spironolactone may be associated with dyspepsia and hypersensitivity to the sun. Flutamide generally has fewer side effects than spironolactone, although it has been reported to rarely result in hepatotoxicity, occasionally fatal. Flutamide is approved by the U.S. food and Drug Administration (FDA) as an adjuvant for the treatment of prostatic carcinoma in men. Cyproterone acetate is not available in the United States, but has strong progestogenic and weak mineralocorticoid activities. While a popular oral contraceptive (Diane or Dianette, Schering AG, Berlin, Germany) containing 2 mg of cyproterone acetate is widely used, usually greater amounts of the CPA (20–80 mg/day) are needed for maximum suppression of hair growth.

Finasteride is an alpha-reductase inhibitor, decreasing the conversion of total testosterone to dihydrotestosterone (DHT) centrally and at the periphery. As DHT is the most potent endogenous androgen, finasteride decreases the overall endocrine and paracrine activity of androgens. Finasteride is somewhat less effective than the other antiandrogens available and potentially has a greater teratogenic potential if the patient were to conceive while taking these medications.

Because all of the antiandrogen medications may be teratogenic and because concomitant suppression of circulating androgens may be of additional therapeutic benefit, the vast majority of patients on antiandrogens are also placed on oral contraceptive medications.

On hormonal therapy, hair growth will begin to improve within 3–8 months following the initiation of antiandrogen therapy, and a maximum effect will generally be obtained at approximately 2 years.

In addition to hormonal medications, various cosmetic modalities are available for the treatment of these women and their use should be encouraged. The use of 13.9% eflornithine hydrochloride (Vaniqa, SkinMedica, Carlsbad, CA) applied topically to the face twice daily may help reduce excess hair growth in this area. Shaving or depilation may also be of value, depending on the degree of skin sensitivity. Waxing and plucking should generally be discouraged as they can cause significant folliculitis and scarring of the treated area. Electrolysis in experienced hands can result in significant decrease in offending hairs on a permanent basis, although treatment may take some time. Laser hair ablation is also available, although it is generally less permanent than electrology and may not be applicable to individuals with darker skin or lighter hairs.

Overall, the treatment of hair growth requires long-term follow-up, and many of these patients will require long-term emotional and/or psychological support. The presence of unwanted hair growth in a male-like pattern in women is distressing, and these patients experience a significant improvement in their quality of life with treatment.

## BIBLIOGRAPHY

Azziz R, Carmina E, Sawaya ME. Idiopathic hirsutism. *Endocrine Rev.* 2000;21:347–362.

Azziz R, Sanchez LA, Knochenhauer ES, Moran C, Lazenby J, Stephens KC, Taylor K, Boots LR. Androgen excess in women: experience with over 1000 consecutive patients. *J Clin Endocrinol Metab.* 2004;89(2):453–462.

Azziz R. The evaluation and management of hirsutism. *Obstet Gynecol.* 2003;101:995–1007.

Azziz R. The time has come to simplify the evaluation of the hirsute patient. *Fertil Steril.* 2000;74:870–872.

Moghetti P, Tosi F, Tosti A, Negri C, Misciali C, Perrone F, Caputo M, Muggeo M, Castello R. Comparison of spironolactone, flutamide, and finasteride. *J Clin Endocrinol Metab.* 2000;85:89–94.

Venturoli S, Marescalchi O, Colombo FM, Macrelli S, Ravaioli B, Bagnoli A, Paradisi R, Flamigni C. A prospective randomized trial comparing low dose flutamide, finasteride, ketoconazole, and cyproterone acetate-estrogen regimens in the treatment of hirsutism. *J Clin Endocrinol Metab.* 1999;84(4): 1304–1310.

# 99 21-HYDROXYLASE DEFICIENT NONCLASSIC ADRENAL HYPERPLASIA

*Ricardo Azziz*

## LEARNING POINT

To understand the prevalence, etiology, diagnosis, screening, and treatment of 21-hydroxylase (21-OH) deficient nonclassic adrenal hyperplasia (NCAH).

## VIGNETTE

A 24-year-old female presents to your office with the complaint of increasingly worsening unwanted hair growth, acne, and irregular menstruation. She states that her irregular menstruation developed at about the age of 15 years and she first noted excess hair growth when she was in high school. Family history is not revealing, although she states that she is of Ashkenazi Jewish descent. Currently she is not sexually active and is not taking any medications.

On examination, she is moderately overweight and has a mild degree of excess hair growth, particularly on the chin and the upper lip, consisting of sparse, coarse, dark hairs. She has inflammatory acne of the cheeks and upper back. Pelvic examination is normal. You obtain an androgen profile including total and free testosterone, dehydroepiandrosterone sulfate (DHEAS), as well as basal levels of 17-hydroxyprogesterone (17-HP), thyroid-stimulating hormone (TSH), and prolactin.

Upon her return visit, you review these tests with her, which indicate that the free testosterone is mildly elevated (0.81 ng/dL), as is the 17-HP (2.75 ng/ mL). All other blood tests are normal. You perform a transvaginal ultrasound, which demonstrates ovaries with many small cysts measuring 2–8 mm in diameter. A acute adrenocorticotropic hormone (ACTH) stimulation test is performed which reveals a peak (post stimulation) 17-HP level of 18.5 ng/mL.

### QUESTION 1

*What is the etiology of 21-OH deficient NCAH, its prevalence in hyperandrogenic women, and ethnic variation?*

### ANSWER 1

21-OH deficient NCAH is an autosomal recessive disorder, which affects approximately 1 in 1000 non-Jewish Caucasian individuals. The prevalence of NCAH among individuals with androgen excess ranges from about 1–10%, depending on ethnicity; in the United States it affects approximately 2% of hyperandrogenic women. It is higher in certain populations, including individuals who are of Ashkenazi Jewish descent.

NCAH results from mutations of the 21-OH gene (*CYP21A2*), which is located in the short arm of chromosome 6 within the HLA histocompatibility complex. A second gene, the inactive pseudogene (*CYP21A1P*), is generally similar to the 21-OH gene but contains a number of mutations that render it nonfunctional and lies in close proximity to the active *CYP21A2* gene. Most deleterious sequence changes present in the active gene occur due to the process of "gene conversion" whereby the active gene picks up abnormal sequences from the proximate pseudogene due to crossover events. Only 1–2% of all affected alleles occur due to spontaneous mutations. If both alleles of *CYP21A2* are mutated, then the resulting protein, after transcription and translation (i.e., the 21-OH enzyme, or P450C21) will also be abnormal or deficient. This then results in decreased functional capacity for 21-OH in these individuals.

Although the exact mechanisms are not clear in nonclassic patients, this deficiency in 21-OH activity results in an increased amount of precursor (17-HP and progesterone) production by the adrenal, although the production of cortisol (the eventual product of 21-OH activity) is maintained normally. In NCAH patients, evidence of overactivation of the hypothalamic-pituitary-adrenal axis (e.g., elevated levels of ACTH) is generally not found.

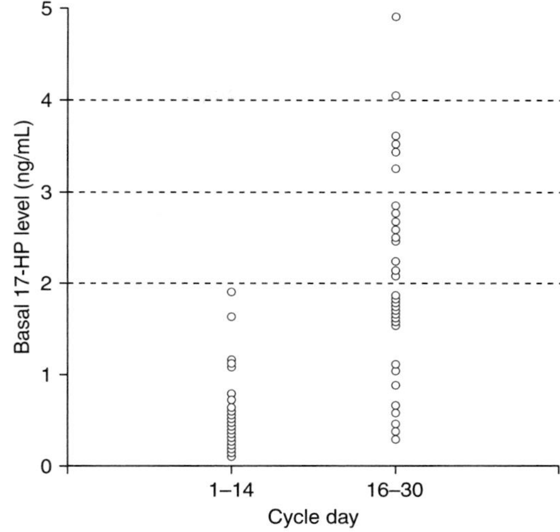


**FIG. 99-1** The variability of the basal 17-hydroxyprogesterone (17-HP) level over the menstrual cycle in eight healthy control women. Of the samples obtained on or before cycle day 14, no subject demonstrated a 17-HP level of ≥2 ng/mL; of those obtained on or after cycle day 16, about 50% of samples had a 17-HP level of >2 ng/mL. SOURCE: Reprinted with permission from Azziz R, et al. Screening for 21-hydroxylase-deficient nonclassic adrenal hyperplasia among hyperandrogenic women: a prospective study. *Fertil Steril.* 1999;72:915–925.

## QUESTION 2

*How do you screen for and diagnose NCAH?*

## ANSWER 2

A good dose of clinical suspicion is critical in selecting patients who may have this inherited disorder. Most frequently, patients will present with irregular menstruation and/or signs of androgen excess (e.g., hirsutism, acne, or androgenic alopecia). However, it is not possible to clinically distinguish women with NCAH from those with the polycystic ovary syndrome (PCOS) and other functional androgen excess disorders. Individuals who are at risk for having NCAH (e.g., those with hyperandrogenic signs or symptoms) can be screened for this disorder by measuring a basal 17-HP level. This hormone should be measured in the immediate postmenstrual period, or following a progestin-induced withdrawal bleed, as the corpus luteum will also produce 17-HP and could result in a false positive test result (Fig. 99-1). Although blood sampling should also preferably be obtained in the morning, this requirement is less critical.

A level of 17-HP of greater than 2 ng/mL (or 3 ng/mL if one does not mind missing a few patients with NCAH) can be used to identify those individuals most likely to have this disorder (Fig. 99-2); individuals whose screening 17-HP level is above this cutoff level should undergo an acute ACTH stimulation test. During the acute ACTH stimulation test, the level of 17-HP will be measured before and approximately 60 minutes after the IV administration of 0.25 mg of 1-24 ACTH (Cortrosyn, Organon, New Orange, NJ). A poststimulation level

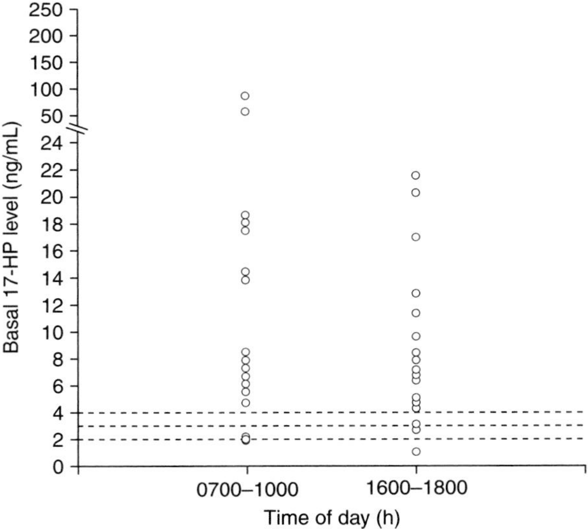


**FIG. 99-2** The basal 17-hydroxyprogesterone (17-HP) level in 20 patients with 21-hydroxylase–deficient nonclassic adrenal hyperplasia, obtained in the morning (7:00–10:00 A.M.) and in the afternoon (4:00–5:30 P.M.). All samples obtained in the morning had 17-HP levels of >2 ng/mL, and 18 of 20 had levels of >3. Of samples obtained in the afternoon, 19 and 18 had levels of >2 ng/mL or >3 ng/mL, respectively. SOURCE: Reprinted with permission from Azziz R, et al. Screening for 21-hydroxylase-deficient nonclassic adrenal hyperplasia among hyperandrogenic women: a prospective study. *Fertil Steril.* 1999;72:915–925.

of 17-HP of greater than 10–12 ng/mL is indicative of the disorder.

## QUESTION 3

*What are the clinical signs and symptoms of NCAH?*

## ANSWER 3

Patients with 21-OH deficient NCAH may occasionally be asymptomatic, although symptoms will generally develop over time in most individuals. Classic symptoms include irregular menstruation, excess hair growth (unwanted hair growth or hirsutism), acne, or androgenic alopecia (Table 99-1). Approximately 40% of these individuals may also demonstrate polycystic-appearing ovaries on ultrasound and could also demonstrate evidence of hyperplasia or nodularity of the adrenals on magnetic resonance imaging (MRI) or computerized tomography (CT) scan. Nonetheless, symptoms are generally mild to moderate, and these individuals cannot be clinically differentiated from patients with other functional androgen excess disorders (e.g., PCOS), hence the importance of the endocrine testing described.

## QUESTION 4

*What treatment options do patients with NCAH have?*

## ANSWER 4

In those patients who do not desire immediate fertility, treatment with replacement dose glucocorticoids can be offered, such as 0.25 mg dexamethasone daily or every other day, or 5–10 mg of prednisone daily. The minimum dose required to maintain the circulating androstenedione levels within the upper normal range (or even slightly above normal) should be used. Nonetheless, we should note that many patients do not tolerate corticosteroids due to development of cushingoid symptoms or weight gain.

Patients who are older (e.g., greater than 20 years of age) and have just been diagnosed with NCAH will often remain oligo-ovulatory despite corticosteroid administration, and will require the use of oral contraceptives for better regulation. Alternatively, patients with this disorder can be treated with oral contraceptives as their first-line agent, since these patients generally do not suffer from cortisol insufficiency, even under stress. Patients who are hirsute would also benefit from the addition of an antiandrogen, such as spironolactone or flutamide.

Patients with NCAH desiring fertility often conceive spontaneously, although up to 50% of these women may require assistance. While most respond quite well to the use of standard ovulation induction regimens such as clomiphene or gonadotropins, in some patients the persistence of elevated levels of 17-HP (and progesterone) of adrenocortical origin may become a problem. In a minority of patients with NCAH, the levels of 17-HP, and often progesterone, remain elevated despite adequate (or even supraphysiologic) doses of glucocorticoids. The exact etiology of this is unclear, but may relate to the persistence of hyperplasia of the adrenal and intrinsic alterations in intra-adrenal enzyme kinetics. In these individuals, the persistence of elevated levels of progestogens in the circulation results in a persistently suppressed and decidualized endometrium and a thickened cervical mucus, both of which can preclude fertility. In these rare patients, either the use of a gestational carrier, or even bilateral adrenalectomy, has been attempted.

**TABLE 99-1. Clinical Features Among 193 Patients with 21-Hydroxylase Deficient Nonclassic Adrenal Hyperplasia**

| FEATURE | PREVALENCE |
|---|---|
| Hirsutism | 114 (59%) |
| Oligomenorrhea | 104 (54%) |
| Acne | 64 (33%) |
| Infertility | 25 (13%) |
| Clitoromegaly | 19 (10%) |
| Alopecia | 15 (8%) |
| Primary amenorrhea | 6 (4%) |
| Premature pubarche | 7 (4%) |

All patients older than 19 years of age.
SOURCE: Adapted from Moran C, et al. 21-hydrolyxase-deficient nonclassic adrenal hyperplasia is a progressive disorder: a multicenter study. *Am J Obstet Gynecol.* 2000;183:1468–1474.

## BIBLIOGRAPHY

Azziz R, Dewailly D, Owerbach D. Clinical Review 56—nonclassic adrenal hyperplasia: current concepts. *J Clin Endocrinol Metab.* 1994;78:810–815.

Azziz R, Hincapie L, Knochenhauer E, Dewailly D, Fox L, Boots L. Screening for 21-hydroxylase-deficient nonclassic adrenal hyperplasia among hyperandrogenic women: a prospective study. *Fertil Steril.* 1999;72:915–925.

Moran C, Azziz R, Carmina E, Dewailly D, Fruzzetti F, Ibanez L, Knochenhauer E, Marcondes J, Mendonca B, Pignatelli D, Pugeat M, Rohmer V, Speiser P, Witchel S. 21-Hydroxylase-deficient nonclassic adrenal hyperplasia is a progressive disorder: a multicenter study. *Am J Obstet Gynecol.* 2000;183:1468–1474.

Speiser PW, White PC. Congenital adrenal hyperplasia. *N Engl J Med.* 2003;349:776–788.

# 100 POLYCYSTIC OVARY SYNDROME: INSULIN RESISTANCE AND USE OF INSULIN SENSITIZERS

*Ricardo Azziz*

## LEARNING POINT

To understand the role of insulin resistance and insulin sensitizers in the pathophysiology and treatment, respectively, of polycystic ovary syndrome (PCOS).

## VIGNETTE

A 32-year-old woman presents to your office with a history of PCOS, diagnosed by her generalist. The diagnosis was apparently based on her history as well as blood testing and ovarian sonography. She has read about insulin sensitizers on the internet and wonders whether this is something she should use.

### QUESTION 1

*What is the prevalence of insulin resistance in PCOS and how is it related to the pathophysiology of the disorder?*

### ANSWER 1

PCOS is a frequent disorder affecting approximately 6–7% of reproductive age women, whose prevalent features include hyperandrogenism and ovulatory dysfunction. However, as it is a heterogeneous disorder, some patients with PCOS may be ovulatory at times. Many of these women also have polycystic-appearing ovaries on ultrasonography. Insulin resistance, namely the deficient response of glucose and lipids to the effect of insulin, is present in 50–70% of all patients with PCOS. In young, healthy women with well-preserved beta-cell function, this results in secondary compensatory hyperinsulinemia. Insulin is a very potent hormone with multiple actions, including regulation of glucose and lipid metabolism, and cellular mitogenic effects.

As insulin also demonstrates gonadotropic properties, the hyperinsulinemia observed in insulin-resistant PCOS patients can result in excessive stimulation of androgen secretion by ovarian theca cells. Insulin, because of its mitogenic (growth-promoting) effect, can stimulate theca cell growth resulting in thecal hyperplasia and/or hyperthecosis.

In addition, insulin regulates the production of sex hormone-binding globulin (SHBG) by the liver; SHBG is the carrier protein for androgens and binds the vast majority of testosterone, among other androgens, in essence regulating the potential activity of androgens. As insulin levels increase in insulin-resistant PCOS patients, SHBG levels drop, increasing the fraction of circulating free testosterone, amplifying the cellular effect of this androgen. Overall, while insulin resistance and hyperinsulinemia are not universal features of PCOS, they are an important factor in the hyperandrogenism of many of these women.

### QUESTION 2

*What is the role of insulin sensitizers in improving fertility in patients with PCOS?*

### ANSWER 2

The use of insulin sensitizers, including the biguanide metformin, and the thiazolidinediones (TZDs) pioglitazone, rosiglitazone, and troglitazone, has been reported to improve ovulatory function in patients with PCOS. The vast majority of studies have examined the use of metformin. Data with TZDs is relatively more limited; the largest trial was carried out with troglitazone, which has since been withdrawn from the market secondary to hepatic complications in some of the patients. These drugs are approved by the U.S. Food and Drug Administration (FDA) for the treatment of diabetes. The beneficial effect of insulin sensitizers on ovulatory function appears to be mediated primarily through an improvement in insulin sensitivity and a decrease in insulin levels, resulting in decreased ovarian androgen production and increase SHBG levels. It is unclear whether insulin sensitizers and their associated insulin reduction also improve the pituitary secretion and regulation of gonadotropins.

In patients with PCOS desiring fertility, the use of metformin alone appears to be effective in improving ovulatory function, with results similar to that of clomiphene in some, but not all, studies (Fig. 100-1). However, clearer guidelines for the treatment of PCOS-related oligo-ovulatory infertility awaits the results of a large multicenter ongoing trial sponsored by the

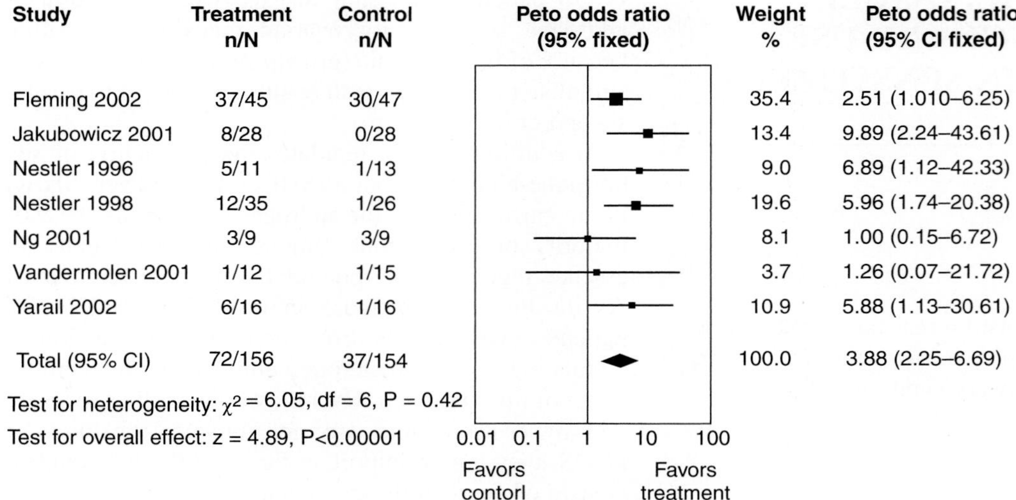


**FIG. 100-1** Meta-analysis of the ovulation rate following the use of metformin compared with placebo or no treatment.

SOURCE: Reprinted with permission from Lord JM, et al. Metformin in polycystic ovary syndrome: systematic review and meta-analysis. *BMJ.* 2003;327:951–953.

National Institutes of Health, which should address the question of whether metformin and clomiphene are equally effective as first-line agents for ovulation induction in PCOS.

Better demonstrated is the use of metformin in PCOS patients who are clomiphene-resistant (i.e., fail to ovulate following the administration of clomiphene citrate up to at least 150 mg/day for 5 days per cycle). The majority of studies suggest that up to 90% of patients who are clomiphene-resistant will ovulate with the addition of metformin and that up to 50% of patients who respond favorably will conceive (Fig. 100-2). In addition, anecdotal studies have suggested that metformin administration during early pregnancy may also decrease the rate of pregnancy loss in patients with PCOS who conceive, although this remains to be verified in prospective studies. The underlying mechanism for this improvement may lie in improved oocyte and ovulatory quality, improved endometrial receptivity, or a decreased detrimental effect of hyperinsulinemia on early pregnancy. While no early detrimental pregnancy effects of metformin have been demonstrated, the possibility that subsequent studies may reveal some mild teratogenic effect of this medication remains.

## QUESTION 3

*What is the role of insulin sensitizers in the long term care of patients with PCOS?*

## ANSWER 3

Although insulin sensitizers appear to improve ovulatory function and short-term fertility in patients with PCOS, less certain is the long-term impact of insulin sensitizers on the risk of metabolic complications in PCOS. Patients with PCOS are at five- to sevenfold greater risk for type 2 diabetes mellitus (DM). Patients with PCOS may also be at increased risk for cardiovascular complications, although only a small increased risk for cerebrovascular disease has been demonstrated to date. Currently there are no long-term data available on the effect of insulin sensitizers on the risk of metabolic complications in PCOS, and recommendations for the use of these drugs in PCOS patients is based on similar findings in other metabolically challenged populations (e.g., those with a family history of diabetes or who already demonstrate impaired glucose intolerance) in combination with the demonstration of a beneficial effect of insulin sensitizers on secondary markers (e.g., circulating levels of insulin, lipids, inflammatory products, or coagulation factors).

For example, in the diabetes prevention program (DPP) the use of metformin in individuals with glucose intolerance at risk for developing type 2 diabetes reduced the risk of developing diabetes within 3 years by 31%, although those subjects treated with lifestyle intervention only experienced a 58% reduction in this risk. We should note that while insulin resistance is an important predictive factor, incipient beta-cell failure

Comparison: Metformin combined with ovulation induction agent versus ovulation induction agent alone (clinical outcomes)
Outcome: Ovulation rate

| Study | Treatment n/N | Control n/N | Peto odds ratio (95% CI fixed) | Wight % | Peto odds ratio (95% CI fixed) |
|---|---|---|---|---|---|
| Polycystic ovary syndrome and clomifene sensitive | | | | | |
| Subtotal (95% CI) | 0/0 | 0/0 | | 0.0 | Not estimable |
| Test for heterogeneity: $\chi^2 = 0.0$, df = 0 | | | | | |
| Test for overall effect: z = 0.0, P = 1 | | | | | |
| Polycystic ovary syndrome and clomifene resistant | | | | | |
| Kocak 2002 | 21/27 | 4/28 | | 35.0 | 12.36 ( 4.32–35.39) |
| Malkawi 2002 | 11/16 | 3/12 | | 17.9 | 5.41 (1.24–23.51) |
| Subtotal (95% CI) | 32/43 | 7/40 | | 52.9 | 9.34 (3.97–21.97) |
| Test for heterogeneity: $\chi^2 = 0.80$, df = 1 p = 0.37 | | | | | |
| Test for overall effect: z = 5.12, P<0.00001 | | | | | |
| Polycystic ovary syndrome and clomifene sensitivity not defined | | | | | |
| El-Biely 2001 | 35/45 | 29/45 | | 47.1 | 1.90 (0.77–4.70) |
| Subtotal (95% CI) | 35/45 | 29/45 | | 47.1 | 1.90 (0.77–4.70) |
| Test for heterogeneity: $\chi^2 = 0.0$, df = 0 | | | | | |
| Test for overall effect: z = 1.39, P = 0.17 | | | | | |
| Total (95% CI) | 67/88 | 36/85 | | 100.0 | 4.41 (2.37–8.22) |
| Test for heterogeneity: $\chi^2 = 7.07$, df = 2 P = 0.029 | | | | | |
| Test for overall effect: z = 4.68, P<0.00001 | | | | | |



**FIG. 100-2** Meta-analysis of the ovulation rate following the use of metformin combined with clomiphene compared with clomiphene alone.
SOURCE: Reprinted with permission from Lord JM et al. Metformin in polycystic ovary syndrome: systematic review and meta-analysis. *BMJ.* 2003;327:951–953.

(i.e., glucose intolerance) is the most important predictor of the future risk of developing frank type 2 DM. Consequently, PCOS women who have a strong family history of diabetes, have developed gestational diabetes in the past, or have current glucose intolerance would probably benefit from the addition of metformin along with lifestyle modifications to their treatment regimen. Less certain is the use of metformin long-term in patients with PCOS who do not have evidence of beta-cell failure, albeit being insulin resistant, or even less so in those patients without measurable evidence of insulin resistance and/or hyperinsulinism.

## QUESTION 4

*What are the risks and side effects of insulin-sensitizing drugs?*

## ANSWER 4

There are two general classes of insulin-sensitizing drugs, the biguanides, of which metformin is the most commonly used, and the TZDs, of which pioglitazone and rosiglitazone are currently available in the United States. The use of metformin has been associated with lactic acidosis infrequently (~1/10,000 patients treated). This complication, however, has a 30% risk of death. More frequently, with metformin use between 5% and 15% of patients will develop gastrointestinal symptoms, principally intestinal cramping, diarrhea and loose stools, and, less frequently, dyspepsia. The incidence of this side effect can be minimized by increasing the dose of the medication slowly over a period of 4–6 weeks. Up to 30% of patients receiving metformin have also been reported to develop vitamin B12 deficiency. Patients treated with metformin also may experience some degree of weight loss, although the exact mechanism underlying this is unclear, although it does not appear to be associated with the development of gastrointestinal side effects.

The TZDs generally have less immediate side effects, although they are associated with the rare development of hepatotoxicity and possible liver failure (1/43,000 patients treated). Because TZDs are PPAR-gamma agonists, they may stimulate adipocyte differentiation and development and patients on therapy may experience a mild increase in weight.

Metformin is classified as a pregnancy category B drug, suggesting that there is no current evidence that it causes any significant problems if administered during pregnancy. Alternatively, TZDs are category C and currently should be used with caution in pregnancy.

## BIBILIOGRAPHY

Barbieri RL. Metformin for the treatment of polycystic ovary syndrome. *Obstet Gynecol.* 2003;101(4):785–793.

Costello MF, Eden JA. A systematic review of the reproductive system effects of metformin in patients with polycystic ovary syndrome. *Fertil Steril.* 2003;79(1):1–13.

De Leo V, la Marca A, Petraglia F. Insulin-lowering agents in the management of polycystic ovary syndrome. *Endocr Rev.* 2003;24(5):633–667.

Ehrmann DA. Polycystic ovary syndrome. *N Engl J Med.* 2005;352(12):1223–1236.

Knowler WC, Barrett-Connor E, Fowler SE, Hamman RF, Lachin JM, Walker EA, Nathan DM. Diabetes Prevention Program Research Group. Reduction in the incidence of type 2 diabetes with lifestyle intervention or metformin. *N Engl J Med.* 2002;346(6):393–403.

Lord JM, Flight IH, Norman RJ. Metformin in polycystic ovary syndrome: systematic review and meta-analysis. *BMJ.* 2003;327(7421):951–953.

Ovalle F, Azziz R. Insulin resistance, polycystic ovary syndrome, and type 2 diabetes mellitus. *Fertil Steril.* 2002;77(6): 1095–1105.

Palomba S, Orio F Jr, Falbo A, Manguso F, Russo T, Cascella T, Tolino A, Carmina E, Colao A, Zullo F. Prospective parallel randomized, double-blind, double-dummy controlled clinical trial comparing clomiphene citrate and metformin as the first-line treatment for ovulation induction in nonobese anovulatory women with polycystic ovary syndrome. *J Clin Endocrinol Metab.* 2005;90(7):4068–4074.

# 101 POLYCYSTIC OVARY SYNDROME: OVULATION INDUCTION

*Ashim Kumar*

## LEARNING POINT

To understand the indications for ovulation induction (OI) for patients with polycystic ovary syndrome (PCOS) and the risks associated with these treatments.

## VIGNETTE

A 27-year-old female, body mass index (BMI) of 34 kg/m$^2$, G0, presents with complaints of a 14-month history of primary infertility. She reports irregular menses every 2–3 months since menarche. She also reports excessive facial and abdominal hair. After excluding other etiologies, you diagnose PCOS. A hysterosalpingogram is obtained and reveals normal uterine contour and bilaterally patent tubes. Semen analysis on her partner is within normal limits.

### QUESTION 1

*What modalities are available to induce ovulation in women with PCOS?*

### ANSWER 1

Although a variety of modalities are available for the induction of ovulation in PCOS, see Table 101-1, initial management plan advocated by the physician should be weight loss (Fig. 101-1). Clomiphene citrate (CC) is advocated as the first line pharmacologic therapy due to a large amount of data indicating efficacy. Insulin-sensitizing agents such as metformin have been proposed as first line therapy, but there is insufficient data at this time to support its use.

### QUESTION 2

*What is the first line of therapy? What is the algorithm should this fail?*

**TABLE 101-1. Ovulation Induction Agents Usable in PCOS**

| AGENTS ACTING ON THE HPO AXIS | INSULIN–SENSITIZING REGIMENS | SELECTIVE ESTROGEN RECEPTOR MODULATORS (SERMs) |
|---|---|---|
| 1. Clomiphene citrate | 1. Metformin | 1. Tamoxifen |
| 2. Gonadotropins | 2. TZDs | 2. Clomiphene citrate |
| 3. Pulsatile GnRH | 3. Life style modifications | |
| **AROMATASE INHIBITORS** | | **SURGICAL** |
| 1. Letrozole | | 1. Ovarian drilling/diathermy |
| | | 2. Wedge resection |

HPO is hypothalamic-ovarian
TZDs is thiazolidinediones
GnRH is ganadotropine releasing hormone

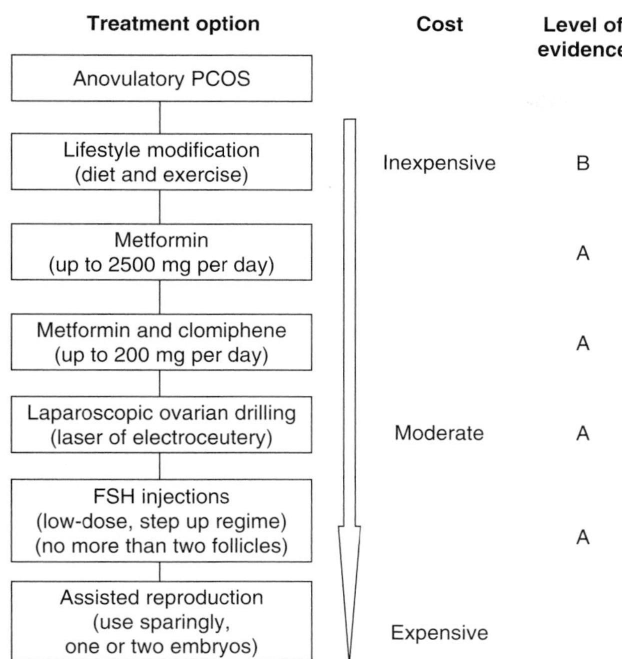


**FIG. 101-1** A cost-effective and evidence-based approach to the anovulatory woman with PCOS who is seeking to become pregnant. SOURCE: Norma RJ. (editorial) Metformin—comparison with other therapies in ovulation induction in polycystic ovary syndrome. *J Clin Endocrinol Metab.* 2004;89(10):4801–4809.

## ANSWER 2

Other selective estrogen receptor modulators (SERMs) have shown less or equivalent efficacy to CC for the treatment of infertility and may be used for specific circumstances (e.g., tamoxifen in a female with history of breast cancer). There is increasing evidence and support for the use of metformin (and possibly other insulin sensitizing agents) as first line of pharmacologic therapy in women; metformin may also play an important adjunctive role in women resistant to CC.

If the patient fails CC with or without metformin therapy, the next step in the algorithm should be gonadotropin administration (Fig. 101-1). Human menopausal gonadotropin (HMG) and recombinant follicle stimulating hormone (rFSH) are equally efficacious. There is a substantial risk of multiple gestations and ovarian hyperstimulation syndrome (OHSS), therefore close monitoring of the stimulation cycle is essential. Pulsatile GnRH is unavailable in the United States.

Ovarian drilling has fallen out of favor with the increasing success of ovulation medications, but it remains an option in women resistant to ovulation on medication regimens. Wedge resection is rarely done as it necessitates a laparotomy, and similar results are obtained with laparoscopic ovarian drilling/diathermy.

## QUESTION 3

*What risks are associated with gonadotropin use for OI in PCOS? How can this risk be minimized?*

## ANSWER 3

The principal risks of OI in PCOS are:

1. High order multiple gestation (HOMG)
2. OHSS

Close monitoring of follicle number (e.g., OHSS) and estradiol levels during stimulation is required to adequately assess the risk for HOMG and OHSS. The risk of both can be minimized by using dose (50 IU) gonadotrophin protocols in an attempt to induce monofollicular development. Withholding human chorionic gonadotropin (hCG) and cycle cancellation when high number of follicle are mature and/or elevated estradiol level is encountered is preferable to either HOMG or OHSS with their attendant risks to the patient.

## QUESTION 4

*What are the success rates for OI and live birth achieved for CC and gonadotrophin threapy?*

## ANSWER 4

Ovulation is achieved in approximately two-thirds of patients with CC (150 mg on CD 3-7) or metformin (1000 mg bid). Per cycle pregnancy rates are 5–10% for CC or cumulative pregnancy rates after 6 months of treatment is. The cumulative pregnancy rate after three cycles gonadotrophin is 45%.

## BIBLIOGRAPHY

Calaf Alsina J, Ruiz Balda JA, Romeu Sarrio A, Caballero Fernandez V, Cano Trigo I, Gomez Parga JL, Gonzalez Batres C, Rodriguez Escudero FJ. Ovulation induction with a starting dose of 50 IU of recombinant follicle stimulating hormone in WHO group II anovulatory women: the IO-50 study, a prospective, observational, multicentre, open trial. *BJOG.* 2003;110: 1072–1077.

Homburg R. The management of infertility associated with polycystic ovary syndrome. *Reprod Biol Endocrinol.* 2003;1(1):109.

Kashyap S, Wells GA, Rosenwaks Z. Insulin-sensitizing agents as primary therapy for patients with polycystic ovarian syndrome. *Hum Reprod.* 2004;19:2474–2483.

Lopez E, Gunby J, Daya S, Parrilla JJ, Abad L, Balasch J. Ovulation induction in women with polycystic ovary syndrome: randomized trial of clomiphene citrate versus low-dose recombinant

FSH as first line therapy. *Reprod Biomed Online.* 2004;9: 382–390.

Lord JM, Flight IH, Norman RJ. Metformin in polycystic ovary syndrome: systematic review and meta-analysis. *BMJ.* 2003; 327:951–953.

Nardo LG. Management of anovulatory infertility associated with polycystic ovary syndrome: tamoxifen citrate an effective alternative compound to clomiphene citrate. *Gynecol Endocrinol.* 2004;19:235–238.

Norman RJ. (editorial) Metformin—comparision with other therapies in ovulation induction in polycystic ovary syndrome. *J Clin Endocrinol Metab.* 2004;89(10):4801–4809.

Palomba S, Orio F Jr, Falbo A, Manguso F, Russo T, Cascella T, Tolino A, Carmina E, Colao A, Zullo F. Prospective parallel randomized double-blind double-dummy controlled clinical trial comparing clomiphene citrate and metformin as the first-line treatment for ovulation induction in non-obese anovulatory women with polycystic ovary syndrome. *J Clin Endocrinol Metab.* 2005; [Epub ahead of print].

Palomba S, Orio F Jr, Nardo LG, Falbo A, Russo T, Corea D, Doldo P, Lombardi G, Tolino A, Colao A, Zullo F. Metformin administration versus laparoscopic ovarian diathermy in clomiphene citrate-resistant women with polycystic ovary syndrome: a prospective parallel randomized double-blind placebo-controlled trial. *J Clin Endocrinol Metab.* 2004;89:4801–4809.

Yildiz BO, Chang W, Azziz R. Polycystic ovary syndrome and ovulation induction. *Minerva Ginecol.* 2003;55:425–439.

# 102 ASHERMAN'S SYNDROME

*Ashim Kumar*

## LEARNING POINT

Describe the clinical features of Asherman's syndrome, response to treatment, and possible pregnancy complications after treatment.

## VIGNETTE

A 28-year-old female, G1P0010, is referred for a 14-month history of infertility. She had one spontaneous abortion 16 months ago requiring dilation and curettage (D&C) due to retained productions of conception. Patient states that she has regular cycles but with minimal flow since her loss 16 months ago. Ovulation predictor kit revealed a luteinizing hormone (LH) surge on cycle day 11 on the previous cycle. Her partner has had two previous semen analysis; the results of both were normal. She reports that her hysterosalpingogram (HSG) revealed an intrauterine filling defect.

### QUESTION 1

*What are the presenting complaints and risk factors for Asherman's syndrome which should alert the physicians?*

### ANSWER 1

Presenting complaints:

1. Menstrual disorders including secondary amenorrhea or decreased menstrual volume after possible uterine insult (62%)
2. Infertility after possible uterine insult (43%)

Risk factors:

1. History of instrumentation of the uterus including D&C
   a. After recent pregnancy (e.g., for continued bleeding after delivery, or retained placental remnants)
   b. For septic abortion
   c. Repeat D&C for retained products of conception after first D&C
2. Uterine infection
   a. Endometritis
   b. Tuberculosis

### QUESTION 2

*What are diagnostic modalities available to diagnose Asherman's syndrome?*

### ANSWER 2

1. HSG—can concurrently diagnose tubal patency (see Fig. 102-1)
2. Sonohysterogram—easily performed office procedure with good sensitivity and specificity
3. Diagnostic office hysteroscopy—allows for direct visualization of uterine cavity
4. Magnetic resonance imaging (MRI)—may be useful in patients who failed attempts at cervical cannulation due to synechiae

### QUESTION 3

*What is the treatment of choice and resulting rates of success for amenorrhea and infertility?*

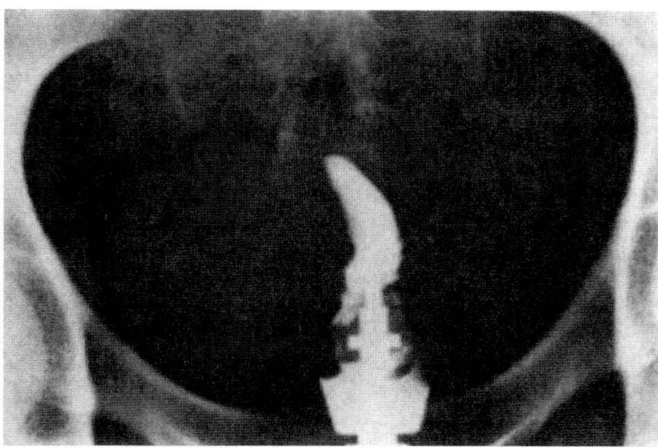

**FIG. 102-1** X-ray film of patient with Asherman syndrome. Patient (33 years, G3PO, abortus 3) had been amenorrhic for 6 months after D&C for most recent therapeutic abortion (TAB). Filling of endocervical canal and nonvisualization of endometrial cavity are consistent with complete obliteration of cavity by adhesions or with obstruction at internal os level by adhesions in lower endometrial cavity. This appearance may also be seen with advanced endometrial tuberculosis.
SOURCE: Reproduced with permission from Richmond JA. Hysterosalpingography. In: Daniel R. Mishell, Jr., Val Davajan, MD (eds.). *Infertility, Contraception and Reproductive Endocrinology*. 4th ed. Malden, Mass: Blackwell Scientific Publications; 1997.

## ANSWER 3

Hysteroscopic resection or ablation of the adhesions is the first line therapy for Asherman's syndrome. The bands can be excised by a variety of instruments including endoshears or electrocautery (resectoscope or bipolar), and laser. The adjunctive use of intrauterine contraceptive device (IUD), intrauterine Foley catheter, postoperative estrogen, and postoperative antibiotics are of uncertain utility except in those that have recurrent disease after previous adhesiolysis. Restoration of menses occurred in greater than 90% of patients. Live births were reported from 30% to 70% depending upon the degree of adhesion and the age of the patient.

## QUESTION 4

*What obstetrical complications are women previously treated for Asherman's syndrome at risk for?*

## ANSWER 4

1. Spontaneous abortion (early and midtrimester)
2. Preterm delivery
3. Placenta accreta with severe hemorrhage

## BIBLIOGRAPHY


Bacelar AC, Wilcock D, Powell M, Worthington BS. The value of MRI in the assessment of traumatic intra-uterine adhesions (Asherman's syndrome). *Clin Radiol.* 1995;50:80–83.

Capella-Allouc S, Morsad F, Rongieres-Bertrand C, Taylor S, Fernandez H. Hysteroscopic treatment of severe Asherman's syndrome and subsequent infertility. *Hum Reprod.* 1999;14: 1230–1233.

Jewelewicz R, Khalaf S, Neuwirth RS, Vande Wiele RL. Obstetric complications after treatment of intrauterine synechiae (Asherman's syndrome). *Obstet Gynecol.* 1976;47:701–705.

Klein SM, Garcia CR. Asherman's syndrome: a critique and current review. *Fertil Steril.* 1973;24:722–735.

Parker JD, Alvero RJ, Luterzo J, Segars JH, Armstrong AY. Assessment of resident competency in the performance of sonohysterography: does the level of training impact the accuracy? *Am J Obstet Gynecol.* 2004;191:582–586.

Sanfilippo JS, Fitzgerald MR, Badawy SZ, Nussbaum ML, Yussman MA. Asherman's syndrome. A comparison of therapeutic methods. *J Reprod Med.* 1982;27:328–330.

Schenker JG. Etiology of and therapeutic approach to synechia uteri. *Eur J Obstet Gynecol Reprod Biol.* 1999;65:109–113.

Westendorp IC, Ankum WM, Mol BW, Vonk J. Prevalence of Asherman's syndrome after secondary removal of placental remnants or a repeat curettage for incomplete abortion. *Hum Reprod.* 1998;13:3347–3350.

Zikopoulos KA, Kolibianakis EM, Platteau P, de Munck L, Tournaye H, Devroey P, Camus M. Live delivery rates in subfertile women with Asherman's syndrome after hysteroscopic adhesiolysis using the resectoscope or the versapoint system. *Reprod Biomed Online.* 2004;8:720–725.


# *103* CUSHING'S SYNDROME

*Ricardo Azziz*

## LEARNING POINT

To understand the screening and diagnostic evaluation of patients suspected of having Cushing's syndrome.

## VIGNETTE

An 18-year-old patient comes to your office complaining of progressive weight gain, abdominal and thigh stretch marks, and the development of irregular menses, occurring over the past 2 years. On evaluation, she has minimal excess hair growth, significant abdominal and centripetal obesity, and evident pink skin striae of the lower abdomen, posterior thighs, and upper arms. You are concerned that this patient may have Cushing's syndrome and proceed to coordinate her evaluation.

## QUESTION 1

*What is the prevalence and clinical features of Cushing's syndrome?*

## ANSWER 1

Cushing's syndrome refers to the clinical presentation of patients who experiences excessive glucocorticoid effect. It is a rare disorder occurring in approximately 1–2/1,000,000 individuals. The principal clinical signs and symptoms arise secondary to the excessive production of glucocorticoids, and include centripetal obesity (with the development of so-called "buffalo hump" to the posterior neck), muscle wasting and thinning of the extremities, osteopenia and osteoporosis, purple striae, easy bruisability, and moon facies with a distinctive reddish rubor of the cheeks (Table 103-1). These patients may also demonstrate glucose intolerance and hyperglycemia, hyperlipidemia (primarily of very low-density lipoproteins [VLDL], low-density lipoproteins [LDL], and total cholesterol and triglycerides), leukocytosis, and derangement of the hemostatic system. Patients may also present with cognitive deficits and psychological alterations, primarily depression, although a minority may present with euphoria, anxiety, and mania.

**TABLE 103-1. Signs and Symptoms in 302 Patients with Cushing's Syndrome**

| SIGN/SYMPTOM | FREQUENCY (%) |
|---|---|
| Truncal obesity | 96 |
| Facial fullness | 82 |
| Diabetes or glucose intolerance | 80 |
| Gonadal dysfunction | 74 |
| Hirsutism, acne | 72 |
| Hypertension | 68 |
| Muscle weakness | 64 |
| Skin atrophy and bruising | 62 |
| Mood disorders | 58 |
| Osteoporosis | 38 |
| Oedema | 18 |
| Polydipsia, polyuria | 10 |
| Fungal infections | 6 |

The mean age of the 239 female and 63 male patients included was 38.4 years (range 8–75 years).
SOURCE: Adapted from Boscaro M., et al. Cushing's syndrome. *Lancet.* 2001;357:783–791.

If the source of the excess glucocorticoids also produces excess mineralocorticoids (e.g., deoxycorticosterone and aldosterone), patients may also present with hypertension. If excess androgens are also produced, then affected women may present with hirsutism and acne. Irregular ovulation develops in a significant majority of patients with Cushing's syndrome, regardless of whether excess androgens are produced or not. We should note that gonadal dysfunction and hirsutism and acne are present in over 70% of patients with the disorder.

## QUESTION 2

*What is the differential diagnosis of Cushing's syndrome?*

## ANSWER 2

Cushing's syndrome can occur secondary to the excessive ingestion, of exogenous glucocorticoids. More commonly, it is secondary to the excessive production of endogenous glucocorticoids. The excess may result from a primary abnormality of the adrenal cortex i.e., adrenocorticotropic hormone (ACTH) independent, such as that due to adrenal adenomas or carcinomas (Table 103-2). Alternatively, excessive glucocorticoids may arise secondary to pituitary neoplasms or extra-adrenal tumor producing excess ACTH (i.e., ACTH or corticotrophin dependent). In essence, there are two general categories of disorders that result in Cushing's syndrome, ACTH dependent (e.g., pituitary or ectopic tumors) and independent (e.g., adrenocortical adenomas or carcinomas, or exogenous glucocorticoid ingestion). Finally, a few disorders may yield persistently abnormal screening tests for Cushing's syndrome, including obesity, depression, alcoholism, and HIV infection, termed "pseudo-Cushing's syndrome."

## QUESTION 3

*How is a patient suspected of having Cushing's syndrome evaluated?*

## ANSWER 3

The evaluation of Cushing's syndrome patients generally involves three steps. First, the presence of excess

**TABLE 103-2. Causes of Hypercortisolism and Cushing's Syndrome**

| |
|---|
| **Corticotropin dependent** |
| Pituitary-dependent Cushing's syndrome (Cushing's disease) |
| Ectopic corticotropin syndrome (bronchial, thymic, pancreatic carcinoids) |
| Ectopic CRH syndrome |
| Macronodular adrenal hyperplasia (autonomous) |
| Latrogenic: treatment with corticotropin or its analogues |
| **Corticotropin independent** |
| Adrenal adenoma |
| Adrenal carcinoma |
| Macronodular adrenal hyperplasia |
| Micronodular adrenal hyperplasia (including the Carney complex) |
| Adrenal hyperplasia caused by abnormal adrenal expression and function of receptors for various hormones (gastric inhibitory polypeptide, vasopressin, β-adrenergic agonists, interleukin 1) |
| **Pseudo-Cushing's syndrome** |
| Major depressive disorder |
| Alcoholism |

SOURCE: Adapted from Boscaro M., et al. Cushing's syndrome. *Lancet.* 2001;357:783–791.

glucocorticoid levels and action are confirmed, such that the patient is then known to actually have Cushing's syndrome (i.e., excess glucocorticoid effect). Second, the etiology of the excess glucocorticoids is elucidated, generally categorizing the disorders into ACTH-dependent and independent. Third, once the etiology of the disorder is established, the lesion, if one is present, must be localized to direct surgical treatment if necessary (Fig. 103-1).

The most common tests used to screen patients suspected of having Cushing's syndrome for hypercortisolism are the overnight dexamethasone suppression test, the 24-hour urinary free cortisol level, and the late evening cortisol level. The overnight dexamethasone suppression test is performed by administering 1.0 mg of dexamethasone at 11:00 P.M. and obtaining a cortisol level in the morning. If the cortisol level is less than 3.6 mcg/dL, there is a high probability that the patient does not have Cushing's syndrome. However, the false positive rate for this test can be as high as 30%, particularly in obese and depressed individuals. Alternatively, screening for excess glucocorticoids can be performed by measuring a 24-hour urine free cortisol level, which generally should be less than 100 mg/24 h. Again, the false positive rate can be significant, particularly in obese individuals. At times, patients may have intermittent glucocorticoid secretion, and up to three repeat

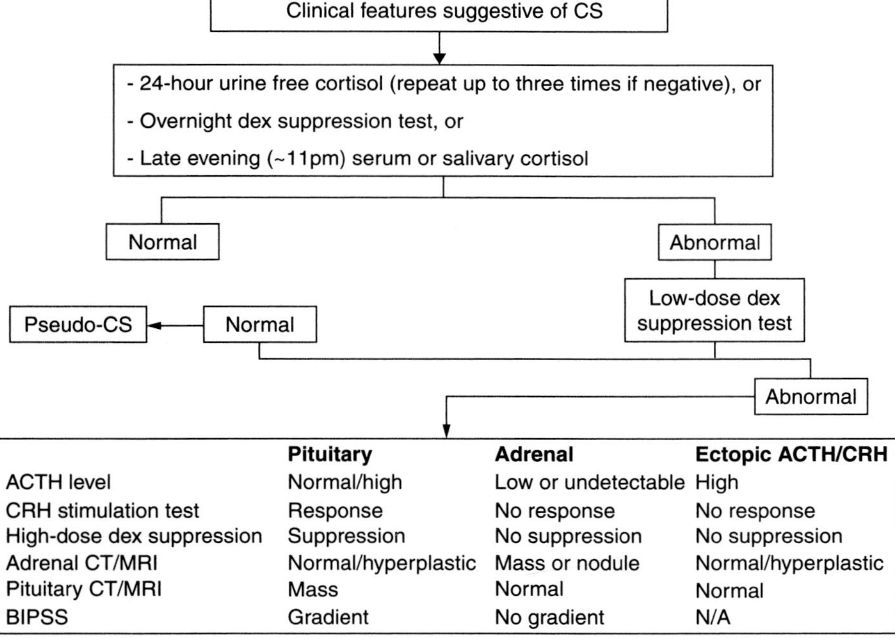


| | Pituitary | Adrenal | Ectopic ACTH/CRH |
|---|---|---|---|
| ACTH level | Normal/high | Low or undetectable | High |
| CRH stimulation test | Response | No response | No response |
| High-dose dex suppression | Suppression | No suppression | No suppression |
| Adrenal CT/MRI | Normal/hyperplastic | Mass or nodule | Normal/hyperplastic |
| Pituitary CT/MRI | Mass | Normal | Normal |
| BIPSS | Gradient | No gradient | N/A |

**FIG. 103-1** Algorithm denoting the evaluation of patients suspected of having Cushing's syndrome. Abbreviations: CS is Cushing's syndrome, Dex is dexamethasone, CRH is corticotrophin-releasing hormone, CT is computerized tomography, MRI is magnetic resonance imaging, and BIPSS is bilateral inferior petrosal sinus sampling. High-dose Dex suppression refers to the administration of 2 mg q. 6 hours for 24 hours, accompanied by the measurement of plasma or urinary cortisol levels.

SOURCE: Adapted from Boscaro M., et al. Cushing's syndrome. *Lancet.* 2001;357:783–791 and Arnaldi G, et al. Diagnosis and complications of cushing's syndrome: a consensus statement. *J Clin Endocrinol Metab.* 2003;88:5593–5602.

24-hour urine free cortisol measurements may be needed to detect the presence of excess glucocorticoid secretion, if the initial results are negative and clinical suspicion is high. The late night salivary cortisol level appears to be a promising new test for the screening of patients suspected of having Cushing's syndrome, and relies on the loss of the normal cortisol circadian rhythm.

If any of these tests is abnormal, then a more exact test to confirm the presence of excess glucocorticoids must be performed. Most clinicians prefer to use the low-dose dexamethasone suppression test. This is performed by administering 0.5 mg of dexamethasone every 6 hours for 48 hours, measuring the 24-hour urine free cortisol before and during the second day of suppression. Serum cortisol levels may also be obtained instead. Individuals who do not have Cushing's syndrome will have dexamethasone-suppressed 24-hour urine free cortisol or serum level that are either undetectable or very low (generally less than 10 mcg/24 h or 1.8 mcg/dL, respectively).

Individuals who persist in having elevated levels of urinary free cortisol in the face of a 2-day low-dose dexamethasone suppression test are now considered to have Cushing's syndrome. The evaluation of these patients for etiology or source generally requires referral to a medical endocrinologist. In brief, the circulating ACTH level is assessed, and if measurable or elevated, the source of the excess ACTH secretion (i.e., in the face of confirmed hypercortisolemia) will need to be located, generally using radiographic or invasive sampling methods. Alternatively, if ACTH is undetectable, the source of the excess glucocorticoids will also need to be radiographically localized, generally imaging the adrenal gland. An ectopic ACTH-producing tumor may at times be quite difficult to locate, as may be the identification of those patients who are ingesting large amounts of exogenous glucocorticoids.

## BIBLIOGRAPHY

Arnaldi G, Angeli A, Atkinson AB, Bertagna X, Cavagnini F, Chrousos GP, Fava GA, Findling JW, Gaillard RC, Grossman AB, Kola B, Lacroix A, Mancini T, Mantero F, Newell-Price J, Nieman LK, Sonino N, Vance ML, Giustina A, Boscaro M. Diagnosis and complications of Cushing's syndrome: a consensus statement. *J Clin Endocrinol Metab.* 2003;88: 5593–5602.

Boscaro M, Barzon L, Fallo F, Sonino N. Cushing's syndrome. *Lancet.* 2001;357:783–791.

Neiman LK. Diagnostic tests for Cushing's syndrome. *Ann NY Acad Sci.* 2002;970:112–118.

Raff H, Findling JW. A physiologic approach to diagnosis of the Cushing syndrome. *Ann Intern Med.* 2003;138:980–991.

# 104 GALACTORRHEA

*Shahin Ghadir*

## LEARNING POINT

To understand the differential diagnosis and workup of galactorrhea.

## VIGNETTE

A 28-year-old, G0, female presents to her gynecologist's office complaining of a milky fluid discharge from both of her breasts for the past month. She is currently sexually active and uses condoms. She does not desire fertility at this time. There is no family history of breast cancer or any other significant medical illness other than hypertension in her father. The patient denies any headaches and has no significant medical problems and denies any previous surgeries. The patient takes a multivitamin daily and has no known drug allergies. The patient also denies the use of tobacco, alcohol, or drugs. She states she has always had regular menstrual cycles every 28 days until 6 months ago. During the past 6 months she has had two normal menses and a few days of spotting last week. She denies any postcoital spotting.

The physical examination reveals a well-nutritioned, well-developed Caucasian female. Vital signs: blood pressure 122/76 mm Hg, pulse 81/min, respiratory rate 18/min, temperature 98.5°F, weight 143 lb, and height is 5 ft 7 in. Thyroid: no enlargement, no masses, lungs: clear to auscultation bilaterally, heart: regular rate and rhythm, no murmurs, abdomen: soft, nontender, no masses. Pelvic examination: external genitalia within normal limits, vagina well estrogenized, no vaginal discharge, normal cervix, uterus anteverted with normal shape and size, adnexa nontender, without palpable masses. Rectovaginal is negative with no masses.

### QUESTION 1

*What is the differential diagnosis of galactorrhea?*

### ANSWER 1

The differential diagnosis of galactorrhea are:

1. Pituitary tumor releasing prolactin.
2. Drugs that inhibit hypothalamic dopamine secretion, including phenothiazine derivatives, reserpine derivatives, amphetamines, and the like.
3. Hypothyroidism.
4. Excessive estrogen, including oral contraceptives, can cause milk secretion via the hypothalamic suppression that causes reduction of dopamine and the release of prolactin.
5. Intensive suckling of the nipples.
6. Stress, including trauma, surgical procedures, and anesthesia.
7. Hypothalamic lesions, stalk lesions, or stalk compression that reduce dopamine and cause excessive prolactin release.
8. Lung and renal tumors causing nonpituitary sources of increased prolactin.

### QUESTION 2

*What should be included in the workup of galactorrhea?*

### ANSWER 2

First, the patient should be excluded from being pregnant. Next, measurement of thyroid stimulating hormone (TSH) in order to rule out primary hypothyroidism and basal prolactin level should be obtained. A magnetic resonance imaging (MRI) to visualize the sella turcica is the best imaging test to diagnose macroadenomas.

### QUESTION 3

*What is the recommended method of treatment for galactorrhea as an isolated symptom of hypothalamic dysfunction in an otherwise healthy person?*

### ANSWER 3

There is no need to treat a patient that has had a negative workup for galactorrhea. If the patient has had periodic prolactin levels checked and all are within the normal limits, the galactorrhea does not need to be treated. However, if symptoms of galactorrhea are bothersome to the patient and there is a need to restore ovarian function and normalize cyclic estrogen production and ovulation, then dopamine agonists can be used.

### QUESTION 4

*What is a prolactinoma and what is the recommended long-term follow-up for microadenomas?*

### ANSWER 4

Prolactinomas are pituitary tumors that secrete prolactin. They are classified as microadenomas if they measure less than 10 mm in diameter. If they are greater than 10 mm in diameter then they are called macroadenomas. In the absence of any symptoms, microadenomas can be evaluated annually for 2 years. At that time a prolactin level and imaging of the sella turcica is recommended.

## BIBLIOGRAPHY

Davis, J. Prolactin and reproductive medicine. *Curr Opin Obstet Gynecol.* 2004;16:331–337.

Hwang PLH, Ng CSA, Cheong ST. Effect of oral contraceptives on serum prolactin: a longitudinal study of 126 normal premenopausal women. *Clin Endocrinol.* 1986;24:127.

Schlechte J. Prolactinoma. *N Engl J Med.* 2003;349:2035–2041.

Speroff L, Fritz MA. *Clinical Gynecologic Endocrinology and Infertility.* 7th ed., Philadelphia, PA: Lipincott Williams & Wilkins; 2005.

# *105* GONADAL DYSGENESIS: TURNER'S SYNDROME

*Ricardo Azziz*

## LEARNING POINT

The diagnosis, counseling, and reproductive prognosis of patients with Turner's syndrome.

## VIGNETTE

A 23-year-old female presents to your office complaining of infertility. Her pediatrician has previously diagnosed her as having "Turner's syndrome." The patient was started on estrogen replacement therapy some 7 years prior with satisfactory development of secondary sexual characteristics. She is sexually active, and she and her husband would like to proceed to have a child. On physical examination, the patient is 4 ft 9 in. in height, weighs 93 lb, has slight webbing of the neck, widely placed nipples, with small breasts Tanner Stage IV, and what appears to be normal pubic and axillary hair.

## QUESTION 1

*What is the epidemiology of Turner's syndrome?*

## ANSWER 1

Turner's (also known as Ullrich-Turner's) syndrome occurs in 1 in 2000 to 1 in 3000 live born girls. Since approximately 1–2% of 45,X female fetuses survive to term, this would raise the estimate of Turner's syndrome to as high as 1 in 20–50 pregnancies. Turner's also accounts for approximately 10% of all spontaneous miscarriages. It is estimated that there are approximately 75,000–80,000 girls and women with Turner's syndrome in the United States alone today.

## QUESTION 2

*How is Turner's syndrome suspected and diagnosed antenatally? Postnatally?*

## ANSWER 2

Antenatally, the diagnosis of Turner's syndrome can be suspected with the finding of generalized fetal edema on ultrasonography, with other ultrasonographic findings that are suggestive of Turner's syndrome including coarctation of the aorta and/or a left-sided cardiac defect, brachycephaly, renal anomalies, polyhydramnios or oligohydramnios, and growth retardation. Beta human chorionic gonadotropin ($\beta$-hCG) levels may be abnormal, as may be the triple or quadruple maternal serum screen (alpha-fetoprotein, $\beta$-hCG inhibin A, and unconjugated estriol). However, none of these features are diagnostic; rather they are suggestive, and diagnosis must be confirmed by karyotypic analysis. Diagnosis may often occur incidentally during prenatal diagnosis for advanced maternal age.

Postnatally, newborns may present with puffy hands or feet, or redundant nuchal skin, the residual effect of cystic hygromas in utero. Turner's syndrome should also be suspected in any newborn girls with generalized edema, those with evidence of a hypoplastic left heart or coarctation of the aorta. Alternatively, the diagnosis in many children is suspected only when they are evaluated for short stature and/or primary or even secondary amenorrhea, often with the lack of development of secondary sexual characteristics, although the phenotype can vary widely (Fig. 105-1). A karyotype in these patients is diagnostic.

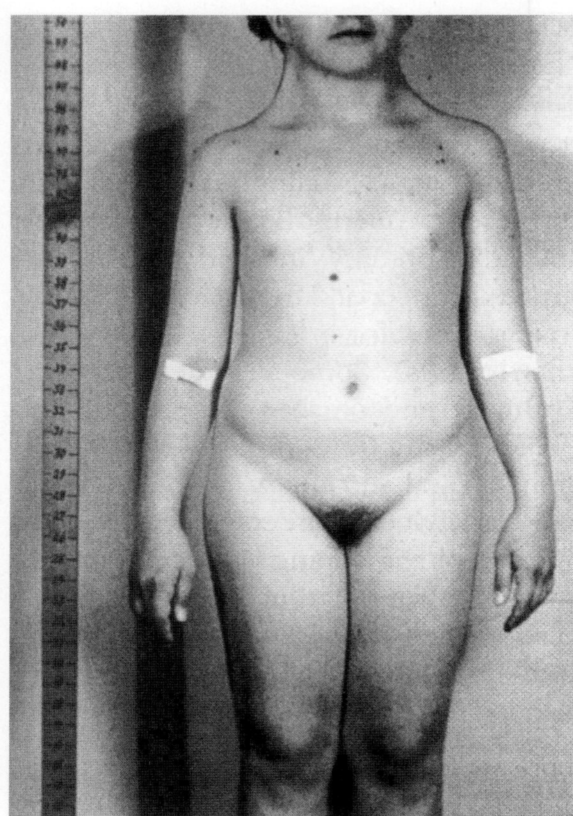

**FIG. 105-1** Patient with stigmata of Turner's syndrome, including short stature, sexual infantilism, webbed neck, and broadly spaced nipples.

SOURCE: From Carr BR. Disorders of the ovaries and female reproductive tract. In Wilson JD, Foster DW, Kronenberg HM, Larsen PR. (eds.). Williams' *Textbook of Endocrinology*. 9th ed., Saunders, Philadelphia, PA; W. B. Saunders; 1998:751–817, with permission.

## QUESTION 3

*What is the genetic defect in Turner's syndrome?*

## ANSWER 3

Approximately one-half of Turner's syndrome newborns will have monosomy X (45,X), approximately 40% will have mosaicism for 45,X, and the remainder will have a duplication (isochromosome) of the long arm of 1,X (46,X,i[Xq]). Both the short and long arms of the X chromosome contain genes important for ovarian function. In general, most Turner's syndrome features are due to reduced dosage of genes on the short arm of the X chromosome (Xp). The loss of interstitial or terminal material from the long arm of the X chromosome (Xq) have less obvious phenotypic implications, but can also result in short stature.

## QUESTION 4

*What are the long-term health risks of patients with Turner's syndrome?*

## ANSWER 4

Children and women with Turner's syndrome are at significant risk for cardiovascular abnormalities. In one study of 179 women with Turner's syndrome, 26% had a cardiovascular malformation, including 10% with aortic coarctation and 18% with aortic valve disease, most often a bicuspid aortic valve. All patients with Turner's syndrome should be evaluated cardiovascularly both by clinical examination and echocardiography, and those patients in whom coarctation of the aorta is discovered should have it corrected surgically. Patients with aortic valve abnormalities should receive antibiotics prophylactically to prevent endocarditis during any surgical or dental procedure.

Girls with Turner's syndrome have an increased incidence of renal abnormalities, including horseshoe kidney and duplication of the collecting system. These abnormalities may be found in up to 40% of affected girls. Ten percent of patients may develop silent hydronephrosis resulting from the obstruction of a duplicated collecting system. Consequently, screening renal ultrasonography and/or an intravenous pyelogram (IVP) should be performed in all patients with Turner's syndrome. Hypertension is common in patients with Turner's syndrome, even in the absence of cardiac or renal malformations, and its etiology remains unclear.

Turner's syndrome patients also suffer from a number of musculoskeletal abnormalities including skeletal dysplasia, with short stature, mild epiphyseal dysplasia, and other bony alternations. Malformation of the head of the ulna results in the typical increased carrying angle of the arm and may result in decreased range of motion. Congenital dislocation of the hip may occur in up to 5% of children, and 10% of adolescents with Turner's syndrome will develop scoliosis. An orthopaedic evaluation should be part of the regular examination.

Recombinant growth hormone therapy has been demonstrated to improve short stature in children with Turner's syndrome (particularly if therapy is begun before the age of 9 years) and should be initiated as soon as the patients begin to fall off their growth curve, even as early as the age of 2 years. For girls who are diagnosed late (i.e., between the ages of 9–12 years) the addition of anabolic steroids (e.g., oxandrolone 0.625 mg/kg/day) to GH therapy should be considered. Nonetheless, the virilizing effect of these agents should be taken into consideration.

Turner's syndrome patients often have a number of structural abnormalities of their inner ear, which results in recurrent otitis media and a hearing loss in between 50–90% of patients. Consequently, many of these children also have speech problems that require treatment and evaluation by an ear, nose, and throat (ENT) specialist, and a speech therapist.

Thyroid abnormalities occur relatively frequently in patients with Turner's syndrome, with hypothyroidism present in 15–30% of affected women. Consequently, the levels of TSH and T4 should be measured at regular intervals (e.g., every 1–2 years) beginning at birth, as up to 10% of hypothyroidism may present prior to adolescent.

While some patients with Turner's syndrome may actually present with limited ovulatory function, the vast majority will present with premature ovarian failure (POF). Consequently, these patients may be at increased risk for osteoporosis secondary to limited bone mass deposition during the critical years. They may also present with lack of secondary sexual characteristics, sexual infantilism, and streak gonads (Figs. 105-1 and 105-2). These individuals will benefit from exogenous hormonal therapy, which should be initiated using low dose unopposed estrogen (e.g., 0.3 mg of conjugated estrogens). After 6–9 months of this treatment, the dose will be increased gradually, with the addition of intermittent doses of cyclic progestins (e.g., medroxyprogesterone acetate, 5 mg 12–14 days every 2–3 months)

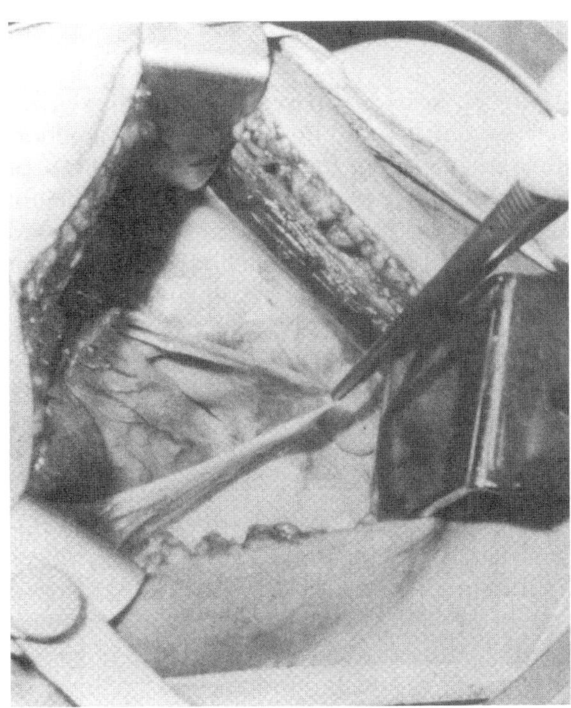

**FIG. 105-2** Streak ovary (held by forceps) seen at laparotomy in a patient with Turner's syndrome (gonadal dysgenesis).

beginning at 6 months of therapy. It should be stressed that estrogenization and development of the secondary sexual characteristics should occur slowly, in order to avoid the poor development of the breasts, resulting in small breasts with widely spaced nipples (the so-called "shield chest").

## QUESTION 5

*What are the reproductive options and obstetrical concerns in patients with Turner's syndrome?*

## ANSWER 5

Spontaneous fertility is rare among patients with Turner's syndrome and has primarily been reported in women with mosaicism, with a normal 46,XX cell lineage. Nonetheless, these women will have increased risks of spontaneous pregnancy loss or aneuploidy in the fetuses that are carried to term. Overall, the most important therapy for achieving fertility in patients with Turner's syndrome is donor oocyte in vitro fertilization.

It should be recognized that Turner's syndrome patients who conceive by oocyte donation would be at increased risk of cardiovascular complications during pregnancy. Approximately 2% of patients with Turner's syndrome will develop aortic dissection or rupture during pregnancy, and the risk of death during pregnancy is increased about 100-fold above normal. Women at the greatest risk for this complication include those exhibiting baseline and progressive aortic root dilation, although aortic dissection may occur in the absence of any of these signs. Prompt recognition of aortic dissection may provide the opportunity for successful surgical intervention in most, but not all, women.

As noted previously, all women with Turner's syndrome should be evaluated periodically for cardiovascular abnormalities, both clinically and by echocardiography, and by magnetic resonance imaging (MRI), if necessary. Women with Turner's syndrome during pregnancy should have their hypertension, if present, aggressively treated. Women in stable condition having an aortic root diameter of less than 4 cm may attempt vaginal delivery under epidural anesthesia; women exhibiting or progressive aortic root dilation should have an elective cesarean section performed prior to the onset of labor, also under epidural anesthesia. Careful monitoring of these patients will often result in a successful pregnancy outcome. Future interventions for the preservation of fertility in patients with Turner's syndrome include the cryopreservation of ovarian tissue containing immature follicles before the onset of premature ovarian failure, with subsequent in vitro maturation of oocytes. Nonetheless, currently these strategies should be considered experimental and should probably only be attempted in those individuals who are mosaic, with a normal 46,XX cell lineage.

## BIBLIOGRAPHY

Abir R, Fisch B, Nahum R, Orvieto R, Nitke S, Ben Rafael Z. Turner's syndrome and fertility: current status and possible putative prospects. *Hum Reprod Update.* 2001;7:603–610.

Bradshaw K, Carr BR. Disorders of puberty and amenorrhea. In: Carr BR, Blackwell RE, Azziz R. (eds.). *Essential Reproductive Medicine*. New York, NY: McGraw-Hill Co;2005:203–238.

Practice Committee, American Society for Reproductive Medicine. Increased maternal cardiovascular mortality associated with pregnancy in women with Turner syndrome. *Fertil Steril.* 2005; 83:1074–1075.

Saenger P, Wikland KA, Conway GS, Davenport M, Gravholt CH, Hintz R, Hovatta O, Hultcrantz M, Landin-Wilhelmsen K, Lin A, Lippe B, Pasquino AM, Ranke MB, Rosenfeld R, Silberbach M. Fifth International Symposium on Turner Syndrome. Recommendations for the diagnosis and management of Turner syndrome. *J Clin Endocrinol Metab.* 2001;86: 3061–3069.

Saenger P. Transition in Turner's syndrome. *Growth Horm IGF Res.* 2004;14 (Suppl. A):S72–S76.

Sybert VP, McCauley E. Turner's syndrome. *N Engl J Med.* 2004; 351:1227–1238.

# 106 HYPERPROLACTINEMIA

*Lee Kao*

## LEARNING POINTS

How to: evaluate for a potential pituitary adenoma, describe the management-treatment for hyperprolactinemia, and describe the long range management plan for medical treatment in hyperprolactinemia.

## VIGNETTE

A 44-year-old, G0, Caucasian female referred for issues of secondary amenorrhea for about 6 months after discontinuing her oral contraceptives presents to your office. On evaluation she was found to have elevated serum prolactin and a head magnetic resonance imaging (MRI) recently revealed a 1.3-cm pituitary tumor. The patient had been on oral contraceptive pills (OCPs) for about 20 years without any problem. During the past year she began to notice some increasing weight gain and breast enlargement, and occasionally she also noticed whitish discharge from her nipples. She also complains of occasional visual blurriness and difficulty sleeping and night sweats. She had discontinued her OCPs with no return of normal spontaneous cycles; subsequently she received Provera withdrawal two times and both failed to result in withdrawal bleeding. What would you do with her now?

## QUESTION 1

*Please describe how you can evaluate for a potential pituitary adenoma, and what are the limitations of the techniques uses. How common is pituitary adenoma and what if you don't find it?*

## ANSWER 1

After other common causes have been excluded, (hyperthyroidism, local breast lesions, use of neuroleptoc drugs) patients with persistent hyperprolactinemia should be investigated for structural pathology of the pituitary/hypothalamus. Clinical examination should include assessment of visual fields as the optic chiasm may be damaged by local mass effect. Direct confrontation visual field testing is important, but may miss subtle defects that should be assessed by formal ophthalmological examination. Pituitary imaging is usually undertaken by MRI or computed tomography (CT). Possible structural abnormalities include: pituitary microadenoma (<10 mm diameter), pituitary macroadenoma (>10 mm diameter, with possible suprasellar invasion, and optic chiasm compression), pituitary stalk lesions, and hypothalamic tumors, granulomas, or other lesions.

MRI produces excellent resolution and displays the optic chiasm and carotid arteries with greater clarity than CT, and can display in both sagittal and coronal formats. CT is helpful when thin slice images are used, and may be necessary in patients known to have intracranial ferromagnetic material, or in occasional highly claustrophobic patients. As repeat scanning is often necessary, care should be taken to avoid excessive exposure of the eyes.

Small pituitary adenomas are picked up with increasing frequency, as sensitivity and resolution increase with the advance of technologies. It is important to remember that such microadenomas may or may not be the reason for the endocrine abnormality. Pituitary microadenomas are found in approximately 20% of the normal population at autopsy, and MRI may reveal possible microadenoma in as many as 50% of cases. On the other hand, some patients with sustained hyperprolactinaemia have no demonstrable lesion even on high-resolution scanning, suggesting either that they harbor a microadenoma less than 2 mm in diameter, or that they have lactotroph hyperplasia, or nontumoral hyperprolactinemia.

## QUESTION 2

*Please describe the management-treatment for hyperprolactinemia.*

## ANSWER 2

The goal of treatment is to restore ovarian function, normalizing both cyclical estrogen production and ovulation, and to suppress abnormal lactation. In patients with prolactinomas, tumor shrinkage may also be an important goal. Treatment for idiopathic hyperprolactinemia has become very similar to that of pituitary prolactinoma.

The management options of pituitary adenomas in general are a medical, surgical, or radiation therapy. In the case of prolactinoma, medical treatment has become so effective and other modalities are now rarely used. Prolactinomas respond dramatically to dopamine agonists, with both the suppression of the abnormal hormone secretion and often dramatic shrinkage of the pituitary mass. Surgical treatment though holds the potential for long-term cure and avoid prolonged medication has yielded relatively poor results for long-term remission of hyperprolactinemia. Surgery now plays a limited role in the management of prolactinoma, unless there is excellent local surgical expertise, or there are resistant mass requiring debulking. External beam radiotherapy plays a very limited part in the management of prolactinoma.

Patients with prolonged hyperprolactinemia may suffer long periods of amenorrhea and hypoestrogenism, and may have considerable reductions in bone mineral density. Protection against the development of osteoporosis therefore is an important facet of the treatment of these women, even if they do not require treatment for other symptoms. Alternatively, women with modest elevations of serum prolactin may retain normal ovarian function and have few symptoms, and they may not require any specific treatment at all. It should be noted that prolactinomas are often indolent over many years, with little if any progression when left untreated, and sometimes they even undergo spontaneous resolution.

Dopamine D2-receptor agonists have demonstrated remarkable success in 80–90% of patients in achieving prolactin suppression and tumor shrinkage. Even in large macroadenomas, approximately 80% of patients can achieve tumor shrinkage by at least 25% of volume. Tumor shrinkage can be extremely rapid, with an improvement in pressure symptoms within 48 hours, although further substantial shrinkage may continue for many months. The restoration of ovarian function occurs in almost 90% of women, although in male patients testicular function is less successful and up to 50% may require testosterone replacement despite an apparently adequate suppression of prolactin. Three dopamine agonist drugs have been licensed for use in the United Kingdom, namely bromocriptine, cabergoline, and quinagolide. In United States, instead of quinagolide, pergolide has been used from time to time.

Bromocriptine was the first dopamine agonist drug introduced, and is still widely used. It is often given two to three times a day and is given with food to avoid the very common side-effect of nausea. Other common side-effects include postural hypotension and dizziness, headache, and constipation. Psychosis is rare, but milder depression may be quite common. With similar efficacy in both prolactin suppression and tumor shrinkage, but fewer adverse reactions than bromocriptine, cabergoline, and quinagolide/pergolide, are now widely used as first choice. Cabergoline has a long action, and is usually given once or twice a week; quinagolide is given as a single daily dose. However, it is still recommended to start treatment with low doses and build up to the dose gradually, to avoid nausea and postural dizziness. In general, patients are maintained on the minimum effective dose that will allow the restoration of ovarian function and the suppression of galactorrhoea. Women starting treatment with dopamine agonists should be warned to expect the restoration of ovulatory cycles within weeks. Those who do not wish to become pregnant should take contraceptive precautions.

### QUESTION 3

*Please describe the long range management plan for medical treatment in hyperprolactinemia. Can you withdraw treatment, and what are the recurrence rates?*

### ANSWER 3

Long-term follow-up studies of untreated patients have demonstrated that prolactinomas are very indolent, with little evidence of progression over many years. In addition, some patients adequately treated with dopamine agonists and later stopped treatment appeared to have gone into remission without recurrent hyperprolactinemia. As some prolactinomas are known to shrink to disappearance, it may be that dopamine agonists are able to exert a more permanent tumor-killing effect than was originally thought. A recent prospective study following the outcome of withdrawing cabergoline therapy in patients with either no visible tumor or small tumor remnants while on treatment, indicated recurrence rates of only 24% for nontumoral hyperprolactinemia, 31% for microprolactinomas, and 36% for macroadenomas, over a 2–5-year period. Longer follow-up would clearly be important, but these results do seem to indicate the possibility of the permanent remission of pituitary disease, and should prompt trial cessation of therapy in most patients who have achieved a period of satisfactory endocrine and radiological control.

## BIBLIOGRAPHY

Colao A, Di Sarno A, Cappabianca P, Di Somma C, Pivonello R, Lombardi G. Withdrawal of long-term cabergoline therapy for tumoral and nontumoral hyperprolactinemia. *N Engl J Med.* 2003;349:2023–2033.

Julian RE, Davis. Prolactin and reproductive medicine. *Curr Opini Obstet Gynecol.* 2004;16:331–337.

Schlechte JA. Clinical practice. Prolactinoma. *N Engl J Med.* 2003;349:2035–2041.

# 107 IN VITRO FERTILIZATION

*Margareta D. Pisarska*

## LEARNING POINT

In vitro fertilization (IVF) is a form of assisted reproductive technologies (ARTs), and is utilized for various causes of infertility.

## VIGNETTE

A 32-year-old, G0P0, comes in to seek information regarding fertility. She states that she and her husband have been actively trying to get pregnant for the past 6 months, having intercourse around the time of ovulation. Prior to this time they have not used any birth control and they never got pregnant. She has tested for ovulation and ovulates on a monthly basis. Additional workup has not been performed.

Gynecologic history: Menarche at age 14 years, cycles every 28–30 days with 4–5 days flow.
No history of fibroids or ovarian cysts. She states she had chlamydia at the age of 21 but was treated with antibiotics.
Obstetrics history: negative.
Medical history and surgical history is negative.
Social history: She does not smoke, drink alcohol, or use illicit drugs. She is not taking any medications and has no allergies to medications. She has two older sisters, both of them have two children each and did not have any problems with fertility.

Her partner is a 33-year-old male who has not fathered any children. He does not have any medical problems or surgeries. He does not take any medications and does not have any allergies to medications. He does not smoke, drink alcohol, or use illicit drugs. His family history is noncontributory.

Physical examination reveals a healthy appearing female. Vital signs: blood pressure 110/70 mm Hg, pulse 80/min, respiratory rate 18/min, and temperature 98.6°F. Thyroid: nonpalpable, lungs: clear, heart: regular rate and rhythm without audible murmurs. Abdomen: normal bowel sounds, soft, nontender, no palpable masses. Pelvic examination: normal external genitalia, cervix multiparous, no lesions, uterus anteverted normal size, adnexa nontender, no masses bilaterally. Rectovaginal confirms.

Hysterosalpingogram: normal uterine cavity, right fallopian tube is blocked at the isthmus and the left fallopian tube is occluded at the distal end.

Semen analysis: count 40 million/mL, motility 70%, morphology 70% (World Health Organization criteria).

## QUESTION 1

*What is ART?*

## ANSWER 1

ART includes all fertility treatments in which both eggs and sperm are handled. ART procedures involve removing eggs from a woman's ovaries, combining them with sperm in the laboratory. Subsequently, the gametes are returned to the female partner. Gametes can either be replaced in the fallopian tube, fertilized in the laboratory and the resultant embryos can be placed either in the fallopian tube or more commonly, replaced in the uterus. ART does not include treatments in which only sperm is handled or involving procedures that involve stimulation of ovaries without the intention of oocyte retrieval.

There are a number of different types of ART, including:

IVF: Oocytes are retrieved, most commonly through a transvaginal approach. The oocytes are fertilized in the laboratory with sperm. In certain circumstances, fertilization can be performed using a technique known as intracytoplasmic sperm injection (ICSI). In ICSI, a single sperm is injected directly into the oocyte and minimizes the amount of sperm needed for fertilization. A number of embryos that develop are selected and transferred into the uterus through the cervix.
Gamete intrafallopian transfer (GIFT): GIFT involves laparoscopic transfer of unfertilized oocytes and sperm (gametes) into the woman's fallopian tubes.
Zygote intrafallopian transfer (ZIFT): ZIFT involves fertilizing oocytes in the laboratory and the fertilized eggs (zygotes) are transferred into the fallopian tubes using a laparoscope.

## QUESTION 2

What are the causes of infertility among couples who use IVF?

## ANSWER 2

There are various different indications for the use of IVF. IVF was originally intended for utilization in women who had tubal damage as a result of scarring from sexually transmitted diseases, pelvic surgery, or endometriosis. Today IVF is utilized for various other causes. In addition, many couples who undergo IVF may have more than one factor affecting fertility. The various different causes for couples presenting to IVF centers in the United States are outlined and defined below:

1. Tubal factor: In women who have scarring as a result of sexually transmitted diseases, pelvic surgery, or endometriosis, fertilization of the oocyte by sperm as well as transport of the embryo to the uterine cavity is affected.
2. Ovulatory dysfunction: There are various different causes of ovulatory dysfunction, including polycystic ovary syndrome, hyperprolactinemia, pituitary, and hypothalamic causes.
3. Diminished ovarian reserve: Diminished ovarian reserve is a term used to describe diminished number and quality of oocytes that are produced by a woman.

Most commonly, this occurs as a function of age, however congenital, medical, or surgical causes can also contribute to diminished ovarian reserve.

4. Endometriosis: Endometriosis involves the presence of tissue similar to the uterine lining to be present in abnormal locations throughout the peritoneal cavity. Decreased fecundity is present in women with endometriosis. This may be due in part to the scarring that develops as a result of endometriosis.
5. Uterine factor: Uterine factors are any structural or functional disorder of the uterus that results in reduced fertility.
6. Male factor: Male factor refers to a low sperm count or problems with sperm function that make it difficult for sperm to fertilize an oocyte.
7. Unexplained: Unexplained infertility is defined when no other causes of infertility has been identified. This affects approximately 15% of couples seeking fertility treatment (Fig. 107-1).

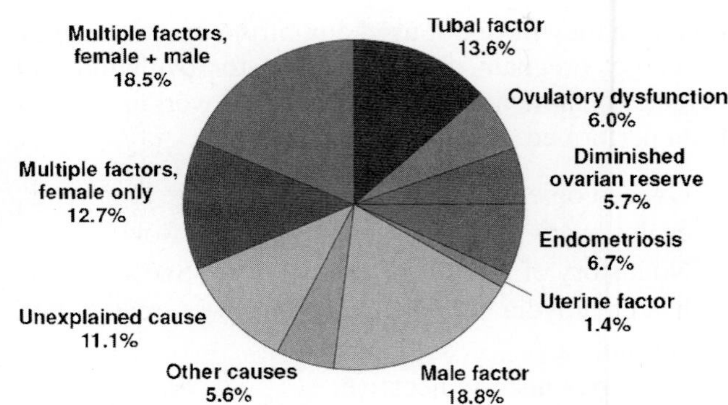


**FIG. 107-1** Diagnoses among couples who had ART cycles using fresh nondonor eggs or embryos, 2002.
SOURCE: From Centers for Disease Control and Prevention, American Society for Reproductive Medicine, Society for Assisted Reproductive Technology, and RESOLVE 2002. *Assisted Reproductive Technology Success Rates*. Atlanta, GA: Centers for Disease Control and Prevention; 2004.

## QUESTION 3

*Does the cause of infertility affect the chances of success using ART?*

## ANSWER 3

In general, couples diagnosed with tubal factor, ovulatory dysfunction, endometriosis, male factor, or unexplained infertility have the best success rates. The lowest success rates are in women with diminished ovarian reserve. In addition, couples with uterine factor, *other* causes, or multiple infertility factors have decreased success rates. (Fig. 107-2).

Age alone also plays a very important and independent role in success rates of IVF. Overall, 37% of cycles started in 2002 among women younger than 35 resulted in live births. This percentage decreased to 31% among women 35–37 years of age, 21% among women 38–40,

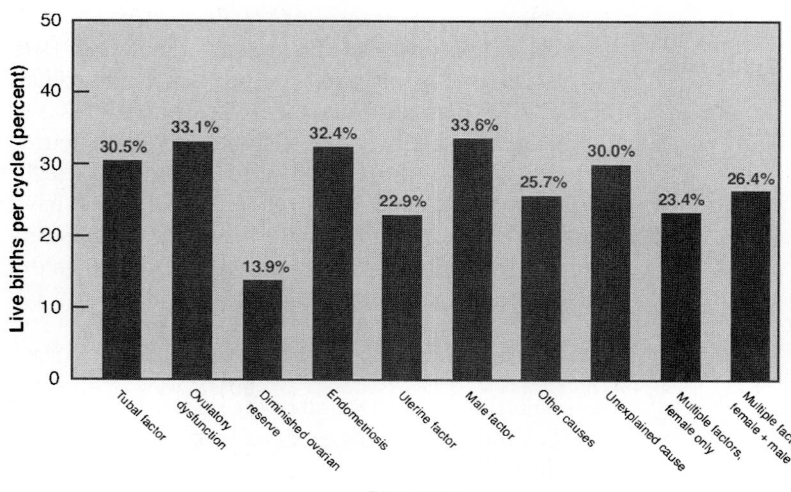


**FIG. 107-2** Live birth rates among women who had ART cycles using fresh nondonor eggs or embryos, by diagnosis, 2002.
SOURCE: From Centers for Disease Control and Prevention, American Society for Reproductive Medicine, Society for Assisted Reproductive Technology, and RESOLVE 2002. *Assisted Reproductive Technology Success Rates*. Atlanta, GA: Centers for Disease Control and Prevention;2004.

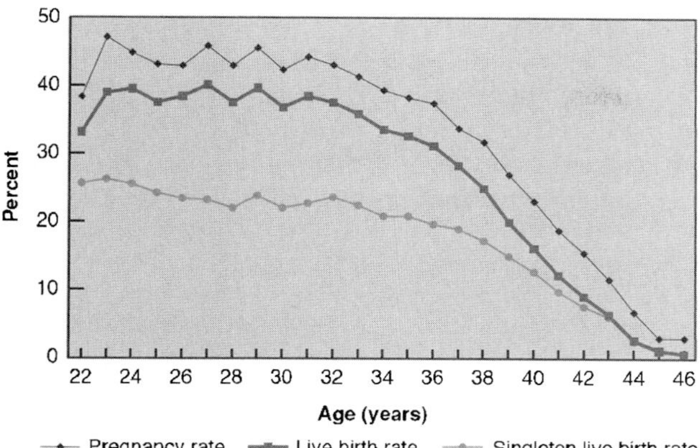


**FIG. 107-3** Pregnancy rates, live birth rates, and singleton live birth rates for ART cycles using fresh nondonor eggs or embryos, by age of woman, 2002.
SOURCE: From Centers for Disease Control and Prevention, American Society for Reproductive Medicine, Society for Assisted Reproductive Technology, and RESOLVE 2002. *Assisted Reproductive Technology Success Rates*. Atlanta, GA: Centers for Disease Control and Prevention;2004.

11% among women 41–42, and 4% among women older than 42. As noted in Figure 107-3, the proportion of cycles that resulted in singleton live births is even lower for each age group.

## BIBLIOGRAPHY

Carr BR, Blackwell RE, Azziz R. Essential reproductive medicine. Assisted reproductive technology. *Clin Aspects.* 2005;22:535–560.

Centers for Disease Control and Prevention, American Society for Reproductive Medicine, Society for Assisted Reproductive Technology, and RESOLVE 2002. *Assisted Reproductive Technology Success Rates.* Atlanta, GA: Centers for Disease Control and Prevention;2004.

# *108* ENDOMETRIOSIS AND INFERTILITY

*Lee Kao*

## LEARNING POINTS

To understand the diagnosis modality for endometriosis, and staging system; describe the benefit, or the lack of, by hormonal therapy only, for minimal/mild endometriosis patients suffering from infertility; and describe the benefit, or the lack of, by surgical therapy only, for minimal/mild endometriosis patients suffering from infertility.

## VIGNETTE

This is a 37-year-old Caucasian female presenting for primary infertility and also with complaints of history of pelvic endometriosis. In 1997 the patient was found to have pelvic endometriosis and underwent diagnostic laparoscopy along with ovarian endometrioma cystectomy of the right ovary done in Massachusetts. The patient relocated to California in 2001 and she subsequently married and is now returning to pursue her fertility issues. On pelvic examination and ultrasound evaluation, she again is found to have bilateral large ovarian cysts consistent with recurrent endometriomas.

### QUESTION 1

*Please describe the diagnostic modality and staging system for endometriosis.*

### ANSWER 1

The current opinion is that a surgical procedure such as laparoscopy is required for definitive diagnosis of endometriosis. Endometriosis is a heterogeneous disease with typical and atypical morphology and spanning a spectrum from a single 1-mm peritoneal implant to 10-cm endometriomas with cul-de-sac obliteration. A history and physical examination can yield a number of significant findings, including affected first degree relatives, chronic pelvic pain and dysmenorrhea, retroverted uterus, adnexal masses, cul-de-sac nodularity, and uterosacral ligament thickening and tenderness, but none is diagnostic. Ultrasound can help the clinician establish a presumptive diagnosis of ovarian involvement with endometriosis, but laparoscopy is necessary to confirm the diagnosis.

A clinical staging system is necessary to allow effective communication regarding prognosis and treatment. The American Society for Reproductive Medicine revised classification system for endometriosis (ASRM 1996) remains the most widely accepted staging system. Unfortunately, it does not correlate well with a woman's chance of conception following therapy. This poor predictive ability is related to the arbitrary assignment of a point score for the observed pathology and the arbitrary cut-off points chosen to establish the stage of disease.

## QUESTION 2

*In minimal/mild endometriosis patients suffering from infertility, please describe the benefit, or the lack of, by treatment with only hormonal therapy, and can you describe the strength of evidence of the studies?*

## ANSWER 2

The hypotheses behind how endometriosis causes infertility or a decrease in fecundity remain controversial. Whereas there is a reasonable body of evidence to demonstrate an association between endometriosis and infertility, a cause and effect relationship has not been established.

Medical therapy is effective in relieving pain associated with endometriosis, and many of these have been suggested for infertility treatment (e.g., danazol, gonadotropin-releasing hormone agonists [GnRH-a] and antagonists, progestins, and combined estrogen-progestin therapy). But there is no evidence that medical treatment of endometriosis improves fecundity. Several randomized control trials (RCTs) have demonstrated that danazol, progestins or GnRH-a, are not effective for minimal/mild endometriosis associated infertility.

*Danazol:* In two RCTs involving 105 infertile women with minimal to mild endometriosis, pregnancy rates were no better with danazol than expectant management.

*GnRH-a:* In an RCT involving 71 infertile women with minimal to mild endometriosis, the 1- and 2-year cumulative pregnancy rates were similar in the groups receiving GnRH-a treatment (6 months) or expectant management.

*Progestin:* In a small RCT involving 37 infertile women with minimal to mild endometriosis treated with progestins or expectant management, pregnancy rates were similar at 1 year in both groups. Also, in a small RCT involving 31 women, pregnancy rates with progestins and expectant management were 41% and 43%, respectively.

In a meta-analysis that included seven studies comparing medical treatment to no treatment or placebo, the common odds ratio for pregnancy was 0.85 (95% confidence interval [CI] 0.95, 1.22).

## QUESTION 3

*In minimal/mild endometriosis patients suffering from infertility, please describe the benefit, or the lack of, by treatment with only surgical therapy, and can you describe the strength of evidence of the studies?*

## ANSWER 3

Two RCTs have reported on the effectiveness of laparoscopic surgery for Stage I or II endometriosis associated with infertility. Both studies permitted surgical discretion in the intervention regarding excision or ablation. The primary outcomes were slightly different: the Italian study analyzed pregnancies, which occurred within 1 year after laparoscopy and proceeded to live births and the Canadian study analyzed pregnancies which occurred within 36 weeks after laparoscopy and proceeded to 20 weeks gestation, an endpoint which is nearly identical to the live birth rate.

In the Italian study, 10/51 (20%) of the ablation/resection, and 10/45 (22%) of the no treatment patients, were successful. In the Canadian study, 50/172 (29%) and 29/169 (17%) of the ablation/resection and no treatment patients, respectively, were successful. The baseline untreated rates were 22% in 52 weeks and 17% in 36 weeks, respectively, in the Italian and Canadian patients, indicating that the patient populations were similar. The main difference was the lower power of the Italian study. When the results are combined, there is no significant statistical heterogeneity and the overall absolute difference is 8.6% in favor of therapy (95% CI 2.1, 15). The number needed to treat is 12 (95% CI 7, 49). Thus, for every 12 patients having Stage I/II endometriosis diagnosed at laparoscopy, there will be one additional successful pregnancy if ablation/resection of visible endometriosis is performed, compared to no treatment. There is no evidence that the outcome is affected by the method of ablation, whether electro-surgery or laser.

A nonrandomized study demonstrated that the cumulative probability of pregnancy in 216 infertile patients with severe endometriosis, followed for up to 2 years after laparoscopy or laparotomy, was significantly increased, 45% and 63%, respectively. These and other observational studies, that are not free from bias, suggest that in women with Stage III/IV endometriosis, without other identifiable infertility factors, conservative surgical treatment with laparoscopy, and possible laparotomy may increase fertility.

## BIBLIOGRAPHY

Marcoux S, Maheux R, Berube S. Laparoscopic surgery in infertile women with minimal or mild endometriosis. Canadian

Collaborative Group on Endometriosis. *N Engl J Med.* 1997; 337:217.

Parazzini F. Ablation of lesions or no treatment in minimal-mild endometriosis in infertile women: a randomized trial. Gruppo Italiano per lo Studio dell'Endometriosi. *Hum Reprod.* 1999; 14:1332.

Practice Committee of the American Society for Reproductive Medicine. Endometriosis and infertility. *Fertil Steril.* 2004;82 (Suppl. 1):S40–S45.

Revised American Society for Reproductive Medicine classification of endometriosis: 1996, American Society for Reproductive Medicine. *Fertil Steril.* 1997;67:817.

# 109 BASIC EVALUATION FOR FEMALE INFERTILITY

*Lee Kao*

## LEARNING POINTS

Who are the candidates for infertility workup; What are included in the general infertility workup; and is routine postcoital testing necessary?

## VIGNETTE

This is a 44-year-old Caucasian female, G1P0010, who presents for secondary infertility consultation with her husband. The patient had a past history of pelvic inflammatory disease and experienced an ectopic pregnancy about 20 years ago. She underwent a laparotomy and she remembers that the evacuation of ectopic pregnancy was performed and also some kind of tuboplasty was performed. The patient denies that there was any salpingectomy of either side involved. In 2000, a hysterosalpingogram (HSG) was performed and a left-sided hydrosalpinx was noted. The right tube was described as normal although without spill and the uterine cavity was described to be normal.

Subsequently, the patient and her husband underwent two cycles of in vitro fertilization (IVF) in 2003. During the first cycle she was told she had a shortened stimulatory cycle under a long suppression with Lupron. Eventually, six oocytes were retrieved, and all were fertilized. On day 3 five embryos were transferred; unfortunately the patient did not achieve pregnancy. A second IVF cycle was also performed using a similar protocol, with five oocytes retrieved, five fertilized and, eventually, a day 3 transfer of four embryos, again without success. Her prolactin at that time was noted to be elevated but, supposedly, she had a head magnetic resonance imaging (MRI), which was negative. She had also long been on thyroxine replacement for her hypothyroidism, and her thyroid stimulating hormone (TSH) and T4 were reported to be normal. On record, the patient's rubella status is immune. Her blood type is A positive. Cystic fibrosis genetic screening was equivical, but the patient's partner was screened as negative. The patient also reports that in the past day 3 FSH levels were reported to be 6.5 and 10.2 m/Iu/mL on two separate occasions. The patient's partner supposedly reports a normal semen analysis, but no records are available.

The couple subsequently went to see another infertility clinic, and a repeat HSG was performed in July 2004. At that time, the report indicated: intrauterine synechia, mass effect in the uterine fundus, the left tube with normal fill and spill and caliber, and the right tube was not visualized, with presumed proximal occlusion. They were recommended to have surgery and then directly move into IVF. Now they are here for a fertility consultation.

### QUESTION 1

*Which patients are candidates for an infertility evaluation?*

### ANSWER 1

Formal evaluation of infertility is generally indicated in women attempting pregnancy who fail to conceive after a year or more of regular, unprotected intercourse. Eighty five percent of couples who will achieve pregnancy without assistance succeed within this interval of time. Earlier evaluation and treatment is indicated in women with: (1) age over 35 years, (2) history of oligo/amenorrhea, (3) known or suspected uterine/tubal disease or endometriosis, or (4) a partner known to be subfertile. Initial consultation with the infertile couple should include a complete medical and menstrual history and physical examination, preconceptional counseling, and instruction on how coital timing might be optimized. Evaluation of both partners should begin at the same time.

### QUESTION 2

*What is included in the general female infertility workup?*

## ANSWER 2

*History and physical examination:*

Relevant history includes: (1) gravidity, parity, pregnancy outcome, and associated complications; (2) age at menarche, cycle length and characteristics, and onset/severity of dysmenorrhea; (3) methods of contraception and coital frequency; (4) duration of infertility and results of any previous evaluation and treatment; (5) past surgery, its indications and outcome, previous hospitalizations, serious illnesses or injuries, pelvic inflammatory disease or exposure to sexually transmitted diseases, and unusual childhood disorders; (6) previous abnormal pap smears and any subsequent treatment; (7) current medications and allergies; (8) occupation and use of tobacco, alcohol, and other drugs; (9) family history of birth defects, mental retardation, or reproductive failure; and (10) symptoms of thyroid disease, pelvic or abdominal pain, galactorrhea, hirsutism, and dyspareunia. Physical examination should note the patient's weight and body mass index and identify the following: (1) thyroid enlargement, nodule, or tenderness; (2) breast secretions and their character; (3) signs of androgen excess; (4) pelvic or abdominal tenderness, organ enlargement, or mass; (5) vaginal or cervical abnormality, secretions, or discharge; (6) uterine size, shape, position, and mobility; (7) adnexal mass or tenderness; and (8) cul-de-sac mass, tenderness, or nodularity.

*Laboratory evaluation:*

The laboratory evaluation should be directed toward identifying the cause(s) of infertility in a systematic, expeditious, cost-effective, and least invasive manner.

*Ovulatory factors:* Evaluation of ovulatory function is important for all infertile couples. The method chosen (menstrual history, basal body temperature [BBT], progesterone determinations during the luteal phase, urinary luteinizing hormone [LH] determinations, endometrial biopsy, or serial transvagina (ultrasound) should be tailored to the needs of the patient. Evidence of dysfunction mandates a hormonal evaluation including TSH, prolactin, and exclusion of androgen excess. Failure to achieve pregnancy within three to six treatment cycles of treatment with ovulation induction agents is an indication to expand diagnostic evaluation or to change treatment strategy. Ovarian reserve testing (cycle day 3 follicle stimulating hormone [FSH] or clomiphene citrate challenge test) should be performed in selected patients; patients who are: (1) age over 35 years, (2) have a single ovary or history of previous ovarian surgery, or (3) have documented poor response to exogenous gonadotropin stimulation, to obtain prognostic information that may have significant influence on treatment recommendations.

*Cervical factors:* It is very rare for abnormal cervical mucus formation or sperm/mucus interaction to be the principal cause of infertility. Postcoital testing methodology and results are subjective and exhibit high variations. Its utility and predictive value has been seriously questioned.

*Uterine factors:* Examination of the uterine cavity is an integral part of a thorough infertility evaluation. The method chosen (ultrasound, HSG, sonohysterography, hysteroscopy) may vary and should be tailored to the needs of the individual patient.

*Tubal factors:* Tubal occlusive disease is highly prevalent and should be specifically excluded. All available methods (HSG, sonohysterography, chromotubation during laparoscopy, fluoroscopic/hysteroscopic selective tubal cannulation) for evaluation of tubal factors have technical limitations. When any one technique yields abnormal results, evaluation with a second, complementary method is prudent.

*Peritoneal factors:* Peritoneal factors, including endometriosis, pelvic/adnexal adhesions, can contribute to reproductive failure. The history and/or physical examination findings are rarely sufficient to exclude peritoneal factors. Ultrasound may reveal otherwise unsuspected pathology that may have reproductive implications. Laparoscopy with direct visual examination of the pelvic anatomy is the only specific diagnostic method for otherwise unrecognized peritoneal factors.

## QUESTION 3

*Is routine postcoital testing and laparoscopy necessary?*

## ANSWER 3

The postcoital test, used to examine a specimen of cervical mucus obtained shortly before expected ovulation under the microscope for the presence of motile sperm within hours after intercourse, is the traditional method for identifying the precence of a cervical factor. But controversies exist regarding technique, timing, and interpretation of the test. Routine postcoital testing is unnecessary nowadays and should be reserved for patients only when results will clearly influence treatment strategy.

Laparoscopy is indicated when there is evidence or strong suspicion of endometriosis, pelvic/adnexal adhesions, or significant tubal disease. Laparoscopy should also be seriously considered before applying aggressive empirical treatments involving significant cost and/or potential risks. Finally, laparoscopy should be considered in oligo-ovulatory patients not conceiving after 4–5 cycles of ovulation.

## BIBLIOGRAPHY

Practice Committee of the American Society for Reproductive Medicine. Optimal evaluation of the infertile female. *Fertil Steril.* 2004;82 (Suppl.1):S169–S172.

# 110 LIFESTYLE IMPLICATIONS (SMOKING) FOR INFERTILITY

*Lee Kao*

## LEARNING POINTS

Does smoking cause infertility, is smoking associated with adverse reproductive outcome and how to provide smoking cessation therapy.

## VIGNETTE

A 37-year-old, G0, Caucasian female, presents by self-referral with her husband to discuss their desire to achieve pregnancy. The couples both consider that they are healthy and hard working, and they had delayed child bearing for career reasons. The patient has been smoking for about 5 years due to her work stress and considers herself a light smoker and "can quit anytime." She is asking you whether smoking poses any risk for her fertility.

### QUESTION 1

*Does smoking cause infertility?*

### ANSWER 1

About 30% of reproductive age women and 35% of reproductive age men in United States smoke cigarettes. Though not generally appreciated, substantial deleterious effects of smoking on reproduction have been established. These include conception delay, ovarion follicular depletion and mutagenesis as follows:

*Conception delays:* Comprehensive reviews support the conclusion that smoking has an adverse impact. Most recent meta-analysis included 12 studies meeting strict inclusion criteria yielded an overall odds ratio of 1.60 (95 percent confidence interval [CI] 1.34–1.91) for infertility in smoking compared to nonsmoking women. The odds ratio (OR) for conception delay over 1 year in smoking versus nonsmoking women was 1.42 (CI 1.27–1.58), and the OR for infertility versus fertility in smokers compared to nonsmokers was 2.27 (CI 1.28–4.02). In some studies, the effects on fertility were only seen in women smoking more than 20 cigarettes per day, but a trend for all levels of smoking was identified. Increasing delay to conception correlated with increasing daily numbers of cigarettes smoked.

*Ovarian follicular depletion:* Smoking may accelerate ovarian follicular depletion as menopause occurs 1–4 years earlier in smoking women than in nonsmokers. Mean basal follicle stimulating hormone (FSH) levels are significantly higher in young smokers than in nonsmokers. Smokers also have higher prevalence of abnormal clomiphene citrate challenge test results than in age-matched nonsmokers. Mean gonadotropin dose used for smokers in in vitro fertilization (IVF) is higher when compared to nonsmokers. Overall, the literature strongly supports an association between smoking and infertility.

*Mutagenic potential:* Gametogenesis is vulnerable to damages from tobacco smoke. Smoking in pregnant women is associated with an increased risk of trisomy 21 offspring. The prevalence of Y chromosome disomy in sperm correlates with a marker of recent exposure to cigarette smoke, urinary cotinine concentrations. Increases in birth defects have also been reported among the offspring of smoking parents.

### QUESTION 2

*Is smoking associated with adverse reproductive outcome?*

## ANSWER 2

Smoking is associated with an increase in spontaneous miscarriage in both natural and assisted cycles. Studies of natural conception in female smokers have found an increased miscarriage risk. Though the mechanisms have not been completely elucidated, vasoconstrictive and antimetabolic properties of cigarette smoke (such as nicotine, carbon monoxide, and cyanide) may lead to placental insufficiency and embryonic and fetal growth restriction and demise. Smoking has also been associated with bacterial vaginosis and preterm labor. The chance of multiple gestations may also be increased in smokers. Women who smoked >20 cigarettes daily had an OR for ectopic pregnancy of 3.5 (95% CI 1.4–8.6) compared to nonsmokers.

An epidemiologic study has suggested an effect of maternal smoking on sperm counts in men; men whose mothers had smoked more than 10 cigarettes per day had lower sperm densities than men; with nonsmoking mothers.

The effect of smoking becomes more detectable in older women as smoking and advancing age may synergize to accelerate the rate of oocyte depletion. No study has specifically examined the effects of cigarette smoking on ovulation induction outcomes. But a meta-analysis of nine studies examining the effects of smoking on the outcome of assisted reproduction identified an OR of 0.66 (95% CI 0.49–0.88) for conception among smokers undergoing IVF. If a woman ever smoked during her lifetime, her risk of failing to conceive via IVF more than doubled (relative risk: 2.5 & 95% CI 1.38–4.55). Overall, it appears that IVF may not necessarily be able to overcome the reduction in natural fecundity associated with smoking.

## QUESTION 3

*How can you help patients quit smoking?*

## ANSWER 3

Smoking cessation rates generally are better for infertile women than for pregnant women. Unfortunately, only 5% of women referred to a specialty smoking cessation clinic actually attend. The recommended approach to smoking cessation for infertile women includes several minutes of counseling, education, and encouragement during each clinic visit, according to their individual stage of readiness to quit. Providing educational materials and websites alone is helpful but unlikely to achieve cessation without other methods of intervention such as: (1) behavior modification, (2) group counseling, (3) feedback, advice, and (4) nicotine weaning with patches and gum. The Public Health Service and National Cancer Institute suggest validated office-based intervention guidelines. A five-step (5-A) approach is suggested: (1) ask about smoking at every opportunity, (2) advise all smokers to stop, (3) assess willingness to stop, (4) assist patients in stopping (including the use of pharmaceuticals and carbon monoxide [CO] monitoring), and (5) arrange follow up visits. When behavioral approaches fail, the use of nicotine replacement therapy (NRT) and/or bupropion (Zyban) has resulted in a two-fold increase in the proportion of nonpregnant women able to quit smoking. NRT can be provided in the form of a gum (category C) or patches (category D) both available over the counter as well as nasal sprays and inhalers. NRT nasal inhalers and sprays are category D agents (adverse effects in animal models) and should be avoided in women attempting to conceive or pregnant. The only non-nicotine approved by the U.S. Food and Drug Administration for smoking cessation agent is the aminoketone bupropion. Bupropion is also available for use as an antidepressant (Wellbutrin), but is marketed differently for smoking cessation with a category B classification. The efficacy of bupropion appears similar to that of NRT.

No studies have directly compared bupropion and NRT in infertile or pregnant women. However, given the relative safety and generally good compliance with prescribed bupropion treatment, it would appear to be an acceptable initial medical intervention, when needed.

## BIBLIOGRAPHY

Practice Committee of the American Society for Reproductive Medicine. Smoking and infertility. *Fertil Steril.* 2004;82 (Suppl. 1:)S62–S67.

# 111 HYDROSALPINX/TUBAL DAMAGE

*Ashim Kumar*

## LEARNING POINT

To understand the ramifications of salpingostomy versus salpingectomy for the treatment of ectopic pregnancy as well as recommendations for the treatment of hydrosalpinx prior to in vitro fertilization-embryo transfer (IVF-ET).

# VIGNETTE

A 27-year-old female, P0010, presents with complaints of a 2-year history of infertility. She reports regular menses every 29 days. Patient reports a history of Chlamydia/pelvic inflammatory disease (PID) in her late teens. She states that she had an ectopic pregnancy two and a half years ago. Removal of the ectopic gestation was done via laparoscopic salpingectomy. A hysterosalpingogram is obtained and reveals normal uterine contour and bilaterally hydrosalpinx. Semen analysis on her partner is within normal limits. The patient has undergone four cycles of clomiphene citrate ovulation induction with intrauterine insemination (IUI) and three cycles of human menopausal gonadotropin (HMG) and IUI without successful conception.

## QUESTION 1

*What are the risk factors for hydrosalpinx or tubal damage? What mechanisms provide protection against these risk factors?*

## ANSWER 1

Risk factors include a history of pelvic surgery, especially tubal surgery. The use of microsurgical technique (e.g., limit tissue damage, avoid desiccation of tissue) and adhesion barriers can decrease the risk. A history of tubal infection, such as pelvic inflammatory disease or tubo-ovarian abscess increases the risk of subsequent hydrosalpinx or tubal damage. The use of barrier contraceptives and oral contraceptives independently decrease the risk.

## QUESTION 2

*Does salpingostomy in lieu of salpingectomy for the treatment of an ectopic gestation increase the likelihood of future fertility?*

## ANSWER 2

Salpingostomy, allowing retention of the fallopian tube, should theoretically be associated with improved future fertility as reported in a study with intrauterine pregnancy rate of 61% versus 38% for salpingostomy and salpingectomy, respectively. However, fertility outcome appears to be more closely associated with the condition of the contralateral tube. Fertility outcome in women without previous history of tubal surgery and normal-appearing contralateral tube was comparable to that observed with conservative management, salpingostomy. The main determinants of future fertility were previous history of tubal surgery and condition of contralateral fallopian tube.

## QUESTION 3

*Should a hydrosalpinx be resected prior to IVF-ET? What mechanisms may be involved in hydrosalpinges decreasing the IVF-ET pregnancy rate?*

## ANSWER 3

There is evidence associating hydrosalpinges with decreased implantation rate (and pregnancy rate) due to embryo cytotoxicity, mechanical flushing of the embryo, and adverse effects of toxins, cytokines, and so on. Investigators have found an increase in implantation rate, pregnancy rate, and live birth rate with removal of hydrosalpinx via laparoscopic salpingectomy prior to IVF-ET (see Fig. 111-1).

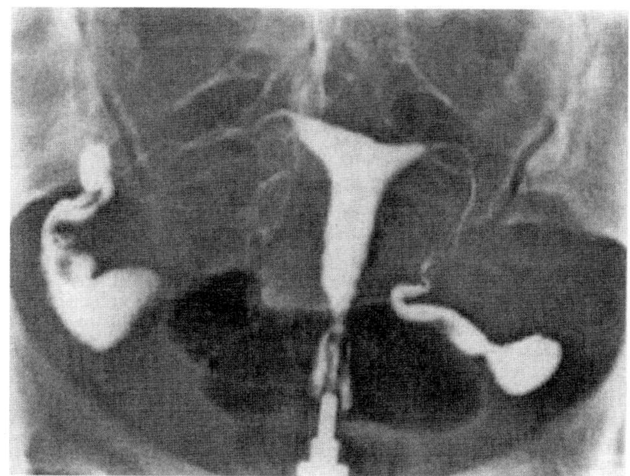

**FIG. 111-1** HSG showing bilateral hydrosalpinges with dilation, clubbing, and obstruction at fimbriated ends. Patient was 32-years-old woman with 10-year history of primary infertility. SOURCE: From Richmod JA. Hysterosalpingography. In: Mishell DR Jr, Davajan V, Lobo RA (eds.). Infertility, Contraception and Reproductive Endocrinology, 3d, ed., Cambridge, MA Blackwell Scientific Publications, 1991, St. Louis, MO: Mosby. Stenchever A. *Comprehensive Gynecology*. 4th ed., 2001: 1082–1084.

## QUESTION 4

*What are additional options if laparoscopic salpingectomy is unfeasible?*

## ANSWER 4

Due to pelvic adhesions as a result of previous abdominopelvic surgery, infection, or endometriosis, laparoscopic salpingectomy can be difficult in some cases. In order to minimize the detrimental effects of hydrosalpinges, tubal interruption is believed to have similar efficacy in returning IVF pregnancy rates to normal. Other options such as salpingostomy, aspiration of the fluid, or antibiotics have insufficient evidence to support their use. Fluid reaccumulation is not uncommon after salpingostomy or fluid aspiration.

## BIBLIOGRAPHY

Ault KA, Faro S. Pelvic inflammatory disease. Current diagnostic criteria and treatment guidelines. *Postgrad Med.* 1993;93: 85–86, 89–91.

Bahamondes L, Bueno JG, Hardy E, Vera S, Pimentel E, Ramos M. Identification of main risk factors for tubal infertility. *Fertil Steril.* 1994;61(3):478–482.

Dubuisson JB, Morice P, Chapron C, De Gayffier A, Mouelhi T. Salpingectomy—the laparoscopic surgical choice for ectopic pregnancy. *Hum Reprod.* 1996;11:1199–1203.

Johnson NP, Mak W, Sowter MC. Laparoscopic salpingectomy for women with hydrosalpinges enhances the success of IVF: a Cochrane review. *Hum Reprod.* 2002;17:543–548.

Practice Committee of the American Society for Reproductive Medicine. Salpingectomy for hydrosalpinx prior to in vitro fertilization. *Fertil Steril.* 2004;82 (Suppl. 1):S117–S119.

Sagoskin AW, Lessey BA, Mottla GL, Richter KS, Chetkowski RJ, Chang AS, Levy MJ, Stillman RJ. Salpingectomy or proximal tubal occlusion of unilateral hydrosalpinx increases the potential for spontaneous pregnancy. *Hum Reprod.* 2003;18: 2634–2637.

Strandell A, Lindhard A, Waldenstrom U, Thorburn J, Janson PO, Hamberger L. Hydrosalpinx and IVF outcome: a prospective, randomized multicentre trial in Scandinavia on salpingectomy prior to IVF. *Hum Reprod.* 1999;14:2762–2769.

Strandell A, Lindhard A. Why does hydrosalpinx reduce fertility? The importance of hydrosalpinx fluid. *Hum Reprod.* 2002;17: 1141–1145.

Yao M, Tulandi T. Current status of surgical and nonsurgical treatment of ectopic pregnancy. *Fertil Steril.* 1997;67: 421–433.

Zeyneloglu HB. Hydrosalpinx and assisted reproduction: options and rationale for treatment. *Curr Opin Obstet Gynecol.* 2001; 13:281–286.

# *112* FIBROIDS

*Catherine M. DeUgarte*

## LEARNING POINT

Submucosal fibroids can be a cause of infertility.

## VIGNETTE

A 34-year-old, G0, female presents to the infertility clinic with her husband. They have attempted to conceive for the past 2 years without success. She has no significant medical problems and denies any previous surgeries. Her husband has had a semen analysis in the past which was normal. She denies any menopausal symptoms, galactorrhea, hirsutism, or heat/cold intolerance. She takes prenatal vitamins and has no allergies. Her menses are regular every 29 days, lasting 7 days and she has occasional spotting midcycle. She denies any smoking, alcohol, or drugs.

The physical examination reveals an overweight African American woman. Vital signs: blood pressure 130/70 mm Hg, pulse 87/min, respiratory rate 16/min, temperature 98.5°F, weight 180 lb, and height of 5 ft 4 in. Thyroid: no enlargement, no masses, lungs: clear to auscultation bilaterally, heart: regular rate and rhythm: no murmurs, abdomen: obese, soft, nontender, no masses. Pelvic examination: External genitalia within normal limits, vagina well estrogenized, no vaginal discharge, normal cervix, uterus anteverted, irregular and enlarged to 10 week size, adnexa no masses and not tender. Rectovaginal examination: possible fibroid palpated.

## QUESTION 1

*Which diagnostic tests would you do to determine the cause of her infertility?*

## ANSWER 1

1. Hysterosalpingogram (HSG): This test uses a dye to evaluate the uterine cavity and assess for tubal patency. It is very specific but not very sensitive.
2. Sonohystogram: Performed placing saline through a special catheter into the uterine cavity. More sensitive

than HSG for the evaluation of uterine cavity, but does not allow for evaluation of tubal patency.
3. Transvaginal ultrasound: A simple method to evaluate the uterus and can also give information about the ovaries.
4. Assess ovulation: In this patient, this is probably not an issue, given the fact that she has regular menses, however it is important to document. Documentation of ovulation can mid-luteal progesterone level.

## QUESTION 2

*Can fibroids cause infertility and if so, which kind?*

## ANSWER 2

Submucosal or intracavitary fibroids are the most common type of fibroids associated with infertility (Fig. 112-1). Occasionally large intramural fibroids that impinge on the uterine lining may also be associated with infertility or miscarriages. Subserosal fibroids are rarely associated with infertility.

## QUESTION 3

*What is the recommended treatment for submucosal fibroids in a patient with infertility?*

## ANSWER 3

Treatment for submucosal fibroids usually involves hysteroscopy with hysteroscopic myomectomy. Occassionally if a large intracavitary fibroid is encountered, abdominal myomectomy may be needed.

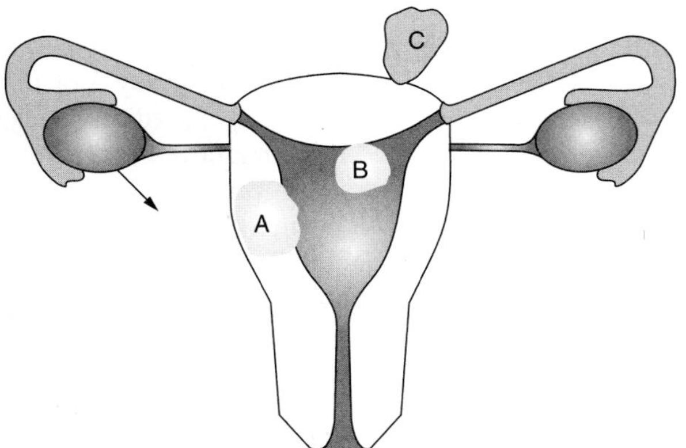


**FIG. 112-1** The types of fibroids by location. A is intramural, B is intracavity (submucus), and C is subserosel.

## BIBLIOGRAPHY

ACOG Practice Bulletin No. 16. 2000.

ACOG Technology Assessment in OB/GYN No. 3. 2003.

Eldar-Geva T, Meagher S, Healy DL, MacLachlan V, Breheny S, Wood C. Effect of intramural, subserosal, and submucosal uterine fibroids on the outcome of assisted reproductive technology treatment. *Fertil Steril.* 1998;70:687.

Speroff L, Fritz MA. *Clinical Gynecologic Endocrinology and Infertility.* 7th ed., Philladelphia, PA: Lippincott Williams & Wilkins; 2005.

# 113 ADVANCED REPRODUCTIVE AGE

*Margareta D. Pisarska*

## LEARNING POINT

Infertility and the risk of spontaneous abortion becomes more pronounced in women after the age of 35 years. This is largely due to diminished ovarian reserve and increasing prevalence of fetal chromosomal abnormalities. Early evaluation and intervention are warranted.

## VIGNETTE

A 38-year-old, G0, presents seeking information regarding fertility. She states that she and her husband have been actively trying to get pregnant for the past 6 months, having intercourse around the time of ovulation. Prior to this time they have not used any birth control and they never got pregnant. She has tested for ovulation and ovulates on a monthly basis. Additional workup has not been performed.

Gynecologic history: Menarche at age 12 years, regular monthly cycles with 3 days flow.

No history of fibroids, ovarian cysts, or sexually transmitted diseases.

Obstetrics history: Negative.

Medical history and surgical history is negative.

Social history: She used to smoke in her early twenties, approximately half pack per day for 10 years. She discontinued at the age of 30. She does not drink alcohol or use illicit drugs. She is not taking any medications and has no allergies to medications. States that her mother has some type of thyroid condition.

Physical examination reveals a healthy-appearing female. Vital signs: blood pressure 110/70 mm Hg, pulse 80/min, respiratory rate 18/min, and temperature 98.6°F. Thyroid: nonpalpable, lungs clear, heart: regular rate and rhythm without audible murmurs. Abdomen: normal bowel sounds, soft, nontender, no palpable masses. Pelvic examination: normal external genitalia, cervix multiparous, no lesions, uterus anteverted normal size, adnexa nontender, no masses bilaterally. Rectovaginal confirms.

The laboratory evaluation reveals the following: Day 3 follicle stimulating hormone (FSH) is 12 mIU/mL, day 3 estradiol 60 pg/mL, thyroid stimulating hormone (TSH) is 2 mIU/mL, prolactin 10 ng/dL.

Semen analysis: Count 40 million/mL, motility 70%, morphology 70% normal (World Health Organization criteria)

Hysterosalpingogram: Normal uterine cavity, bilateral tubal patency.

## QUESTION 1

*What is the definition of advanced reproductive age? What causes reduced fecundity in women as they age?*

## ANSWER 1

Although there is no strict definition of advanced reproductive age in women, infertility becomes more pronounced after the age of 35. The risk of a spontaneous abortion also increases with female age. From the 2002 assisted reproductive technology success rates, the miscarriage rate is relatively stable at 13% in women under the age of 35, above the age of 35 the rate of loss increases, between 35, and 37 years, it is 15–16%, at age 38, it increases to 22%, and by the time a women is 40, the miscarriage rate is 30% (Fig. 113-1). This continues to increase and by age 42 years the miscarriage rate is greater than 40%.

The decline in female fecundity and increased risk of spontaneous abortion as a result of age are predominantly due to diminished ovarian reserve. Diminished ovarian reserve is attributed to a decrease in the number and quality of the oocytes. There are age related abnormalities in the meiotic spindle in oocytes of older women leading to abnormalities of chromosomal alignment and a higher rate of aneuploidy. This leads to an increased rate spontaneous abortions and a decreased rate of live birth with increased reproductive age.

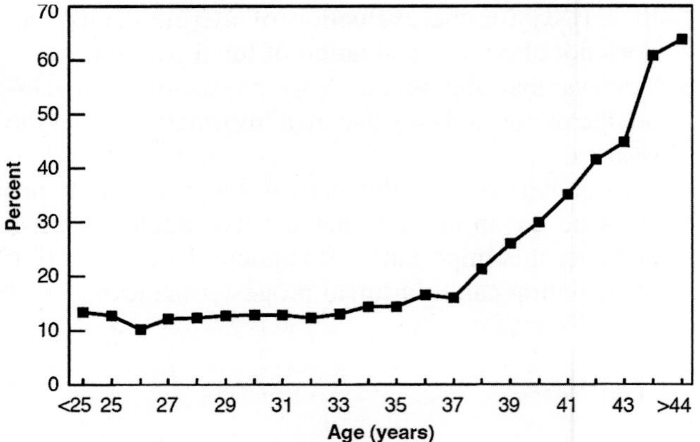


**FIG. 113-1** Miscarriage rate in women undergoing ART.
SOURCE: Centers for Disease Control and Prevention, American Society for Reproductive Medicine, Society for Assisted Reproductive Technology, and RESOLVE 2002. *Assisted Reproductive Technology Success Rates*. Atlanta, GA: Centers for Disease Control and Prevention;2004.

In addition, older women have had more opportunity to acquire conditions, such as endometriosis, pelvic infection, or fibroids, which may contribute to reduced fecundity. Success of fertility treatment in women with these conditions is significantly influenced by maternal age.

## QUESTION 2

*How do you test for ovarian reserve?*

## ANSWER 2

In women over the age of 35 years it is prudent to consider an infertility evaluation after a couple has been trying for 6 months instead of waiting for a full year. The infertility evaluation in women of advanced reproductive age should include an assessment of ovarian reserve. The most commonly used test for ovarian reserve is the serum FSH and estradiol on day 3 of the menstrual cycle. Elevated FSH and estradiol levels, which constitute accelerated follicular development, are independent predictors of poor prognosis in older women. Common criteria for normal ovarian reserve are an early follicular phase FSH level of <10 mIU/mL and an estradiol level of <80 pg/mL. A single elevated day 3 FSH value is an indicator of poor prognosis, regardless of normal values in subsequent cycles.

The clomiphene citrate challenge test (CCCT) is another test of ovarian reserve. A basal day 3 serum FSH is obtained followed by administering clomiphene citrate 100 mg orally on cycle days 5–9, and then measuring FSH on cycle day 10. The CCCT is abnormal if either the day 3 or the day 10 FSH is above the normal value for the laboratory.

The prognosis for women with diminished ovarian reserve, diagnosed by an abnormal basal FSH, estradiol, or CCCT is poor. They have lower live birth rates with ovulation induction and intrauterine insemination, decreased responses to ovulation induction, require higher doses of gonadotropin, have higher IVF cycle cancellation rates, and experience lower pregnancy rates through IVF.

## QUESTION 3

*What treatment options are available for women of advanced reproductive age?*

## ANSWER 3

There are no treatment options available that will improve the quality of a woman's eggs as she ages. Thus, treatment options available to women of advanced reproductive age are aimed accelerating the time to conception. These options include controlled ovarian hyperstimulation with intrauterine insemination (COH/IUI) and IVF. Alternatively, oocyte donation is an effective option for women over the age of 40 and women with diminished ovarian reserve.

Women who undergo COH/IUI are treated with gonadotropins in order to induce growth and maturation of more than one oocytes at a given time. Once the oocytes are mature, a timed IUI is performed (sperm is washed and then placed in the uterine cavity through the cervix using a small catheter). In a large single center review of pregnancy outcome in women over the age of 40 who underwent IUI, the ongoing pregnancy rates were 9.6, 5.2, and 2.4 per cycle for women aged 40, 41, and 42 years, respectively. There were no viable pregnancies in women over the age of 43. Other studies demonstrate a delivery rate per cycle of 5% or less (range 1.4–5.2%) in women over the age of 40. This is in contrast to live birth rates per cycle of 17–22% for women under 35 and 8–10% for women aged 35–40.

Live birth rates for women with IVF also decline with age. From the CDC SART database for 2002, success rates with IVF, in women less than 35 years of age, is 35–40%. This is in contrast to the diminished live birth rates in women with each advancing age, at age 35–37 the rate is 28–32%, age 38–39, the success rate is 20–25%, age 40–41, the rate is 12–16%, at age 42 the success is 9%, and continues to decline steadily (see Fig.107-3).

Oocyte donation is a very effective treatment option for women over the age of 40 and women with diminished ovarian reserve. Success rates are dependent on the age of the donor and not the recipient. Since most donors are in their early twenties, success rates with egg donation are approximately 50–60% (Fig.113-2).

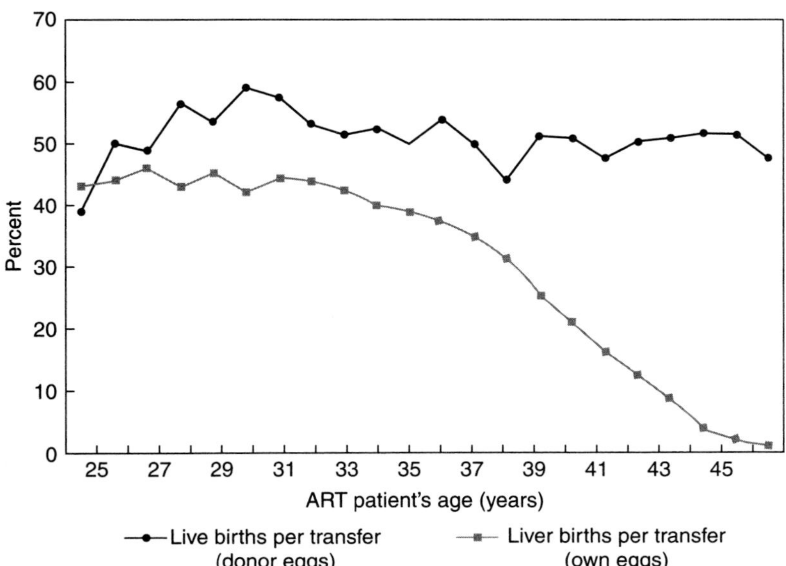


**FIG. 113-2** Live birth rates in ART patients using own egg versus donar eggs. SOURCE: Centers for Disease Control and Prevention, American Society for Reproductive Medicine, Society for Assisted Reproductive Technology, and Resolve 2002. *Assisted Reproductive Technology Success Rates.* Atlanta, GA: Centers for Disease Control and Prevention;2004.

## BIBLIOGRAPHY

American Society for Reproductive Medicine Practice Committee Report. Aging and Infertility in Women. 2002;1–6.

Battaglia DE, Goodwin P, Klein NA, Soules MR. Influence of maternal age on meiotic spindle assembly in oocytes from naturally cycling women. *Hum Reprod.* 1996;11:2217–2222.

Centers for Disease Control and Prevention, American Society for Reproductive Medicine, Society for Assisted Reproductive Technology, and Resolve 2002. *Assisted Reproductive Technology Success Rates*. Atlanta, GA: Centers for Disease Control and Prevention;2004.

Corsan, G, Trias, A, Trout, S, Kemmann, E. Ovulation induction combined with intrauterine insemination in women 40 years of age and older, is it worthwhile? *Hum Reprod.* 1996;11:1109.

# 114 MALE INFERTILITY

*Catherine M. DeUgarte*

## LEARNING POINT

Male infertility is often treated with intracytoplasmic sperm injection (ICSI).

## VIGNETTE

A 29-year-old, G0, female presents to the infertility clinic with her 50-year-old husband. They have attempted to conceive for the past 3 years without success. She has no significant medical problems and denies any previous surgeries. She denies any menopausal symptoms, galactorrhea, hirsutism, or heat/cold intolerance. She takes no medications and has no allergies. Her menses are regular every 28 days, lasting 5 days and denies any smoking, alcohol, or drugs. Her husband is a truck driver and has no medical problems. He smokes one pack of cigarettes per day and has occasional alcohol on the weekends.

The physical examination reveals a healthy Caucasian female. Vital signs: blood pressure 120/70 mm Hg, pulse 80/min, respiratory rate 18/min, temperature 98.5°F, weight 120 lb, and height is 5 ft 6 in. Thyroid: no enlargement, no masses, lungs: clear to auscultation bilaterally, heart: regular rate and rhythm: no murmurs, abdomen: soft, nontender, no masses. Pelvic examination: external genitalia within normal limits, vagina well estrogenized, no vaginal discharge, normal cervix, uterus anteverted, normal size, adnexa no masses and nontender.

Labs: day 3 follicle stimulating hormone (FSH) 6 mIU/mL, thyroid stimulating hormone (TSH) 6 μU/mL
Ultrasound: within normal limits
Semen analysis: vol 2 mL, sperm concentration 3 million/mL, motility 20%, normal morphology 20% (by World Health Organization [WHO] criteria).

### QUESTION 1

*What are normal sperm parameters using WHO criteria?*

### ANSWER 1

| | |
|---|---|
| Volume | ≥2.0 mL |
| Sperm concentration | ≥20 million/mL or more |
| Motility | ≥50% with forward progression |
| Morphology | ≥30% or more normal forms |
| White blood cells | <1 million/mL |

### QUESTION 2

*Should a karyotype be ordered on the couple?*

### ANSWER 2

Initially the semen analysis should be repeated. If similar results are revealed, a karyotype should be ordered for the male. Given his sperm count, a karyotype would be wise since low sperm counts can be associated with abnormal karyotypes. It is important to know if the male harbors a genetic abnormality before treatment, since there is a chance of transmission of the mutation. It is usually recommended that if semen analysis demonstrates severe oligospermia or (<5 million/mL), a karyotype should be obtained. In infertile men the prevalence of chromosomal abnormalities is about 7%; it is higher for those with azospermia (no sperm) than in those with oligospermia (decreased sperm).

## QUESTION 3

*What is the recommended treatment for this couple?*

## ANSWER 3

Intrauterine insemination can be attempted for one to two cycles. However it is very unlikely that it would result in pregnancy. Therefore IVF with ICSI is more appropriate (Fig. 114-1).

## QUESTION 4

*What are the indications for ICSI?*

## ANSWER 4

1. Male factor infertility
   a. Severe oligospermia: <5 million sperm/mL
   b. Asthenospermia: <5% progressive motility
   c. Teratospermia: <4% normal morphology
2. Surgically retrieved sperm
3. Cryopreserved oocytes
4. HIV male patients with a sero discordant female partner
5. Rescue ICSI in cases where fertilization fails

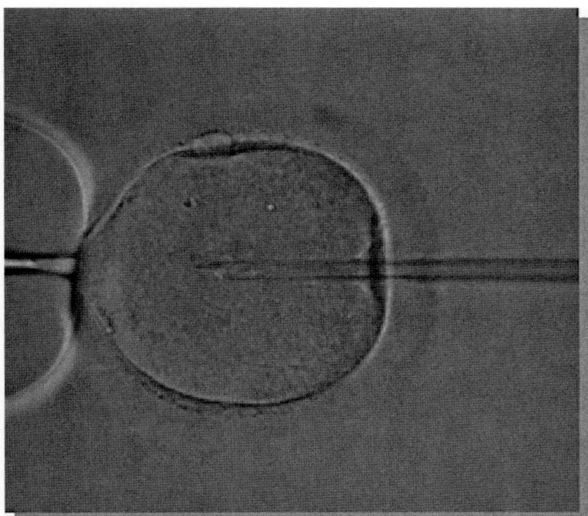

**FIG. 114-1** ICSI procedure. The oocyte is held in place with a holding pipette (9 o'clock) while injection of sperm is performed (3 o'clock), staying away from the polar body (12 o'clock)

## BIBLIOGRAPHY

Sharlip ID, Jarow JP, Belker AM, Lipshultz LI, Sigman M, Thomas AJ, Schlegel PN, Howards SS, Nehra A, Damewood MD, Overstreet JW, Sadowsky R. Best practice policies for male infertility. *Fertil Steril.* 2002;77:873.

Shlegel PN, Girardi SK. Clinical Review 87: In Vitro Fertilization for male factor infertility. *J Clin Endocrinol Metab.* 1997;82:709.

Speroff L, Fritz MA. *Clinical Gynecologic Endocrinology and Infertility*. 7th ed., Philladelphia, PA: Lippincott Williams & Wilkins; 2005.

World Health Organization. *Laboratory Manual for the Examination of Human Semen and Sperm-Cervical Mucus Interaction*. 4th ed. Cambridge University Press; 1999.

# *115* MENOPAUSE: SEXUALITY AND ANDROGEN DEFICIENCY

*Catherine M. DeUgarte*

## LEARNING POINT

Menopause can be associated with androgen deficiency.

## VIGNETTE

A 58-year-old, G3P3, female presents with complaints of vaginal dryness and decreased libido. She has been postmenopausal for 6 years and is not taking any hormone replacement therapy. She has diabetes and hypertension and denies any previous surgeries. She denies any menopausal symptoms, galactorrhea, hirsutism, or heat/cold intolerance. She takes insulin for her diabetes and captopril for hypertension. She denies any allergies. She has a history of three vaginal births without complications and she denies any urinary symptoms.

Her husband is 55 and has no trouble with erections. Neither of them smoke or drink.

The physical examination reveals a Caucasian female. Vital signs: blood pressure 130/85 mm Hg, pulse 85/min, respiratory rate 18/min, temperature 98.6°F, weight 140 lb, and height of 5 ft 6 in. Thyroid: no enlargement, no masses, lungs: clear to auscultation bilaterally, heart: regular rate and rhythm: no murmurs, abdomen: soft, nontender, no masses. Pelvic examination: external genitalia within normal limits with sparse pubic hair, vagina not well estrogenized, no vaginal discharge, normal cervix, uterus midposition, normal size, adnexa no masses and not tender.

Labs: total testosterone 15 ng/dL, hematocrit 37, TSH of 7 μU/mL.

## QUESTION 1

*What happens to androgens after menopause?*

## ANSWER 1

Androgen levels decrease with age but there is not a dramatic drop as there is with estradiol after menopause. After menopause, estradiol decreases by 80% whereas androgens decrease by 50% (androstenedione and dehydroepiandrosterone sulfate [DHEAS] decrease the most). Testosterone production is near normal 5 years after menopause at which time it begins to decrease. Sex hormone binding globulin (SHBG) also decreases after menopause.

## QUESTION 2

*What is androgen insufficiency syndrome?*

## ANSWER 2

Women with this syndrome usually present with fatigue, low energy, decreased or absent sexual motivation, and desire in conjunction with decreased testosterone levels and normal estradiol levels. Other conditions need to be ruled out such as depression, anemia, hypothyroidism and adrenal unsufficiency. Before treatment, the physician should determine if the patient is well estrogenized. If there is evidence of decreased estrogen, then estrogen therapy should be administered first; if there is no improvement, androgen treatment may follow.

**TABLE 115-1. Sources of Testosterone in Women**

| | OVARY | ADRENAL | PERIPHERAL CONVERSION FROM ANDROSTENEDIONE |
|---|---|---|---|
| Before menopause | 25% | 25% | 50% |
| After menopause | 50% | 10% | 40% |

## QUESTION 3

*What are the possible treatments for this patient?*

## ANSWER 3

1. Combined conjugated estrogen and methyltestosterone (Estratest)
2. Methyltestosterone
3. Testosterone gel, cream, or intramuscular injection

Although this patient may benefit from androgen replacement, it should be noted that none of these treatments approved by the U.S. Food and Drug Administration (FDA) and estrogen treatment should still be considered first line for these patients.

## QUESTION 4

*Where is testosterone produced in females?*

## ANSWER 4

Before menopause, testosterone is produced from peripheral conversion of androstenedione. After the menopause, as adrenal product decreases, the ovary becomes relatively more important (Table 115-1).

# BIBLIOGRAPHY

ACOG Committee Opinion No. 244. 2000.

Bachman G, Bancroft J, Braunstein G, et al. Female androgen insufficiency: The Princeton Consensus Statement on definition, classification, and assessment. *Fertil Steril.* 2002; 77:660.

Cameron DR, Braunstein GD. Androgen replacement therapy in women. *Fertil Steril.* 2004;82:273.

Speroff L, Fritz MA. *Clinical Gynecologic Endocrinology and Infertility.* 7th ed., Philladelphia, PA: Lippincott Williams & Wilkins; 2005.

# 116 CLOMIPHENE AND OVULATION INDUCTION

*Lee Kao*

## LEARNING POINTS

To understand the pharmacophysiology, indictions, side effects and risks of clomiphene citrate (CC)?

## VIGNETTE

A 34-year-old, G0, Caucasian female, presents by self-referral with her husband due to their inability to achieve pregnancy. Although they are anxious, they both believe that she's still very young and does not want to take any strong fertility medication or do the "test tube baby." The patient was told by her friends that she can take a pill to improve their chance of getting pregnant, and she would like to have it so that they can try on their own for the next year or so.

### QUESTION 1

*What is CC and how does it work?*

### ANSWER 1

Clomiphene is a nonsteroidal triphenylethylene derivative that exhibits both estrogen agonist and antagonist properties. Its agonist properties are only seen when endogenous estrogen level is extremely low. Clomiphene acts mainly as a competitive estrogen antagonist. About 85% of a single dose is eliminated after approximately 6 days. As currently manufactured, CC is a racemic mixture of two distinct stereoisomers, en-clomiphene and zu-clomiphene. Available evidence indicates that en-clomiphene is more potent and the primary isomer responsible for the ovulation inducing actions of CC.

The drug's effectiveness in ovulation induction is attributed to its actions at the hypothalamic level. Clomiphene binds to estrogen receptors (ERs) throughout the reproductive system for a longer period of time than estrogen and ultimately depletes receptor concentrations by interfering with receptor replenishment. Depletion of hypothalamic ER prevents correct interpretation of circulating estrogen levels. Reduced levels of estrogen negative feedback trigger normal compensatory mechanisms that alter pulsatile hypothalamic gonadotropin-releasing hormone (GnRH) secretion to stimulate increased pituitary gonadotropin release that, in turn, drives ovarian follicular activity. In ovulatory women, CC treatment increases GnRH pulse frequency. In anovulatory women with polycystic ovary syndrome (PCOS), in whom the GnRH pulse frequency is already abnormally high, CC treatment increases pulse amplitude, but not frequency. In successful treatment cycles, one or more dominant follicles emerge and mature, generating a rising tide of estradiol that ultimately triggers midcycle luteinizing hormone (LH) surge and ovulation.

### QUESTION 2

*What are the indications for CC treatment?*

### ANSWER 2

The indications for CC treatment are:

*Anovulation:* The causes of anovulation are many and varied. Thyroid disease, pituitary tumors, eating disorders, extremes of weight loss and exercise, hyperprolactinemia, PCOS, and obesity may be identified, but often the immediate cause of anovulation cannot be identified. Clomlphene is the initial choice for most anovulatory or oligo-ovulatory infertile women. Because of its hypothalamic site of action, it is often ineffective in hypothalamic amenorrhea (hypogonadotropic hypogonadism). Women with other endocrinopathies (diabetes mellitus, thyroid disorders, hyperprolactinemia, congenital adrenal hyperplasia) should first receive specific treatment, and be offered CC only when that therapy fails to restore ovulation.

*Luteal phase deficiency:* Corpus luteum is derived from the follicle that ovulates. Its functional capacity is at least in part dependent on the quality of preovulatory follicle development. In such context, CC is a logical choice for luteal phase deficiency. Progesterone levels are typically higher after CC treatment than in spontaneous cycles, reflecting improved preovulatory follicle and corpus luteum development and/or the combined hormone production of more than one corpus luteum.

*Unexplained infertility:* In couples with unexplained infertility, empiric CC, particularly in young couples with a short duration of infertility and in those unwilling or unable to pursue more aggressive therapies may be justified. The efficacy of empiric CC treatment may be attributed to correction of subtle and unrecognized ovulatory dysfunction and/or superovulation of more than a single oocyte. CC treatment is most effective when it is combined with properly timed intrauterine insemination (IUI).

## QUESTION 3

*What are the side effects and risks of CC treatment?*

## ANSWER 3

Clomiphene is generally very well tolerated. Some side effects are relatively common, but rarely persistent or severe enough to threaten completion of the usual 5-day course.

Hot flashes occur in approximately 10% of CC treated women. Mood swings are also common. Visual disturbances, including blurred or double vision, scotomata, and light sensitivity, are seen <2% and are reversible. Cases of persistent and more severe complications such as optic neuropathy have been reported. Whenever visual disturbances are identified, clomiphene use should be stopped. Less specific side effects, including breast tenderness, pelvic discomfort, and nausea, are seen in about 2–5% of CC-treated women.

Studies have suggested antiestrogenic effects (endocervix, endometrium, ovary, ovum, and embryo) be responsible for the discrepancy between successful ovulation and conception rates, observed in CC-treated patients. However, there is little or no compelling evidence to support these. When reduced endometrial thickness is observed, tamoxifen or letrozole can be offered as an alternative. Taken together, available evidence support that any adverse antiestrogenic effects of CC present no significant obstacle in the majority of treated women.

*Multiple gestation:* Overall multifollicular development is common for CC treatment and the risk of multiple gestation is approximately 8%. The overwhelming majority of multiple pregnancies from CC treatment are twins; with triplet and higher order pregnancies being rare.

*Congenital anomalies:* There is no evidence that CC treatment increases the overall risk of birth defects or of any one anomaly in particular.

*Spontaneous abortion:* Early studies suggested that the incidence of pregnancy losses in CC pregnancies was higher than in spontaneous pregnancies. However, more recent studies have described abortion rates that are no different from those of losses pregnancies conceived spontaneously (10–15%).

*Ovarian hyperstimulation syndrome (OHS):* The incidence of OHSS in CC-treated women is difficult to determine, as definitions of OHSS vary widely. The mild form with moderate ovarian enlargement is relatively common while severe OHSS with massive ovarian enlargement, progressive weight gain, severe abdominal pain, nausea and vomiting, hypovolemia, ascites, and oliguria is rare.

*Ovarian cancer:* Two epidemiologic studies had suggested significantly increased risk of ovarian cancer in women exposed to ovulation-inducing drugs, but subsequent studies have failed to corroborate. Recent pooled data of eight studies concluded that neither fertility drug use nor use for more than 12 months was associated with invasive ovarian cancer. Patients should be counseled that no causal relationship between ovulation-inducing drugs and ovarian cancer has been established. However, prolonged treatment with CC is generally futile and should be avoided.

## BIBLIOGRAPHY

Practice Committee of the American Society for Reproductive Medicine. Use of clomiphene citrate in women. *Fertil Steril.* 2003;80(5):1302–1308.

# 117 PREMATURE OVARIAN FAILURE

*Margareta D. Pisarska*

## LEARNING POINT

Although most cases of premature ovarian failure (POF) are idiopathic, a complete workup should be performed.

## VIGNETTE

A 32-year-old, G0, comes in because she has not had a period in 4 months. She states that she is sexually active but uses a condom. She did a home pregnancy test and it was negative. She also complains that she has been feeling irritable and occasionally wakes up in a cold sweat. She states that her job has become more stressful in the past 6 months and she is working 10 hour days.

Gynecologic history: Menarche occured at age 12 years and cycles were regular until they ceased.
No history of fibroids, ovarian cysts or sexually transmitted diseases.
Obstetrics history: none.
Medical history and surgical history is negative.
Social history: She does not smoke, drink alcohol, or use illicit drugs. She is not taking any medications and has no allergies to medications. She states that her mother went through menopause in her late thirties.
Physical examination reveals a healthy appearing female.
Vital signs: blood pressure 110/70 mm Hg, pulse 80/min, respiratory rate 18/min, and temperature 98.6°F. Thyroid: nonpalpable, lungs: clear, heart: regular rate and rhythm without audible murmurs. Abdomen: normal bowel sounds, soft, nontender, no palpable masses. Pelvic examination: normal external genitalia, cervix nulliparous, no lesions, uterus anteverted normal size, adnexa nontender, no masses bilaterally. Rectovaginal confirms.
Blood work reveals the following: beta-human chorionic gonadotropin ($\beta$-hCG) is negative, follicle stimulating hormone (FSH) is 50 mIU/mL, thyroid stimulating hormone (TSH) is 2 mIU/mL, and prolactin of 10 ng/mL.

## QUESTION 1

*What is the definition and prevalence of POF?*

## ANSWER 1

POF is defined as amenorrhea, hypoestrogenism, and elevated gonadotropins before the age of 40 years. A commonly used definition is at least 4 months of amenorrhea-associated with serum FSH concentrations in the menopausal range on two occasions. Ovarian failure does not always mean permanent cessation of ovarian function. Up to 50% of young women can experience some ovarian function following the diagnosis. Coulam et al. estimated the age-specific incidence of POF to be 1 in 100 by age 40 and 1 in 1000 by age 30. In women with primary amenorrhea, the prevalence of POF is 10–28%; in those with secondary amenorrhea, POF occurs in 4–18%.

## QUESTION 2

*What are the etiologies of POF?*

## ANSWER 2

Although most cases of POF are considered to be idiopathic, there are several known causes. In 90% of cases no etiology for spontaneous POF will be identified, even after a thorough evaluation. An abnormal karyotype was present in only 13% of a select group of young women who developed secondary amenorrhea due to POF (at age 30 years or less). Many of these chromosome abnormalities are X-chromosome defects. These include complete absence of one X chromosome (i.e., Turners syndrome), Turners mosaics, translocations and deletions within two critical regions on the X chromosome, designated POF1 (Xq21.3–q27) and POF2 (Xq13.3–q21.1). Approximately 14% of women with familial POF will have a premutation in the fragile X syndrome (*FMR1*) gene as compared with 2% of women with isolated POF.

There are other rare genetic causes of familial POF such as mutations involving the FSH receptor (*FSHR*), galactose-1-phosphate uridylytransferase associated with galactosemia (*GALT*), a forkhead transcription factor associated with the blepharophimosis/ptosis/epicantus inversus syndrome (*FOXL2*), inhibin alpha gene (*INHA*), *EIF2B* (a family of genes associated with central nervous system leukodystrophy and ovarian failure), bone morphogenetic protein 15 (*BMP15*), and autoimmune regulator gene (*AIRE*) associated with the autoimmune polyendocrinopathy-candidiasis-ectodermal dystrophy syndrome.

Other causes of spontaneous POF include autoimmune lymphocytic oophoritis. Up to 4% of women will have steroidogenic cell autoimmunity leading to autoimmune lymphocytic oophoritis. These women are at risk of developing adrenal insufficiency.

Chemotherapeutic agents and radiation therapy increase risk of POF. Alkylating agents are the most likely to induce ovarian failure. The effects of radiation therapy are dose- and age-dependent. There is also an increased risk of ovarian failure in women who undergo uterine artery embolization for fibroids.

## QUESTION 3

*What is the initial evaluation of POF?*

## ANSWER 3

Menstrual irregularity for 3 or more consecutive months warrants evaluation in a young woman. Pregnancy needs to be ruled out first with a $\beta$-hCG. Further evaluation includes measurement of serum prolactin, FSH, and TSH. If the FSH is in the menopausal range in a woman less than 40 years of age, the test should be repeated, along with measurement of serum estradiol. A progestin withdrawal test is not a substitute to measure serum FSH and estradiol levels since up to 50% of women with POF will respond to the progestin challenge due to the presence of some ovarian function and the presence of estrogen. This can lead to a delay in the diagnosis.

## QUESTION 4

*Once the diagnosis of POF has been made, what are some of the additional tests that should be performed?*

## ANSWER 4

A karyotype should be performed for all women with POF. Although more prevalent in women with primary amenorrhea, the presence of Y chromosomal material requires extirpation of the gonadal tissue secondary to an increased risk of gonadal tumors. A karyotype will also determine if there is an X chromosome abnormality. Of particular importance, are chromosomal abnormalities resulting in Turner's syndrome. These women should be screened for associated abnormalities.

Following appropriate genetic counseling, testing for premutations in the *FMR1* gene should be considered. Women found to have a premutation in the *FMR1* gene are at risk of having a child with mental retardation. The prevalence of premutations in the *FMR1* gene is approximately 14% in women with familial POF. The prevalence in sporadic cases is approximately 2%. Thus, it is important to consider testing individuals with a family history of POF. In addition, a family history of fragile X syndrome, mental retardation, developmental delay, intension tremor, ataxia, or dementia should also warrant testing, after appropriate genetic counseling.

Approximately 20% of women with spontaneous POF will develop autoimmune hypothyroidism. Therefore TSH, free T4, and serum peroxidase autoantibodies should be tested.

Up to 4% of women with spontaneous POF will be found to have antiadrenal antibodies. They are at increased risk of developing autoimmune adrenal insufficiency. Adrenal antibody testing will help identify women who should be followed closely for subsequent development of adrenal insufficiency through an ACTH stimulation test.

POF can occur in association with other autoimmune diseases such as systemic lupus erythematosis (SLE) or myasthenia gravis. Although they are less common than hypothyroidism and adrenal insufficiency, laboratory evaluation should be considered based on clinical indications.

## QUESTION 5

*What is the potential reproductive outcome for women with POF?*

## ANSWER 5

The chance of spontaneous conception is 5–10% in women with POF. Occult ovarian function is intermittent and unpredictable. There are no therapies available that may improve ovarian function and increase rates of spontaneous conception. Alternative family planning should also be considered in these women desiring children, such as oocyte donation, embryo donation, and adoption.

## BIBLIOGRAPHY

Anasti JN. Premature ovarian failure: an update. *Fertil Steril.* 1998;70(1):1–15. Review.

Bakalov VK, Vanderhoof VH, Bondy CA, Nelson LM. Adrenal antibodies detect asymptomatic auto-immune adrenal insufficiency in young women with spontaneous premature ovarian failure. *Hum Reprod.* 2002;17(8):2096–2100.

Baker, TG. Radiosensitivity of mammalian oocytes with particular reference to the human female. *Am J Obstet Gynecol.* 1971;110:746.

Coulam CB, Adamson SC, Annegers JF. Incidence of premature ovarian failure. *Obstet Gynecol.* 1986;67(4):604–660.

Kim TJ, Anasti JN, Flack MR, Kimzey LM, Defensor RA, Nelson LM. Routine endocrine screening for patients with karyotypically normal spontaneous premature ovarian failure. *Obstet Gynecol.* 1997;89(5 Pt. 1):777–779.

Nelson LM, Covington SH, Rebar RW. An update: spontaneous premature ovarian failure is not an early menopause. *Fertil Steril.* 2005;83:1327–1332.

Olive DL, Lindheim SR, Pritts EA. Non-surgical management of leiomyoma: impact on fertility. *Curr Opin Obstet Gynecol.* 2004;16(3):239–243. Review.

Rebar RW, Erickson GF, Yen SSC. Idiopathic premature ovarian failure: clinical and endocrine characteristics. *Fertil Steril.* 1982;37:35–41.

Sherman SL. Premature ovarian failure in the fragile X syndrome. *Am J Med Genet.* 2000;97(3):189–194. Review.

Stenchever MA, Droegemueller W, Herbst AL, Mishell DRJ. Primary and secondary amenorrhea. In: Stenchever MA, Droegemueller W, Herbst AL, Mishell DRJ (eds.). *Comprehensive Gynecology*. St. Louis, MO: Mosby; 2001: 1099–1123.

van Kasteren YM, Schoemaker J. Premature ovarian failure: a systematic review on therapeutic interventions to restore ovarian function and achieve pregnancy. *Hum Reprod Update*. 1999;5(5):483–492. Review.

# *118* UTERINE ANOMALY

*Ricardo Azziz*

## LEARNING POINT

The evaluation and management of the infertile women with a uterine anomaly.

## VIGNETTE

A 24-year-old, female presents to your office with a history of having had two miscarriages over the past 18 months, with the last pregnancy occurring approximately 1 year ago. She and her husband have been attempting pregnancy for 3 years. They have regular sexual intercourse, and the patient has regular and predictable episodes of vaginal bleeding with symptoms suggestive of premenstrual molimina and ovulatory function. Physical examination, including a pelvic examination, is essentially normal. The husband's semen analysis is normal, and the hysterosalpingogram reveals a "double uterus."

### QUESTION 1

*What is the epidemiology of uterine anomalies and their relationship to infertility?*

### ANSWER 1

Müllerian anomalies affect 3–5% of the general population. The primary classification of Müllerian anomalies in use today stems from a report by the American Fertility Society (now the American Society for Reproductive Medicine) in 1988 (Fig. 118-1). The vast majority of Müllerian anomalies are uterine in origin, and of these approximately 35% are septate (type V), 25% bicornuate (type IV), and 20% are arcuate (type VI). Between 5% and 25% of women with recurrent miscarriages, late abortions, or preterm deliveries demonstrate uterine anomalies.

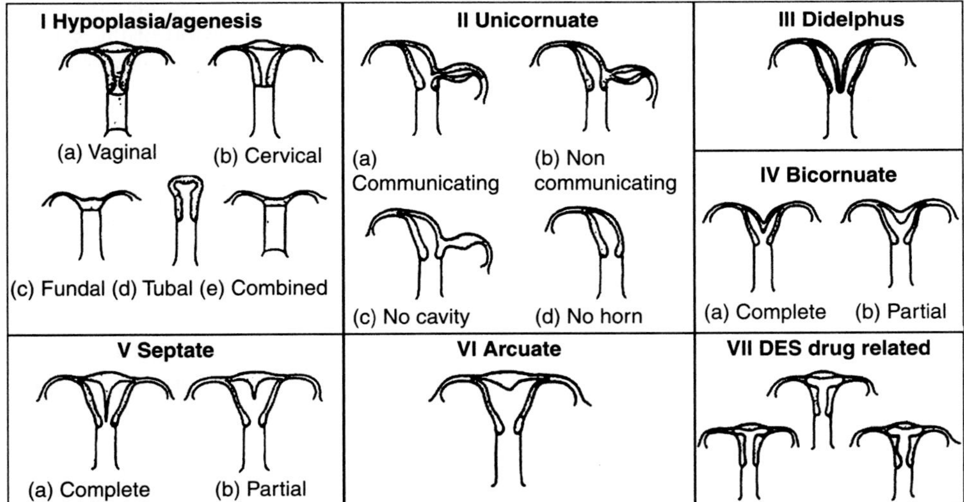


**FIG. 118-1** Classification system of müllerian duct anomalies proposed by the American Fertility Society (now the American Society for Reproductive Medicine) in 1988

SOURCE: Reprinted with permission from Anonymous. The American Fertility Society classifications of adnexal adhesions, distal tubal occlusion, tubal occlusion secondary to tubal ligation, tubal pregnancies, mullerian anomalies and intrauterine adhesions. *Fertil Steril.* 1988;49:944–55.

The majority of current data suggests that uterine anomalies do not decrease overall fertility, but affect primarily the maintenance of pregnancy and obstetrical outcome. The incidence of Müllerian defects in women who are infertile is similar to that of women with normal reproductive histories, however, it appears to be two- to threefold higher in women with first trimester recurrent miscarriages and fivefold higher in women with late first trimester and early second trimester miscarriages and preterm deliveries. In patients with a uterine septum, implantation on the relatively avascular septum and abnormal development of pregnancy-related vascularization has been implicated in the early pregnancy loss of these patients. Late pregnancy losses and preterm deliveries are more likely associated with the overall uterine deformation present.

Paradoxically, the less severe the defect is the higher the spontaneous miscarriage rate. Overall, the frequency of miscarriages is highest in patients with a partial uterine septum, followed by those with a bicornuate uterus, complete uterine septum, and finally didelphic uteri. The overall miscarriage rate is 20–30% for all Müllerian anomalies. However, we should note that the arcuate uterus is not associated with an adverse impact on reproductive outcome.

## QUESTION 2

*How are uterine malformations diagnosed?*

## ANSWER 2

The diagnosis of a uterine malformation may occur incidentally in up to 50% of patients in whom this is identified (e.g., during hysterectomy or cesarean section) or may be diagnosed during the evaluation for infertility or recurrent pregnancy loss. The process of evaluating a uterine anomaly generally involves two steps. Firstly, the interior appearance of the uterine cavity is delineated, and secondly definition of the appearance of the uterine serosal surface. Delineation of the uterine cavity is usually performed by hysterosalpingography (HSG).

Once a double uterus is identified, frequently the next step is to proceed to a combination of laparoscopy and hysteroscopy, which will permit both the evaluation of the uterine fundus, with the diagnosis of a septate versus a bicornuate or didelphic uterus, and will also provide an opportunity for immediate uterine septum resection hysteroscopically (see later on). It should be noted that, while the uterine fundus is smooth across in the majority of patients with a septate uterus, a small midline indentation is often observed at the fundus.

A number of investigators have suggested that the type of double uterus can be identified preoperatively using abdominal or transvaginal ultrasonography, sonohysterography, or magnetic resonance imaging (MRI). This latter technique can effectively classify up to 100% of all patients with Müllerian anomalies.

## QUESTION 3

*What is the treatment of a uterine septum?*

## ANSWER 3

Uterine septae are treated by surgical resection, primarily using the hysteroscopic route. Transection can be done safely with hysteroscopic rigid scissors, or less optimally by laser or electrosurgery. Dissection should be carried up to the point near the uterine fundus where the myometrium begins to demonstrate increased vascularity. Residual uterine septae of less than 1 cm after hysteroscopic metroplasty do not appear to impair reproductive outcome. For patients with a complete uterine septum, resection may involve puncturing the septum wall, close to the uterine cervix, and then dissecting upward. Although evidence is limited, it is preferable not to damage the uterine septae that involves the cervical os as anecdotally this may result in a greater incidence of cervical incompetence.

The hysteroscopic metroplasty entails incising rather than excising the septum. Secondary to the muscular structure of the septum, it will tend to pull apart toward the uterine walls as it is incised. Excision of the septum will simply lead to a larger defect in the uterine wall and the chance for increased bleeding. A concomitant laparoscopy may be performed in patients undergoing hysteroscopic resection of the septum, particularly if it was already in place during a simultaneous diagnostic and therapeutic procedure. Otherwise, it is not absolutely necessary to perform a laparoscopy while performing a hysteroscopic resection of the septum, as long as it is known that the uterine fundus is smooth. It is preferable to perform the hysteroscopic resection in the early follicular phase of the menstrual cycle. Some surgeons advocate the preoperative thinning of the endometrium using progestins, danazol, or a long-acting gonadotropin-releasing hormone (GnRH) analog, although most do not consider routine preoperative preparation of the endometrium essential.

Most reports documenting the effects of a hysteroscopic metroplasty on pregnancy outcome in patients with recurrent pregnancy loss indicate that postoperatively between 60% and 80% of these women will be able to carry a pregnancy close to term. Alternatively, hysteroscopic metroplasty does not appear to be of great value in improving patients' overall infertility. Finally, it should be clear that the finding of a uterine septum should not curtail the evaluation of the patient with recurrent pregnancy loss or infertility for the presence of other causes of these problems.

## BIBLIOGRAPHY

Anonymous. The American Fertility Society classifications of adnexal adhesions, distal tubal occlusion, tubal occlusion secondary to tubal ligation, tubal pregnancies, müllerian anomalies and intrauterine adhesions. *Fertil Steril.* 1988;49: 944–955.

Grimbizis GF, Camus M, Tarlatzis BC, Bontis JN, Devroey P. Clinical implications of uterine malformations and hysteroscopic treatment results. *Hum Reprod Update.* 2001;7: 161–174.

Homer HA, Li TC, Cooke ID. The septate uterus: a review of management and reproductive outcome. *Fertil Steril.* 2000; 73:1–14.

Lin PC, Bhatnagar KP, Nettleton GS, Nakajima ST. Female genital anomalies affecting reproduction. *Fertil Steril.* 2002; 78:899–915.

Troiano RN, McCarthy SM. Müllerian duct anomalies: imaging and clinical issues. *Radiology.* 2004;233:19–34.

## Section 7

# GYNECOLOGIC ONCOLOGY

## 119 ATYPICAL GLANDULAR CELLS OF UNCERTAIN SIGNIFICANCE

*Alison Axtell*

### LEARNING POINT

The appropriate triage and evaluation for patients with atypical glandular cells (AGC) pap smears.

## VIGNETTE

A 53-year-old, G2P2002, presents to the office complaining of metrorrhagia for the past year. She has spotting every other week with a normal period once every 3 months. In addition, she has noticed hot flashes, five to ten times a day, and night sweats. Her medical history is significant for diet-controlled diabetes and moderate obesity. She has no prior history of abnormal pap smears and had two cesarean-sections for a large for gestational age fetuses. A pap smear and endometrial biopsy are performed. The pap returns as AGC, and the endometrial biopsy was insufficient for diagnosis.

### QUESTION 1

*What is the sensitivity of cervical cytology screening for glandular neoplasia?*

### ANSWER 1

In general, pap smears are better at detecting squamous abnormalities than they are at detecting glandular abnormalities. The sensitivity of the pap smear to detect glandular dysplasia ranges from 50% to 72%.

### QUESTION 2

*What is the most likely histologic abnormality with an AGC pap smear?*

### ANSWER 2

AGC of uncertain significanies (formerly referred to as AGUS) are associated with premalignant or malignant lesions in 10–39% of cases. The abnormality is most frequently cervical intraepithelial neoplasia (CIN). In premenopausal women, an AGC pap smear is more likely to be related to CIN II to CIN III or adenocarcinoma in situ (AIS), while in postmenopausal women the abnormality is usually related to endometrial pathology.

### QUESTION 3

*What is the appropriate evaluation for patients with AGC pap smears?*

### ANSWER 3

1. Immediate referral to colposcopy with endocervical curettage (ECC) and an endometrial biopsy in patients

with complaints of irregular bleeding. Human papilloma virus (HPV) testing does not play a role in the management of AGC pap smears.

2. In patients with AGC due to cervical neoplasia, a cold knife conization should be performed. Women with AGC and no obvious site (NOS) can be followed conservatively if the colposcopy and biopsies are normal. Pap smears should be performed every 4–6 months, and any abnormality dictates repeat colposcopy or excisional procedure, while persistent AGC NOS requires a cone biopsy.
3. Consider transvaginal ultrasound, CT scan, or laparoscopy if the workup is negative, given the small risk of finding significant ovarian or tubal pathology.

## BIBLIOGRAPHY

Koonings PP, et al. Evaluation of atypical glandular cells of undetermined significance: is age important: *Am J Obstet Gynecol.* 2001;184:1457.

Solomon D, et al. The 2001 Bethesda System. *JAMA.* 2002; 287:2114.

Veljovich DS, et al. Atypical glandular cells of undetermined significance: a five-year retrospective histopathologic study. *Am J Obstet Gynecol.* 1998;179:382.

Wright IC Jr, et al. 2001 consensus guidelines for the management of women with cervical cytological abnormalities. *JAMA.* 2002; 287:2120–2129.

Zweizig S, et al. Neoplasia associated with atypical glandular cells of undetermined significance on cervical cytology. *Gyn Oncol.* 1997;65:314–318.

# 120 ADNEXAL MASSES IN YOUNG WOMEN

*Ilana Cass*

## LEARNING POINT

To understand the common etiologies of adnexal masses in young women.

## VIGNETTE

A 25-year-old, G0, presents with left lower quadrant pain. She reports a sharp pain with associated discomfort most severe when she lies on her left side that has progressed over the past 2–3 months. She is sexually active using oral contraceptive pills in a monogamous relationship. Her last menstrual period was 2 weeks ago. She denies any change in her bowel habits, urination, or weight.

She has no significant past medical or gynecologic history, and no prior surgeries. She denies any family history of cancer, but reports a maternal history of cardiovascular disease.

The physical examination reveals a thin woman in no apparent distress. Vitals signs: pulse 68/min, BP 100/60 mm Hg, and afebrile. Head, eyes, ears, nose, and throat examination reveals no adenopathy; chest is clear to auscultation, cardiac examination shows regular rate and rhythm; abdominal examination shows no ascites of distention, there is slight tenderness to deep palpation in the left lower quadrant without any masses or inguinal adenopathy; and pelvic examination reveals normal anatomy with a palpable, slightly tender, mobile mass approximately 6 cm on bimanual examination on the left, with no masses in the rectovaginal septum.

A pelvic ultrasound is performed 3 days after her next menses begins which shows a complex left adnexal mass of 8 cm × 5 cm × 6 cm, a normal size uterus and right ovary, without any pelvic fluid noted in the cul-de-sac.

### QUESTION 1

*What is the likely differential diagnosis of a pelvic mass in a young patient, <30 years of age.*

### ANSWER 1

Ovarian—functional ovarian cyst, benign neoplasm (benign mature cystic teratoma, endometrioma, cystadenoma, tubo-ovarian abscess, malignant neoplasm)
Uterine—fibroid
Tubal—hydrosalpinx, ectopic pregnancy
Colon—periappendiceal abscess

### QUESTION 2

*What is the most common ovarian neoplasm in young women <30 years of age? What tumor markers may be useful in the assessment of a young patient with a presumed ovarian neoplasm?*

### ANSWER 2

Germ cell tumors are the most common neoplasms in young women. The mature cystic teratoma is the most common benign neoplasm, and malignant germ cell tumors are the most common malignant neoplasm, of which the dysgerminoma is the most common. Specific tumor markers that are useful include human chorionic gonadotropin (hCG), lactate dehydrogenase (LDH), and alpha-fetoprotein (AFP).

## QUESTION 3

*What is the appropriate evaluation for an adnexal mass in a symptomatic young patient?*

## ANSWER 3

A detailed history and physical examination are essential. Particular attention should be paid to past medical history, any related gastrointestinal symptoms, including hematochezia, diarrhea, history of fevers, past gynecologic, and sexual history including any history of infertility, dysmenorrhea. Family history of malignancy is also important. The examination should include a lymph node survey, abdominal and rectovaginal examination with careful attention to the presence of any ascites, nodularity of the uterosacral ligaments, stool guaiac if any gastrointestinal symptoms, cervical motion tenderness, and presence of cervical discharge or bleeding. The size, mobility, mass contour, and the laterality of the mass should be noted.

Ultrasound assessment is valuable to provide information regarding the size and morphologic features of the mass. Ultrasound features that have been associated with ovarian malignancy include solid areas/nodules and thick septations, bilateral involvement, and the presence of ascites. Tumor markers that may be of some utility in suspicious adnexal masses include hCG, LDH, and AFP, which may be elevated in germ cell tumors. Cancer antigen-125 (CA 125) has been shown to have limited utility in premenopausal women. Clinical examination and transvaginal ultrasound are the most useful modalities to discriminate benign from malignant ovarian neoplasm.

## BIBLIOGRAPHY


Berek JS. Epithelial ovarian cancer. Chapter 11. In: Berek JS, Hacker NF (eds.). *Practical Gynecologic Oncology*. 4th ed. Philadelphia, PA: Lippincott Williams & Wilkins;2005: 443–509.

CP Morrow, JP Cutrin. Tumors of the ovary: soft tissue and secondary (metastatic) tumors; tumor-like conditions. Chapter 12. In: CP Morrow, JP Cutrin (eds.). *Synopsis of Gynecologic Oncology*. 5th ed. Philadelphia PA: Churchill Livingstone; 1998:307–314.

Malkasian GD, et al. Preoperative evaluation of serum CA 125 in premenopausal and postmenopausal women with pelvic masses: discrimination of benign from malignant disease. *Am J Obstet Gynecol.* 1988;159:341–346.

Roman LD, et al. Pelvic examination, tumor marker level, and gray-scale and Doppler sonography in the prediction of pelvic cancer. *Obstet Gynecol.* 1997;89:493–500.

Sassone AM, et al. Transvaginal sonographic characterization of ovarian disease:evaluation of a new scoring system to predict ovarian malignancy. *Obstet Gynecol.* 1991;78:70–76.


# 121 BORDERLINE OVARIAN TUMOR

*Andrew John Li*

## LEARNING POINT

No further therapy is indicated in women with low malignant potential (LMP) tumors after surgical resection. While surgical staging may not impact survival, frozen section is unreliable to confirm a diagnosis of LMP and patients with this result on frozen section should be staged in case a frank carcinoma is found on permanent analysis.

## VIGNETTE

A 45-year-old, G3P2, presents with increasing abdominal girth. She reports mild abdominal cramping and discomfort for the past 3 months. She denies nausea or vomiting, but has experienced early satiety. She denies irregular vaginal bleeding or dyspareunia. She had gained 10 lb over the last 3 months.

Her past gynecologic history is significant for two spontaneous vaginal deliveries and one spontaneous abortion. She has a medical history significant for borderline diabetes. She denies any past surgical history, use of tobacco or regular alcohol, or history of abnormal pap smears. Review of systems reveals no urinary symptoms, but she reports chronic constipation.

The physical examination reveals a slightly obese Caucasian female. Vital signs: blood pressure 120/70 mm Hg; pulse 80/min, respiratory rate 14/min; and temperature 98.6°F. Chest is clear to auscultation; cardiac shows regular rate and rhythm; abdomen reveals a 20 cm pelvic mass extending to the umbilicus that is nontender. No fluid wave is appreciated. On pelvic examination, she has normal external female genitalia without lesions, no blood or discharge in the vaginal vault, a parous cervix, a 6 cm size mobile anteverted uterus, and a large left mass. Rectal examination is confirmatory.

Abdominal/pelvic CT reveals an 18 × 15 × 13 cm complex pelvic mass. No free fluid or lymphadenopathy is identified. Chest x-ray is clear. At exploratory laparotomy, a large left adnexal mass is identified without evidence of carcinomatosis. The contralateral ovary appears normal. Frozen section reveals a mucinous tumor of LMP.

## QUESTION 1

*What is a borderline ovarian tumor (i.e., of LMP) and what is the management of women with this disease?*

## ANSWER 1

Borderline tumors are histologically serous or mucinous, and are characterized by the presence of complex, branching papillae, epithelial stratification, nuclear atypia, mitotic activity, and the absence of stromal invasion in the primary tumor. These tumors have a more indolent course than frank ovarian carcinomas, and are characterized by an earlier stage at presentation, longer survival, and late recurrences.

The principal treatment of borderline ovarian tumors is surgical resection. Total abdominal hysterectomy and bilateral salpingo-oophorectomy is typically recommended given a higher incidence of recurrence with unilateral adenxectomy. There are no prospective data to suggest that either adjuvant chemotherapy or radiation therapy improves survival. When peritoneal implants are identified (either invasive or noninvasive) adjuvant chemotherapy is controversial; while no data suggest a survival advantage with treatment, many oncologists will offer chemotherapy with the finding of invasive implants.

## QUESTION 2

*Do borderline tumors require surgical staging? And if so, why?*

## ANSWER 2

Current guidelines recommend surgical staging for borderline tumors identical to those for frankly invasive ovarian cancers. This includes biopsy of the pelvic and abdominal peritoneum, omentum, and retroperitoneal lymph nodes. In a large study of 225 patients, Lin et al found that 66% of patients had at least one staging biopsy performed. The overall frequency of a positive staging biopsy was 37%, and 47% of patients who underwent biopsies were upstaged as a result of positive biopsies, with 41% having extrapelvic spread.

Winter et al found no difference in survival (93% at 5 years) between patients who did and did not undergo surgical staging. However, the frozen section diagnosis of LMP was changed to invasive carcinoma in 8/93 patients (9%). A larger review of 140 cases correlating frozen and permanent histopathologic diagnoses found that diagnoses of borderline tumors by frozen and permanent pathology were consistent in 60% of cases. A true invasive cancer was interpreted as LMP in 29.3% of cases. Due to the risk of upstaging at time of final pathology, women with the frozen section diagnosis of borderline tumor should undergo surgical staging.

## QUESTION 3

*What is the role of conservative fertility-sparing surgery in patients with LMP tumors?*

## ANSWER 3

Unilateral ovarian cystectomy or oophorectomy has been described in several case series for LMP tumors. In the largest cohort of women under age 45 years who had fertility sparing surgery for LMP tumors, recurrence was more frequent in patients treated with ovarian cystectomy than in those treated with oophorectomy alone (58% compared with 23%, $P < 0.04$). The risk of recurrence is higher after fertility-sparing surgery (35/189 cases) than after radical surgery (7/150 cases); all but one patient with recurrence of LMP after conservative treatment were salvaged.

## BIBLIOGRAPHY

Berek JS, Hacker NF (eds.) *Practical Gynecologic Oncology*. 3rd ed. Philadelphia, PA: Lippincott Williams & Wilkins; 2000.

Gershenson DM. Contemporary treatment of borderline ovarian tumors. *Cancer Invest.* 1999;17:206–210.

Houck K, et al. Borderline tumors of the ovary: correlation of frozen and permanent histopathologic diagnosis. *Obstet Gynecol.* 2000; 95:839–843.

International Federation of Gynecology and Obstetrics. Annual report and results of treatment in gynecologic cancer. *Int J Gynecol Obstet.* 1989;28:189–190.

Lin PS, et al. The current status of surgical staging of ovarian serous borderline tumors. *Cancer.* 1999;85:905–911.

Morris RT, et al. Outcome and reproductive function after conservative surgery for borderline ovarian tumors. *Obstet Gynecol.* 2000;95(4):541–547.

Winter WE, et al. Surgical staging in patients with ovarian tumors of low malignant potential. *Obstet Gynecol.* 2002;100:671–676.
Zanetta G, et al. Behavior of borderline tumors with particular interest to persistence, recurrence, and progression to invasive carcinoma: a prospective study. *J Clin Oncol.* 2001;19: 2658–2664.

# 122 SQUAMOUS CELL CARCINOMA OF THE CERVIX

*Andrew John Li*

## LEARNING POINT

Cervical cancer shares the same risk factors as its precursor lesion cervical dysplasia; cervical cancers should be managed with radical hysterectomy in early stage disease and chemoradiation in advanced stage disease.

## VIGNETTE

A 23-year-old, G2P2, presents with vaginal spotting and a foul-smelling vaginal discharge. She reports heavier bleeding with sexual intercourse. She denies any back pain, hematuria, or bright red blood per rectum. She reports no fevers or nausea.

Her past medical history is not significant for any chronic conditions. Her gynecologic history is significant for coitarche at age 13 with more than 15 sexual partners. She had an abnormal Pap smear several years ago but has not been seen by a medical professional since that time. She reports a history of gonorrhea that was treated at age 18. The patient reports smoking a pack of cigarette per day for the past 5 years.

The physical examination reveals a thin Caucasian female. Vital signs: blood pressure 120/60 mm Hg, pulse 70/min, respiratory rate 16/min, and temperature 96.8°F. Chest is clear to auscultation; cardiac shows regular rate and rhythm; abdomen is obese, nontender, without masses or fluid wave. On pelvic exam, she has normal external female genitalia. There is dark blood in the vaginal vault with a foul-smelling discharge. There is a large 5 cm fungating lesion at the proximal vagina that encompasses the entire cervix. No lesion is seen encroaching onto the vaginal mucosa. Rectovaginal examination does not reveal parametrial or sidewall tumor.

A cervical biopsy is performed, which returns as a moderately differentiated squamous cell carcinoma.

### QUESTION 1

*What are risk factors and symptoms for cervical cancer?*

### ANSWER 1

Cervical cancer develops from untreated cervical dysplasia, and thus shares the same risk factors. These include demographic factors, such as low socioeconomic state, African-American race, and older age; behavioral and sexual factors, such as multiple sexual partners, early age at coitarche, and cigarette smoking; and medical/gynecologic factors, such as a history of sexually transmitted diseases, infection with the human papillomavirus (high risk types), lack of routine Pap smear screening, and immunosuppression.

Early stage cervical cancers may be asymptomatic and are diagnosed on pelvic examination or Pap smear. As the disease progresses, women frequently develop irregular vaginal bleeding, especially after sexual activity, and vaginal discharge. Symptoms of late stage disease include back or pelvic pain, hematuria, and rectal bleeding; these reflect growth of the primary tumor into the surrounding parametria or sidewall, or into the bladder or rectum.

### QUESTION 2

*What treatment modalities may be considered for women with cervical cancer?*

### ANSWER 2

Treatment of cervical cancer depends on the stage of disease; remember that advanced cervical cancer is staged clinically. For microinvasive squamous cell carcinomas (stage IA1, defined as less than 3 mm invasion through the basement membrane), cold knife conization is safe for women desiring future fertility. For those who have completed childbearing, an extrafascial hysterectomy is appropriate. For macroscopic stage I disease with tumor size less than 4 cm (stages IA2–IB1), modified radical hysterectomy with pelvic and para-aortic lymph node dissection is appropriate. Patients with macroscopic disease greater than 4 cm but limited to the cervix or involving the upper third of the vagina (stage IB2–IIA) treatment may either entail radical hysterectomy or primary radiation with chemosensitization. For advanced stage disease (stage IIB–IV) chemoradiation is recommended. In 1999, the results of five randomized studies were published and a clinical announcement by the National Cancer Institute was published strongly recommending the addition of sensitizing chemotherapy to standard radiation; these studies found a statistically significant survival benefit with the addition of chemotherapy.

## QUESTION 3

*What role is there for ovarian preservation for women undergoing radical hysterectomy for cervical cancer?*

## ANSWER 3

In stage I disease, the risk of ovarian metastases is low and ovarian preservation is a benefit to treatment with surgery rather than chemoradiation. For squamous cell cancers, the risk of ovarian metastasis has been shown in two large studies to be less than 1%. These same studies identify a 1.7–3.6% risk of ovarian metastasis with adenocarcinomas of the cervix.

In advanced stage disease, chemoradiation is typically recommended, with ablation of ovarian function by radiation. In stage IIB disease and higher, squamous cell histology is associated with a 4.5% risk of ovarian spread, while the risk is 23.5% with advanced stage adenocarcinomas of the cervix.

## BIBLIOGRAPHY

American College of Obstetricians and Gynecologists. ACOG Practice Bulletin No. 35 Diagnosis and treatment of cervical carcinomas. 2002. American College of Obstetricians and Gynecologists. *Int J Gynecol Obstet.* 2002;78:79–91.

Berek JS, Hacker NF (eds). In: *Practical Gynecologic Oncology.* 4th ed. Philadelphia, PA: Lippincott Williams & Wilkins; 2005.

Creasman WT, Zaino RJ, Major FJ, DiSaia PJ, Hatch KD, Homesley HD. Early invasive carcinoma of the cervix (3 to 5 mm invasion): risk factors and prognosis. A Gynecologic Oncology Group study. *Am J Obstet Gynecol.* 1998;178:62–65.

Landoni F, Maneo A, Colombo A, Placa F, Milani R, Perego P, Favini G, Ferri L, Mangioni C. Randomised study of radical surgery versus radiotherapy for stage Ib-IIa cervical cancer. *Lancet.* 199;350:535–540.

Morris M, Eifel PJ, Lu J, et al. Pelvic radiation with concurrent chemotherapy compared with pelvic and para-aortic radiation for high-risk cervical cancer. *N Engl J Med.* 1999;340:1137–1143.

Nakanishi T, Wakai K, Ishikawa H, Nawa A, Suzuki Y, Nakamura S, Kuzuya K. A comparison of ovarian metastasis between squamous cell carcinoma and adenocarcinoma of the uterine cervix. *Gynecol Oncol.* 2001;82:504–509.

Rose PG, Bundy BN, Watkins EB, et al. Concurrent cisplatin-based radiotherapy and chemotherapy for locally advanced cervical cancer. *N Engl J Med.* 1999;340:1144–1153.

Sutton GP, Bundy BN, Delgado G, Sevin BU, Creasman WT, Major FJ, Zaino R. Ovarian metastases in stage IB carcinoma of the cervix: a Gynecologic Oncology Group study. *Am J Obstet Gynecol.* 1992;166:50–53.

Whitney CW, Sause W, Bundy BN, et al. A randomized comparison of fluorouracil plus cisplatin versus hydroxyurea as an adjunct to radiation therapy in stages IB-IVA carcinoma of the cervix with negative para-aortic lymph nodes. A Gynecologic Oncology Group and Southwest Oncology Group Study. *J Clin Oncol.* 1999;17:1339–1348.

# 123 NEOADJUVANT CHEMOTHERAPY

*Christine Walsh*

## LEARNING POINT

Definition of neoadjuvant chemotherapy, adjuvant chemotherapy, and interval cytoreduction. Use of neoadjuvant chemotherapy in epithelial ovarian cancer.

## VIGNETTE

A 62-year-old Caucasian woman presents to the emergency room with increasing abdominal girth over the last 3 weeks and shortness of breath over the last 3 days. Other than a history of hypertension that is well controlled on medications, she is otherwise healthy. On physical examination, she is found to have ascites, omental caking, and a complex pelvic mass. CT scan confirms your examination findings and also demonstrates a 5 cm tumor plaque along the right diaphragm and the absence of a pleural effusion or pulmonary embolus. Her cancer antigen 125 (CA 125) is elevated at 550 IU/mL. You suspect a diagnosis of epithelial ovarian cancer.

## QUESTION 1

*What is the difference between neoadjuvant chemotherapy and adjuvant chemotherapy?*

## ANSWER 1

Neoadjuvant chemotherapy refers to the use of chemotherapy *before* any other treatment. Neoadjuvant chemotherapy is generally used to treat cancers where initial treatment with surgery or radiation therapy is not likely to be curative or where the initial use of chemotherapy could make subsequent surgical treatment less morbid by shrinking the size of the tumor. Because neoadjuvant chemotherapy is given as the first treatment modality, it is also referred to as "primary chemotherapy," "induction chemotherapy," or "anterior chemotherapy." In contrast, adjuvant chemotherapy is used *after* an initial treatment with curative intent has been attempted. Adjuvant chemotherapy is generally chosen to further treat a cancer that has been initially managed by a local treatment modality, but is thought to remain at a high risk for recurrence due to particular high-risk features (see Table 123-1).

## QUESTION 2

*Why is it appropriate to use neoadjuvant chemotherapy?*

## ANSWER 2

Neoadjuvant chemotherapy has been used in the treatment of locally advanced cancers that are not easily resected, or to make an unresectable cancer resectable. This approach has also been used in patients with comorbid medical conditions where an initial operative procedure is considered too risky. Neoadjuvant chemo-therapy has been applied to the treatment of breast cancer, head and neck cancer, cervical cancer, bladder cancer, and ovarian cancer with variable results.

**TABLE 123-1. Important Definitions**

| | |
|---|---|
| Neoadjuvant chemotherapy | Chemotherapy is used as the primary treatment. This is sometimes followed by subsequent attempt at surgical resection. |
| Adjuvant chemotherapy | Chemotherapy is used after primary local treatment (surgery or radiation) to decrease risk of recurrence in high-risk disease. |
| Interval cytoreduction | Surgical resection is performed after chemotherapy. This terminology implies initial attempt at surgical resection was unsuccessful. |

## QUESTION 3

*What is the role of neoadjuvant chemotherapy in the management of epithelial ovarian cancer?*

## ANSWER 3

It is important to establish a definitive histologic diagnosis before choosing a chemotherapeutic regimen. Most patients with epithelial ovarian cancer have this diagnosis made at the time of exploratory laparotomy. The majority of these patients undergo the current standard of care treatment, which consists of aggressive surgical cytoreduction to the smallest volume residual disease possible followed by six cycles of adjuvant chemotherapy, most commonly with carboplatin and paclitaxal (Taxol). Some authors have advocated for the alternative use of neoadjuvant chemotherapy followed by standard cytoreductive surgery, suggesting comparable survival to patients who receive the standard of care treatment. This concept remains controversial. The Gynecologic Oncology Group (GOG) began a randomized clinical trial to try to determine the role of neoadjuvant chemotherapy compared to standard therapy, but had difficulty accruing patients, and ultimately closed the trial without an answer.

The European Organization for the Research and Treatment of Cancer (EORTC) is currently conducting a trial randomizing patients between neoadjuvant chemotherapy (three cycles of platinum and taxane, followed by aggressive cytoreduction, then three additional cycles of chemotherapy) versus conventional treatment (aggressive cytoreduction followed by 6 cycles of platinum and taxane chemotherapy). The results of this trial may provide some insights. In the meantime, most gynecologic oncologists reserve the use of neoadjuvant chemotherapy to those patients with too many medical comorbidities to safely attempt a surgical procedure (i.e., severe malnourishment, severe cardiac, pulmonary, or thromboembolic disease, poor performance status) or to those judged to have unresectable disease.

## QUESTION 4

*Is neoadjuvant chemotherapy followed by surgery the same concept as interval cytoreduction?*

## ANSWER 4

No. Interval cytoreduction implies that an initial surgical procedure was performed where the tumor was judged to be unresectable. Because an unsuccessful attempt to surgically remove the tumor preceded the use of chemotherapy, this does not meet the definition of neoadjuvant chemotherapy. In one trial, it was suggested that patients who have undergone an initial suboptimal cytoreduction fare better if they undergo an interval cytoreduction between the third and fourth cycles of cisplatin and cyclophosphamide chemotherapy than if they do not undergo the interval debulking surgery. These results were not reproduced in another trial that differed by requiring maximal surgical efforts at the time of initial surgery and by using cisplatin and paclitaxol as the chemotherapeutic agents.

## BIBLIOGRAPHY

Bookman MA, Young RC. Principles of chemotherapy in gynecologic cancer. In: Hoskins WJ, Perez CA, Young RC (eds.). *Principles and Practice of Gynecologic Oncology*. 3rd ed. Philadelphia, PA: Lippincott Williams & Wilkins; 2000:413.

Kuhn W, Rutke S, Spathe K, et al. Neoadjuvant chemotherapy followed by tumor debulking prolongs survival for patients with poor prognosis in International Federation of Gynecology and Obstetrics Stage IIIC ovarian carcinoma. *Cancer.* 2001; 92:2582–2591.

Neijt JP, Omura GA. Primary chemotherapy for advanced-stage disease. In: Gershenson DM, McGuire WP (eds.). *Ovarian Cancer: Controversies in Management*. New York, NY: Churchill Livingstone Inc.; 1998:129–130.

Rose PG, Nerenstone S, Brady MF, et al. Secondary surgical cytoreduction for advanced ovarian carcinoma. *N Engl J Med.* 2004;351:2489–2497.

Schwartz PE, Rutherford TJ, Chambers, Kohorn EI, Thiel RP. Neoadjuvant chemotherapy for advanced ovarian cancer: long-term survival. *Gynecol Oncol.* 1999;72:93–99.

van der Berg MEL, van Lent M, Buyse M, et al. The effect of debulking surgery after induction chemotherapy on the prognosis in advanced epithelial ovarian cancer. Gynecological Cancer Cooperative Group of the European Organization for Research and Treatment of Cancer. *N Engl J Med.* 1995;332:629–634.

# 124 ENDOMETRIAL CANCER

*Andrew John Li*

## LEARNING POINT

All endometrial cancers should be staged, with the exception of stage IA/B grade 1 tumors; progestin therapy is a viable option in limited patients with endometrial cancer.

## VIGNETTE

A 55-year-old, G0, presents with symptoms of vaginal bleeding. She reports undergoing menopause 4 years ago, with hot flashes at that time that resolved without medication. She now reports having persistent bright red spotting over the last month. She denies hematuria or bloody stools; she also denies fevers, weight changes, nausea, or anorexia.

Her past medical history is significant for adult-onset diabetes and hypertension, both controlled with medication. Her past gynecologic history is significant for a long history of irregular menses and infertility. She denies tobacco use.

The physical examination reveals a moderately obese Caucasian female. Vital signs: blood pressure 140/80 mm Hg, pulse 70/min, respiratory rate 16/min, and temperature 96.8°F. Chest is clear to auscultation, cardiac shows regular rate and rhythm; abdomen is obese, nontender, without masses or fluid wave. On pelvic exam, she has normal external female genitalia. There is dark blood in the vaginal vault. Her cervix is nulliparous and without lesions. Uterus and adnexa are difficult to examine secondary to her habitus.

A pelvic ultrasound shows an endometrial stripe of 7 mm. An endometrial biopsy returns as grade 1 endometrioid adenocarcinoma.

### QUESTION 1

*What are risk factors for endometrial cancer?*

### ANSWER 1

Obesity and unopposed estrogen are the most common risk factors for endometrial carcinoma. Adipose tissue converts circulating androgens to estrone, and the constant stimulation of the endometrium with endogenous estrogens promotes hyperplasia and malignant transformation. Similarly, women who take unopposed estrogens exogenously risk hyperplasia of the endometrium. Other risk factors include nulliparity, hypertension, and diabetes.

Tamoxifen is a selective estrogen receptor agonist used as adjuvant treatment and chemoprevention for breast cancer. While tamoxifen has an antiestrogenic effect on breast tissue, it functions as an estrogen agonist on the endometrium. Women who take tamoxifen have an increased risk for endometrial cancer (approximately 0.1%). Anastrazole, a more recently developed adjuvant agent for breast cancer, is equally effective in reducing breast cancer risk, and has no increased risk of endometrial cancer.

## QUESTION 2

*When should endometrial cancers be staged and why?*

## ANSWER 2

A small subset of endometrial cancers may not require lymph node dissection due to the low incidence of metastases. These data were reported in Gynecologic Oncology Group (GOG), which identify 0–3% lymph node metastases in patients with grade 1 tumors with no inner or midthird myometrial involvement, and in grade 2 tumors with no invasion. Of note, they also did not see any lymph node metastases in grade 3 tumors with no invasion, but there were only 11 patients in this subgroup.

Otherwise preoperative/intraoperative factors that should guide you to stage include: grade 3 lesions; grade 2 lesions >2 cm; nonendometrioid histologies, like clear cell or papillary serous; greater than 50% myometrial invasion; cervical extension of disease.

Schink and colleagues reported that in grade 2 lesions larger than 2 cm with less than 50% myometrial invasion, 12% had lymph node metastases as opposed to no lymph node metastases in grade 2 lesions <2 cm.

## QUESTION 3

*What options are there for patients with endometrial cancer seeking future fertility?*

## ANSWER 3

In selected (young) patients seeking fertility, endometrial cancer may be managed with progestin therapy. These patients must have grade 1 tumors on endometrial biopsy (EMB) with no myometrial invasion (magnetic resonance imaging [MRI] best imaging modality). As many as 75% will demonstrate regression of carcinoma, but 1/3 will recur after progestins are stopped. Some studies have reported a fecundity rate of 20%, with most patients needing assisted reproductive techniques. Of note, any abnormal adnexal finding should be investigated, as 15% will have ovarian metastases or synchronous ovarian cancers.

## BIBLIOGRAPHY


Berek JS, Hacker NF (eds). In: *Practical Gynecologic Oncology*. 4th ed. Philadelphia, PA: Lippincott Williams & Wilkins; 2005.

Cass I, Walsh CS, Holschneider CH, Tieu K, et al. Coexisting ovarian malignancy in young women with endometrial cancer (Abstract No. 136). Abstract book of the 34th annual meeting of the Society of Gynecologic Oncologists, 2003;138.

Creasman WT, Morrow CP, Bundy BN, Homesley HD, Graham JE, Heller PB. Surgical pathologic spread patterns of endometrial cancer. A Gynecologic Oncology Group Study. *Cancer.* 1987;60:2035–2041.

Fisher B, et al. Endometrial cancer in tamoxifen-treated breast cancer patients: findings from the National Surgical Adjuvant Breast and Bowel Project (NSABP) B-14. *J Natl Cancer Inst.* 1994;86:527–537.

Hoskins WJ, et al. (eds.) *Principles and Practice of Gynecologic Oncology*. 2nd ed. Lippincott-Raven; Philadelphia, PA: 2005.

Howell A, Cuzick J, Baum M, Buzdar A, Dowsett M, Forbes JF, Hoctin-Boes G, Houghton J, Locker GY, Tobias JS. ATAC Trialists' Group. Results of the ATAC (Arimidex, Tamoxifen, Alone or in Combination) trial after completion of 5 years' adjuvant treatment for breast cancer. *Lancet.* 2005;365(9453): 60–62.

Kim YB, Holschneider CH, Ghosh K, Nieberg RK, Montz FJ. Progestin alone as primary treatment of endometrial carcinoma in premenopausal women. Report of seven cases and review of the literature. *Cancer.* 1997;79(2):320–327.

Randall TC, Kurman RJ. Progestin treatment of atypical hyperplasia and well-differentiated carcinoma of the endometrium in women under age 40. *Obstet Gynecol.* 1997;90:434–440.

Schink JC, Lurain JR, Wallemark CB, Chmiel JS. Tumor size in endometrial cancer: a prognostic factor for lymph node metastasis. *Obstet Gynecol.* 1987;70:216–219.


# 125 GESTATIONAL TROPHOBLASTIC DISEASE

*Andrew John Li*

## LEARNING POINT

Complete and incomplete moles are distinct clinical entities with different risks of malignant sequelae; persistent disease should be recognized and referred for chemotherapy.

## VIGNETTE

A 15-year-old, G1P0, presents to your office reporting abdominal distension. Her last menstrual period was 2 months ago, and she denies any vaginal bleeding. She reports nausea and vomiting over the last several weeks, but denies weight changes. She has had no fevers or changes in her bowel or bladder habits. She denies dizziness or palpitations.

Her past gynecologic history is negative for sexually transmitted diseases, and she has not had a Pap smear. She has been sexually active for 1 year, and denies use of any contraception.

The physical examination reveals a young Caucasian female. Vital signs: blood pressure 90/60 mm Hg, pulse 80/min, respiratory rate 16/min, and temperature 98.6°F. Chest is clear to auscultation, cardiac examination shows a regular rate and rhythm; and her abdomen is soft with a gravid uterus and a fundal height of 20 cm. Pelvic examination demonstrates normal female genitalia without evidence of blood in the vagina. Her cervix is closed. Laboratory work demonstrates a serum beta-human chorionic gonadotropin ($\beta$-hCG) of 219,000 mIU/ml, and a pelvic ultrasound demonstrates no viable intrauterine pregnancy, but shows dilated vesicles consistent with a "snowstorm" pattern.

## QUESTION 1

*Describe the genetic and clinico-pathologic differences between complete and incomplete molar gestations.*

## ANSWER 1

Complete hydatidiform mole is identified macroscopically by edema and swelling of virtually all chorionic villi, without identifiable fetal parts or amniotic membranes. Complete moles are almost uniformly diploid with completely paternal chromosomal composition (most are 46 XX). The most common origin of complete mole is fertilization of an empty egg by a haploid sperm with reduplication. One-third to half of women will have uterine size greater than dates. Theca lutein cysts are detected clinically in 20%. Ultrasound is characteristically a mixed echogenic snowstorm image filling the uterus.

Incomplete moles are associated with identifiable fetal parts or membranes. Grossly, the placental is a mixture of normal and hydropic villi. Partial moles are almost always associated with one haploid maternal and two haploid paternal sets of chromosomes, thought to result from dispermic fertilization of a haploid ovum or fertilization of a haploid ovum with a diploid sperm. Initial hCG levels are lower than those with complete moles.

Fewer than 5% of patients with partial moles develop criteria requiring chemotherapy, while women with complete moles have a 10–30% incidence of malignant sequelae.

## QUESTION 2

*What is the management of women after a diagnosis of molar pregnancy, and when is chemotherapy indicated?*

## ANSWER 2

Suction curettage is the method of choice for evacuation of molar pregnancy. Sharp curettage is not recommended due to possibility of uterine perforation and of increasing the risk of Asherman's syndrome. Medical termination should be avoided when possible. There is a theoretical concern over the routine use of oxytocin because of the possibility of forcing trophoblastic tissue into the venous spaces of the placental bed and disseminating disease to the lungs. Hysterectomy is an alternative for women not seeking future fertility, with subsequent decrease in risk of malignant sequelae (20–10%).

Women should undergo surveillance with weekly $\beta$-hCG testing until zero, then twice a month to monthly testing for 1 year. Women should avoid pregnancy for 6–12 months. Persistent disease is an indication for further treatment with chemotherapy (methotrexate or actinomycin-D). Persistent disease is defined as a plateau of $\beta$-hCG levels for 3 weeks or more, a rise of $\beta$-hCG for 2 weeks or more, or elevated $\beta$-hCG levels at 6 months or more.

## QUESTION 3

*Why is $\beta$-hCG useful to follow molar pregnancies, and how would you evaluate a possible false-positive value?*

## ANSWER 3

Human chorionic gonadotropin is a glycoprotein hormone composed of two dissimilar subunits. Common hCG-related molecules include hCG, hyperglycosylated hCG, nicked hCG, hCG missing the $\beta$-subunit C-terminal peptide, free $\alpha$-subunit, free $\beta$-subunit, nicked free $\beta$-subunit and urine $\beta$-core fragment.

Almost all tests today utilize a multiantibody sandwich assay. All tests use at least one antibody directed against the $\beta$-subunit. Labs will use antibodies to different sites on the $\beta$-subunit together with antibodies directed to alternate sites on the $\beta$- and $\alpha$-subunit. Thus different tests may measure different hCG related molecules.

False-positive hCG tests have led to many incidences in which the presence of gestation trophoblastic disease (GTD) has been erroneously diagnosed and needlessly treated. When false-positive tests are suspected, the USA hCG Reference Service recommends urine hCG testing for detection of the $\beta$-core fragment (the terminal degradation product of hCG and its variants). Evaluation should include serum testing by a lab using a different $\beta$-hCG assay.

## BIBLIOGRAPHY


Cole LA, Butler S. Detection of hCG in trophoblastic disease. *J Reprod Med.* 2002;47:433–444.

Diagnosis and Treatment of Gestational Trophoblastic Disease. ACOG Practice Bulletin, No. 53. 2004.

Hancock BW, Tidy JA. Current management of molar pregnancy. *J Reprod Med.* 2002;47:347–354.

Kohorn EI. What we know about low-level hCG: definition, classification and management. *J Reprod Med.* 2004;49(6): 433–437.

Li AJ, Karlan BY. Gestational trophoblastic neoplasms. In: Scott JR, Gibbs RS, Karlan BY, Haney AF (eds.). *Danforth's Obstetrics and Gynecology*. 9th ed. Philadelphia, PA: Lippincott Williams & Wilkins;2003:1019–1030.

Suzuka K, Matsui H, Iitsuka Y, Yamazawa K, Seki K, Sekiya S. Adjuvant hysterecotmy in low-risk gestational trophoblastic disease. *Obstet Gynecol.* 2001;97:431–434.


# 126 OVARIAN TERATOMAS

*Ilana Cass*

## LEARNING POINT

To understand the histologic features that distinguish a mature from immature teratoma, and the histopathological features that allowing grading of immature teratomas.

## VIGNETTE

A 17-year-old, G0, presents with right lower quadrant pain. She reports progressive pain over the past 3 weeks that is most severe at night when she is sleeping on her side. She has never been sexually active and is using no birth control. She reports previously normal menses, but has had no menses for the past 2 months. She denies any change in her bowel habits, urination, or weight.

She has no significant past medical or gynecologic histories, but she had a laparoscopic appendectomy at age 9 without associated complications or peritonitis. She denies any family history of cancer, but reports a maternal history of diabetes.

The physical examination reveals a thin woman in no apparent distress. Vitals signs: pulse 68/min, BP 100/60 mm Hg, and is afebrile. Head, eyes, ears, nose, and throat examination reveals no adenopathy; chest is clear to auscultation, cardiac examination shows regular rate and rhythm; abdominal examination shows no ascites or distention, there is slight tenderness to deep palpation in the right lower quadrant without any masses or inguinal adenopathy; and pelvic examination reveals normal anatomy with a palpable, tender, solid mass approximately 5 cm on bimanual examination on the right, without any masses in the rectovaginal septum.

A pelvic ultrasound is performed which demonstrates a complex right adnexal mass 4 cm × 5 cm × 5 cm mostly solid; a normal size uterus and right ovary, with a moderate amount of pelvic fluid noted in the cul-de-sac.

Labs: Beta-human chorionic gonadotropin ($\beta$-hCG) negative, alpha fetoprotein (AFP) is 7.5 μg/mL, and lactate dehydrogenase (LDH) 135 U/L.

### QUESTION 1

*What are the components of an ovarian teratoma and which of the components is most commonly immature and therefore used to grade the tumor?*

### ANSWER 1

Ovarian teratomas are thought to arise from a single germ cell, with tissues derived from the ectoderm, endoderm, and mesoderm. The immature elements are typically of neuroectodermal origin, and the grading system of Thurlbeck and Scully, later modified by Norris and Colleagues, assigns a grade to the tumor based upon the amount of immature neuroepithelium present.

Grade 1: Some immaturity present, neuroepithlium is absent or limited to one or less high power fields (40X) in any slide
Grade 2: Immaturity and neuroepithelium present greater than grade 1, but does not exceed three low-power fields in any one slide
Grade 3: Immaturity and neuroectoderm prominent; neuroectoderm occupies greater than four or more low-power fields within individual sections

## QUESTION 2

*How often is an immature teratoma bilateral? What is the appropriate surgical procedure for a patient with an immature teratoma who desires future fertility?*

## ANSWER 2

Immature teratomas are bilateral in less than 5% of cases, however benign cystic teratomas are seen in the other ovary in 5–10% of patients. Fertility-sparing surgical staging is appropriate in young patients who desire future fertility without clinical evidence of uterine or contralateral ovarian involvement. These patients should have a unilateral oophorectomy, peritoneal washings, biopsies, omentectomy, and pelvic and para-aortic lymph node dissection. Patients with more advanced disease benefit from surgical cytoreduction, and every attempt should be made to optimally cytoreduce these patients to less than 1 cm residual disease and preserve fertility. Mature glial implants of the peritoneum do not advance the stage of disease.

## QUESTIONS 3

*Which patients with immature teratomas are candidates for adjuvant chemotherapy?*

## ANSWER 3

The rationale used to advise adjuvant chemotherapy for patients with immature teratomas is based upon the data described by Norris et al. in which the malignant potential of an immature teratoma was related to the stage and grade at presentation. Survival was most significantly correlated with tumor stage and grade. Patients with low-stage, low-grade tumors do not require adjuvant chemotherapy, all others benefit from combination cisplatin-based chemotherapy regimens. The additional presence of other more malignant germinal elements, such as an endodermal sinus tumor, also adversely affects patient survival.

## BIBLIOGRAPHY

Bonazzi C, et al. Immature teratoma, a unique and curable disease: 10 years' experience of 32 prospectively treated patients. *Obstet Gynecol.* 1994;84:598–604.

Norris HJ, et al. Immature malignant teratoma of the ovary. *Cancer.* 1976;37:2359.

Peccatori F, et al. Surgical management of malignant ovarian germ-cell tumors: 10 years experience of 129 patients. *Obstet Gynecol.* 1995;86:367–372.

SD Williams, DM Gershenson, CJ Horowitz, RE Scully. Ovarian germ-cell tumors. Chapter 33. In: Hoskins WJ, Perez CA, Young RC (eds.). *Principles and Practice Gynecologic Oncology.* 2nd ed. Philadelphia, PA: Lippincott-Raven;1997:987–1001.

Tewari K, et al. Malignant germ cell tumors of the ovary. *Obstet Gynecol.* 2000;95:128–133.

Thurlbeck WM, Scully RE. Solid teratoma of the ovary. *Cancer.* 1960;13:804–811.

# 127 HEREDITARY OVARIAN CANCER SYNDROME

*Andrew John Li*

## LEARNING POINT

Women with family histories suggestive of a hereditary ovarian cancer syndrome should undergo genetic screening and possible testing.

## VIGNETTE

A 35-year-old, G2P2, presents for evaluation after her mother was diagnosed with epithelial ovarian cancer. She reports having normal menses, and denies any pelvic pain, bloating, nausea, vomiting, or anorexia. She is healthy and does not desire future fertility.

Her past medical history is not significant for any chronic conditions. Her gynecologic history is significant for two spontaneous vaginal deliveries and no history of abnormal Pap smears. She denies any tobacco or regular alcohol use. Her family history is significant for a mother with ovarian cancer, and a grandmother who was diagnosed with breast cancer at age 45 years. She also has a maternal aunt with breast cancer diagnosed at age 42 years. The patient is of Ashkenazi Jewish descent.

The physical examination reveals a thin Caucasian female. Vital signs: blood pressure 120/60 mm Hg; pulse 70/min; respiratory rate 16/min; and temperature 96.8°F. Chest is clear to auscultation, cardiac shows regular rate and rhythm; abdomen is obese, nontender, without masses or fluid wave. On pelvic exam, she has normal external female genitalia. Her vagina and cervix are unremarkable. The uterus is 6 cm in size, mobile, and anteverted; her adnexae are palpable bilaterally and are without masses. Recto-vaginal examination is confirmatory.

On follow-up visit, the patient reports that her mother tested positive for a mutation in the breast cancer gene 1 (*BRCA1*).

## QUESTION 1

*What are hereditary syndromes associated with epithelial ovarian cancer?*

## ANSWER 1

Hereditary etiologies of epithelial ovarian cancer are responsible for 10% of all cases. The affected genes are most commonly *BRCA1, BRCA2*, and mutations in the DNA mismatch genes responsible for hereditary nonpolyposis colon cancer (HNPCC). The BRCA genes are breast and ovarian cancer susceptibility genes on chromosomes 17 and 13, respectively. The lifetime risk of developing ovarian cancer is 54% with mutations in *BRCA1* and 23% with mutations in *BRCA2*. The DNA mismatch repair genes (e.g., human mutS homolog 2 [*hMSH2*], human mutL homolog 1 [*hMLH1*]) associated with HNPCC are also linked to an increased risk of endometrial and ovarian cancers; the lifetime risk of developing ovarian cancer is 10–12% with HNPCC (see Fig. 127-1).

These hereditary cancers are typically diagnosed 10–15 years earlier than their sporadic counterparts.

## QUESTION 2

*What intervention strategies may be utilized to minimize risk in women with a family history of hereditary ovarian cancer?*

## ANSWER 2

In patients with known mutations in *BRCA1, BRCA2*, or the HNPCC genes, several strategies may be considered to minimize risk of developing ovarian cancer. These include surveillance, chemoprevention, and prophylactic surgery. Surveillance guidelines for these patients are not well established; typically gynecologic oncologists recommend screening with transvaginal ultrasounds and serum cancer antigen-125 (CA-125). An National Institute of Health (NIH) consensus statement reported that while no data exists to suggest screening decreases mortality in women with genetic susceptibility to ovarian cancer development, at least annual recto-vaginal exam, transvaginal ultrasound, and serum CA-125 is recommended. Chemoprevention is also controversial; studies have not demonstrated consensus regarding the protective role of oral contraceptives against ovarian carcinogenesis in women with BRCA mutations. Prophylactic bilateral salpingo-oophorectomy in women who have completed childbearing is a third option, and studies suggest significant reductions in risk for both development of ovarian as well as breast cancers, with a risk reduction of 0.15 for BRCA mutation carriers who undergo prophylactic surgery.

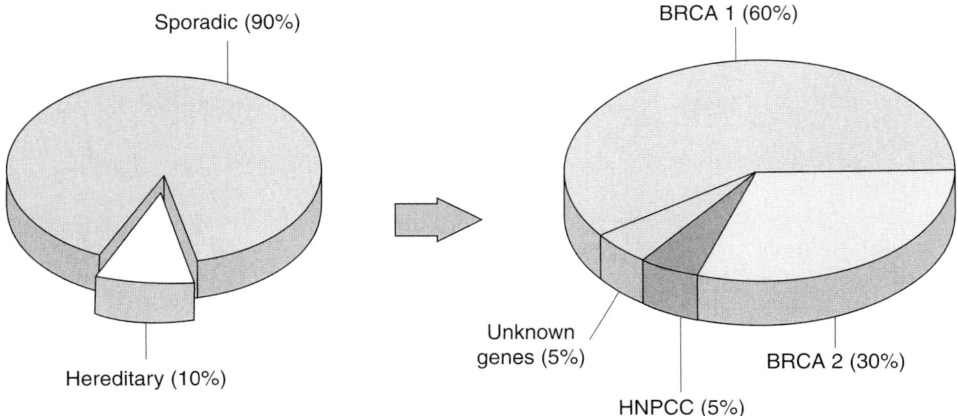


**FIG. 127-1** Percentages of hereditary ovarian neoplasia.

## QUESTION 3

*Are there clinical differences in prognosis in women with hereditary ovarian cancers?*

## ANSWER 3

Several studies suggest an improvement in overall survival when patients with epithelial ovarian cancer and a BRCA mutation are compared to their counterparts with sporadic disease. In a retrospective series, some have identified median survival differences as wide as 77 months for those with *BRCA1* mutations compared to only 29 months for those without BRCA mutations; other data, including patients with both *BRCA1* and *BRCA2* mutations, have supported these findings, with overall survivals of 45 months for those with BRCA mutations compared to 25 months for those without such mutations. In a separate analysis, other investigators suggested that patients who develop ovarian cancer from BRCA mutations have greater sensitivity to chemotherapy, as determined from drug resistance assays.

## BIBLIOGRAPHY

Berek JS. Epithelial ovarian cancer. Chapter 11. In: Berek JS, Hacker NF (eds.). *Practical Gynecologic Oncology*. 4th ed. Philadelphia, PA: Lippincott Williams & Wilkins; 2005:443–509.

Boyd J, Sonoda Y, Federici MG, et al. Clinicopathologic features of BRCA-linked and sporadic ovarian cancer. *JAMA*. 2000; 283(17):2260–2265.

Cass I, Baldwin RL, Varkey T, Moslehi R, Narod SA, Karlan BY. Improved survival in women with BRCA-associated ovarian carcinoma. *Cancer.* 2003;97:2187–2195.

Kauff ND, Satagopan JM, Robson ME, et al. Risk-reducing salpingo-oophorectomy in women with a BRCA1 or BRCA2 mutation. *N Engl J Med.* 2002;346:1609–1615.

King MC, Marks JH, Manell JB. The New York Breast Cancer Study Group. Breast and ovarian cancer risks due to inherited mutations in BRCA1 and BRCA2. *Science.* 2003;302: 643–646.

Modan B, Hartge P, Hirsh-Yechezkel G, et al. Parity, oral contraceptives, and the risk of ovarian cancer among carriers and noncarriers of a BRCA1 or BRCA2 mutation. *N Engl J Med.* 2001;345:235–240.

Narod SA, Risch H, Moslehi R, et al. Oral contraceptives and the risk of hereditary ovarian cancer. Hereditary Ovarian Cancer Clinical Study Group. *N Engl J Med.* 1998;339:424–428.

Ovarian cancer: screening, treatment, and followup. *NIH Consens Statement.* 1994;12(3):1–30.

Rubin SC, Benjamin I, Behbakht K, et al. Clinical and pathological features of ovarian cancer in women with germ-line mutations of BRCA1. *N Engl J Med.* 1996;335:1413–1416.

Watson P, Butzow R, Lynch HT, et al. The clinical features of ovarian cancer in hereditary nonpolyposis colorectal cancer. *Gynecol Oncol.* 2001;82:223–228.

# 128 GRANULOSA CELL TUMOR

*Andrew John Li*

## LEARNING POINT

Ovarian granulosa cell tumors (GCTs) should undergo surgical staging; due to secretion of estrogen, endometrial hyperplasia and cancer should be ruled out.

## VIGNETTE

A 64-year-old, G4P4, female presents with intermittent severe abdominal pain and vaginal bleeding. She reports a 3-month history of bloating with occasional nausea but no vomiting. She denies any weight changes. She reports increased breast tenderness but denies any breast masses or nipple discharge.

The patient's family history is negative for breast, uterine, colon, or ovarian cancer. She denies any tobacco or regular alcohol use. Her obstetrical history is significant for four term pregnancies all of which delivered vaginally. She denies any history of sexually transmitted diseases or abnormal Pap smears.

The physical examination reveals a thin African-American female. Vital signs: blood pressure 100/60 mm Hg, pulse 80/min, respiratory rate 16/min, and temperature 98.6°F. Chest is clear to auscultation, cardiac demonstrates a regular rate and rhythm; abdomen is soft, nondistended, with a tender mass palpable in the left lower quadrant. On pelvic exam, she has normal external female genitalia without lesions. Dark blood is identified in her vaginal vault, and the cervix is normal without fungating lesions. Her uterus is 6 cm in size and mobile; adnexal examination reveals a mobile and tender 6 cm left sided mass. Rectal examination is confirmatory.

## QUESTION 1

*What histologic characteristics are described for GCTs? What are the different classifications of GCTs?*

## ANSWER 1

The microfollicular pattern is the most common histologic finding in adult GCTs, with small cavities lined by granulosa cells and filled with fluid and degenerating desquamated cells. These structures are known as Call-Exner bodies and recapitulate a developing follicle. Other patterns, which may be pure or coexistent, are macrofollicular, trabecular, insular, and "watered silk." The characteristic appearance of the nuclei is the best key for the diagnosis: they are uniform, pale, with longitudinal grooves, and are commonly called "coffee bean" nuclei. Cytologic atypia and mitotic figures are uncommon.

Juvenile GCTs are seen predominantly in patients younger than 20 years of age, and most present with sexual pseudoprecocity. Histologically, these tumors demonstrate a macrofollicular pattern with frequent mitoses and atypical cells. Juvenile GCTs behave less aggressively than the adult type.

## QUESTION 2

*What markers are useful in following patients with GCTs?*

## ANSWER 2

Estradiol and inhibin are useful markers to follow women for recurrence. Estradiol is responsible for some of the clinical manifestations of GCTs, but it remains an unreliable marker due to variability in secretion from patient to patient. No consistent correlation has been shown between estradiol levels and progression or recurrence of disease. Inhibin is a heterodimeric polypeptide hormone produced by granulosa cells of normal ovarian follicles and is a potent negative feedback regulator of follicle-stimulating hormone. The alpha subunit of inhibin may associate with one of two distinct beta subunits, leading to the formation of either inhibin A or inhibin B. Inhibin B is typically more frequently elevated in patients with GCTs, and subsequent elevations have been shown to predate diagnosis of recurrent disease.

## QUESTION 3

*What other gynecologic neoplasms should be ruled out in patients with GCTs of the ovary?*

## ANSWER 3

Theca cells are responsible for estrogen production by the tumor. Vaginal bleeding is a common presenting sign, indicating potential endometrial pathology. Endometrial hyperplasia and carcinoma must be evaluated in women diagnosed with GCT. The incidence of endometrial hyperplasia has been shown to be 30–40% and the incidence of concurrent endometrial carcinoma is 5–10%.

## QUESTION 4

*Why should GCTs undergo surgical staging? What are prognostic factors for survival?*

## ANSWER 4

Over 90% of GCTs are confined to the ovary and have an excellent prognosis. In a review of 92 GCTs, factors predictive of overall survival included age over 40 at the time of diagnosis, a presentation with abdominal symptoms, a palpable mass, a solid large tumor, bilateral tumors, extraovarian spread, and numerous mitotic figures in the tumor. In stage I disease, factors associated with higher risk of recurrence include large tumor size, high mitotic index, or tumor rupture. In a more recent analysis of 47 patients with GCTs, only stage remained statistically significant as an independent predictor of overall survival in a multivariate analysis. Surgery is indicated as first-line management of these tumors for definitive tissue diagnosis, staging, and tumor debulking. In older women, a total abdominal hysterectomy and bilateral salpingo-oophorectomy is recommended; in patients desiring future fertility, unilateral salpingo-oophorectomy is acceptable provided that staging does not identify metastatic disease and a dilation and curettage (D&C) is performed to exclude endometrial carcinoma. With advanced stage disease, adjuvant chemotherapy is indicated, a combination of bleomycin, etoposide, and cisplatin should be considered as first-line treatment.

## BIBLIOGRAPHY

Berek JS, Hacker NF (eds.). In: *Practical Gynecologic Oncology.* 4th ed. Philadelphia, PA: Lippincott Williams & Wilkins; 2005.

Boggess JF, Soules MR, Goff BA, et al. Serum inhibin and disease status in women with ovarian granulosa cell tumors. *Gynecol Oncol.* 1997;64:64–69.

Fox H, Agrawal K, Langley FA. A clinicopathologic study of 92 cases of granulosa cell tumor of the ovary with special reference to the factors influencing prognosis. *Cancer.* 1975; 35(1):231–241.

Homesley HD, Bundy BN, Hurteau JA, Roth LM. Bleomycin, etoposide, and cisplatin combination therapy of ovarian granulosa cell tumors and other stromal malignancies:a Gynecologic Oncology Group Study. *Gynecol Oncol.* 1999;72:131–137.

Lal A, Bourtsos EP, Nayar R, DeFrias DV. Cytologic features of granulosa cell tumors in fluids and fine needle aspiration specimens. *Acta Cytol.* 2004;48:315–320.

Malmstrom H, Hogberg T, Risberg B, Simonsen E. Granulosa cell tumors of the ovary:prognostic factors and outcome. *Gynecol Oncol.* 1994;52:50–55.

Rey RA, Lhomme C, Marcilliac I, et al. Antimullerian hormone as a serum marker of granulosal cell tumors of the ovary: comparative study with serum alpha inhibin and estradiol. *Am J Obstet Gynecol.* 1996;174:958–965.

Schumer ST, Cannistra SA. Granulosa cell tumor of the ovary. *J Clin Oncol.* 2003;21:1180–1189.

Stenwig, et al. Granulosa cell tumors of the ovary. A clinicopathological study of 118 cases with long-term follow-up. *Gynecol Oncol.* 1979;11:261–274.

Unkila-Kallio L, Tiitinen A, Wahlstrom T, Lehtovirta P, Leminen A. Reproductive features in women developing ovarian granulosa cell tumour at a fertile age. *Hum Reprod.* 2000;15(3): 589–593.

Uygun K, Aydiner A, Saip P, et al. Granulosa cell tumor of the ovary:retrospective analysis of 45 cases. *Am J Clin Oncol.* 2003;26:517–521.

# 129 PELVIC EXENTERATION

*Ilana Cass*

## LEARNING POINT

To understand appropriate patient selection and morbidity associated with pelvic exenteration.

## VIGNETTE

A 60-year-old, G3P2, female with a history of squamous cell carcinoma presents with vaginal bleeding over the past 4 weeks. She was diagnosed with a stage IB2 squamous cell carcinoma 2 years ago for which she was treated with a modified radical hysterectomy, bilateral salpingo-oophorectomy, and bilateral pelvic lymphadenectomy. She was treated with adjuvant chemoradiation using cisplatin chemotherapy because of a 4 cm tumor with extensive lymphvascular-space invasion despite no lymph node metastases. She has been followed regularly and has had normal Pap smears.

She does not take hormone replacement therapy. She has a significant medial history of hypertension. She is an ex-smoker, but had a prior 30 pack-year history. She is sexually active in a monogamous relationship.

Physical examination reveals a woman of medium body habitus in no distress. Vitals signs: pulse 88/min, BP 130/80 mm Hg. Head, eyes, ears, nose, and throat examination reveals no adenopathy, chest is clear to auscultation, cardiac examination shows regular rate and rhythm, abdominal examination is consistent with a well-healed low transverse abdominal incision. She has no evidence of any ascites, masses, or inguinal adenopathy. Pelvic examination reveals an atrophic external genitalia. There is a small friable mass at the apex of the vagina which is bleeding. The remainder of the vagina is smooth, but there is a firm area posterior to the mass involving the left vagina on rectovaginal exam. Extremities reveal no edema. A biopsy of the mass is performed which is consistent with recurrent squamous cell carcinoma of the cervix.

### QUESTION 1

*How is the pelvic exenteration procedure classified?*

### ANSWER 1

The essential components of a pelvic exenteration are excision of the rectum or bladder with the distal ureters in conjunction with removal of the vagina and uterus. The pelvic organs that are removed and whether the resection extends below the levator ani muscles classify the operation.

Anterior—bladder and ureters
Posterior—rectum
Total—both bladder and rectum
Supralevator/infralevator—above or below the levator muscles, infralevator exenteration includes a total vaginectomy and urethrectomy
Extended—includes resection of the levator muscles, partial or total vulvectomy, groin node dissection, or partial pubectomy (see Fig. 129-1).

### QUESTION 2

*What percent of patients explored for exenteration are deemed unresectable and the procedure abandoned?*

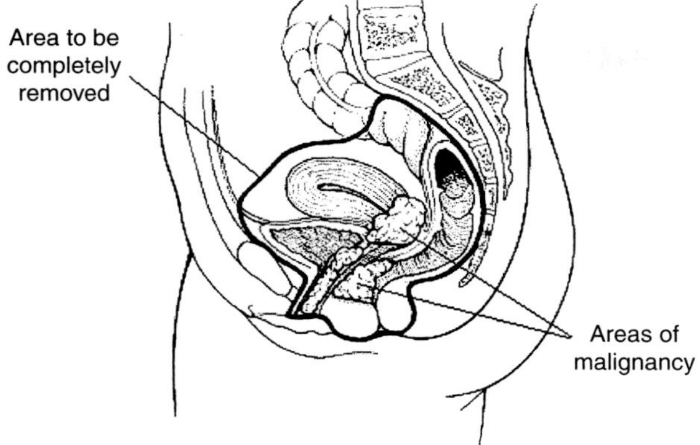


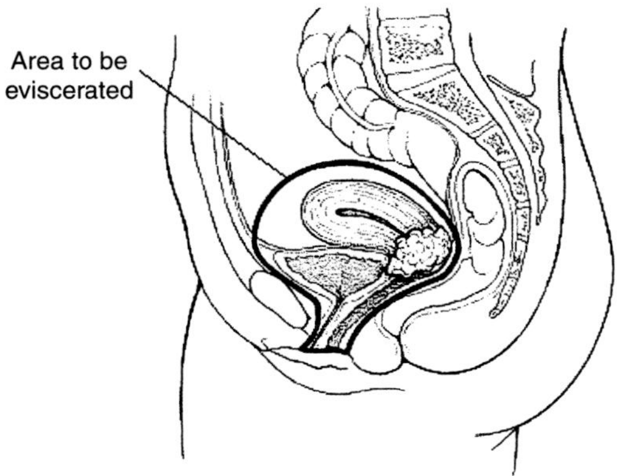


**FIG. 129-1** Schematic representation of lines of resection. Hatch KD, Mann WJ. Exenteration for gynecologic cancer. In: Rose BD (ed.). *UpToDate*. Waltham, MA:UpToDate;2006. www.Uptodate.com.

*What are the major medical and surgical complications associated with a pelvic exenteration procedure?*

## ANSWER 2

Figures vary by institution, but in general 1/3 to 1/2 of exenterations are aborted because of unresectable pelvic sidewall disease, liver or abdominal metastases, or nodal disease. Mortality from exenteration ranges between 2% and 15%, but should be <5% in most institutions. Approximately 1/2 of patients will have a major acute complication including: prolonged hospital stay (>15 days), large blood loss (median 3000 cc), wound infection and dehiscence, urinary fistula, intestinal leak and or anastomosis breakdown, small bowel obstruction, pulmonary embolus, sepsis, deep vein thrombosis, flap or stomal necrosis, renal failure, or pneumonia.

## QUESTION 3

*What is the 5-year survival for patients with recurrent cervical cancer following a pelvic exenteration?*

## ANSWER 3

Five-year survival rates are 40–60%. Large series have found that the clinical and pathologic factors most predictive of outcome include: duration from initial therapy to the exenteration procedure, size of the central mass, presence of preoperative pelvic sidewall fixation, margin status of resection, histology of the primary tumor, and lymph node metastases at the time of pelvic exenteration. Patients at the lowest risk of recurrence were those who had: long duration (>1 year between completion of therapy and exenteration), <3 cm central tumor recurrence, squamous histology, no sidewall fixation, negative margins, and negative lymph nodes with a 70–82% 5-year survival. Patients with any pelvic lymph node metastases had a median survival of 12 months.

## BIBLIOGRAPHY

CP Morrow, JP Curtin (eds.). Surgery for cervical neoplasia. In: *Gynecologic Cancer Surgery*. Philadelphia, PA: Churchill Livingstone; 1996:531–557.

Hatch KD, Mann WJ. Exenteration for gynecologic cancer. In: Rose BD (ed.) UpToDate. Waltham, MA:UpToDate;2006. www.Uptodate.com

Houvenaeghel G, Moutardier V, Karsenty G, Bladou F, Lelong B, Buttarelli M, Delpero JR. Major complications of urinary diversion after pelvic exenteration for gynecologic malignancies. *Gynecol Oncol.* 2004;92:680–683.

Mirashemi R, Avrette HE, Estape R, Angioli R, Mehran R, Mednez L, Cantuaria G, Penalver M. Low colorectal anastomosis after radical pelvic surgery: a risk factor analysis. *Am J Obstet Gynecol.* 2000;183:1375–1380.

Morley GW, Hopkins MP, Lindenauer SM, Roberts JA. Pelvic exenteration, University of Michigan: 100 patients at 5 years. *Obstet Gynecol.* 1989;74(6):934–943.

Ramirez PT, Modesitt SC, Morris M, Creighton EL, Bevers MW, Wharton JT, Wolf JK. Functional outcomes and complications of continent urinary diversions in patients with gynecologic malignancies. *Gynecol Oncol.* 2002;85:285–291.

Shingelton HM, Soong S, Gelder MS, Hatch KD, Baker VV, Austin JM. Clinical and histopathologic factors predicting recurrence and survival after pelvic exenteration for cancer of the cervix. *Obstet Gynecol.* 1989;73:1027–1034.

# 130 PRIMARY PERITONEAL CANCER

*Amer K. Karam*

## LEARNING POINT

To understand the epidemiology, presentation, classification, and treatment of primary peritoneal cancer.

## VIGNETTE

A 55-year-old female presents with progressive abdominal distension, early satiety, nausea, and vomiting. Her past medical history is only notable for hypertension that is well controlled and hyperlipidemia. Her last menstrual period was 4 years prior to presentation and she denies any hormone replacement therapy. Her obstetrical history is significant for one full-term cesarean section. She does not smoke or drink any alcohol. On abdominal examination, a fluid wave and shifting dullness, as well as a palpable omental cake are noted. A computed tomography of the abdomen and pelvis reveals peritoneal carcinomatosis and moderate ascites. The patient's cancer antigen-125 (CA-125) level is 2500 IU/mL. On exploratory laparotomy diffuse peritoneal carcinomatosis with a large omental cake are noted, the ovaries are, however not enlarged.

### QUESTION 1

*What are some of the clinical manifestations of primary peritoneal cancer?*

### ANSWER 1

Primary peritoneal carcinoma is a malignancy that arises primarily from peritoneal cells. The mesothelium of the peritoneum and the germinal epithelium of the ovary arise from the same embryologic origin; therefore, the peritoneum may retain the multipotentiality of the müllerian system, allowing the development of a primary carcinoma. As in patients with ovarian cancer, most women with primary peritoneal cancer have nonspecific symptoms including abdominal discomfort, bloating, constipation, nausea, early satiety, indigestion, and urinary frequency.

### QUESTION 2

*What are the pathologic criteria used to diagnose primary peritoneal cancer?*

### QUESTION 2

The Gynecologic Oncology Group (GOG) has established criteria to define primary peritoneal carcinoma (see Fig. 130-1):

1. Ovaries normal in size.
2. Extraovarian involvement greater than ovarian involvement.
3. Surface involvement of less than 5 mm in depth and width.

### QUESTION 3

*What are some of the risk factors for primary peritoneal cancer?*

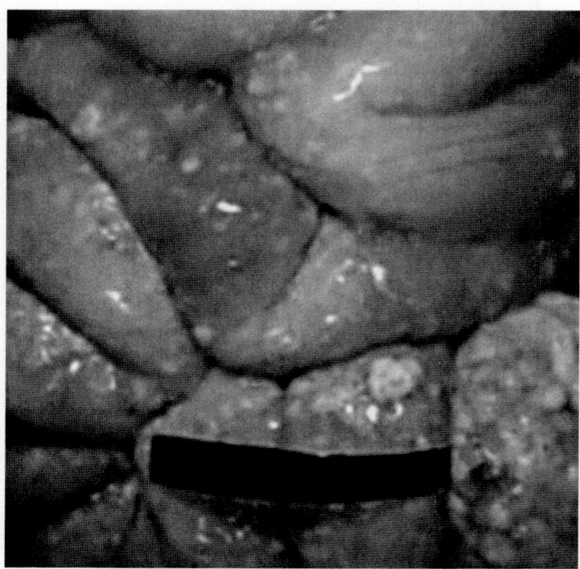

**FIG. 130-1** Peritoneal carcinomatosis.

## ANSWER 3

The strongest known risk factor for primary peritoneal cancer is a family history. Breast cancer gene (*BRCA*) mutations occur more commonly in patients with primary peritoneal cancer with up to 28–41% of Ashkenazi Jewish patients carrying the mutation. There is also evidence that primary peritoneal cancer occur more commonly in patients with *BRCA1* mutations. The incidence of primary peritoneal cancer increases with age, whereas the use of oral contraceptives and pregnancy may exert a protective effect.

## QUESTION 4

*What are the essentials of management of primary peritoneal cancer?*

## ANSWER 4

Patients with primary peritoneal cancer are treated similarly to those with epithelial ovarian cancer. Surgical cytoreduction remains the cornerstone of surgical management, followed by combination chemotherapy using platinum and taxane drugs. These women respond well to surgery and chemotherapy with 15–20% achieving long-term remission.

## BIBLIOGRAPHY


Barda G, et al. Comparison between primary peritoneal and epithelial ovarian carcinoma: a population-based study. *Am J Obstet Gynecol.* 2004;190:1039–1045.

Bloss JD, et al. Extraovarian peritoneal serous papillary carcinoma: a case-control retrospective comparison to papillary adenocarcinoma of the ovary. *Gynecol Oncol.* 1993;50:347–351.

Bloss JD, et al. Extraovarian peritoneal serous papillary carcinoma: a phase II trial of cisplatin and cyclophosphamide with comparison to a cohort with papillary serous ovarian carcinoma-a Gynecologic Oncology Group Study. *Gynecol Oncol.* 2003; 89:148–154.

Fromm GL, et al. Papillary serous carcinoma of the peritoneum. *Obstet Gynecol.* 1990;75:89–95.

Levine DA, et al. Fallopian tube and primary peritoneal carcinomas associated with BRCA mutations. *J Clin Oncol.* 2003;21: 4222–4227.

Menczer J, et al. Frequency of BRCA mutations in primary peritoneal carcinoma in Israeli Jewishwomen. *Gynecol Oncol.* 2003; 88:58–61.

Schorge JO, et al. Molecular evidence for multifocal papillary serous carcinoma of the peritoneum in patients with germline BRCA1 mutations. *J Natl Cancer Inst.* 1998;90:841–845.


# 131 UTERINE SARCOMA

*Amer K. Karam*

## LEARNING POINT

To understand the epidemiology, presentation, classification, and treatment of uterine sarcomas.

## VIGNETTE

A 62-year-old female presents with a recent onset of postmenopausal bleeding and a growing pelvic mass. She had been menopausal for the past 11 years and denies any history of oral contraceptive use or hormone replacement therapy. On pelvic exam, a fleshy tumor is seen protruding through the cervical os. A biopsy of the mass returns as heterologous mixed malignant mullerian tumor.

## QUESTION 1

*What are some risk factors for uterine sarcomas?*

## ANSWER 1

1. Uterine sarcomas occur mostly in postmenopausal women between 40 and 60 years of age.
2. Black women have a two- to threefold increased risk of developing uterine sarcomas as compared to White women.
3. A history of pelvic radiation has been noted in 5–10% of patients with uterine sarcomas.
4. Some studies suggest that the long-term adjuvant use of tamoxifen in women with breast cancer is associated with an increased risk of developing uterine sarcomas particularly mixed malignant mullerian tumors.

## QUESTION 2

*What are the pathologic criteria used to diagnose leiomyosarcomas?*

## ANSWER 2

1. Frequent mitotic figures
2. Significant nuclear atypia
3. Presence of coagulative necrosis of tumor cells

## QUESTION3

*What are the essentials of management of uterine sarcomas?*

## ANSWER 3

Extrafascial abdominal hysterectomy with bilateral salpingo-oophorectomy is the primary treatment of uterine sarcoma and may be curative for tumors confined to the uterus. Radiation therapy and chemotherapy are used as adjunctive modalities to surgery and in patients with advanced disease. Complete surgical staging of patients with mixed malignant mullerian tumors may be useful as occult metastases to the adnexae, omentum, pelvic and paraaortic nodes are common in these patients (see Fig. 131-1). On the other hand, patients with leiomyosarcoma apparently confined to the uterus have a much lower risk of occult adnexal and nodal disease.

## QUESTION 4

*What is the prognosis for uterine sarcomas?*

## ANSWER 4

The prognosis for uterine sarcomas is poorer than that for other uterine malignancies. The 5-year survival for stage I uterine sarcoma is 50% and falls to 20–30% when the tumor has spread beyond the uterus. Factors adversely affecting outcome in cases of mixed malignant mullerian tumors include the depth of myometrial involvement, adnexal extension, lymph node metastasis, and positive peritoneal washings. For leiomyosarcomas, a high mitotic index, large tumors, and advanced age have been associated with lower survival.

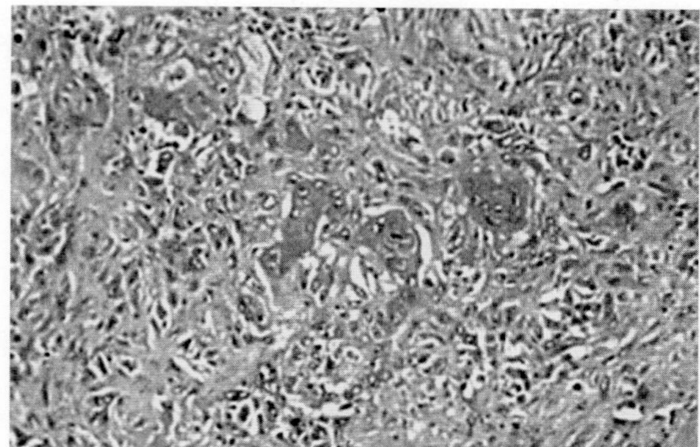

**FIG. 131-1** Mixed malignant mullerian tumor.

## BIBLIOGRAPHY

Brooks SE, et al. Surveillance, epidemiology, and end results analysis of 2677 cases of uterine sarcoma 1989–1999. *Gynecol Oncol.* 2004;93:204–208.

Disaia, PJ Creasman, WT. *Clinical Gynecologic Oncology.* 5th ed. Mosby; St. Louis, MO: 1993:177.

Kurman RJ. *Pathology of the Female Genital Tract.* 4th ed. New York: Springer-Verlang; 499.

Major FJ, et al. Prognostic factors in early-stage uterine sarcoma. *Cancer.* 1993;71:1702–1709.

Meredith RF, et al. An excess of uterine sarcomas after pelvic irradiation. *Cancer.* 1986;58:2003–2007.

Wysowski, et al. Uterine sarcoma associated with tamoxifen use. *N Engl J Med.* 2002;346:1832.

Yamada SD, et al. Pathologic variables and adjuvant therapy as predictors of recurrence and survival for patients with surgically evaluated carcinosarcoma of the uterus. *Cancer.* 2000; 88:2782–2786.

# 132 VULVAR CARCINOMA

*Andrew John Li*

## LEARNING POINT

Smoking is a significant risk factor for vulvar cancer; vulvar lesions should be biopsied to rule out malignant disease.

## VIGNETTE

A 68-year-old, G1P1, presents with vaginal spotting. She reports severe pruritus of her left labia, and scratches herself constantly. She denies any nausea, fevers, or abdominal distension. She has no hematuria or bright red blood per rectum.

Her past medical history is significant for hypertension. Her gynecologic history is negative for any abnormal Pap smears. The patient reports smoking a pack of cigarettes per day for the last 35 years.

The physical examination reveals a thin Caucasian female. Vital signs: BP 140/90 mm Hg, pulse 70/min, respiratory rate 16/min, and temperature 96.8°F. Chest is clear to auscultation; cardiac shows regular rate and rhythm; abdomen is obese, nontender, without masses or fluid wave. On pelvic exam, her vulva demonstrates a $3 \times 5$ cm lesion on her left labia that does not involve the urethra. The lesion is 2 cm away from the midline. A 1 cm mobile lymph node is palpated in the left inguinal region. The remainder of her gynecologic examination is unremarkable.

A vulvar biopsy is performed and results are consistent with an invasive squamous cell carcinoma.

## QUESTION 1

*What are risk factors and symptoms of vulvar cancer?*

## ANSWER 1

Risk factors are not as clearly defined for vulvar cancer as they are for cervical cancer. The malignant potential of vulvar dystrophies is controversial, although the precursor lesion (i.e., vulvar intraepithelial neoplasia [VIN]) is more likely to progress to invasive disease if untreated. Infection with the human papillomavirus (HPV) and tobacco use has also been implicated in case-control studies. These studies suggest two different etiologic types of vulvar cancer: one in younger patients, related to smoking and HPV infection, and a second in older patients, related to concurrent VIN and dystrophic lesions.

Most patients with vulvar cancer present with a pruritic lesion. Less common symptoms include vulvar bleeding, discharge, or dysuria. More rarely will patients present with a large mass in the groin region, representing a lymph node metastasis. Vulvar cancers may occur on the labia majora, labia minora, clitoris, and perineum.

## QUESTION 2

*What treatment modalities may be considered for women with vulvar cancer?*

## ANSWER 2

For most patients with resectable disease, radical vulvectomy and bilateral inguinal-femoral lymphadenectomies are indicated for invasive squamous cell carcinomas of the vulva. Several advances have improved morbidity and quality of life for women undergoing surgery for vulvar cancer. These include use of the "triple" incision; instead of a wide en bloc resection of the bilateral groin lymph nodes and vulva, three separate incisions are used to separately resect disease and lymph nodes at each site. Furthermore, with small lesions (e.g., less than 2 cm) radical local excision is favored over complete bilateral vulvectomy, sparing the contralateral normal labia and reducing postoperative complications. For advanced stage disease that is not resectable (or involves the urethra or bladder), neoadjuvant chemotherapy and radiation may be utilized to shrink the disease prior to surgery. Phase II trials have identified a complete response in 48% of patients treated with this approach.

## QUESTION 3

*What is the significance of "microinvasive" squamous cell carcinoma of the vulva?*

## ANSWER 3

Microinvasive squamous cell carcinoma of the vulva (stage IA) is a distinct subcategory of stage 1 disease defined by an invasive lesion to less than 1 mm below the basement membrane. This must be distinguished from microinvasive squamous cell carcinoma of the cervix, which is defined as less than 3 mm invasion. Patients with stage IA vulvar cancer have a negligible risk of metastases to the inguinal-femoral lymph nodes, and thus do not need to undergo groin lymph node dissection. Similarly, they should be excised with a radical local excision rather than a radical vulvectomy.

## BIBLIOGRAPHY


Brinton LA, Nasca PC, Mallin K, et al. Case control study of cancer of the vulva. *Obstet Gynecol.* 1990;75:859–866.

Farias-Eisner R, Cirisano FD, Grouse D, Leuchter RS, Karlan BY, Lagasse LD, Berek JS. Conservative and individualized surgery for early squamous carcinoma of the vulva: the treatment of choice for stage I and II (T1-2N0-1M0) disease. *Gynecol Oncol.* 1994;53:55–58.

Gotlieb WH. The assessment and surgical management of early-stage vulvar cancer. *Best Pract Res Clin Obstet Gynecol.* 2003;17:557–569.

Hacker NF. Vulvar cancer. Chapter 13. In: Berek JS, Hacker NF (eds). *Practical Gynecologic Oncology.* 4th ed. Philadelphia, PA: Lippincott Williams & Wilkins; 2005;543–583.

Jones RW, Baranyai J, Sables S. Trends in squamous cell carcinoma of the vulva: the influence of vulvar intraepithelial neoplasia. *Obstet Gynecol.* 1996;174:929–933.

Magrina JF, Gonzalez-Bosquet J, Weaver AL, Gaffey TA, Leslie KO, Webb MJ, Podratz KC. Squamous cell carcinoma of the vulva stage IA: long-term results. *Gynecol Oncol.* 2000;76:24–27.

Moore DH, Thomas GM, Montana GS, Saxer A, Gallup DG, Olt G. Preoperative chemoradiation for advanced vulvar cancer: a phase II study of the Gynecologic Oncology Group. *Int J Radiat Oncol Biol Phys.* 1998;42:79–85.

Rusk D, Sutton GP, Look KY, Roman A. Analysis of invasive squamous cell carcinoma and papillomaviruses: indications for two different etiologies. *Gynecol Oncol.* 1994;52:241–246.

# 133 VULVAR INTRAEPITHELIAL NEOPLASIA

*Christine Walsh*

## LEARNING POINT

Classification, risk factors, recognition, and treatment of vulvar intraepithelial neoplasia (VIN).

## VIGNETTE

A 32-year-old female comes into your office for evaluation of an area of pruritis on her vulva. On history, you find out that she had a loop electrosurgical excisional procedure (LEEP) for cervical dysplasia 2 years previously and that she smokes 1 pack of cigarettes per day. On examination, you detect several raised, white, lesions on the right labia minora. You suspect VIN and proceed to biopsy the abnormal areas.

### QUESTION 1

*What are the histopathologic characteristics that define VIN and what are the similarities and differences to cervical intraepithelial neoplasia (CIN)?*

### ANSWER 1

VIN lesions are graded based on the level of nuclear atypia, cellular disarray, and mitotic activity in the squamous epithelium of the vulva. The grading scale parallels that of CIN with involvement of the lowest third classified as VIN I (mild dysplasia), the lower two-thirds as VIN II (moderate dysplasia), and greater than two-thirds as VIN III (severe dysplasia or carcinoma in situ). However, there are important clinical differences between VIN and CIN. Whereas CIN I is a very common lesion of the cervix, VIN I of the vulva is rare and, when seen, is often in the context of higher grades of VIN. In contrast to CIN, which develops in an area of active metaplasia called the transformation zone of the cervix, VIN develops in mature squamous epithelium, and so more closely resembles premalignant lesions of the oral cavity and vocal cords than those of the cervix. Similar to CIN, VIN lesions are associated with high-risk HPV, particularly HPV 16. However, there is a distinct subset of VIN in which the HPV virus is not associated.

### QUESTION 2

*What is the current classification system for VIN? What are the two subtypes and their different clinical and pathologic characteristics?*

### ANSWER 2

The VIN terminology was developed to encompass the spectrum of lesions believed to be precursors to invasive vulvar squamous cell carcinoma (SCC). The VIN classification system has been widely adopted since the 1980s–1990s and replaces outdated terminology such as Bowen's disease, erythroplasia of Queyrat, simplex carcinoma in situ, and atypia. There are two distinct subtypes: classic (bowenoid) VIN and simplex (differentiated) VIN. Table 133-1 demonstrates the different clinical and pathologic features of the two subtypes.

### QUESTION 3

*What are the risk factors associated with VIN?*

### ANSWER 3

The incidence of VIN is increasing worldwide due to the changes in the epidemiology of HPV. In particular, HPV 16 infection had led to an increased incidence of VIN III and a parallel increased incidence of invasive vulvar cancer in young women. Invasive vulvar cancer now has a bimodal age distribution with peaks at 40–50 years and at 70–80 years. Other risk factors for VIN include multiple

**TABLE 133-1. Characteristics of Two Subtypes of VIN**

| | CLASSIC "BOWENOID" VIN | SIMPLEX "DIFFERENTIATED" VIN |
|---|---|---|
| Frequency | Most commonly described VIN | 2–10% of VIN |
| Demographics | Young women, 30s–40s | Postmenopausal women, mean age 67 |
| Association with HPV | Positive | Negative |
| Associated genital pathology | Associated with multicentric lower genital tract neoplasia (cervix/vagina) in 18–52%, condylomas, herpes, HIV | Associated with lichen sclerosis and/or squamous hyperplasia in 83%, often found adjacent to or overlying invasive SCC |
| Association with smoking | 60–80% | 25% |
| Clinical appearance | Bulky, white or erythematous plaques, may be pigmented, verruciform, polypoid, or papular. 40% multifocal. | Less bulky, focal gray-white discoloration with roughened surface, ill-defined raised plaque. May be multifocal. |
| Microscopic appearance | "Wind-blown" disorganization of keratinocytes. Nuclear enlargement with hyperchromatism, pleomorphism, mitotic figures. | Highly differentiated, absence of widespread architectural disarray or nuclear atypia. Enlarged squamous cells . with very eosinophilic cytoplasm. Positive p53 staining. |
| Association with invasive SCC | 6–19% occult invasive SCC. 3–10% subsequent invasive SCC. Risk of progression greatest if age >40, immunocompromised. | Frequently coexists with invasive SCC. |

VIN is vulvar intraepithelical neoplasia.
SCC is squamous cell carcinoma.

sexual partners, a history of genital warts, preinvasive cervical cancer, smoking, HIV infection, or any other immunosuppressive condition. Other epidemiologic risk factors that have been linked to invasive vulvar cancer include hypertension, diabetes, and obesity.

## QUESTION 4

*What are the presentation, workup, and management of VIN?*

## ANSWER 4

VIN often causes symptoms of pruritis or dyspareunia. The lesions may be white, red, or brown in color and are often located in the hairless skin of the interlabial grooves, the posterior fourchette, or the perineum. The workup involves the liberal and timely use of biopsy in order to make the diagnosis and to rule-out invasive carcinoma. Colposcopy with 5% acetic acid application to the vulva can be helpful in deciding the best areas to biopsy. Toludine blue application to the vulva has also been described, but is not commonly used due to a high false negative rate of 40%. Biopsies can be performed easily in the office under local anesthesia. It is important not to delay the diagnostic biopsy by the use of topical treatments. Management involves the use of surgery to control symptoms and prevent progression to invasive carcinoma. A local superficial excision with 5 mm disease-free margins is adequate treatment and results in minimal morbidity. In cases of extensive, multifocal disease, laser ablation can be used. However, this approach should be limited to those with particular expertise in treating vulvar disease to avoid the catastrophic possibility of ablating an occult invasive malignancy. The laser is used to treat to a depth of 1–2 mm in nonhair bearing areas, and to 2–3 mm in hair-bearing areas. There have been several reports describing the use of topical treatments such as 5-fluorouracil, imiquimod (Aldara), and 1% cidofovir. Further studies on the use of these topical agents are necessary.

## BIBLIOGRAPHY

Ghurani GB, Penalver MA. An update on vulvar cancer. *Am J Obstet Gynecol.* 2001;185:294–299.

Hart WR. Vulvar intraepithelial neoplasia: historical aspects and current status. *Int J Gynecol Pathol.* 2001;20:16–30.

Joura EA. Epidemiology, diagnosis and treatment of vulvar intraepithelial neoplasia. *Curr Opin Obstet Gynecol.* 2002;14: 39–43.

Joura EA, Losch A, Haider-Angeler MG, et al. Trends in vulvar neoplasia. Increasing incidence of vulvar intraepithelial neoplasia and squamous cell carcinoma of the vulva in young women. *J Reprod Med.* 2000;45:613–615.

Mimi Zieman, M. Overview of contraception. In: Rose BD (ed.) *UpToDate.* Waltham, MA: UpToDate;2006. www.Uptodate.com

Speroff L, Fritz MA. *Clinical Gynecologic Endocrinology and Infertility*. Philadelphia, PA: Lippincott Williams & Wilkins; 2005.

Stone IK, Wilkinson EJ. Benign and preinvasive lesions of the vulva and vagina. In: Copeland LJ, Jarrell JF (eds.). *Textbook of Gynecology.* 2nd ed. Philadelphia, PA: WB Saunders Company; 2000:1177–1179.

Townsend DE, Morrow CP. Premalignant and related disorders of the lower genital tract. In: Morrow CP, Curtin JP (eds.). *Synopsis of Gynecologic Oncology.* 5th ed. New York, NY: Churchill Livingstone; 1998:24–30.

# LIST OF ABBREVIATIONS

| | |
|---|---|
| 17-HP | 17-hydroxyprogesterone |
| ACOG | American College of Obstetricians and Gynecologists |
| AFLP | Acute fatty liver of pregnancy |
| AFP | alpha-fetoprotein |
| ALT | Alanine aminotransferase (a.k.a. serum glutamic pyruvic transaminase or SGPT) |
| ARDS | Acute respiratory distress syndrome |
| ART | Advanced reproductive techniques |
| ASC-US | Atypical squamous cells of undetermined significance |
| ASD | Atrial septal defect |
| AST | Aspartate aminotransferase (a.k.a. serum glutamic-oxaloacetic transaminase or SGOT) |
| $\beta$hCG | Beta human chorionic gonadotropin |
| BBT chart | Basal body temperature chart |
| BCG | Bacillus Calmette-Guerin vaccine |
| bpm | Beats per minute |
| BRCA | Breast cancer mutations |
| BUN | Blood urea nitrogen |
| CBC | Complete blood count |
| CDC | U.S. Center for Disease Control & Prevention |
| CIN | Cervical intraepithelial neoplasia |
| CMV | Cytomegalovirus |
| CNS | Central nervous system |
| COH | Controlled ovarian hyperstimulation |
| CPP | Chronic pelvic pain |
| CT | Computerized tomography |
| D&C | Dilatation and curettage |
| DES | Diethylstilbestrol |
| DHEA | Dehydroepiandrosterone |
| DHEAS | Dehydroepiandrosterone sulfate |
| DIC | Disseminated intravascular coagulation |
| DUB | Dysfunctional uterine bleeding |
| EKG | Electrocardiogram |
| FDA | U.S. Food and Drug Administration |
| FSH | Follicle stimulating hormone |
| GnRH | Gonadotropin releasing hormone |
| GTD | Gestational trophoblast disease |
| HBcAb | Hepatitis B core antibody |
| HBeAg | Hepatitis B core e antigen |
| HBIG | Hepatitis B immunoglobulin |
| HBsAb | Hepatitis B surface antibody |
| HBsAg | Hepatitis B surface antigen |
| hCG | Human chorionic gonadotropin |
| HCV | Hepatitis C virus |
| HELLP | Hypertension-elevated liver-low platelets syndrome |
| HIV | Human immunodeficiency virus |
| HPV | Human papilloma virus |
| HSV | Herpes simplex virus |
| HTN | Hypertension |
| IUD | Intrauterine device |
| IUI | Intrauterine insemination |
| IV | Intravenous |
| IVF | In vitro fertilization |
| IVF-ET | In vitro fertilization and embryo transfer |
| LDH | Lactate dehydrogenase |
| LH | Luteinizing hormone |
| LMP | Low malignant potential |
| LSD | Lysergic acid diethylamide |
| MRI | Magnetic resonance imaging |
| NCAH | Non-classic congenital adrenal hyperplasia |
| NICHD | U.S. National Institute of Child Health and Human Development |

| | |
|---|---|
| NIH | U.S. National Institutes of Health |
| NSAID | Non-steroidal anti-inflammatory drugs |
| OCP | Oral contraceptive pill |
| PCOS | Polycystic ovary syndrome |
| PCP | Phencyclidine |
| PCR | Polymerase chain reaction |
| POF | Premature ovarian failure |
| PROM | Premature rupture of membranes |
| RPR | Rapid plasma reagin |
| SHBG | Sex hormone-binding globulin |
| SSRI | Selective serotonin reuptake inhibitor |
| TB | Tuberculosis |
| TSH | Thyroid stimulating hormone |
| VBAC | Vaginal birth after cesarean section |
| VDRL | Venereal diseases research laboratory test |
| VIN | Vulvar intraepithelial neoplasia |
| VSD | Ventral septal defect |
| WBC | White cell blood count |

# INDEX

Page numbers followed by *f* or *t* indicate figures or tables, respectively.


**A**

abortion
- death risk from, 156
- fibroids and, 170–171
- midtrimester, 155–157
- recurrent, 170–171, 205–206, 206*t*
- spontaneous, 251

abruption, 111–112
- cesarean section and, 112
- risk and, 111–112

abuse, CPP and, 38–39, 39*t*

acute fatty liver (AFLP), of pregnancy, 120–122, 121*t*
- physical exam for, 121

adenomyosis
- MRI of, 161*f*–162*f*
- prevalence of, 159–160
- risk factors for, 160–161
- signs of, 160, 160*f*–162*f*
- treatment options for, 161–162

adjuvant chemotherapy
- for immature ovarian teratomas, 268
- neoadjuvant v., 262–263, 263*t*

adnexal masses
- in pregnancy, 90–92, 91*f*–92*f*, 95–96
  - risks of, 95–96
- in young women, 258–259

adnexal torsion, 182–183

adolescence, DUB in, 17

adrenal hyperplasia, 21-hydroxylase deficient nonclassic, 214–216, 215*f*, 216*t*

advance directive, 6, 6*t*

advanced reproductive age, 244–246, 245*f*

AFLP. *See* acute fatty liver

amenorrhea
- Asherman's syndrome and, success rates for, 222–223
- evaluation of, 207–208, 208*f*
- hypothalamic
  - causes of, 209
  - diagnosis of, 210
  - therapies of, 208*f*, 210

American College of Obstetricians and Gynecologist, medical screening evaluation by, 4*t*

American Society for Reproductive Medicine, 35*f*

amniocentesis fluid, intra-amniotic infection and, 116

anal incontinence
- diagnosis of, 52–53, 53*t*
- neurologic injury in, 53*t*
- risk of, 53–54, 53*t*
- SUI and, 52–53
- treatments available for, 53, 54*f*

anatomic pregnancy loss, 206*t*

androgen deficiency, menopause and, 247–248

androgen insufficiency syndrome, 248

androgen therapy, systemic, 213

anesthesia complications
- in epidural, 113, 113*f*
- with hysteroscopy, 178
- regional, 114–115, 115*f*
- vignette for, 112

anovulatory
- bleeding, treatment of, 169
- causes of, 249
- cycles, 17
- with PCOS, pregnancy in, 221*f*

antenatal diagnosis
- of IUGR, 134
- of Turner's syndrome, 228, 229*f*

anterior exenteration, 273*f*

anticonvulsants, maternal/fetal effects of, 102–103

antiemetic drugs, during pregnancy, 64, 66

antiviral suppression, in late third trimester, HSV and, 70

appendicitis, in pregnancy, diagnosis of, 104–105
- differential, 104, 104*t*

ART. *See* assisted reproductive technology

arthropathy, 76

ASC-US pap smear, 16, 16*t*

Asherman's syndrome
- amenorrhea and, success rates for, 222–223
- diagnostic modalities for, 222–223, 223*f*
- infertility and, success rates for, 222–223
- obstetrical complications with, risk of, 223
- risk factors for, 222–223
- x-ray film of, 223*f*

assess ovulation, 243

assisted reproductive technology (ART)
- infertility and, 233–234, 234*f*
- live birth rates of, 234*f*, 245*f*
- success of, 233–234, 234*f*
- types of, 233

asthma
- in pregnancy
  - effects of, 98–99
  - pulmonary physiologic changed with, 98, 98*t*
  - understanding of, 97
- pulmonary function testing for, 99

atypical glandular cells
- evaluation of, 257–258
- on pap smear, 257–258
- of uncertain significance, 257

autonomy, 5

**B**

bacterial colonization, choriodecidual, potential pathways from, to preterm delivery, 117*f*

bacterial vaginosis
- clinical features of, 56–57
- diagnostic criteria for, 57, 58*f*
- in pregnancy, 59
- treatment options for, 57
- trichomonas and, 56–59, 58*f*
- vaginitis, 56–59, 58*f*
- vignette for, 56

bariatric surgery, 144–146, 145*f*
- long-term risks of, 146
- obesity and, 144–145
- pregnancy and, 146

Bartholin's gland mass
appropriate management of, 163, 164*f*
carcinoma, clinical features of, 163
incision/drainage of, 164*f*
risk factors for, 163
vignette for, 162–163
BCG vaccination
PPD and, 79
for TB infection, 78–79
beneficence, 6
Bethesda Classification of Cervical Cytology, 15
βhCG, 266–267
birth. *See also* vaginal birth
injuries, minimization of, 53–54
live, rates, 245, 245*f*
in ART, 234*f*, 245*f*
Bishop Scoring System, 133*t*
bone mineral density classification, 32*t*
borderline ovarian tumor
conservative fertility-sparing surgeryof, 260
management of, 260
surgical staging of, 260
vignette for, 259–260
BRCA. *See* breast cancer mutations
breast cancer
breast feeding and, 97
physical exam and, 1
pregnancy after, 96–97
risk factors for, 1
screening for, 4*t*, 5
breast cancer mutations (BRCA), 1
breast feeding
advantages of, 61
contraceptive methods recommended during, 62
contraindications to, 61, 62*t*
mastitis and, 61
breast mass
management of, 1–2
physical exam and, 1
broadly spaced nipples, 229*f*
Burch procedure, 187*f*

**C**

Candida albicans vaginitis, 55f
candida, recurrent, 54–56, 55*f*
cardiac disease
cesarean section and, 107
New York Heart Association classification of, 106–107, 106*t*
in pregnancy, 105–107, 106*t*
risk of, 106–107, 106*t*
cardiopulmonary resuscitation guidelines, during pregnancy, 150–151, 150*t*
cardiovascular disease, hormone replacement therapy for, 37
CCCT. *See* clomiphene citrate challenge test
cephalhematoma formation, 137*f*
cerclage
elective, 131
emergency, 131
incompetent, 129–131
urgent, 131
cerebral palsy, chorioamnionitis and, 116–117
cervical cancer
following pelvic exenteration, 273
screening for, 4*t*, 5
squamous cell carcinoma, 261–262
vignette for, 5
cervical cytology
classification of, 15
pap smear, abnormal and, 15–16, 16*t*
screening, for glandular neoplasia, 257
cervical insufficiency, three categoriesof, 130
cervical intraepithelial neoplasia (CIN), 15–16, 16*t*
VIN v., 278
cervical ripening
labor induction and, 132–133, 133*t*
methods used for, 132–133
cervical stump carcinoma, 176
cervix
hooded, 165*f*
incompetent, 129–131
normal, 165*f*
squamous cell carcinoma of, 261–262
cesarean section
abruption and, 112
cardiac disease and, 107
perimortem, 150–151
postpartum hemorrhage after, 126
vaginal birth after, 153–155, 154*t*
chancre lesions, in syphilis, 68, 68*f*
chemotherapy
after surgical therapy, 263–264
for gestational trophoblastic disease, 266
types of, 262–263, 263*t*, 268
cholestasis, of pregnancy
diagnosis of, 93
risks associated with, 93–94
treatment options for, 94
vignette for, 93, 93*t*
cholesterol screening, 4*t*, 5
chorioamnionitis
cerebral palsy and, 116–117
histologic findings in, 116, 117*f*
risk factors for, 116
choriodecidual bacterial colonization, potential pathways from, to preterm delivery, 117*f*
chronic obstructive pulmonary disease (COPD), smoking cessation in, 9
chronic pelvic pain. *See* pelvic pain, chronic
CIN. *See* cervical intraepithelial neoplasia
cirrhosis, HCV and, 72
clomiphene, 219*f*
ovulation induction and, 248–250, 249*t*
risks of, 249–250
side effects of, 249–250
clomiphene citrate challengetest (CCCT), 244
coaxial technique, 113, 113*f*
COH/IUI. *See* controlled ovarian hyperstimulation with intrauterine insemination
colon cancer screening, 4*t*, 5
complete molar gestation, 266
complete vaginal eversion, 200*f*
congenital anomalies, 250
congenital heart defects, pregnancy and, risk of, 107
conservative fertility-sparing surgery, of borderline ovarian tumor, 260
continuous fetal heart rate monitoring, fetal heart rate patterns and, 122–123, 123*f*
contraception. *See also* emergency contraception; oral contraception
during breast feeding, 62
depo-provera, 21–23, 23*f*
estrogen, 28*t*
IUD and, 18–20
postpartum, for seizure disorders, 103, 103*t*
progestin, 27*t*–29*t*
seizure disorders and, 103, 103*t*
smoking and, 239–240
controlled ovarian hyperstimulation with intrauterine insemination (COH/IUI), 246
corticotropin, 225*t*
CPP. *See* pelvic pain, chronic
cryomyolysis, myomectomy and, uterine artery embolism versus, for fibroids, 173–175, 174*f*
Cushing's syndrome
clinical vignette for, 223–224
differential diagnosis of, 224, 224*t*
evaluation of, 224–226, 225*f*
hypercortisolism and, 225–226, 225*t*
prevalence of, 224
signs of, 224, 224*t*
cystitis, acute, recurrence of, in young women, 193
cystometrogram, 190, 190*f*
multichannel, 195–196, 196*f*
cystometry, complex, 196*f*

**D**

danazol, 236
"Date Rape Drug," 45
delivery. *See also* cesarean section; operative vaginal delivery
in DKA, 120
of HELLP syndrome patient, 125–126
HIV risk during, 75
postpartum hemorrhage after, 126
preterm, choriodecidual bacterial colonization and, 117*f*
depo-provera contraception
advantages of, 22
contraindications to, 22–23
side effects of, 23, 23*f*
vignette for, 21
depression, after pregnancy, 100–102, 100*t*–101*t*
prophylactic treatment of, 102
recommended treatment of, 101–102
risk of, 101*t*
dermatome chart, 115*f*
des exposure, 165–166, 165*f*–166*f*
daughters of, 166, 166*f*
risk of, 166, 166*f*
detrusor overactivity (DO), 189–191, 191*t*
diabetes
obesity and, 7*t*
screening for, 4*t*, 5
diabetic ketoacidosis (DKA), in pregnancy, 118–120, 119*f*
acute treatment of, 119–120
delivery recommendations for, 120
fetal risks in, 120
laboratory findings for, 118
pathophysiology of, 118–119, 119*f*
diethylstilbestrol (DES), 165–166, 165*f*–166*f*
distention media, 177–178, 178*t*

DKA. *See* diabetic ketoacidosis
DNR. *See* do not resuscitate
DO. *See* detrusor overactivity
do not resuscitate (DNR), 6*t*
domestic violence
behaviorally specific questions regarding, 3*t*
cases, obstetrician-gynecologist responsibility in, 3, 3*t*
definition of, 2–3
impact of, 2–3
physician screening responsibility for, 3*t*
potential barriers to, 3
prevalence of, 2–3
vignette of, 1
dominant estrogen, 97
Doppler flow studies, in adnexal torsion diagnosis, 183
DUB. *See* uterine bleeding, dysfunctional

**E**

eclampsia, 142
ectopic gestation, 241–242
ectopic pregnancy, methotrexate for, surgery versus, 166–168, 168*t*
elective induction, 133
electrolyte content, of hysteroscopic distention media, osmolalityand, 178*t*
emergency contraception, 24–26, 24*t*–25*t*
action mechanism of, 24–25
contraindications to, 25–26
oral contraceptives for, 25, 25*t*
potential indications for, 24*t*
providing of, 25, 25*t*
side effects of, 25–26
endocrine changes, during perimenopause, 34–35
endocrine pregnancy loss, 206*t*
endometrial ablation, surgical techniques for, 169–170
endometrial cancer
risk factors for, 264–265
staging of, 265
endometrial glands, 159–160, 160*f*–162*f*
endometrial histology, abnormal, uterine bleeding and, 17
endometriosis
CPP and, 38–39
infertility and, 234–237, 235*f*
staging system for, 235–236
vignette for, 42
epidural anesthesia, needle insertion in, 113, 113*f*
epithelial ovarian cancer
hereditary ovarian cancer syndrome and, 269, 269*f*
neoadjuvant chemotherapy for, 263
erythema infectiosum, 76
estradiol, dominant estrogen and, 97
estrogen
contraceptive, 28*t*
dominant, 97
synthetic, 165
estrogen/progestin therapy (HT), 37

**F**

fatty liver, acute. *See* acute fatty liver
fecal incontinence, 52–54, 53*t*, 54*f*
fecundity, reduction of, 244
Ferriman-Gallwey hirsutism scoring system, 211, 211*f*–212*f*
fertility
after immature ovarian teratomas, 268
conservative fertility-sparing surgery, of borderline ovarian tumor, 260
future, after endometrial cancer, 265
PCOS and, insulin sensitizers and, 217–218, 218*f*–219*f*
fetal heart rate patterns
alterations of, 124
continuous fetal heart rate monitoring and, 122–123, 123*f*
nonreassuring, treatment options for, 124
vignette for, 122
fetal heart rate tracing, reassuring, 123–124
fetal maturity, assessment criteria for, 133
fibroids
abortion and, 170–171
after myomectomy, risk, 170–171
hysteroscopic treatment of, 171–173, 172*f*
infertility and, 242–243, 243*f*
UAE for, cryomyolysis and, 173–175, 174*f*
finasteride, 213
fine needle aspiration biopsy, 12
follicle stimulating hormone (FSH), 34, 34*f*
forceps delivery. *See* operative vaginal delivery
"four As," of smoking cessation, 9
Friedman labor curve, 109–110, 110*f*
frog-leg position, for pediatric patient evaluation, 202*f*
FSH. *See* follicle stimulating hormone

**G**

galactorrhea
differential diagnosis of, 226–227
treatment recommendations for, 227
gamete intrafallopian transfer (GIFT), 233
gamma-hydroxybutyrate (GHB), 45
gastric procedures, 145*f*
gastrointestinal disease, CPP and, 39*t*
gastrointestinal system, injuries to, during laparoscopy, 181–182, 182*f*
GCT. *See* granulosa cell tumor
genetic pregnancy loss, 206*t*
genital lesions, HSV and, 69–70
gestation, multiple, 250
gestational hypertension, 142
gestational trophoblastic disease, 265–267
βhCG after, 266–267
chemotherapy for, 266
false positives of, 266–267
GHB. *See* gamma-hydroxybutyrate
GIFT. *See* gamete intrafallopian transfer
glandular neoplasia, cervical cytology screening for, 257
GnRH. *See* gonadotropin-releasing hormone
gonadal dysgenesis, Turner's syndrome and, 227–230, 229*f*–230*f*
gonadotropin, for ovulation induction, with PCOS, 221
gonadotropin-releasing hormone(GnRH), 236
granulosa cell tumor (GCT)
gynecologic neoplasms and, 271
markers of, 271
surgical staging of, 271
vignette for, 270
Graves' disease
optimal tests for, 89*f*
in pregnancy, 88–89
transient hyperthyroidism, hyperemesis gravidarum and, 87
gynecologic neoplasms, GCT and, 271
gynecology. *See also* obstetrician-gynecologist
CPP and, 39*t*
office management for, 15–61

**H**

hair shaft diameter, in hirsutism patient, 212*f*
HAIRAN syndrome, 211–213, 213*f*
HBV. *See* hepatitis B
HCV. *See* hepatitis C virus
Health Care Proxy, Living Will, and DNR Advance Directives in the State of New York, 6*t*
HELLP syndrome, 142
differential diagnosis of, 125
neonatal complications associated with, 125*t*
preeclampsia and, 144
risks associated with, 125, 125*f*
vignette for, 124–125
hemorrhage
hysteroscopy and, 178
postpartum, 126–128, 127*f*
hepatitis B virus (HBV)
acute, serologic picture of, 83, 83*f*
chronic, serologic picture of, 84, 84*f*
global health concerns of, 83, 83*f*
mortality of, 83–84
neonatal prophylaxis of, 84
in pregnancy, 82–84, 83*f*–84*f*
risk factors for, 83–84, 83*f*–84*f*
screening for, 84
hepatitis C virus (HCV)
cirrhosis and, 72
long term sequelae of, 71–72, 72*f*
in pregnancy, 71–73
HIV and, 73–74
risk associated with, 71–72, 72*f*
hereditary ovarian cancer syndrome
epithelial ovarian cancer and, 269, 269*f*
prognosis of, clinical differencesin, 270
risk of, 269–270
vignette for, 268–269
herniation, of small intestine, 181*f*
herpes simplex virus (HSV)
classification system for, 70, 70*t*
genital
lesions, 69–70
seroprevalence rate of, 70
incidence rate for, 70
neonatal infection and, 70
in pregnancy, 69–71, 69*f*–70*t*
vignette for, 69, 69*f*
hidradenitis suppurativa (HS)
differential diagnosis for, 30
etiology of, 30
stages of, 30, 30*t*
treatment for, 30–31
vignette for, 29–30
hirsutism
clinical vignette for, 210
differential diagnosis of, 211
hair shaft diameter in, 212*f*
hormonal therapy for, 213–214

hirsutism (*Cont.*)
patient evaluation for, 211–213, 212*f*
PCOS and, 211–213
prevalence of, 210–211, 211*f*
therapy for, 212*f*, 213–214
histamine, 153*f*
HIV. *See* human immunodeficiency virus
hormone replacement therapy counseling (HRT), 35–37
for menopause, 35–37
vignette for, 35–36
hormone therapy
endometriosis infertility and, 236
for hirsutism, 213–214
hormones
FSH, 34, 34*f*
TSH, 11–13
17-HP. *See* 17-hydroxyprogesterone
HPV. *See* human papillomavirus
HRT. *See* hormone replacement therapy counseling
HS. *See* hidradenitis suppurativa
HSG. *See* hysterosalpingogram
HSV. *See* herpes simplex virus
HT. *See* estrogen/progestin therapy
human immunodeficiency virus (HIV)
lowering risk of, during delivery, 75
in pregnancy
HCV and, 73–74
risk factors associated with, 74–75, 74*f*
vertical transmission of, 74–75, 74*f*
vignette for, 73–74
human papillomavirus (HPV), testing for, 16
hydrops
fetalis, 128, 129*t*
nonimmune, 128–129, 129*t*
hydrosalpinges, 241*f*
hydrosalpinx/tubal damage
additional treatment options for, 242
IVF-ET and, 241–242, 241*f*
risk factors of, 241
vignette for, 241
21-hydroxylase deficient nonclassic adrenal hyperplasia
diagnosis of, 214–216, 215*f*
in hyperandrogenic women, 214–215
signs of, 216, 216*t*
17-hydroxyprogesterone, 215–216, 215*f*
hypercholesterolemia, obesity and, 7*t*
hypercortisolism, Cushing's syndrome and, 225–226, 225*t*
hyperemesis gravidarum
Graves' disease transient hyperthyroidism and, 87
during pregnancy, 63–66, 65*f*
treatment options for, 64, 65*f*
vignette for, 63
hyperplasia, adrenal, 21-hydroxylase deficient nonclassic, 214–216, 215*f*, 216*t*
hyperprolactinemia
management of, 231–232
reocurrence rates of, 232
vignette for, 230–231
hypertension
chronic, 143
in pregnancy, 85–86
gestational, 142
obesity and, 7*t*
hypertensive disorders, in pregnancy, 142–143
hyperthyroidism
causes of, 11
diagnosis of, 11–12, 12*f*
informed consent/refusal, 5–6
in perimenopause, 17
transient, 87
treatment of, 12–13
vignette for, 10–11
hypogastric artery ligation, 127, 127*f*
hypothalamic amenorrhea, 208*f*, 209–210
hysterectomy
ovarian preservation after, with cervical cancer, 262
supracervical, 175–176
total abdominal, 176
hysterosalpingogram (HSG), 242
hysteroscopic myomectomy, 171–173, 172*f*
hysteroscopy
air emboli during, 179–180
anesthesia complications with, 178
complications of, 177–180, 178*t*
infection and, 178
media for, 177–178, 178*t*
perforated uterus during, 179–180

**I**
IC. *See* interstitial cystitis
ICS. *See* International Continence Society
ICSI. *See* intrauterine insemination
immature ovarian teratomas, 267–268
immunologic pregnancy loss, 206*t*
in vitro fertilization (IVF)
infertility causes and, 233–234, 234*f*
vignette for, 232–233
incompetent cervix/cerclage, 129–131
incomplete molar gestation, 266
infection
hysteroscopy and, 178
intra-amniotic, amniocentesis fluidand, 116
neonatal, HSV and, 70
TB, 78–80, 79*f*
urinary tract, 191–194, 193*t*
infertility
ART and, 233–234, 234*f*
Asherman's syndrome and, success rates for, 222–223
des exposure and, 166
diagnostic test for, 242–243
endometriosis and, 234–237, 235*f*
female, 237–239
fibroids and, 242–243, 243*f*
lifestyle implications in, 239–240
male, 246–247, 247*f*
physical examination for, 238
routine laparoscopy for, 238–239
routine postcoital testing for, 238–239
smoking and, 239
unexplained, 249
uterine anomaly and, 253, 253*f*
in vitro fertilization and, 233–234, 234*f*
work up of, candidates for, 237–238
INH. *See* isoniazid
insulin resistance, PCOS and, prevalence of, 217
insulin sensitizers
PCOS and, fertility and, 217–218, 218*f*–219*f*
risks of, 219–220
International Continence Society (ICS), 189
interstitial cystitis (IC)
confirming diagnosis of, 40–41, 41*f*
CPP and, 38
interval cytoreduction, 263*t*
neoadjuvant chemotherapy versus, after surgery, 263–264
intra-amniotic infection, amniocentesis fluid and, 116
intrauterine device (IUD)
contraception and, 18–20
currently available, 18
insertion complications of, 19, 19*t*
pregnancy prevention and, 18–19
pregnancy risks with, 19
intrauterine growth restriction (IUGR)
mortality/morbidity in, 134–135
risk factors for, 134, 134*t*
intrauterine insemination (ICSI),246–247, 247*f*
isoniazid (INH), 79–80
IUD. *See* intrauterine device
IUGR. *See* intrauterine growth restriction
IVF. *See* in vitro fertilization
IVF-ET, 241–242, 241*f*

**J**
Jarisch-Herxheimer reaction, implications of, in pregnancy, 68–69

**K**
karyotype, 208
for male infertility, 246

**L**
labia, laceration of, 202*f*
labor
abnormal, 109–111, 110*f*
induction of, cervical ripening and, 132–133, 133*f*
stages of, 109–110, 110*f*
pain pathways associated with, 112
laparoscopy
complications with, 180–182, 182*f*
gastrointestinal injuries during, 181–182, 181*f*
to laparotomy, 180–181
of ovarian masses, in pregnancy, 92
routine, for female infertility, 238–239
laparotomy, laparoscopy to, 180–181
latent syphilis, 67
leak point pressure (LPP), 195
leiomyosarcoma, pathological diagnosis of, 275–276
lichen sclerosus, 59–60
lifestyle implications, in infertility, 239–240
living will, 6, 6*t*
low malignant potential tumors, 259–260
LPP. *See* leak point pressure
lumbar epidural puncture, 113, 113*f*
luteal phase deficiency, 249

**M**
maculopapular pruritic rash, 80–81, 80*f*
magnetic resonance imaging (MRI), of adenomyosis, 161*f*–162*f*
male infertility, 246–247, 247*f*
male progeny, smoking effects on, 240
malignant Müllerian tumor, 276*f*

MAS. *See* meconium aspiration syndrome
mastitis
breast feeding and, 61
*Staphylococcus aureus* and, 63
treatment of, 62–63
meconium aspiration syndrome (MAS)
consistency of, 135–136
occurence of, 135, 135*t*
prevention of, 136
medical ethics, 5
medical screening
general, 3–4, 4*t*
for obesity, 8
specific, 4*t*, 5
menarche, anovulatory cycles and, 17
menopause
androgen deficiency and, 247–248
HRT counseling for, 35–37
osteoporosis and, 31–33, 32*t*
perimenopause and, 33–35, 34*f*
sexuality and, 247–248
menses, anovulatory cycles and, 17
metformin, 219–220, 219*f*–220*f*
methotrexate, for ectopic pregnancy, surgery versus, 166–168, 168*t*
microadenomas, long-term follow up of, 227
microbiologic pregnancy loss, 206*t*
microinvasive squamous cell carcinoma, 277
midtrimester abortion, 155–157
miscarriage, smoking and, 240
molar gestations, 265–267
morbidity, in IUGR, 134–135
mortality
in breast cancer, pregnancy after, 97
of HBV, 83–84
in IUGR, 134–135
of obesity, 7
of women, 4
motor vehicle accident (MVA), 111
MRI. *See* magnetic resonance imaging
müllerian agenesis, 208
müllerian duct anomalies, 253*f*
multichannel cystometrogram,195–196, 196*f*
multichannel urodynamic testing, 190*f*
indications for, 196
multigravida, 110
musculoskeletal disease, CPP and, 39*t*
MVA. *See* motor vehicle accident
Mycobacterium tuberculosis, PPD and, 78–79, 79*f*
myolysis, candidates for, 175
myomectomy
advantages/disadvantages of, 174
fibroids after, risk, 170–171
hysteroscopic, 171–173, 172*f*
laparoscopic, alternative therapies to, 172–173
UAE v., for fibroids, cryomyolysis and, 173–175, 174*f*
myometrium, 159, 160*f*–162*f*

**N**

nausea, during pregnancy, 63–64
treatment of, 64, 65*f*, 66
neoadjuvant chemotherapy
adjuvant v., 262–263, 263*t*
interval cytoreduction versus, after surgery, 263–264
role of, for epithelial ovariancancer, 263
vignette for, 262
neonatal
complications, from shoulder dystocia, 148
complications, with HELLP syndrome, 125*t*
infection, with HSV, 70
prophylaxis, of HBV, 84
neurologic injury, in anal incontinence, 53*t*
New York Heart Association, of cardiac disease classification, 106–107, 106*t*
nicotine replacement therapy (NRT), 240
nipples, broadly spaced, 229*f*
nitroglycerin, 153*f*
noncontraceptive effects, 27–29, 28*t*
nonimmune hydrops
differential diagnosis of, 128, 129*t*
overall prognosis of, 128–129
vignette for, 128
nonmaleficence, 6
nonreassuring fetal heart rate patterns, treatment options for, 124
nonsteroidal triphenylethylene derivative, 250
NRT. *See* nicotine replacement therapy

**O**

obesity
bariatric surgery and, 144–145
definition of, 7, 145
diabetes and, 7*t*
health risks associated with, 7–8, 7*t*
hypercholesterolemia and, 7*t*
hypertension and, 7*t*
measurement of, 7
medical screening for, 8
mortality of, 7
pregnancy and, 145
prevalence of, 7
primary care for, 7–8, 7*t*
treatment options for, 8, 145, 145*f*
"*Obstetrical Emergency,*" 151
obstetrician-gynecologist. *See also* gynecology
preventative health care suggestion by, 4
responsibility of, in domestic violence cases, 3, 3*t*
obstetrics
complications, Asherman's syndrome risk of, 223
office management for, 61–107
Turner's syndrome and, 229–230
office management
for gynecology, 15–61
for obstetrics, 61–107
for primary care, 1–13
oocyte donation, 246
operative vaginal delivery
indications for, 136
low, classification for, 137
risk associated with, 138
success rate of, 138
oral contraception
administration of, 29
contraindications to, 26, 28
cost of, 27*t*–28*t*
for emergency contraception, 25, 25*t*
noncontraceptive effects of, 28
pharmacology of, 26
risks with, 28
selected, 27*t*–28*t*
side effects of, 27
types of, 27*t*–28*t*
oral lesions, HSV and, 69–70
osmolality, of hysteroscopic distention media, 178*t*
osteoporosis
characterizations of, 31
diagnosis of, 32, 33*t*
menopause and, 31–33, 32*t*
risk factors for, 31–32
treatment options for, 32–33
ovarian cancer, 250, 263
hereditary, syndrome, 268–270, 270*f*
ovarian follicular depletion, smoking and, 239
ovarian hyperstimulation syndrome, 250
ovarian masses
benign, ultrasound of, 91*f*–92*f*, 92
malignant, ultrasound of, 91, 91*f*–92*f*
in pregnancy, 90–92
laparoscopy of, 92
risks of, 92
surgery of, 92
ovarian neoplasia, percentages of, 269*f*
ovarian neoplasm, in young women, tumor markers for, 258–259
ovarian reserve, 244
ovarian teratomas, 267–268
immature, 267–268
ovarian tumor, borderline, 259–260
ovary, streak, 230*f*
ovulation
assess, 243
rate, meta-analysis of, 218*f*–219*f*
super, 250
ovulation induction
clomiphene and, 248–250, 249*t*
in PCOS, 220–221, 220*f*–221*f*

**P**

pap smear, abnormal
ASC-US, 16, 16*t*
atypical glandular cells on, 257–258
cervical cytology and, frequencies of, 15–16, 16*t*
parvovirus, in pregnancy
B19 producing, 76
diagnosis of, 77
forms of, 76, 76*f*
management of, 77
PCOS. *See* polycystic ovarian syndrome
pediatric patients
evaluation of, frog-leg position for, 202*f*
vulvar lacerations in, 201–203, 202*f*
pelvic artery embolization, common major complications of, 127–128
pelvic examination, POP technique for, 51
pelvic exenteration
anterior, 273*f*
cervical cancer following, 273
classification of, 272–273, 273*f*
total, 273*f*
pelvic floor support disorders, risk factors for, 51
pelvic inflammatory disease (PID),48–49, 48*f*
pelvic organ prolapse (POP)
gradings for, 50–51, 50*f*–51*f*
nonsurgical management of, 49–51, 50*f*–51*f*
pelvic examination technique for, 51
risk of, 51
staging of, 198, 198*f*, 200, 200*f*
treatment options for, 51–52

pelvic organ prolapse quantification (POPQ), 200, 200*f*
pelvic organ support quantification, 198*f*
pelvic pain, chronic (CPP), 37–40, 39*t*
abuse and, 38–39, 39*t*
clinical vignette for, 38
common causes of, 42–43
current treatment recommendations for, 43–44
differential diagnosis of, 40
diseases associated with, 39*t*
endometriosis and, 38–39
gastrointestinal disease, 39*t*
gynecology and, 39*t*
IC and, 38
musculoskeletal disease and, 39*t*
prevalence of, 38, 42
treatment of, 42–43
urologic disease and, 39*t*
perimenopause
abnormal uterine bleeding and, 35
endocrine changes during, 34–35
hyperthyroidism and, 17
menopause and, 34–35, 34*f*
symptoms of, 34–35, 34*f*
perimortem cesarean delivery, 150–151
peritoneal cancer, primary
clinical manifestations of, 274
management of, 275
pathological diagnosis of, 274, 274*f*
risk factors for, 274–275
peritoneal carcinomatosis, 274*f*
pharmacological therapy, for smoking cessation, 9, 10*t*
physical examination. *See also* pelvic examination
of AFLP, in pregnancy, 121
for anal incontinence, 52–53
for breast cancer, 1
for breast mass, 1
for infertility, 238
physician, responsibility of, in domestic violence cases, 3, 3*t*
PID. *See* pelvic inflammatory disease
pituitary adenoma, 231
placenta accreta
complications arising from, 139–140
risk of, 139, 139*t*
ultrasonographic abnormalities associated with, 139
vignette for, 138–139
placenta increta, 139–140
placenta percreta, 139–140
placenta previa
common complications associated with, 141
common risk factors for, 140–141, 141*t*
vaginal bleeding episode in, 141, 141*t*
vignette for, 140
POF. *See* premature ovarian failure
polycystic ovarian syndrome (PCOS)
clinical vignette for, 217
fertility and, insulin sensitizers and, 217–218, 218*f*–219*f*
hirsutism and, 211–213
insulin resistance and, 217
ovulation induction in, 220–221, 220*f*–221*f*
POP. *See* pelvic organ prolapse
POPQ. *See* pelvic organ prolapse quantification
postcoital testing, for female infertility, 238–239
postnatal diagnosis, of Turner's syndrome, 228, 229*f*
"postpartum blues," 100*t*
postpartum contraception, for seizure disorders, 103, 103*t*
postpartum hemorrhage
after cesarean section, 126
differential diagnosis of, 126–127, 127*f*
UAE and, 127–128
postpartum psychological reactions, 100–102, 100*t*–101*t*
differential diagnosis of, 101
risk factors for, 100
postpartum sterilization procedure counseling, 21
PPD. *See* purified protein derivative
preeclampsia
diagnostic criteria for, 143, 143*t*
HELLP syndrome and, 144
prevention of, 143–144
severe, diagnosis of, 143, 143*t*
vignette for, 142
pregnancy. *See also* risk
adnexal masses in, 90–92, 91*f*–92*f*, 95–96
AFLP and, 120–122, 121*t*
after breast cancer, 96–97
antiemetic drugs during, 64, 66
appendicitis and, 104–105, 104*t*
asthma and, 97–99, 98*t*
bacterial vaginosis during, 59
bariatric surgery and, 146
cardiac disease in, 105–107, 106*t*
cardiopulmonary resuscitation guidelines during, 150–151, 150*t*
cholestasis of, 93–94
chronic hypertension, 85–86
congenital heart defects in, 107
congenital heart disease and, 107
depression after, 100–102, 100*t*–101*t*
DKA in, 118–120, 119*f*
domestic violence prevalence in, 3
ectopic, 166–168, 168*t*
Graves' disease in, 88–89
HBV, 82–84, 83*f*–84*f*
HCV, 71–73, 72*f*
hepatitis B, 82–84, 83*f*–84*f*
HIV, 73–75, 74*f*
HSV, 69–71, 69*f*, 70*t*
hyperemesis gravidarum during, 63–66, 65*f*
hypertensive disorders in, 142–143
Jarisch-Herxheimer reaction implications in, 68–69
loss, recurrent, 205–206, 206*t*
nausea during, 63–64
treatment of, 64, 65*f*, 66
obesity and, 145
ovarian masses, 90–92, 91*f*–92*f*
parvovirus, 76–77, 76*f*
in PCOS, anovulatory women with, 221*f*
PPD, 78–80, 78*f*–79*f*
prevention of, IUD's and, 18–19
psychosis after, 101
pulmonary system during, 98*t*
seatbelt safety during, 150, 150*f*
seizure disorders and, 102–103, 103*t*
surgical therapy in, 92, 166–168, 168*t*
syphilis in, 66–69, 67*f*–68*f*, 68*t*
TB infection, 79–80
teratogenicity during, 64, 66
thyroid disease in, 87–90, 89*f*
thyroid storm in, 89–90, 89*f*
trauma during, 148–151, 150*f*, 150*t*
varicella, 80–82, 80*f*–81*f*
vomiting during, 63–64
treatment of, 64, 65*f*, 66
VSV in, 80–82, 80*f*–81*f*
premature ovarian failure (POF), 250–252
additional testing for, 251–252
etiologies of, 251
initial evaluation of, 251
prevalence of, 251
reproductive outcome of, 252
vignette for, 250–251
preterm premature rupture, 130
preventative health care, obstetrician-gynecologist suggestion of, 4
primary care
for obesity, 7–8, 7*t*
office management for, 1–13
primary syphilis, 66–67
primigravida, 110
progestin, 236
contraceptive, 27*t*–29*t*
prolactinoma, long-term follow up of, 227
pulmonary function testing, forasthma, 99
pulmonary system, during pregnancy, 98*t*
purified protein derivative (PPD)
active/latent risk factors for, 78, 78*f*
BCG vaccination and, 79
Mycobacterium tuberculosis and, 78–79, 79*f*
in pregnancy, 78–80, 78*f*–79*f*
PZA. *See* rifampin/pyrazinamide

**Q**

Q-tip test, 188*t*, 190

**R**

recurrent abortion, 170–171
causes of, 205–206, 206*t*
recurrent vaginal candidiasis, 54–56, 55*f*
regional anesthesia, 114–115, 115*f*
reproductive age, advanced
reduction of, 244
treatment options for, 245, 245*f*
reproductive outcome
adverse, smoking and, 239–240
of POF, 252
resectoscope, 172*f*
retropubic colposuspensions, 187
rifampin/pyrazinamide (PZA), 79–80
risk
of abruption, 111–112
of active/latent PPD, 78, 78*f*
of adenomyosis, 160–161
of anal incontinence, 53–54, 53*t*
of Asherman's syndrome, 222–223
of Bartholin's gland mass, 163
of breast cancer, 1
of chorioamnionitis, 116
of clomiphene, 249–250
of death, from abortion, 156
of des exposure, 166, 166*f*
of endometrial cancer, 264–265
fetal, in DKA, 120

of fibroids, after myomectomy, 170–171
of HBV, 83–84, 83*f*–84*f*
of HCV, 71–72, 72*f*
with HELLP syndrome, 125, 125*f*
of hepatitis B, 83–84, 83*f*–84*f*
of hereditary ovarian cancer syndrome, 269–270
of HIV, 75
of hydrosalpinx/tubal damage, 241
with insulin sensitizers, 219–220
of IUGR, 134, 134*t*
long-term, of bariatric surgery, 146
maternal, in uterine inversion, 152, 152*f*
of noncontraceptive effects, 27, 29
in obesity, 7–8, 7*t*
in operative vaginal delivery, 138
with oral contraception, 28
of osteoporosis, 31–32
in PCOS, with ovulation induction, 221
of pelvic floor support disorders, 51
of peritoneal cancer, primary,274–275
of placenta accreta, 139, 139*t*
of placenta previa, 140–141, 141*t*
of POP, 51
of postpartum depression, 101*t*
of postpartum psychologicalreactions, 100
in pregnancy
of adnexal masses, 95–96
of cardiac disease, 106–107, 106*t*
of cholestasis, 93–94
in chronic hypertension, 86
of congenital heart defects, 107
of congenital heart disease, 107
of HIV, 74–75, 74*f*
with IUD, 19
of ovarian masses, 92
of shoulder dystocia, 147, 147*t*
of sphincter laceration, 53*t*
of squamous cell carcinoma, cervical, 261
of Turner's syndrome, long term, 228–229, 229*f*–230*f*
of uterine rupture, 154
of uterine sarcoma, 275
of VIN, 278–279
of vulvar carcinoma, 277

**S**
SAB. *See* Staphylococcus aureus bacteremia
salpingectomy, 241–242
salpingitis
acute, 48*f*
current treatment guidelines for, 49
vignette for, 48
salpingostomy, 241–242
sandwich assay, 267
seatbelt use, during pregnancy, 150, 150*f*
secondary syphilis, 67
seizure disorders
postpartum contraception for, 103, 103*t*
preconception counseling for, 103, 103*t*
vignette for, 102
serologic screening, for VZV, in pregnancy, 81
sexual assault, 44–45
sexual infantilism, 229*f*
sexuality, menopause and, 247–248
sexually transmitted diseases, salpingitis, 48–49, 48*f*
short stature, 229*f*
shoulder dystocia
complications from, 148
management of, 147
risk of, 147, 147*t*
vignette for, 146–147
"Slapped-cheek" rash, 76*f*
small intestine, herniation of, 181*f*
smoking
adverse reproductive outcome and, 239–240
cessation of, 8–10, 10*t*
contraception and, 239–240
effects of, on male progeny, 240
helping patient quit, 240
infertility and, 239
miscarriage and, 240
ovarian follicular depletion and, 239
withdrawal from, 9
sonohystogram, 242–243
sperm parameters, 246
sphincter laceration, risk of, 53*t*
sphincteroplasty, overlapping, 54*f*
spirochete, darkfield examination of, 68*f*
spontaneous abortion, 251
squamous cell carcinoma
of cervix, 261–262
microinvasive, 277
*Staphococcus aureus*, mastitis and, 63
*Staphylococcus aureus* bacteremia (SAB), 96
sterilization procedure counseling, 20–21
postpartum, methods for, 21
straddle injury, 202*f*
streak ovary, 230*f*
stress urinary incontinence (SUI)
anal incontinence and, 52–53
causes of, 186–187
nonsurgical treatment options for, 187
surgical treatment options for, 187–188, 187*f*, 188*t*
stroma, 159, 160*f*–162*f*
subcutaneous edema, 137*f*
subgaleal hematoma, 137*f*
submucous myoma, treatment of, 171
SUI. *See* stress urinary incontinence
superovulation, 250
supracervical hysterectomy, 175–176
surgical therapy
bariatric, 144–146, 145*f*
chemotherapy after, 263–264
conservative fertility-sparing, for borderline ovarian tumor, 260
for DO, 190–191, 191*t*
for ectopic pregnancy, methotrexate versus, 166–168, 168*t*
for endometrial ablation, 169–170
endometriosis and, infertility and, 236
for ovarian masses, in pregnancy, 92
for SUI, 187–188, 187*f*, 188*t*
surrogate decision maker, 6, 6*t*
syphilis
antibody development during, time course of, 67*f*
chancre lesions in, 68, 68*f*
diagnosis of, 45–47
in pregnancy, 66–68, 67*f*–68*f*, 68*t*
routine screening for, 47
stages of, 66–67
treatment of, 47, 47*t*
in nonpregnant adults, 68*t*
systemic antiandrogen therapy, 213

**T**
TB. *See* tuberculosis infection
teratogenicity, during pregnancy, 64, 66
teratoma. *See* ovarian teratomas
tertiary syphilis, 67
testosterone, in females, 248
TH-HEG. *See* transient hyperthyroidism hyperemesis gravidarum
thyroid disease
diagnosis of, 11–12, 12*f*
in pregnancy, 87–90, 89*f*
treatment of, 12–13
thyroid peroxidase antibodies, 12*f*
thyroid storm, in pregnancy, 89–90
thyroid-stimulating hormone (TSH), 11–13
tocolysis, 111–112
total exenteration, 273*f*
transient hyperthyroidism hyperemesis gravidarum (TH-HEG), Graves' disease and, 87
trans-vaginal ultrasound, 243
Tratner double-balloon catheter, 185*f*
trauma, during pregnancy, 148–151, 150*f*, 150*t*
*Treponema pallidum*, 46–47
trichomonas
diagnostic criteria for, 57, 58*f*
treatment recommendations for, 58–59
vaginitis, 56–59, 58*f*
TSH. *See* thyroid-stimulating hormone
tubal damage, 241–242, 241*f*
tubal ligation, 20–21, 21*f*
tuberculosis infection (TB), 78–79, 79*f*
during pregnancy, 79–80
tumor markers, for ovarian neoplasm, in young women, 258–259
Turner's syndrome
antenatal diagnosis of, 228, 229*f*
gonadal dysgenesis and, 227–230, 229*f*–230*f*
long term health risks of, 228–229, 229*f*–230*f*
obstetrical concerns with, 229–230
postnatal diagnosis of, 228, 229*f*
reproductive options for, 229–230
signs of, 229–230, 229*f*–230*f*
stigmata of, 229*f*

**U**
UAE. *See* uterine artery embolization
ultrasound
abnormalities, placenta accreta and, 139
of benign ovarian mass, 91*f*–92*f*, 92
of malignant ovarian mass, 91, 91*f*–92*f*
trans-vaginal, 243
unexplained infertility, 249
UPP. *See* urethral pressure profile
urethral diverticulum
diagnosis of, 184–186, 185*f*
treatment of, 185–186
urethral function, procedure choice based on, 188*t*
urethral pressure profile (UPP), 195
urge incontinence, 189
urinal incontinence
evaluation of, 190–191, 190*f*, 191*t*
treatment of, 190–191, 190*f*, 191*t*
types of, 189–190, 190*f*
urinary tract infections (UTI)
diagnosis of, 191–193
prevention of, 193–194
therapy for, 193, 193*t*

urodynamic testing, 194–196, 196*f*
urologic disease, CPP and, 39*t*
US Preventative Services Task Force (USPSTF), 8
USPSTF. *See* US Preventative Services Task Force
uterine anomaly
  clinical vignette for, 252–253
  diagnosis of, 253–254
  epidemiology of, 253, 253*f*
  infertility and, 253, 253*f*
uterine artery embolization (UAE)
  myomectomy v., for fibroids, cryomyolysis and, 173–175, 174*f*
  postpartum hemorrhage and, 127–128
uterine bleeding, abnormal
  abnormal endometrial histology and, 17
  perimenopause and, 35
  understanding of, 16
  vignette for, 16–17
uterine bleeding, dysfunctional (DUB), 17
  in adolescence, 17
uterine devascularization procedures, 127, 127*f*
uterine inversion
  etiology of, 152
  incidence of, 152
  management of, immediate steps for, 151–152
  maternal risk in, 152, 152*f*
  treatment methods for, 152–153, 153*f*
  vignette for, 151
uterine ligation, 127, 127*f*
uterine malformations, diagnosis of, 253–254
uterine prolapse, 196–198, 198*f*
  treatment options for, 197–198
uterine rupture
  reported rates of, 154*t*
  risk of, 154
  vaginal birth after, cesarean section and, 153–155, 154*t*
uterine sarcoma
  management of, 276, 276*f*
  pathologic diagnostic criteria of, 275–276
  prognosis for, 276
  risk factors for, 275
  vignette for, 275
uterine septum, treatment of, 254
uterus
  perforated, during hysteroscopy, 179–180
  "T" shaped, 165*f*
UTI. *See* urinary tract infections

**V**

vaginal birth, after cesarean section, 153–155, 154*t*
  uterine rupture and, 153–155, 154*t*
vaginal bleeding, in placenta previa, 141, 141*t*
vaginal candidiasis
  diagnosis of, 55, 55*f*
  differential diagnosis of, 55
  recurrent, 54–56, 55*f*
  treatment of, 55
  vignette for, 54–55
vaginal cystic lesions, benign, differential diagnosis of, 184–185
vaginal vault prolapse, 199–201, 200*f*
  POPQ for, 200, 200*f*
  treatment options for, 200–201
vaginitis
  bacterial vaginosis, trichomonas and, 56–59, 58*f*
  vaginal candida, 54–56, 55*f*
varicella pneumonia, 81*f*
varicella zoster virus (VSV), 80–82, 80*f*–81*f*
  incubation period of, 80–81, 80*f*
  in pregnancy
    concerns for, 81, 81*f*
    natural course of, 80–81, 80*f*
    serologic screening for, 81
    treatment of, 82
    vignette for, 80
vault prolapse. *See* vaginal vaultprolapse
vertical transmission, of HIV, 74–75, 74*f*
VIN. *See* vulvar intraepithelial neoplasia
vomiting, during pregnancy, 63–66, 65*f*
VSV. *See* varicella zoster virus
vulvar carcinoma
  risk factors of, 277
  symptoms of, 277
  treatment of, 277
  vignette for, 276–277
vulvar disease, 59–60
vulvar intraepithelial neoplasia (VIN)
  bowenoid, 279*t*
  CIN versus, 278
  current classification of, 278
  differentiated, 279*t*
  histopathologic characteristics of, 278
  management of, 279
  presentation of, 279
  risk factors of, 278–279
  subtypes of, 278, 279*t*
  vignette for, 278
  workup of, 279
vulvar lacerations, in pediatric patients, 201–203, 202*f*
  evaluation of, 202–203, 202*f*
  treatment of, 202–203

**W**

webbed neck, 229*f*
WHI. *See* Women's Health Initiative
women
  hyperandrogenic, 21-hydroxylase deficient nonclassic adrenal hyperplasia in, 214–215
  mortality causes in, 4
  smoking cessation in, 9
  testosterone in, 248
  young
    acute cystitis in, 193
    adnexal masses in, 258–259
Women's Health Initiative (WHI), 35–37
World Health Organization, osteoporosis definition of, on bone mineral density, 32*t*

**X**

x-ray film, of Asherman's syndrome, 223*f*

**Z**

ZIFT. *See* zygote intrafallopian transfer
zygote intrafallopian transfer (ZIFT), 233